Quick
Core

Quick Core

A high-yield radiology core exam review for residents

400+ Disease Processes | 800+ Images

Albus Severus Potter, M.D.

Purpose: I used this guide in studying for the 2021 core. I have edited it to high yield material that I encountered, although of course the tests will likely be very different. Images are KEY – this is radiology after all. While Crack the Core remains the best core prep, I was frustrated that a lot of diseases listed did not have images. So I set out to create this supplement.

Suggestion: Read through this twice. The first, take your time. Cross of things you know 100% so you don't waste time on this the second time around. Days before your exam, read through this again. Don't spend more than one day on it.

Disclaimer: This book is not to be used for clinical decision making. Human error will occur and it is your responsibility to double check all facts provided. The author assumes no responsibility for any injury and/or damange to persons or property arising out of or related to any use of the material contained in this book.

Dedicated to the hardest working residents out there. Thank you for making attending life easier. Keep working hard – you're almost there.

My suggested study materials: this study guide, Crack the Core, Core Radiology, TeleRad Physics review, the Radiology Review podcast, RadPrimer question bank.
This essentially guarantees you'll be seeing this:

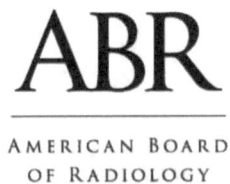

ABR

AMERICAN BOARD
OF RADIOLOGY

Core Exam
February 2021

Result: Pass

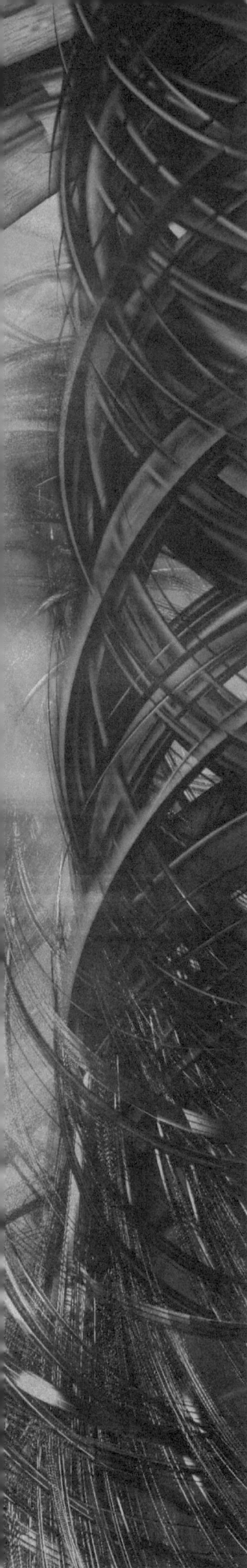

TABLE OF CONTENTS

Chest

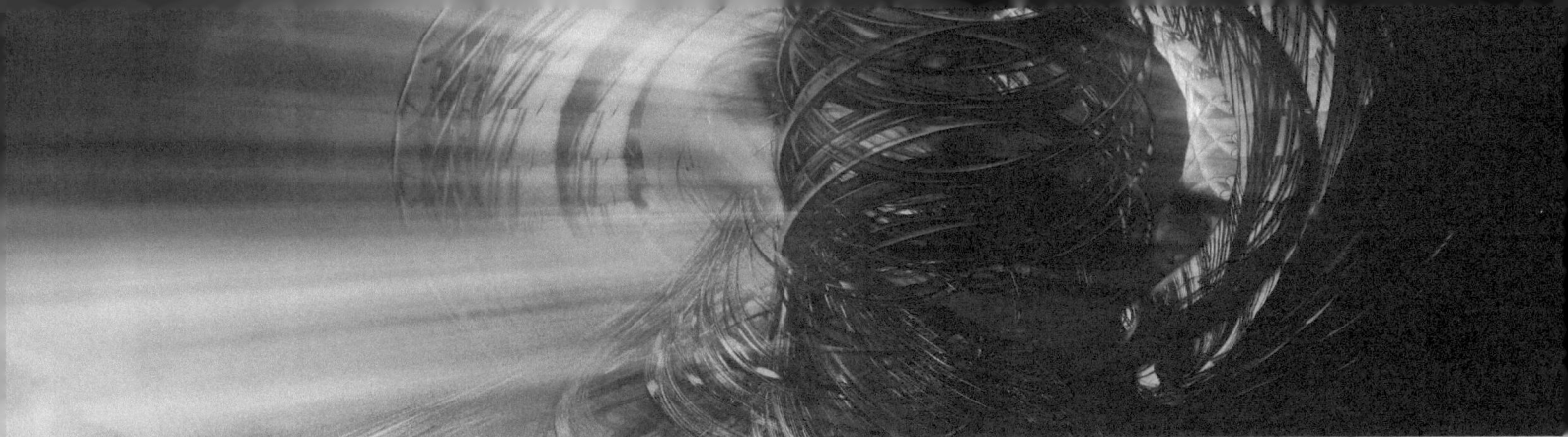

For this section we will start from the outside and work our way in. Topics that will be covered include chest wall and pleura, insterstitial diseases of the lungs, lung masses, central airways, mediastinum, and heart.

PLEURA AND CHEST WALL:

Never miss a pneumothorax, okay? In ICU patients it's trickier because they are sick and supine, so clues are deep sulcus sign, hyperlucent lung, and really sharp border of the heart. Always look for signs of tension.

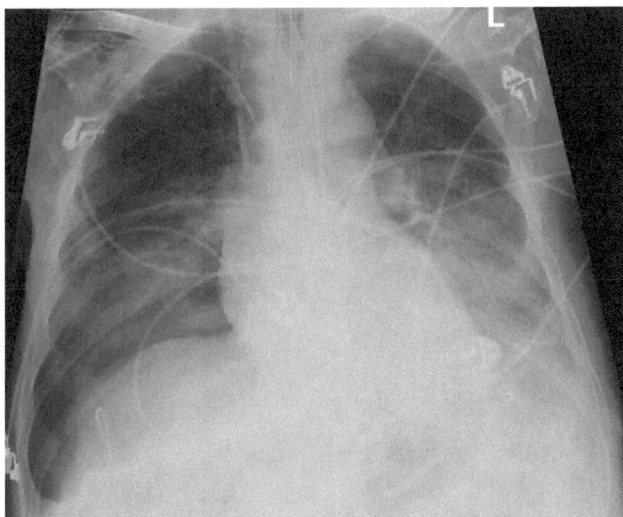

How do you tell if a mass is in the parenchyma or arising from the pleura/chest wall?

Parenchyma	Pleura or Chest Wall
Spherical	Elliptoid (real word? I dunno)
Well-defined	Part of the boder is ill-defined
Acute angles with the pleura	Obtuse angles with pleura

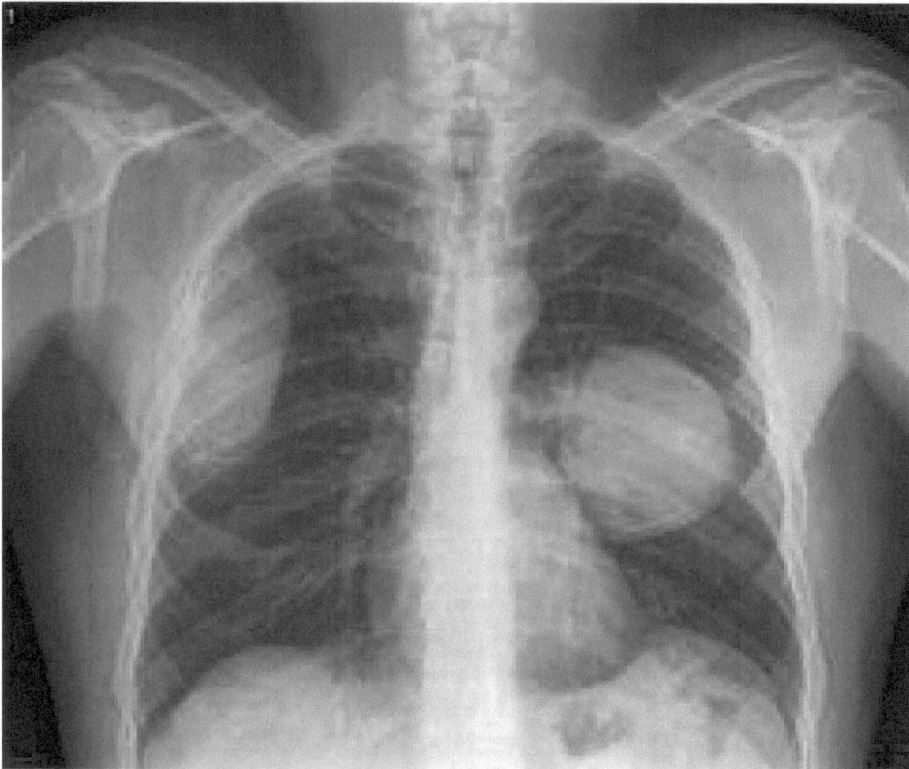

This image demonstrates the difference between the two types of masses really well. Cutaneous chest wall masses such as neurofibromas and moles demonstrate a characteristic incomplete, sharp border.

Mesothelioma: the most dreaded tumor of the pleura; it is a death sentence. Aggressive uncommon tumor associated with asbestosis (not dose dependent). There is a latent period of 20+ years. Patient presents with dyspnea and low posterior non-pleuritic chest pain and pleural effusion.

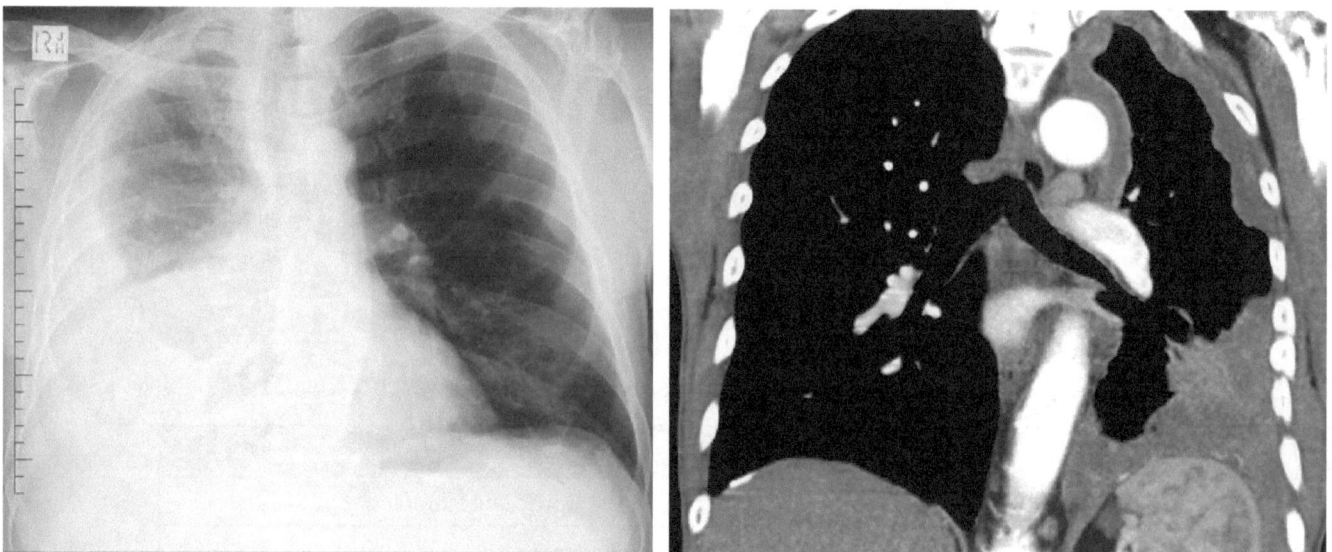

Asbestos pleural plaques: this is a high-density, raised lesion pathognomonic for asbestos exposure. Plaque can be calcified or not. Can see round atelectasis adjacent to sites of plaque (discussed in later sections).

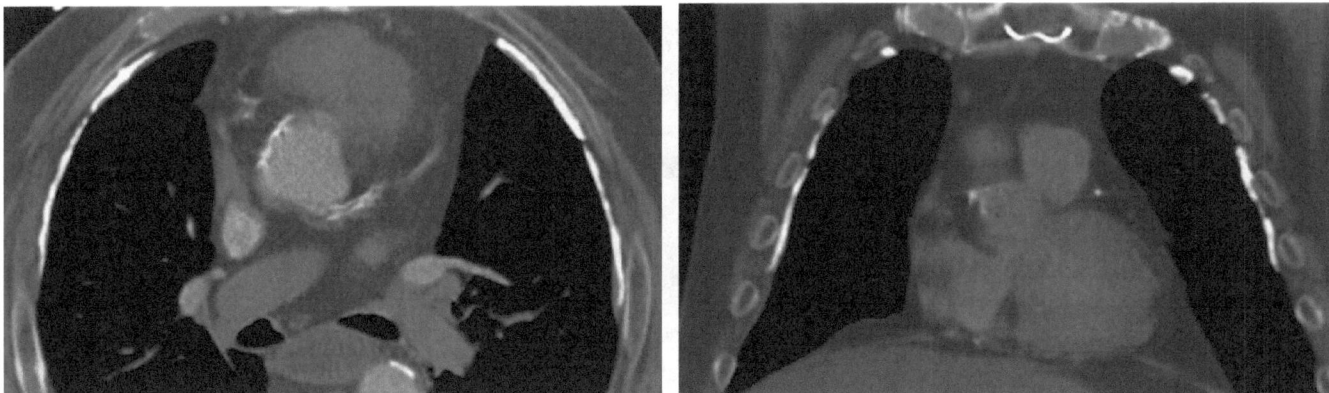

Solitary Fibrous Tumor of Pleura (SFTP): a rare, usually benign tumor. Can be associated with hypertrophic osteoarthropathy or episodic hypoglycemia. Cured by resection. These are very large vascular masses with intense enhancement.

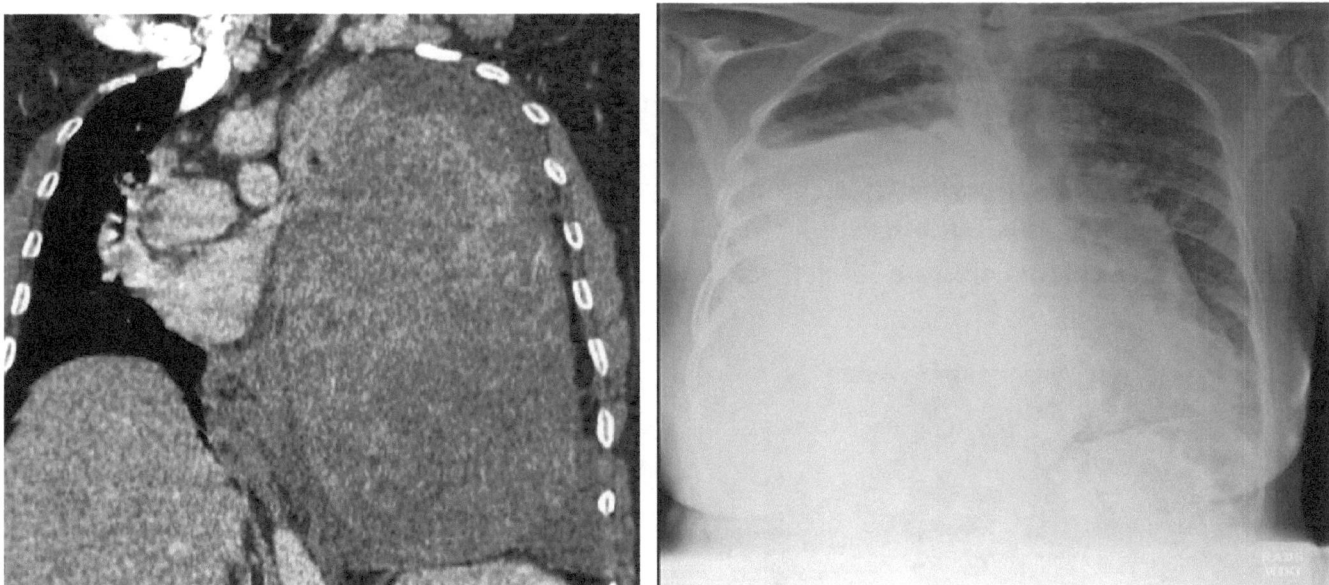

Fibrothroax: characterized by relatively smooth pleural thickening and may be calcified. The mediastinal pleura is usually spared and there is marked volume loss in the affected hemithorax. Associated with TB, empyema, asbestosis, and rheumatoid.

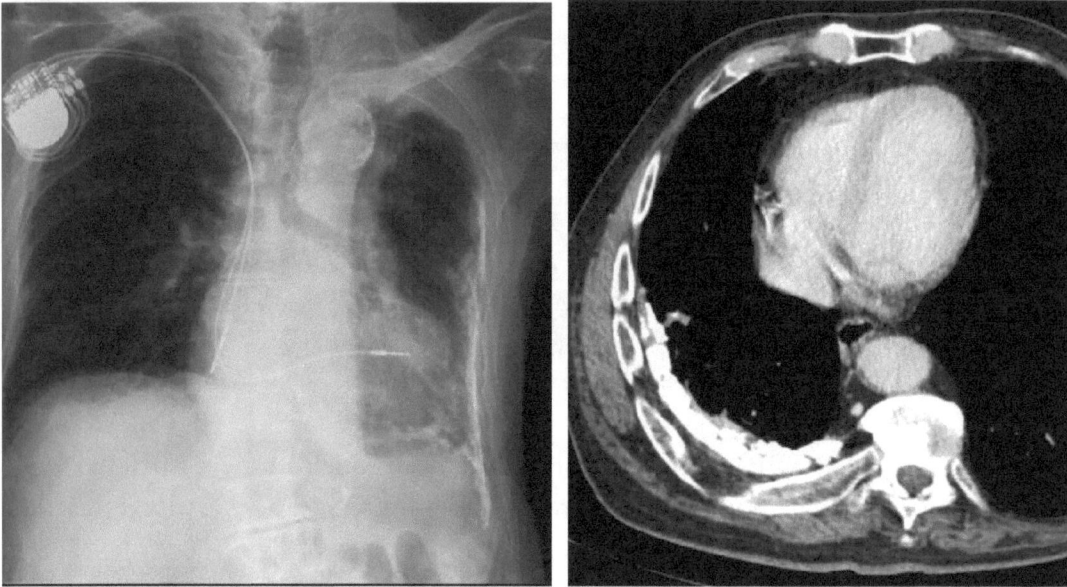

Metastatic disease also affects the pleura, look for nodules and exudative fluid effusions. Enhancing pleura is a bad sign as well. Tumors can eat into the pleura from the outside in (i.e. rib lesions).

Empyema Necessitans (Necessitatis): a chronic empyema that invades through the chest wall in order to try and decompress it self. Rib sclerosis or periosteal reaction is secondary to chronic osteomyelitis. Organisms responsible for this are Blastomyces, Actinomyces, TB, Mucor, Aspergillus, and Nocardia (BATMAN).

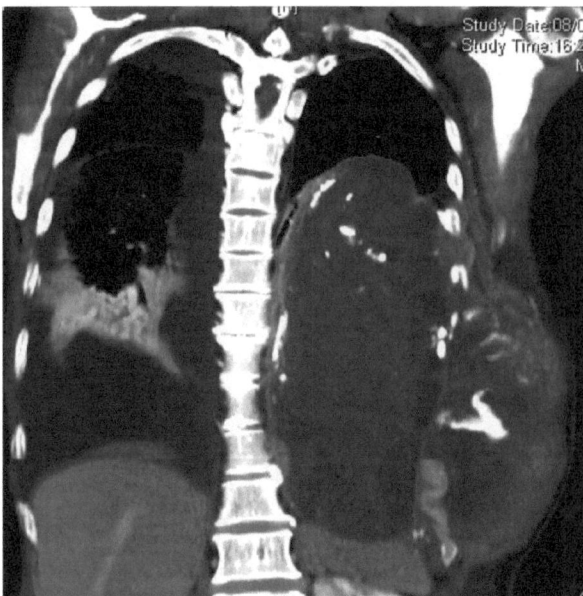

Diaphragm contour can help predict disease process:

- Lateral peak: fluid – 200 cc to blunt lateral angle and 75 to blunt posterior angle
- Medial peak: lobe collapse
- Central peak: phrenic nerve paralysis

Interstitial lung disease: to understand diseases of the lung, you have to understand the anatomy of the secondary pulmonary lobule.

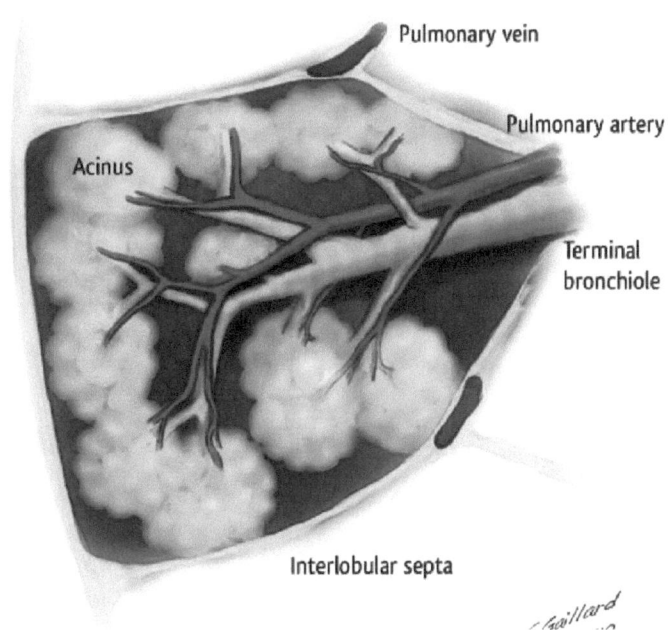

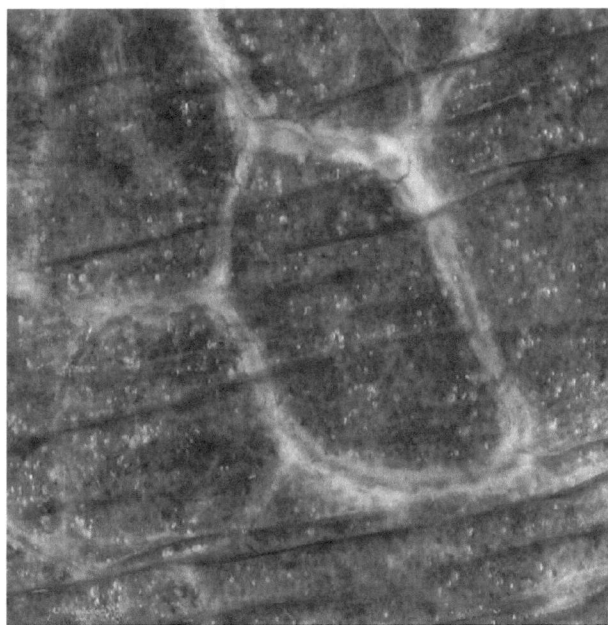

Interstitial pneumonia is a response of the lung to injury. It has several patterns with variable inflammation and fibrosis. Can be caused by: collagen vascular diseases, idiopathic, drugs, or inhalation injury.

Common: UIP, NSIP, COP, DIP, RB-ILD
Uncommon: LIP, AIP

Histology	Clinical Syndrome	Ass. Diseases
UIP	IPF	CVD, Drugs, Asbestosis
NSIP	NSIP	CVD, Drugs
COP	COP	Infection
DIP	DIP	Smoking

UIP: very common disease pattern. It is the imaging appearance corresponding to the clinical diagnosis of IPF. This is considered the dominant pattern in those with RA and concurrent interstitial lung disease. This has a basal posterior, lower lobe, subpleural predominance. Look for reticular opacities with traction bronchiectasis, honeycombing, architectural distortion and GGO.

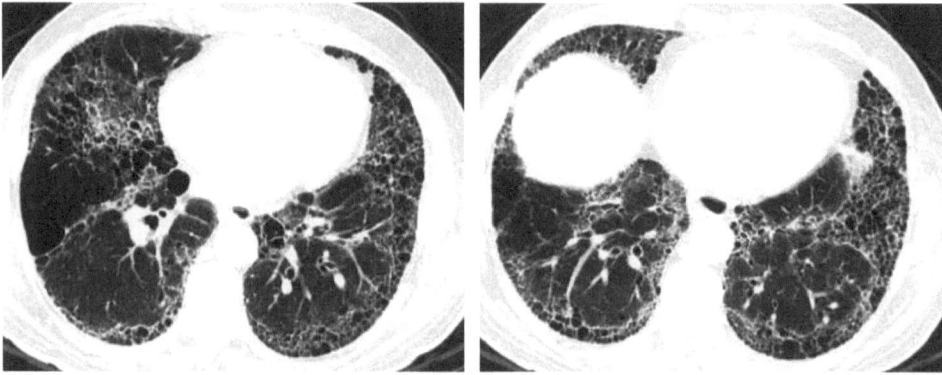

IPF is the most common cause of UIP. Mean survival is 3 years. Patient has progressive dyspnea. This is a diagnosis of exclusion. Need UIP findings on HRCT, lung biopsy not needed.

NSIP: less common than UIP. Demonstrates homogeneous fibrosis and is associated with CVD, drug reactions. Good 5-year survival. Imaging findings demonstrate GGO, reticular opacities with a lower lobe posterior peripheral predominance. This spares the subpleural lung.

If you see fibrosis or honeycombing it is fibrotic NSIP.

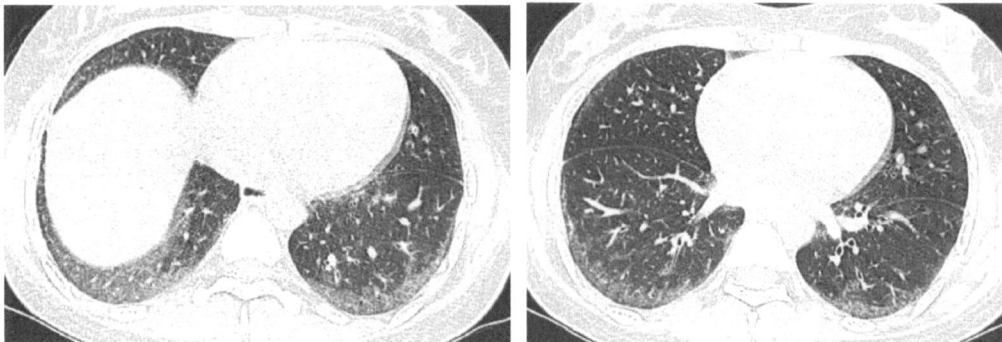

RB-ILD & DIP: strong association with smoking. These are less common than UIP or NSIP. Treated with smoking cessation and steroids. GGO with patchy centrilobular nodules. RB-ILD is upper lobe GGO and nodules. DIP is lower lobe predominantly GGO (15% have upper lung involvement).

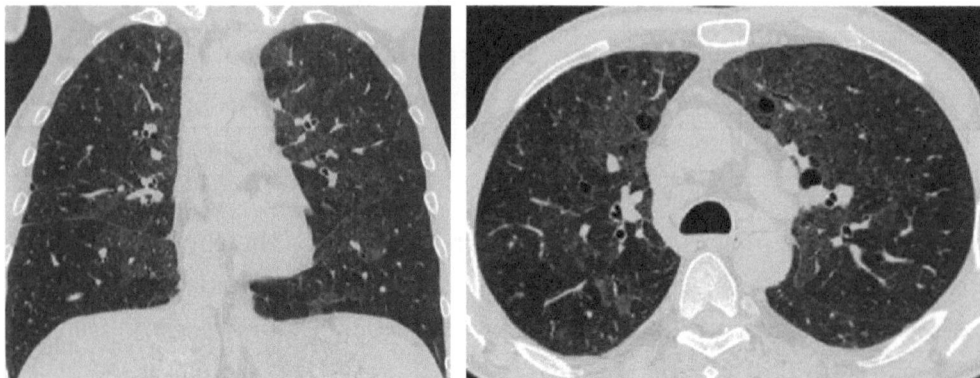

COP: chronic process in which patients present with months of low grade fever, cough, and dyspnea. COP is treated with steroids. Patchy bilateral consolidations and GGO in a peripheral and peribronchovascular distribution are noted on imaging. Look for the "reversed halo" or "atoll" signs.

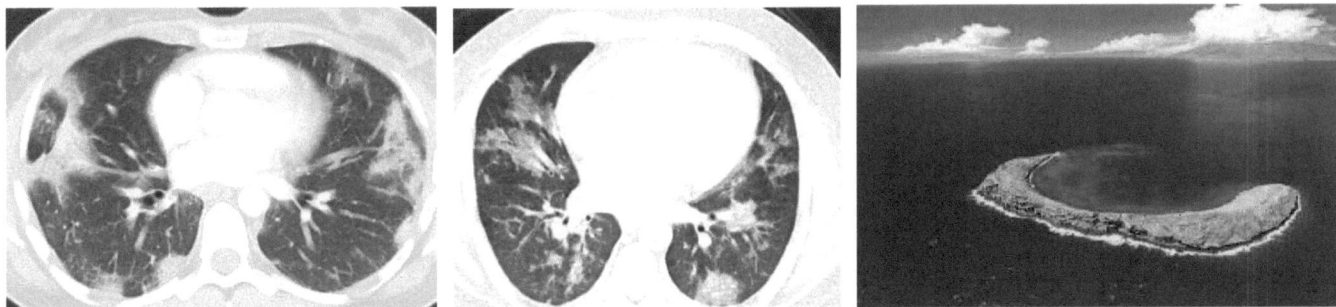

Chronic Eosinophilic Pneumonia: looks a lot like COP. Patient will have peripheral eosinophilia and asthma. They will present with months of cough and SOB. This has upper lobe predominance with peripheral consolidations and GGO. Treated with steroids.

HSP: due to inhalation of organic antigens. Patient has progressive SOB. Diffuse or patchy GGO with illdefined centrilobular nodules and air trapping are the imaging characteristics. Can be diffuse or just involve the mid lung zones with entire cross section of lung involved. "Bird fancier's lung."

When chronic, upper zone fibrotic changes do happen. Below are two images, left is classical picture, right is the chronic form.

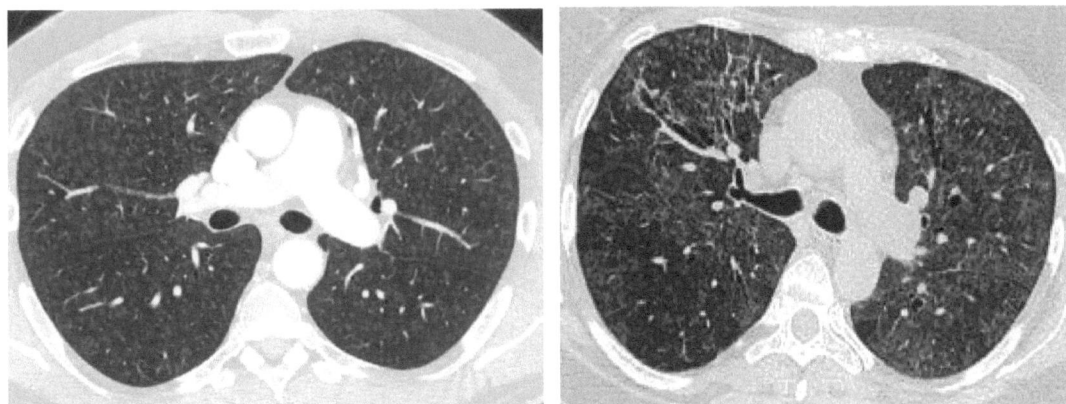

<u>Nodules</u>: 3 delicious flavors, discussed below

Perilymphatic: related to the lymphatics, subpleural and peri-bronchovascular in location, patchy distribution. Differential is classic: sarcoid, silicosis, and lymphangetic spread of tumor.

Sarcoid can look like silicosis, the history of exposure is key, and look for egg-shell calcifications of mediastinal nodes in silicosis.

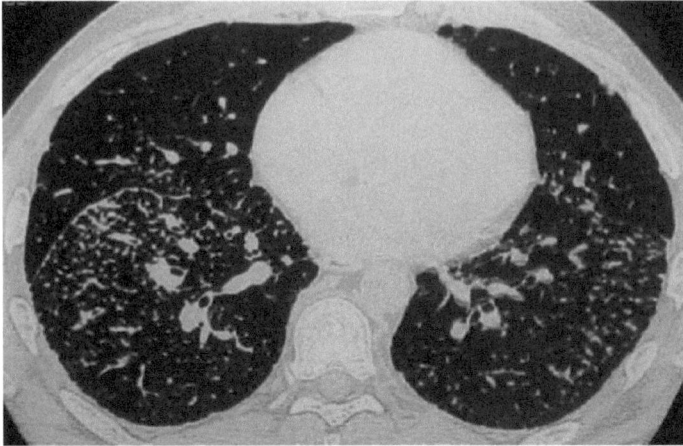

Silicosis: upper lobe predominance of nodules that can coalesce and form soft tissue masses – PMF, be careful not to confuse this with cancer (I know I've done it before).

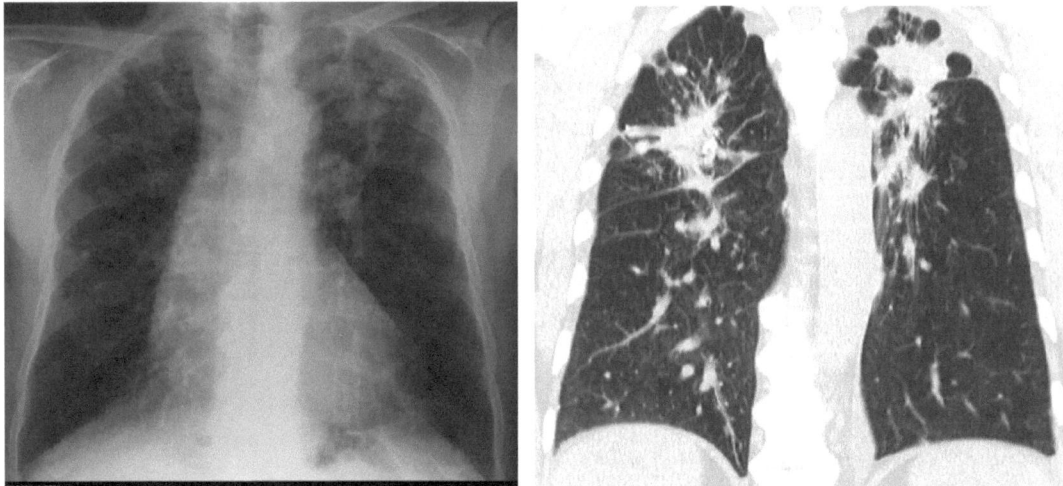

Sarcoid: has four stages and don't forget the potato nodes in the mediastinum
1. LAD
2. LAD + pulmonary changes
3. Pulmonary changes only
4. Fibrosis

Centrilobular: diffuse, uniform, 5-10 mm from the pleura. Differential is: HSP, small airways disease, vasculitis, and RB-ILD. We saw HSP and RB-ILD above.

Random: can be anywhere and everywhere and of varying sizes. Differential is: miliary TB, hematogeneous metastases.

Miliary spread can also be due to pneumoconiosis, eosinophilic granulomas, sarcoidosis, and metastases.

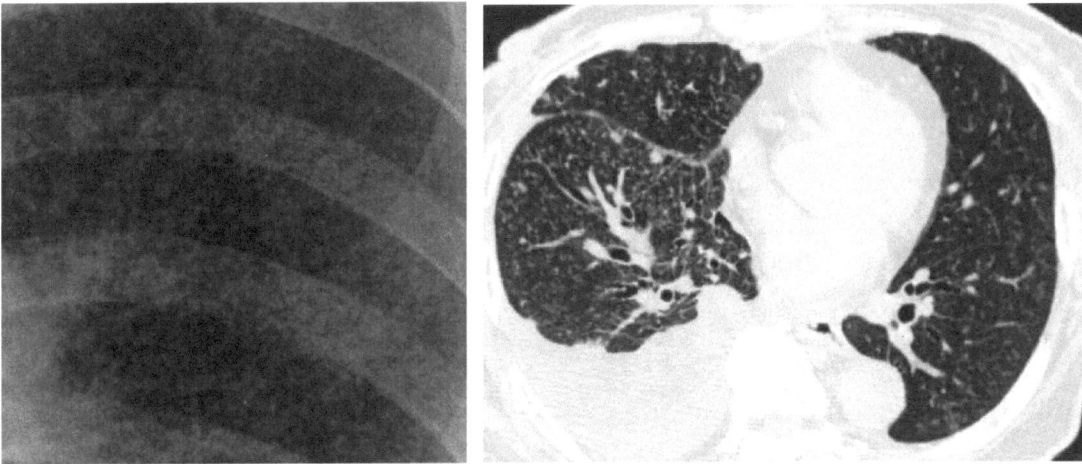

Tree-in-bud nodularity is dilation and impaction of the centrilobular airways, most likely due to infection.

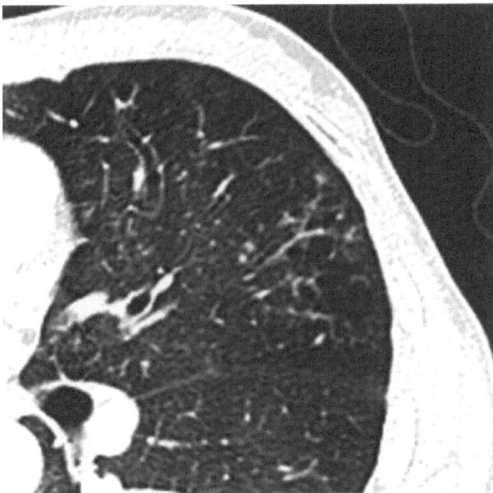

Emphysema: comes in three forms, my favorite is paraseptal
Centrilobular: upper lobe patchy lucencies related to smoking

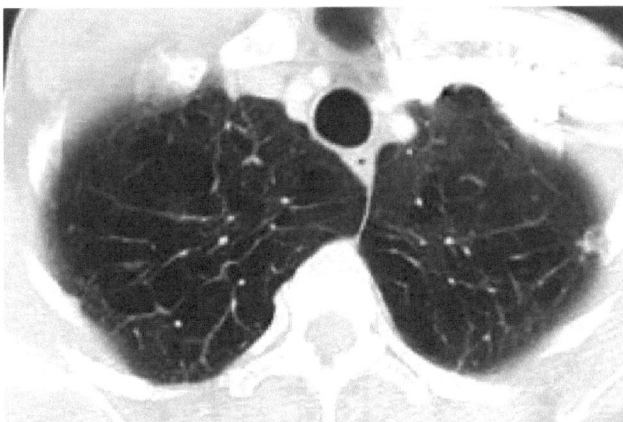

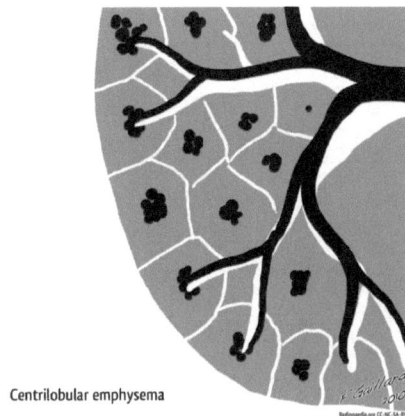

Centrilobular emphysema

Panlobular: predominantly in the lower lobes, total obliteration of the lobule and the lung just appears to be too big

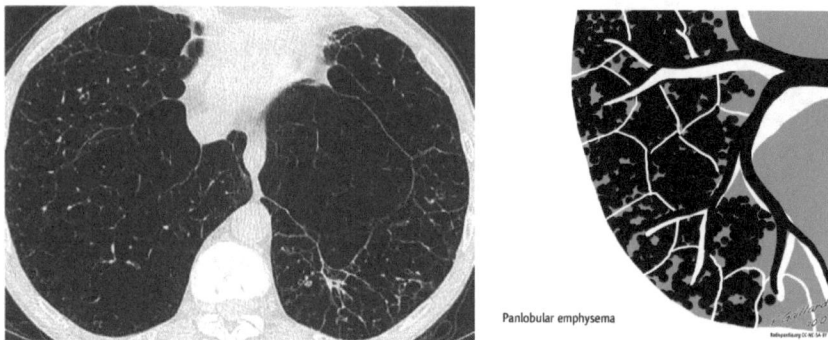

Panlobular emphysema

Paraseptal: is located adjacent to the pleura and septal lines with a peripheral distribution. Looks like a pearl necklace.

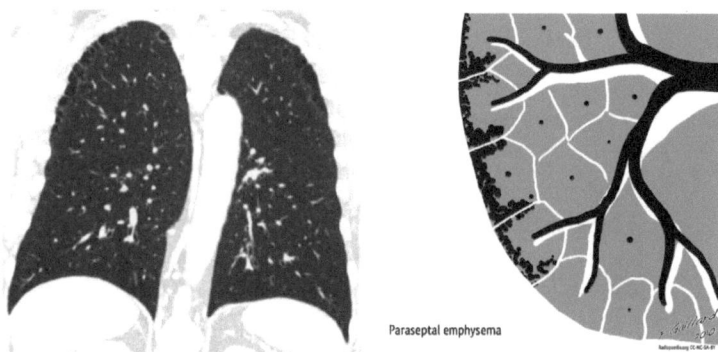

Paraseptal emphysema

<u>**Lung Masses**</u>: size is the number one determinant of malignancy; use the Fleischner Criteria to help with follow-up (only for incidental nodules).

Recommendations for Follow-up and Management of Nodules Smaller than 8 mm Detected Incidentally at Nonscreening CT		
Nodule Size (mm)*	Low-Risk Patient†	High-Risk Patient‡
≤4	No follow-up needed§	Follow-up CT at 12 mo; if unchanged, no further follow-up‖
>4–6	Follow-up CT at 12 mo; if unchanged, no further follow-up‖	Initial follow-up CT at 6–12 mo then at 18–24 mo if no change‖
>6–8	Initial follow-up CT at 6–12 mo then at 18–24 mo if no change	Initial follow-up CT at 3–6 mo then at 9–12 and 24 mo if no change
>8	Follow-up CT at around 3, 9, and 24 mo, dynamic contrast-enhanced CT, PET, and/or biopsy	Same as for low-risk patient

Note.—Newly detected indeterminate nodule in persons 35 years of age or older.
 * Average of length and width.
 † Minimal or absent history of smoking and of other known risk factors.
 ‡ History of smoking or of other known risk factors.
 § The risk of malignancy in this category (<1%) is substantially less than that in a baseline CT scan of an asymptomatic smoker.
 ‖ Nonsolid (ground-glass) or partly solid nodules may require longer follow-up to exclude indolent adenocarcinoma.

Breakdown of lung cancer is as follows –majority is adenocarcinoma (50%), with squamous cell carcinoma (25%) and small cell cancer (20%) making up the bulk of the rest.

- **AdenoCA** is seen in smokers and non-smokers as a peripherally located pulmonary nodule usually picked up on screening. Has low affinity for glucose on PET scans.
- **Squamous cell CA** is a cavitary nodule seen in smokers. Can be central or peripheral with a very high SUV.
- **Small cell CA** is and infiltrative mass that invades the mediastinum and hila. It is a big mass that can be inseparable from LAD.

Staging of CA – key things to know IIIA is operable and IIIB is inoperable
T4 tumors invade the mediastinum or anything in it or can have a satellite nodule in a different lobe of the same lung.

Multiple Masses	Cannonball Mets	Multiple Ca 2+ Nodules	Multiple Cavitary Nodules
Mets	Colon CA	Granulomas	SCC
Fungal	RCC	Amyloid	Septic Emboli
Septic Emboli	Testis/Ovarian CA	Ossified Mets	Cavitary Infection
COP	Osteosarcoma – Ca2+	Alveolar Microliths	Tracheobronchial Papillomatosis – can transform to SCC
PMF			

Round Atelectasis: has very strict criteria to diagnose.
1. Volume loss
2. Contacts the pleura
3. Underlying pleura is abnormal
4. Comet tail

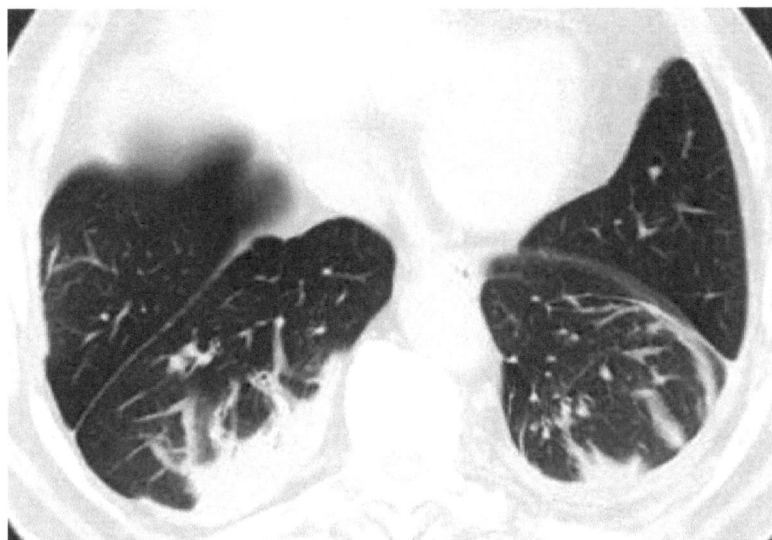

Central Airways Disease: Ask yourself, which airway is involved (trachea, large airway, small airway) and then narrow your differential by category.

Trachea: focal vs. diffuse

Diffuse – circumferential SAW (through the trachea)	Diffuse – spares posterior wall	Focal
Sarcoidosis	Relapsing Polychondritis	Post-Intubation – most common
Amyloidosis	Tracheobronchopathia osteochondroplastica	Post-inflammation
Wegner's		Tumor
		Vascular ring

Relapsing Polychondritis: rare condition with recurrent inflammation of cartilaginous structures. The posterior wall is not cartilage, that's why it is spared.

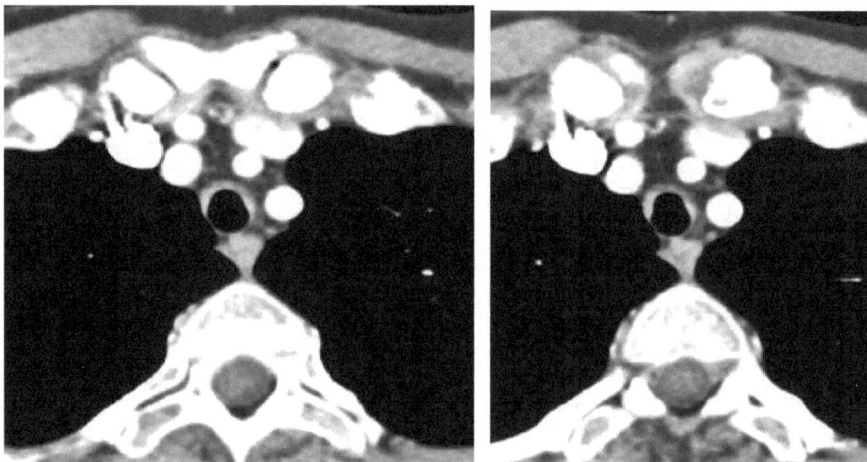

Tracheobronhopathia Osteochondroplastica: rare disease in older males with most people being asymptomatic.
Clasically in the lower 2/3rd of the trachea (anterior and lateral walls only)

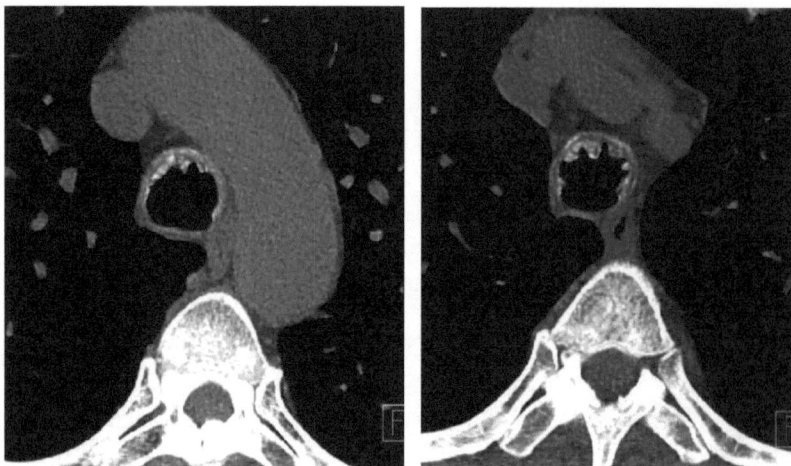

Tracheobronchial Papillomatosis: occurrence of multiple squamous cell papillomas involving trachea and bronchi. It is the most common benign tumor in laryngo-tracheal region.

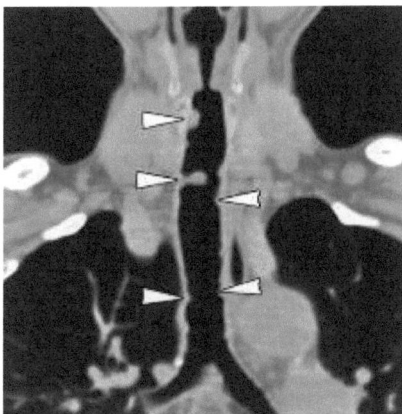

Squamous cell cancer is the most common laryngeal or tracheal tumor and is associated with smoking.

Adenoid Cystic Carcinoma: the most common type of lung cancer of salivary gland origin in the airway. ACC tends to occur in the central airway and have a tendency for submucosal extension manifesting with circumferential growth.

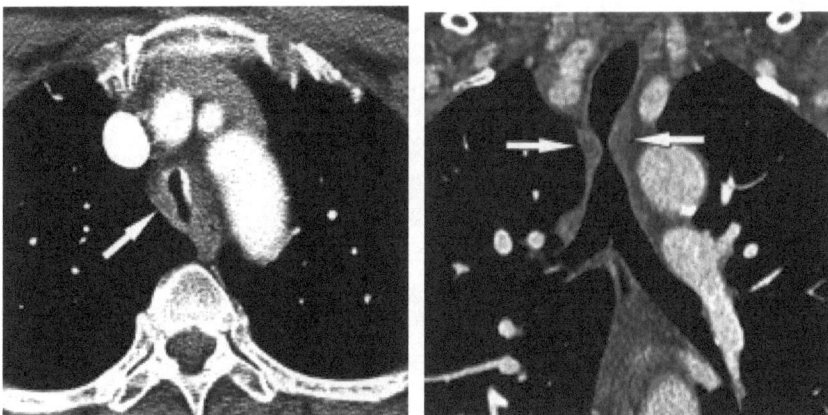

Carcinoid: pulmonary carcinoid accounts for ¼ of all carcinoid tumors and likes to cause obstructive atelectasis. It manifests as a small nodule in the airway demonstrating intense enhancement. Mild FDG uptake on PET.

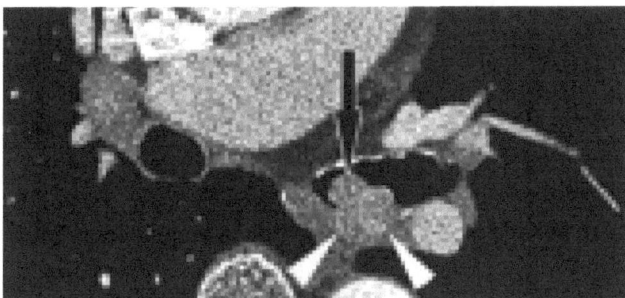

<u>**Large Airway:**</u> mainly thinking of bronchiectasis which comes in four varieties

Cylindrical: the mildest form (Signet Ring sign)
Varicose: enlarged beaded appearance
Cystic: very large dilated sacs
- the above three are a response to inflammatory conditions
Traction: due to adjacent lung fibrosis

Cystic: this is the most severe of the inflammatory bronchiectases and is a sign of long standing infection.

In the lower lungs it can be seen with childhood viral infections, Kartaganer's, Williams-Campbell (absence of cartilage in 4th-6th order airway).

In the upper lungs it will be a symmetric process associated with CF, ABPA, TB, Bronchial atresia.

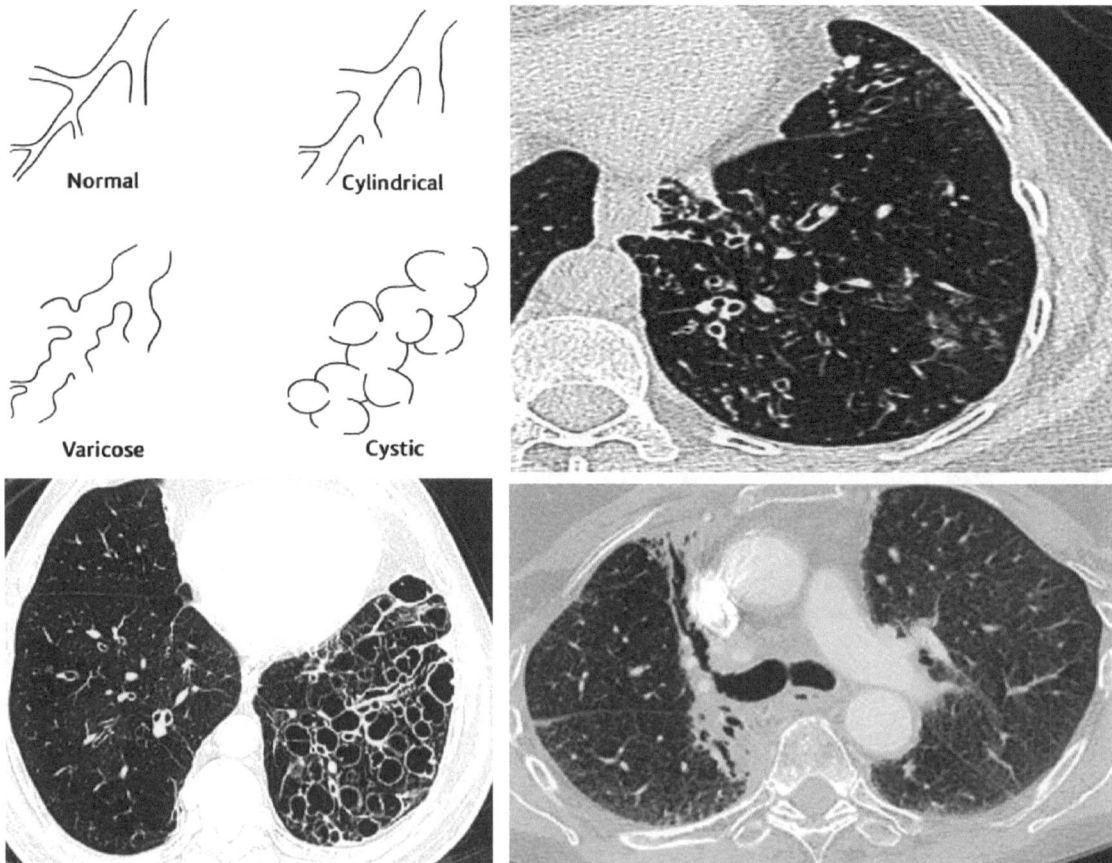

Cylindrical (top right), Cystic (bottom left), and Traction Bronchiectasis (bottom right)

<u>**Small airways:**</u> the causes of disease processes here were discussed in the interstitial lung disease chapter above.

Mosaic perfusion: the key here is to decide if the lucent lung is abnormal or if the opaque lung is abnormal. 50% of the lung's density is based on blood flow. Mosaic perfusion is a geographic area of abnormal perfusion causing lucent lung.

DDX: bronchiolitis, asthma, HSP, chronic PE
1. Geographic lucent lung
2. Small vessels in the lucent lung as compared to opaque lung because of decreased flow
3. Air trapping – abnormal lung stays dark on expiration

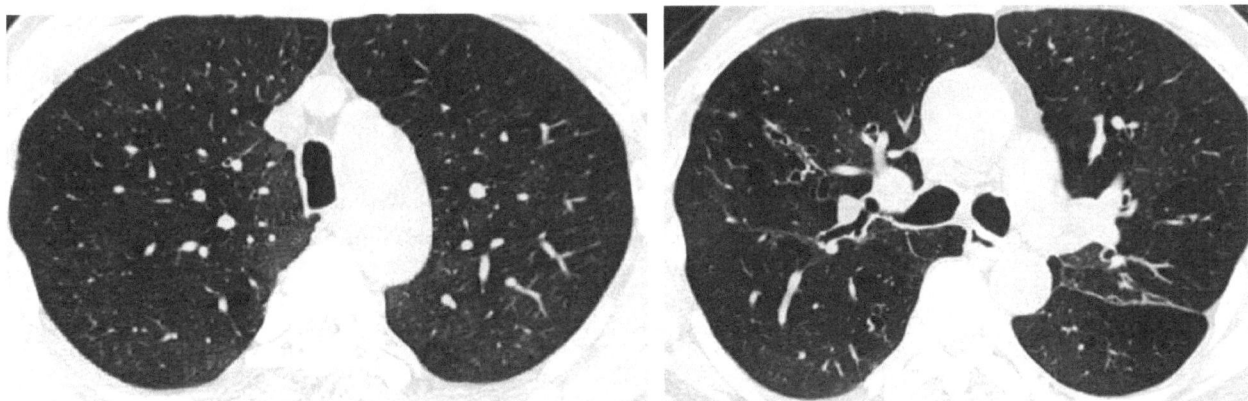

Inspiration on left and expiration on right

Right Middle Lobe Syndrome: is characterized by recurrent or chronic right middle lobe atelectasis without an underlying obstructing lesion. Proximal right middle lobe bronchiectasis is often present, and recurrent atelectasis may result from intermittent mucoid impaction in the abnormal bronchi.

MEDIASTINAL MASSES:

ANTERIOR	MIDDLE	POSTERIOR
Thymoma	LAD	Neurogenic
Teratoma	Vascular	Foregut Cysts
Lymphoma	Esophagus	Vertebral Body Tumors
Thyroid	Foregut Cysts	Aortic Aneurysm
Tons of other things	Tracheal Tumors	LAD
		Extramed Hematopoesis

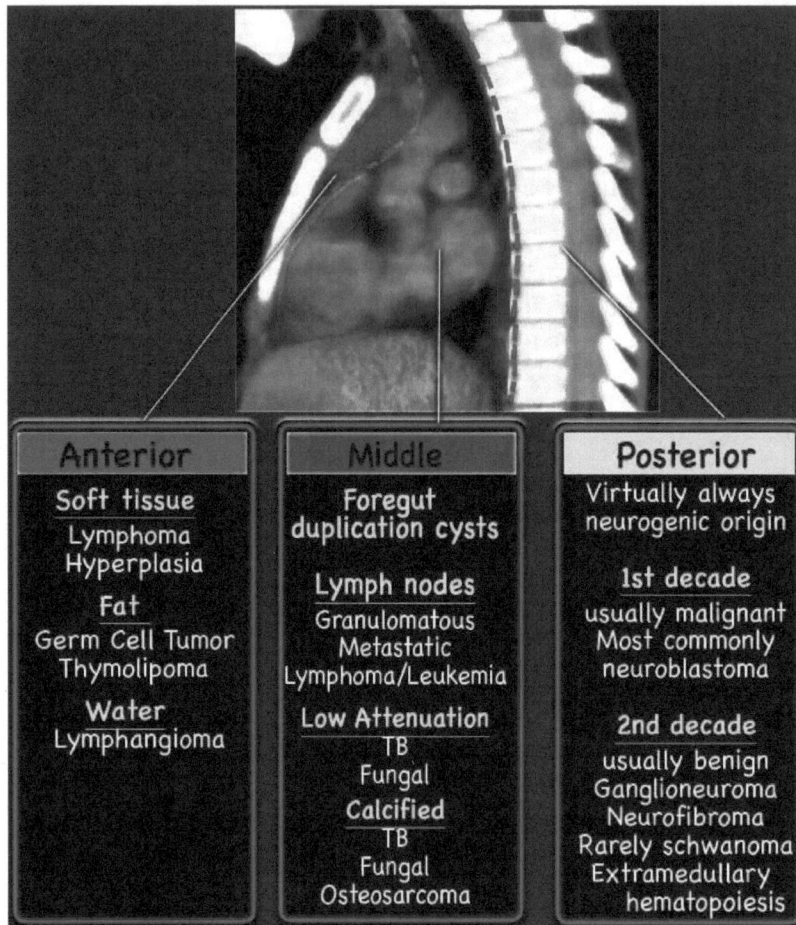

Anterior	Middle	Posterior
Soft tissue Lymphoma Hyperplasia **Fat** Germ Cell Tumor Thymolipoma **Water** Lymphangioma	**Foregut duplication cysts** **Lymph nodes** Granulomatous Metastatic Lymphoma/Leukemia **Low Attenuation** TB Fungal **Calcified** TB Fungal Osteosarcoma	**Virtually always neurogenic origin** **1st decade** usually malignant Most commonly neuroblastoma **2nd decade** usually benign Ganglioneuroma Neurofibroma Rarely schwanoma Extramedullary hematopoiesis

ANTERIOR:

Thymic Tumors: epithelial type is the most common and associated with myasthenia gravis. Seen in patients over 40 years old. Local spread > pleura >> extra-thoracic. Look for clean fat planes around the tumor and no adenopathy or effusions; suggesting non-invasive thymoma.

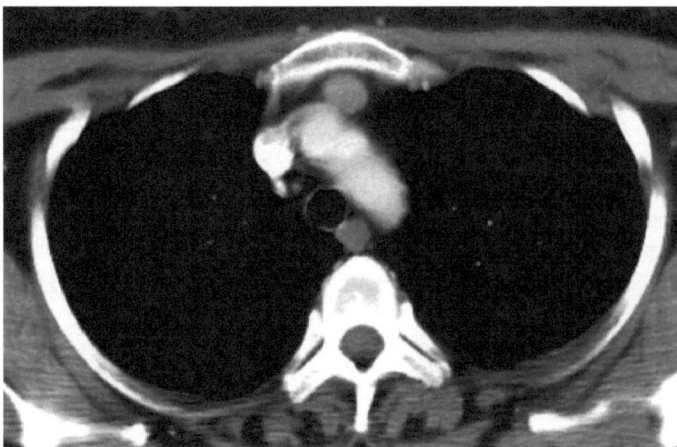

Benign

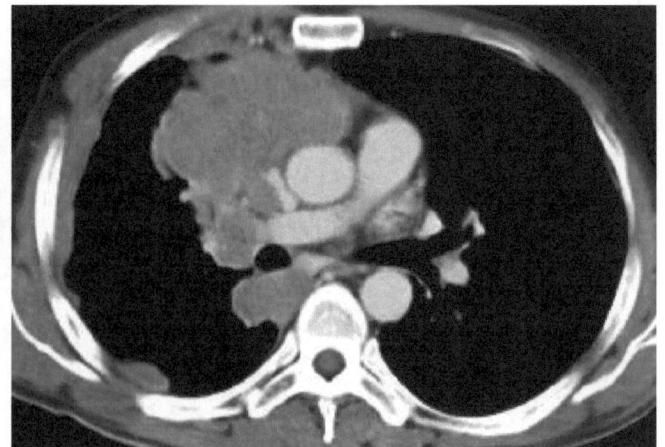

Invasive (malignant)

Germ Cell Tumor: mixed tissue types occurring in less than 40 year old patients. 80% are benign mature teratomas.

1. Mature elements (fat and Ca2+)
2. Seminoma is a homogeneous mass in young males with good prognosis
3. Non-Seminomatous GCT is a large infiltrative mass

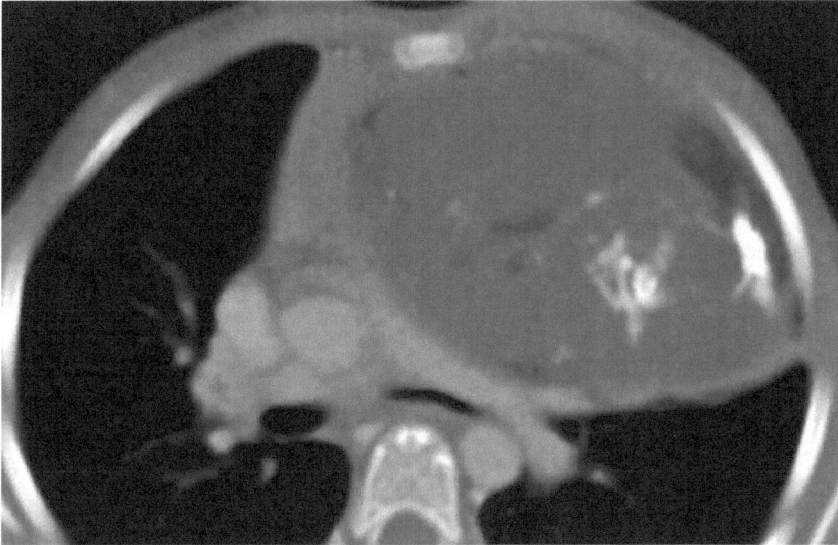

Lymphoma: will appear as a large infiltrative mass. HL is predominantly in the anterior nodes and NHL is going to involve all of the mediastinal nodes.

<u>MIDDLE:</u> look for nodes and vascular malformations

Thoracic Aortic Aneurysm: depicted below, but discussed in much greater detail in the vascular section.

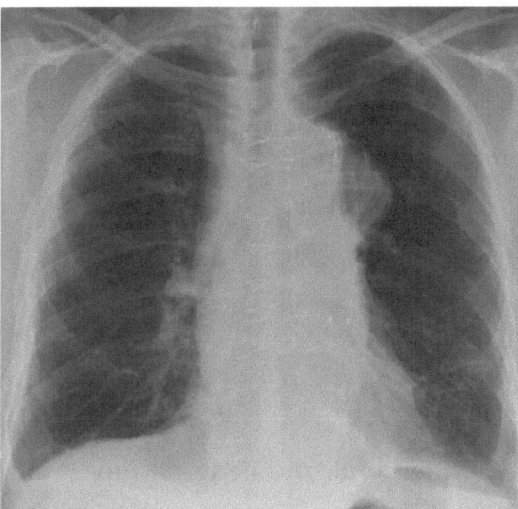

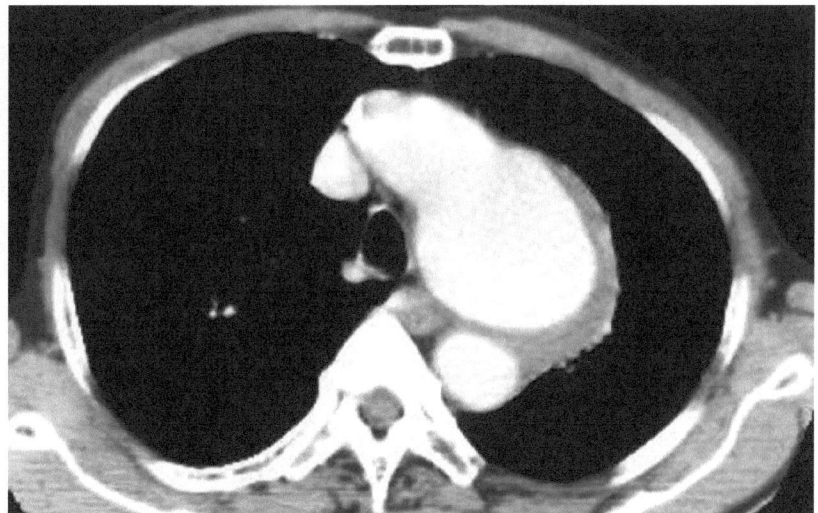

Bronchogenic Cyst: is typically located in the subcarinal region with splaying of the carina. Can also be seen in the paratracheal location and is a solitary lesion.

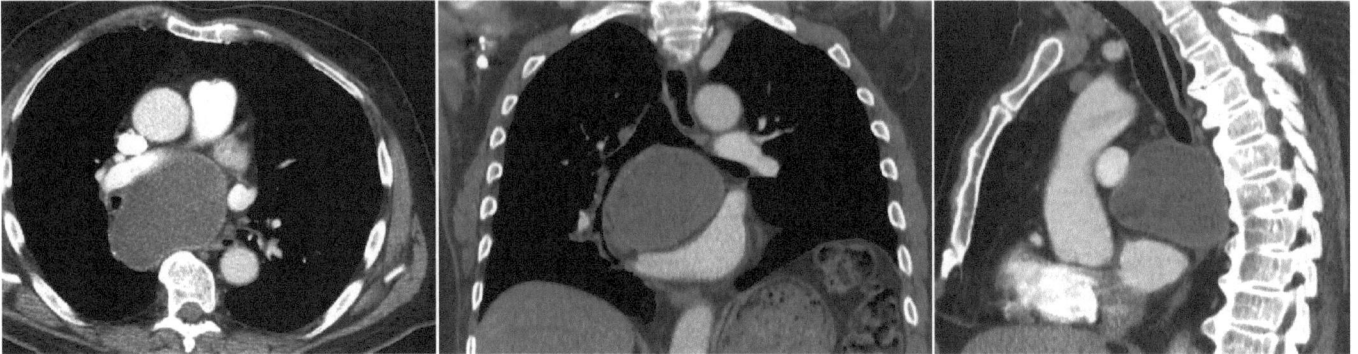

Lymph node characteristics can help categorize the disease:

1. Dense Calcifications - granulomas
2. Egg Shell – silicosis, sarcoid, treated lymphoma
3. Necrotic – TB, fungus, metastatic disease
4. Enhancing – vascular mets (RCC and thyroid)

POSTERIOR: look for widening of the paraspinal lines and extension of mass above the level of the clavicles.

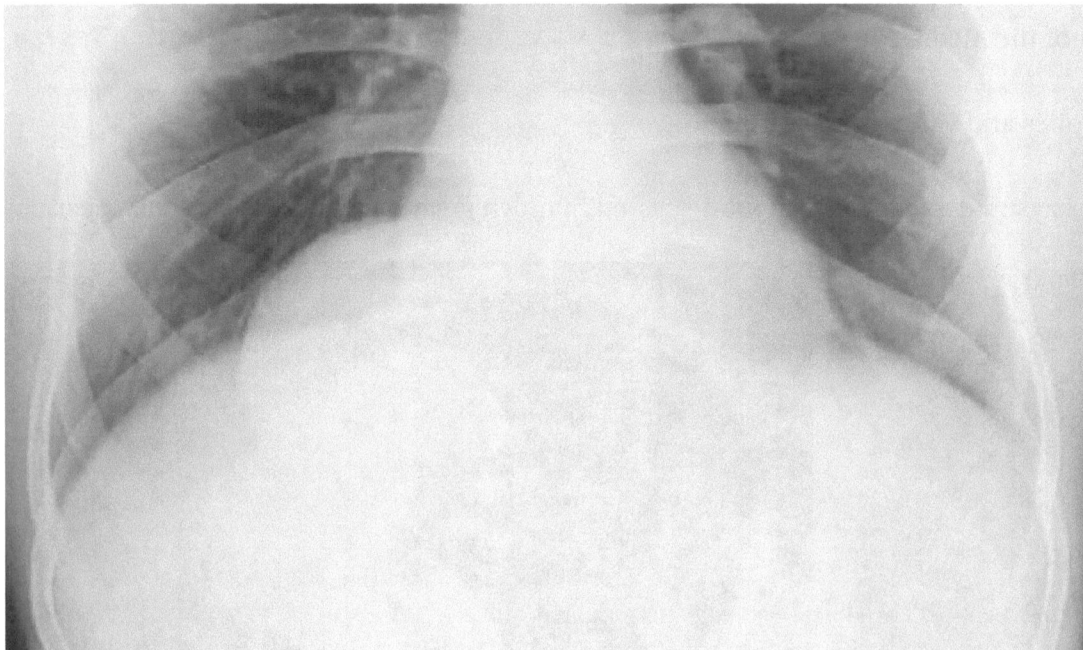

Neurogenic Tumors: this includes a wide differential of benign (schwannoma and neurofibromas) and malignant (neuroblastoma, malignant peripheral nerve sheath tumor) masses. Vertebral body masses (metastases and pannus from osteomyelitis discitis) and extramedullary hematopoiesis (EHM).

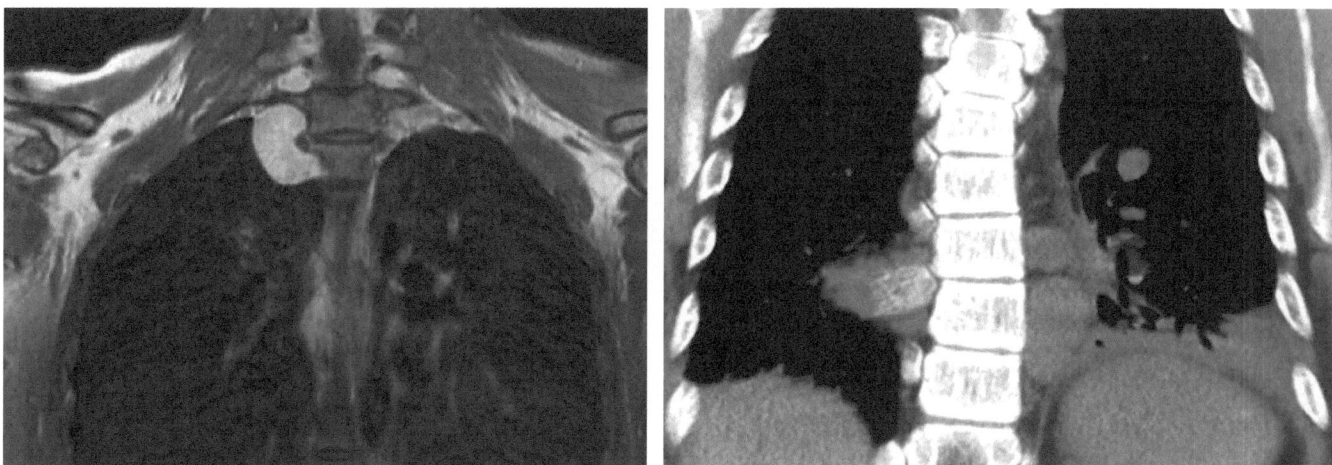

Schwannoma   Extramedullary Hematopoesis

Remember that **EMH** is a response to erythropoiesis failure in bone marrow. It occurs in anemia, hemoglobinopathies, and myeloproliferative disorders. EMH usually happens in the spleen and liver.

Mediastinal Lipomatosis: is a process seen in obesity, Cushing's and steroid use.

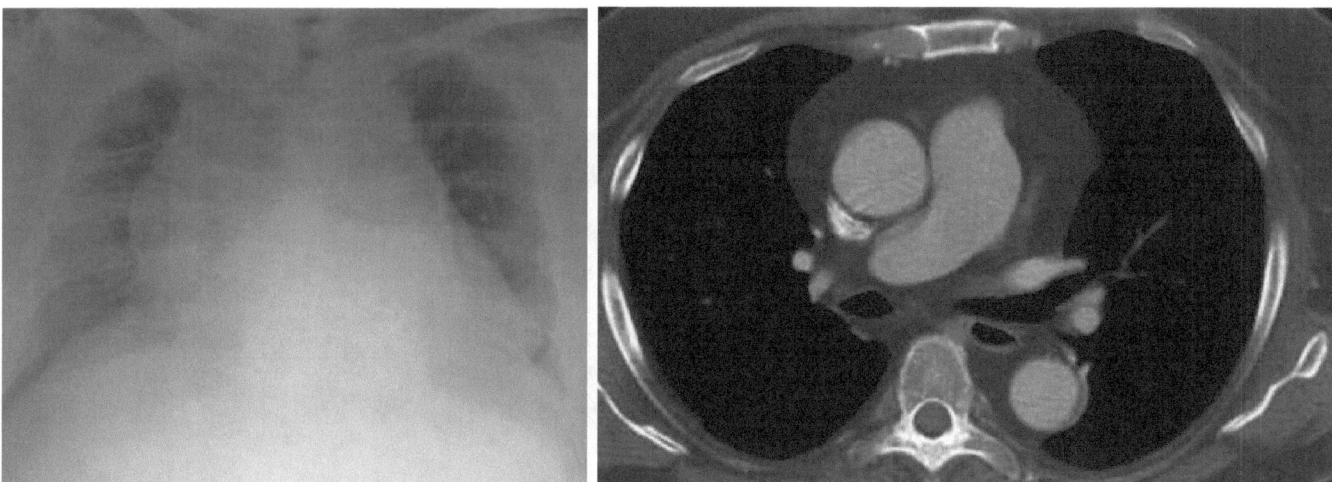

SVC Syndrome: in adults it's due to malignancy but in younger people it's due to fibrosing mediastinitis. Fibrosing mediastinits is a proliferative condition of the mediastinum with infiltration of acellular collagen and fibrous tissue.

VASCULAR:

Widened Mediastinum: in the setting of trauma the number one cause of this is not aortic injury, but that's the first thing you have to exclude. Most mediastinal bleeds are venous, but hematomas can also be due to fractures of the sternum and manubrium.

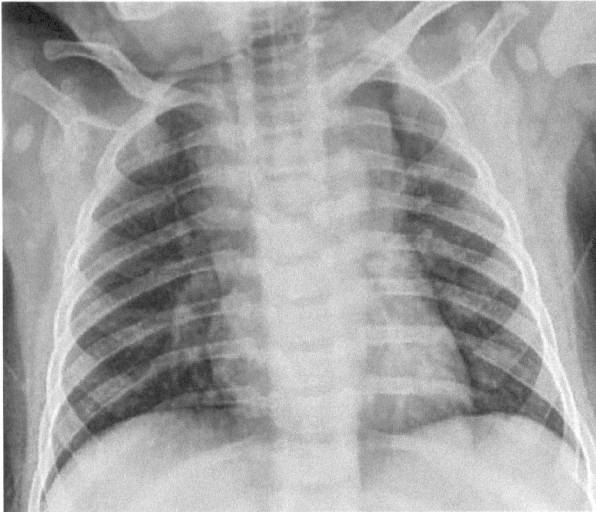

Aortic injury most often occurs at the isthmus, aortic root, and esophageal hiatus. If you see any of the following, send them to the OR:
– Contrast extravasation
– Pseudoaneurysm
– Intimal flap
– Wall irregularity

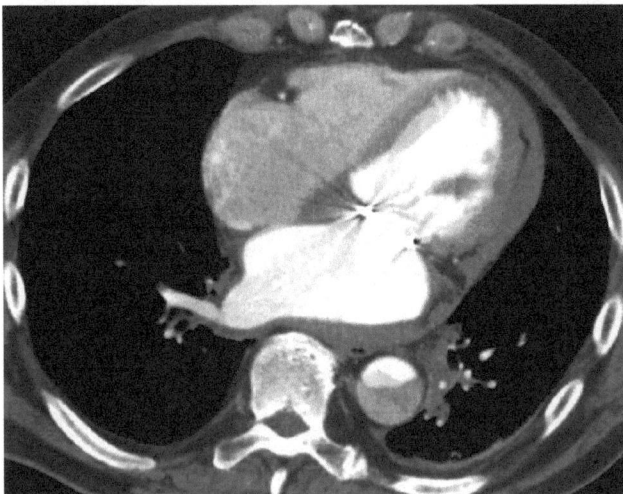

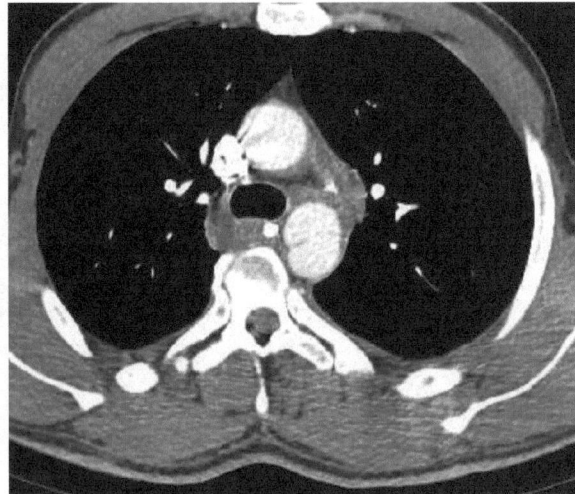

What to do if there is a mediastinal hematoma without direct signs of aortic injury?
– If isolated hemorrhage that doesn't touch the aortic wall, don't need to angio
– If the hematoma touches the aortic wall follow-up with angio

Aortic Aneurysm: The normal aorta should be less than 4 cm; surgery when > 6 cm. True aneurysms will be fusiform. If they involve the ascending aorta, think, annuloarotic ectasia, Marfan's, Ehler-Danlos, and syphilis. False aneurysms will be saccular, likely iatrogenic, traumatic, or mycotic.

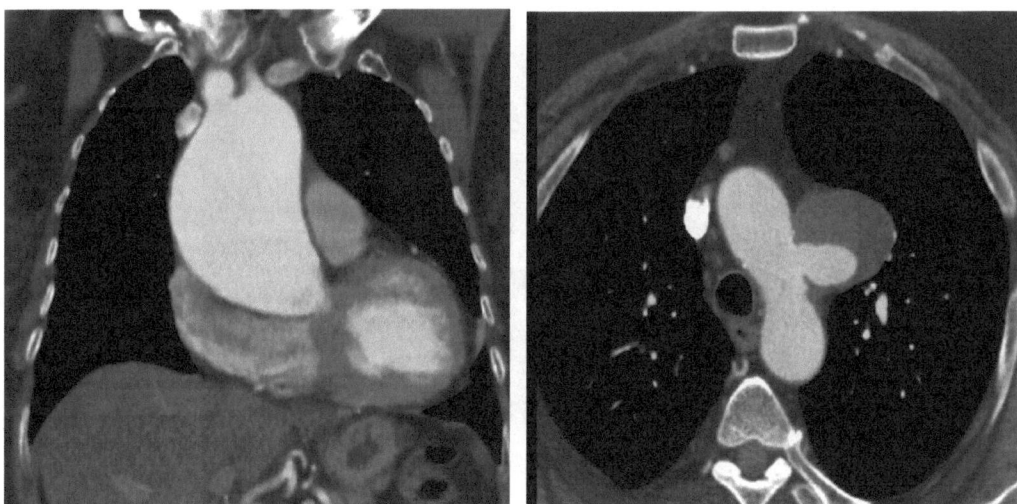

Intramural Hematoma: is on a spectrum of dissection as it is a hemorrhage into the wall from the vasa vasorum. Commonly due to HTN, connective tissue disease, and penetrating ulcer. If it involves the ascending aorta, surgery is needed to fix it.

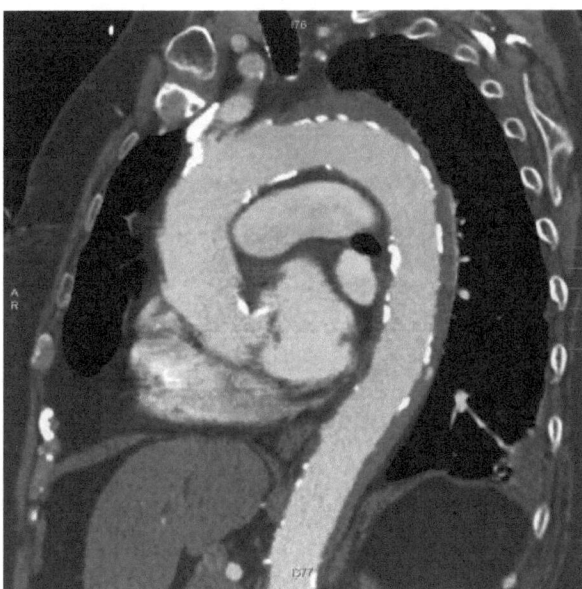

Aortic Dissection: need to separate the true and false lumens and describe what organ is fed by each. The false lumen tends to be larger and contains different blood densities.

Stanford A – ascending aorta; surgical emergency
Stanford B – descending aorta distal to the left subclavian origin; treat with meds to control HTN

Debakey I – ascending and descending aorta
Debakey II – ascending only
Debakey III – descending only

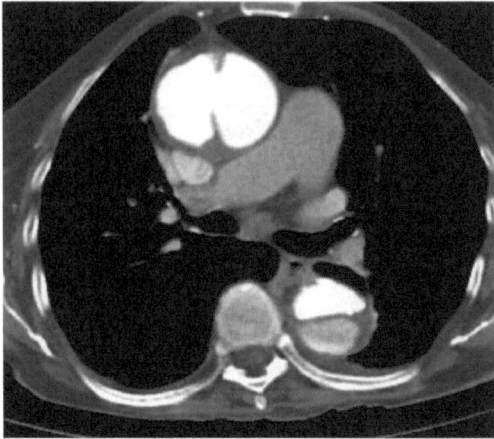

Stanford A/ Debakey I   Stanford B/ Debakey III

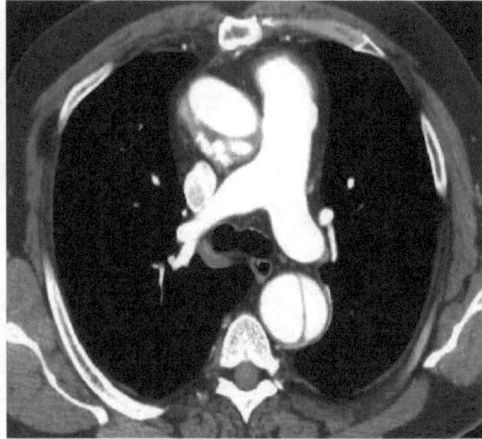

RINGS AND SLINGS:

Aberrant Right Subclavian Artery: the subclavian artery passes posterior to the esophagus if the origin is dilated it's called a diverticulum of Kommerell. Can be associated with dysphagia lusoria. More often caused by R-arch with aberrant left subclavian.

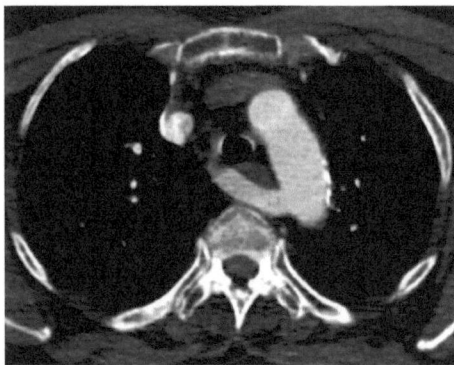

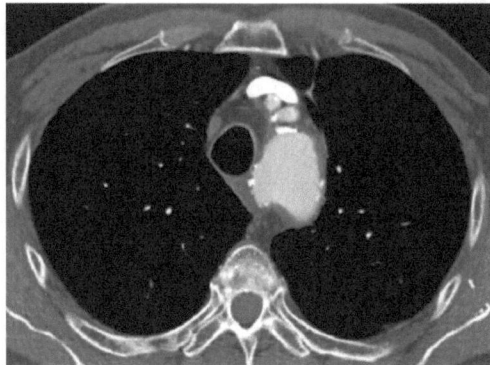

Double Aortic Arch: the most common complete ring. The right arch is typically larger and positioned higher than the left.

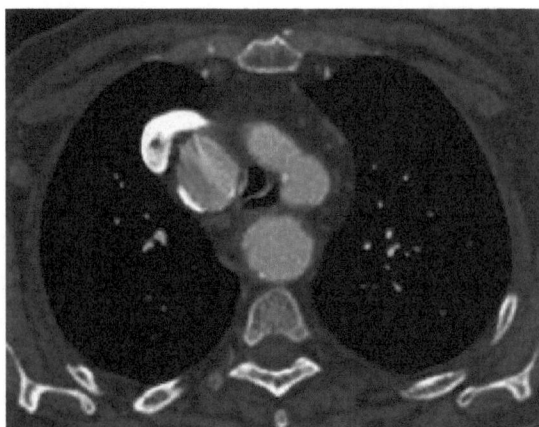

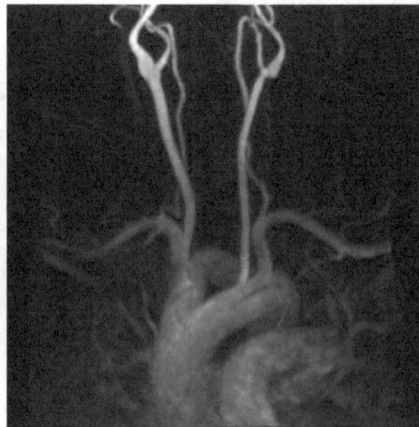

Pulmonary Sling: is a left pulmonary artery arising from the right pulmonary artery. Look for a mass between the trachea and esophagus.

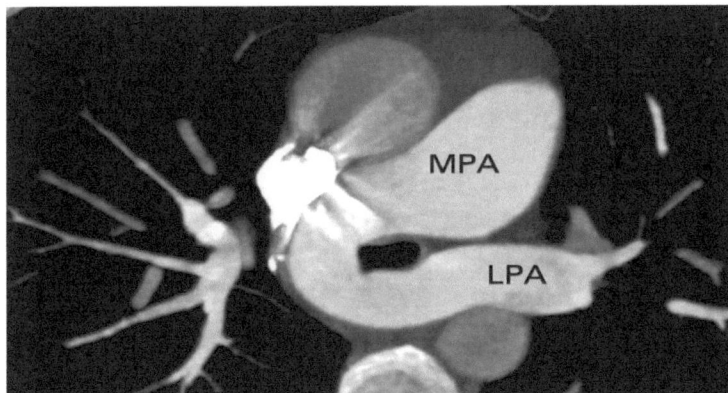

Coarctation: in adults it's more common to see a focal narrowing (juxtaductal) and in a child it'll be a tubular narrowing. Older patients will present with HTN. Coarctation is often associated with a bicuspid aortic valve.

- Look for IMA and intercostal collaterals (rib notching)
- Remember that a pseudocoarctation will be tortuous and longer, not stenotic
- Intercostal collaterals if hemodynamically significant will cause greater flow near the diaphragm than just distal to the coarctation
- Takayasu's can cause long segment coarctation

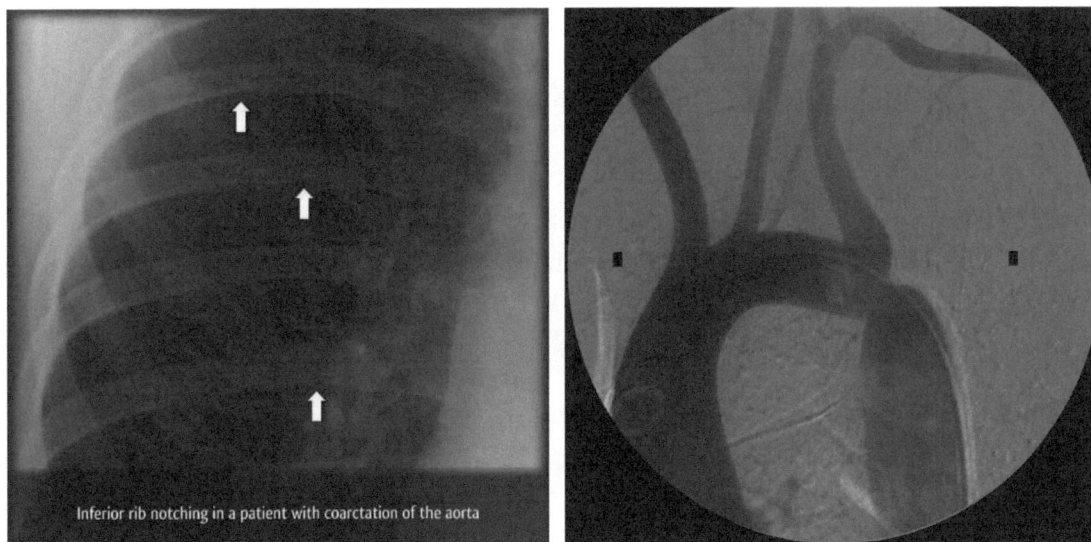

Inferior rib notching in a patient with coarctation of the aorta

CARDIAC:

Coronary CTA (indications): CAD, grafts, stents, anomalous coronaries. Significant stenosis is > 50% in LAD and > 70% elsewhere. If < 50% no more work up needed. If > 50% send patient to cath lab to confirm and or treat.

Left Coronary Artery: LAD, LCX
Right Coronary Artery: infundibular, RCX, inferior interventricular artery

Anomalous Course: can be benign or malignant depending on the course. The aberrant artery is usually a benign course. However, sometimes it can have an inter-arterial course (malignant). This course compresses the artery during systole and can cause sudden death.

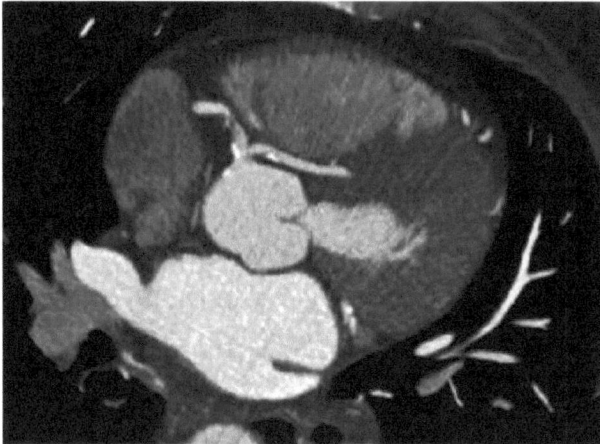

Cardiac MRI: used as a viability study with pre and delayed post CE exams. Inversion recovery sequence blackens the myocardium.

Enhancement – infection, inflammation, scar
No-enhancement – normal, stunned, hibernating

Look at the enhancement pattern: ischemia will be in a vascular territory, non-ischemic is patchy and not in a vascular territory.

– if > 50% enhances, the myocardium is scarred and not reperfusable
– wall motion abnormality without enhancement is hibernating

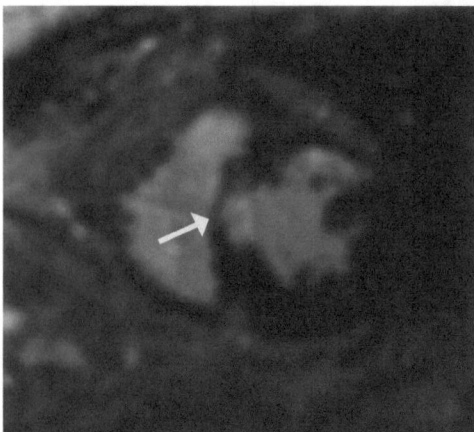

Greater than 50% septal enhancement consistent with infarct in the LAD territory.

Arrhythmogenic Right Ventricular Dysplasia: presents as recurrent ventricular tachycardia originating from a site in the RV. The pathologic process is due to replacement of RV myocardium by fat. Need to have clinical signs and symptoms and often also have familial history. RV wall thins and can have focal aneurysms.

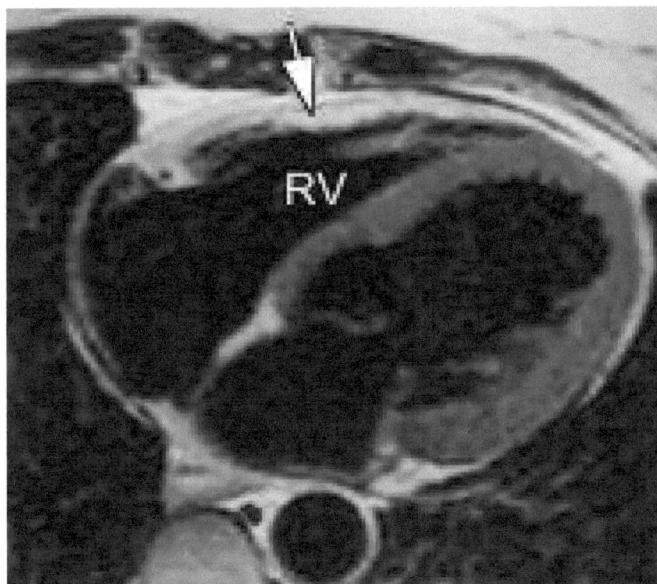

CARDIAC MASSES: both primary and secondary cardiac malignancies are rare. Myxomas are the most common tumor encountered with other benign tumors including papillary fibroelastoma, rhabdomyoma, and lipoma to name a few. Lymphoma and melanoma are malignancies that can go to the heart.

Myxoma: is a benign neoplasm that represents the most common primary tumor of the heart. It is an endocardial mass occupying a portion of the cardiac chamber. Most myxomas are attached to the fossa ovalis of the interatrial septum and 75% are in the left atrium. Patients can present with valvular obstruction, embolic disease, and be asymptomatic. Surgical resection is the treatment. Post-contrast enhancement is how we differentiate from thrombus.

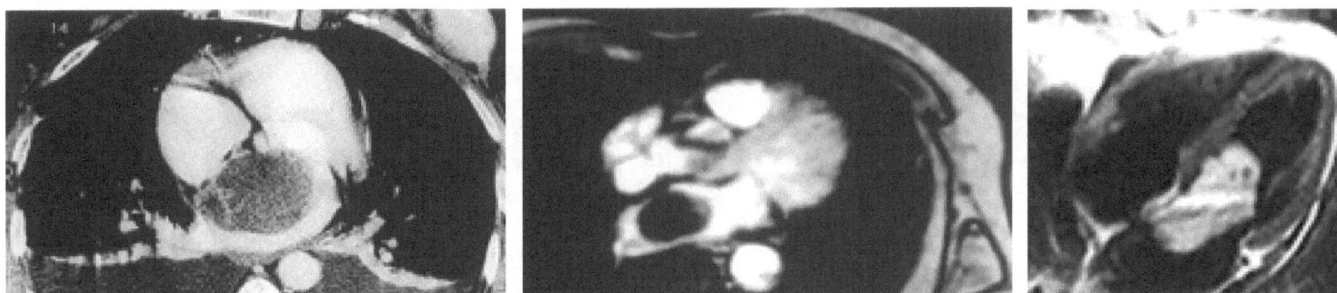

Papillary Fibroelastoma: is a benign endocardial papilloma that affects the cardiac valves and is the most common valvular tumor. These are the second most common primary benign cardiac tumor. Like myxomas it can cause obstructive and embolic symptoms.

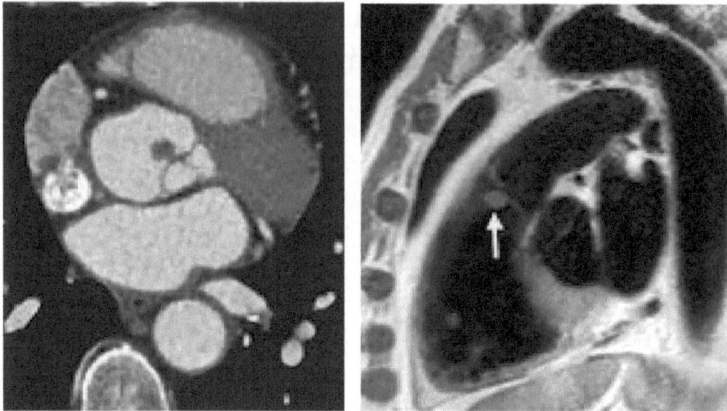

Rhadomyoma: the most common cardiac tumor in infants and children (up to 90%). They are benign myocardial hamartomas strongly associated with tuberous sclerosis. These demonstrate spontaneous regression as the child ages. Surgery is performed if the tumor is causing symptoms. These tumors are located within the myocardium or ventricular septum.

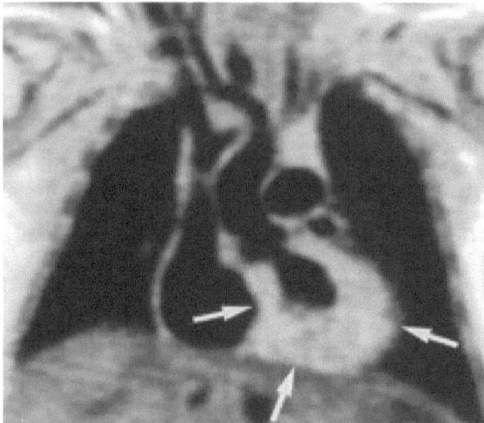

Lipoma: is a rare but benign tumor composed of adipose tissue, it is easy to identify on all modalities. Low density well defined mass on CT, high T1 signal, fat-suppresses out on out of phase imaging. These do not contain brown fat.

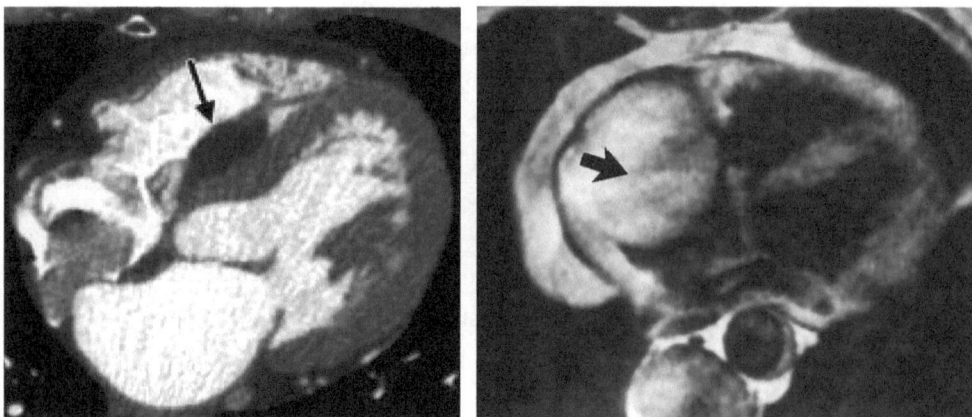

Sarcoma: these are rare, malignant tumors and by definition are confined to the heart or pericardium with no evidence of extra-cardiac metastasis. The most common cell type is angiosarcoma. Dyspnea is the most common presenting clinical symptom. The majority of these occur in the right atrium and involve the pericardium, symptoms of cardiac tamponade due to inflow obstruction are common.

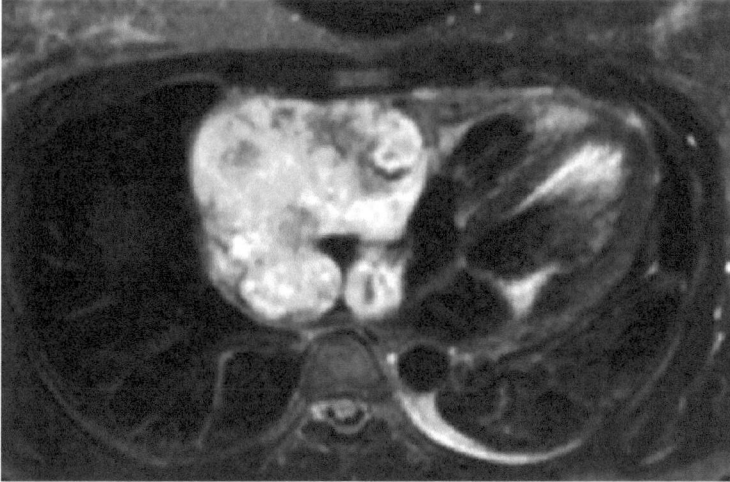

Gastrointestinal

ESOPHAGUS

Zenker's Diverticulum: an outpouching of mucosa in the hypopharynx between the circular and oblique fibers of the cricopharyngeus muscles (Kilian dehiscence). Most often seen in the elderly. Patients have dysphagia, globus, and halitosis (food gets stuck). Look for it around C5-C6.

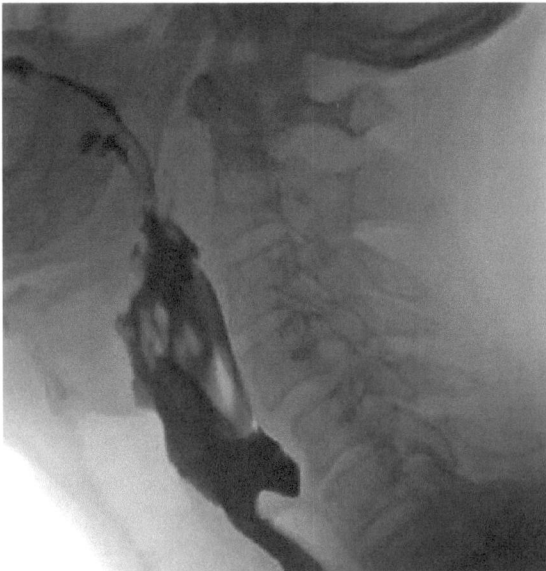

Cricopharyngeal bar: look for a posterior shelf-like impression on the esophagus at the C5-C6 level. Failure of the cricopharyngeus muscle to relax. If you see this anteriorly, it's an esophageal web.

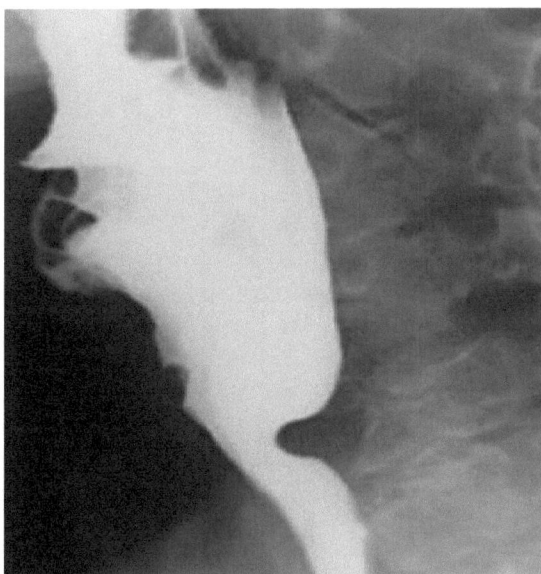

Killian-James Diverticulum: this is a true diverticulum located just below the cricopharyngeus muscle, anteriorly and laterally on the left, usually smaller than Zenker's (<1.5 cm).

Epiphrenic Diverticulum: pulsion diverticula of the distal esophagus just above the LES, more frequently on the right. Symptoms of dysphagia and regurgitation are common. Associated with achalasia and hiatal hernia.

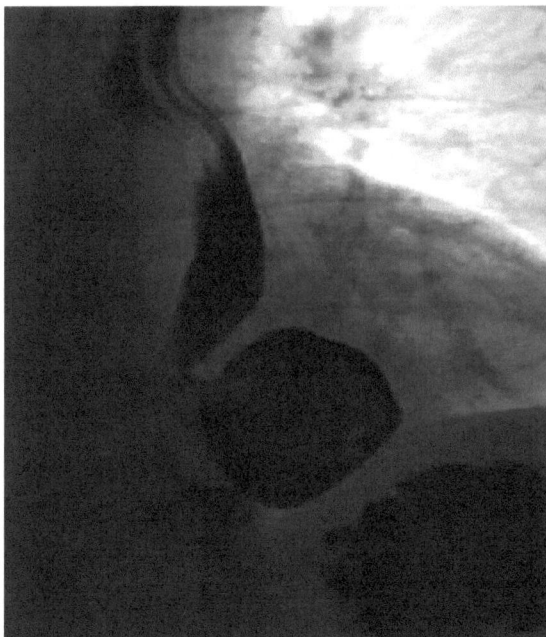

Strictures: can be cancer, peptic (distal), caustic (acid is worse on the stomach than base), erosive, and radiation induced. Barrett's causes mid to upper stricture and if you see filling defect in Barrett's start to worry about CA. Upper esophagus CA – SCC and lower esophagus CA – AdenoCA.

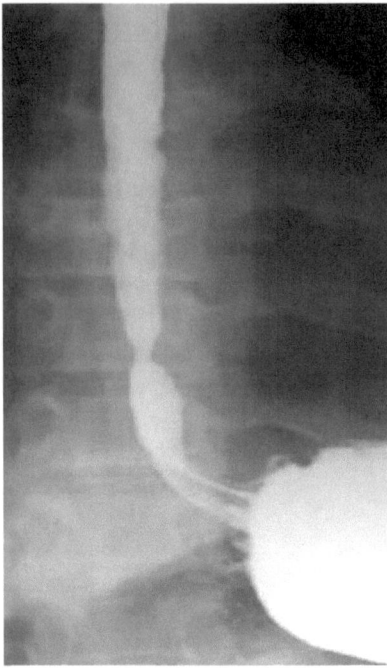

Peptic Stricture   Malignant Stricture

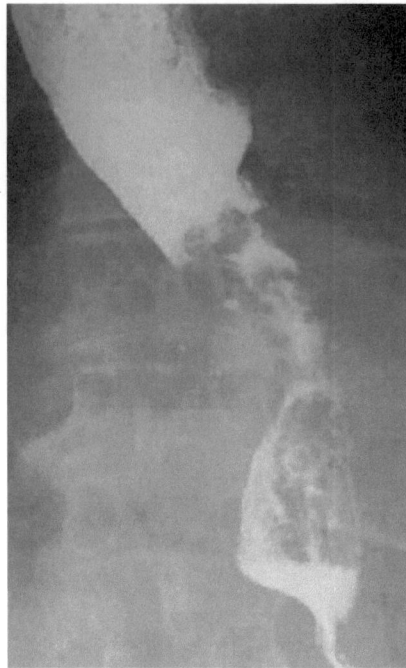

Achalasia: failure of relaxation at the LES with marked upstream dilation and stasis. Middle to late adulthood disease and is most often idiopathic. Chaga's disease (*T. cruuzi*) has a similar appearance. Most dreaded complication is esophageal CA, due to chronic irritation of the mucosa.

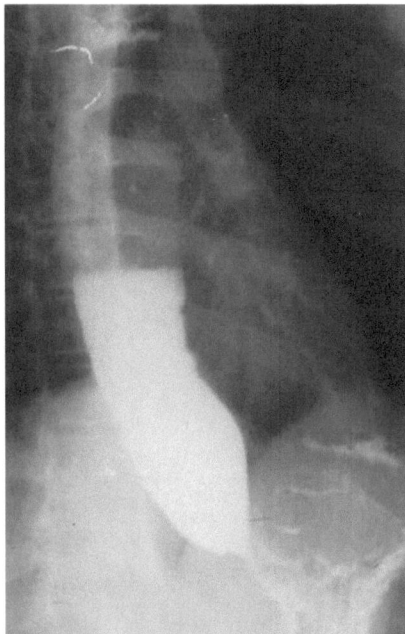

Scleroderma: connective tissue disease that most often involves the esophagus when it affects the GI tract. Patulous LES with chronic reflux, can have malignancy due to chronic mucosal irritation. Just look for a long dilated esophagus, filled with air, and basilar lung fibrosis.

Candida Esophagitis: most common cause of infectious esophagitis. Odynophagia in an immune compromised patient (AIDS). Look for discrete plaque like lesions in the esophagus in a linear configuration separated by normal intervening mucosa. Can cause pseudodiverticula.

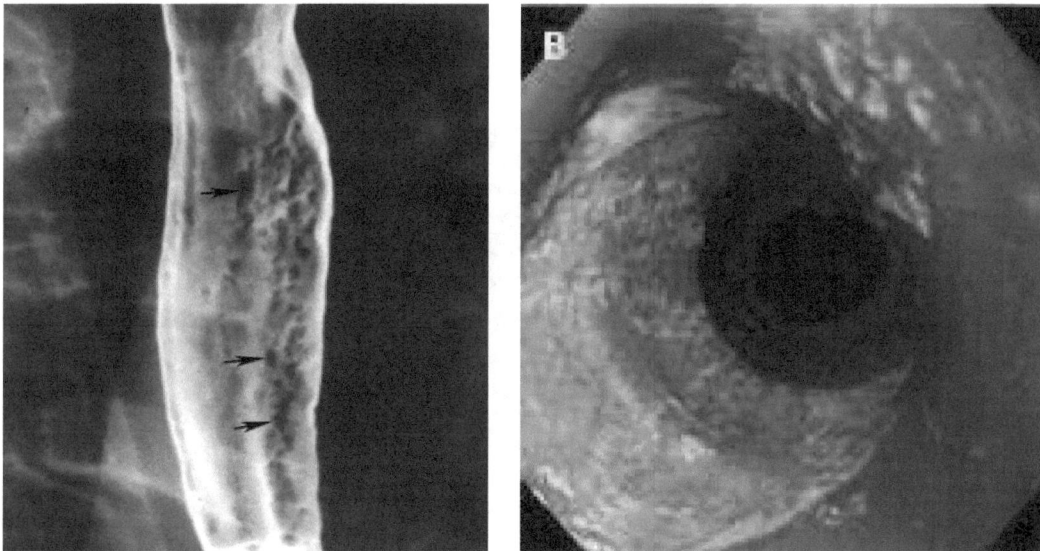

Diffuse Esophageal Spasm: symptoms include chest pain and dysphagia, look for a cork-screw esophagus.

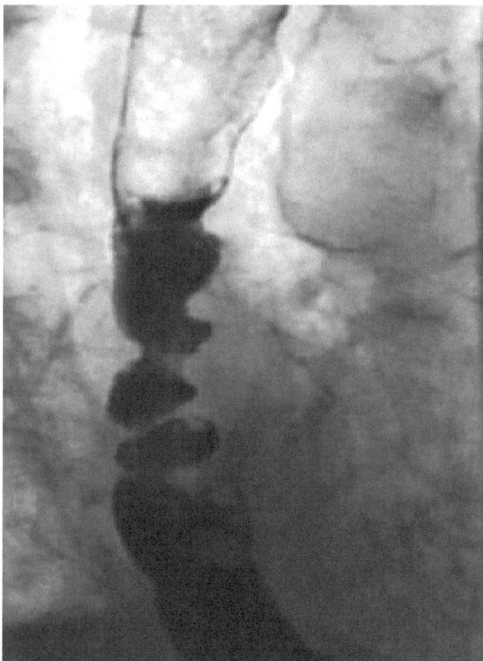

Feline Esophagus: transient transverse bands seen in the esophagus, almost always seen in patients with GERD, folds are 1-2 mm thick and circumferential. Caused by contraction of the longitudinal muscularis mucosa.

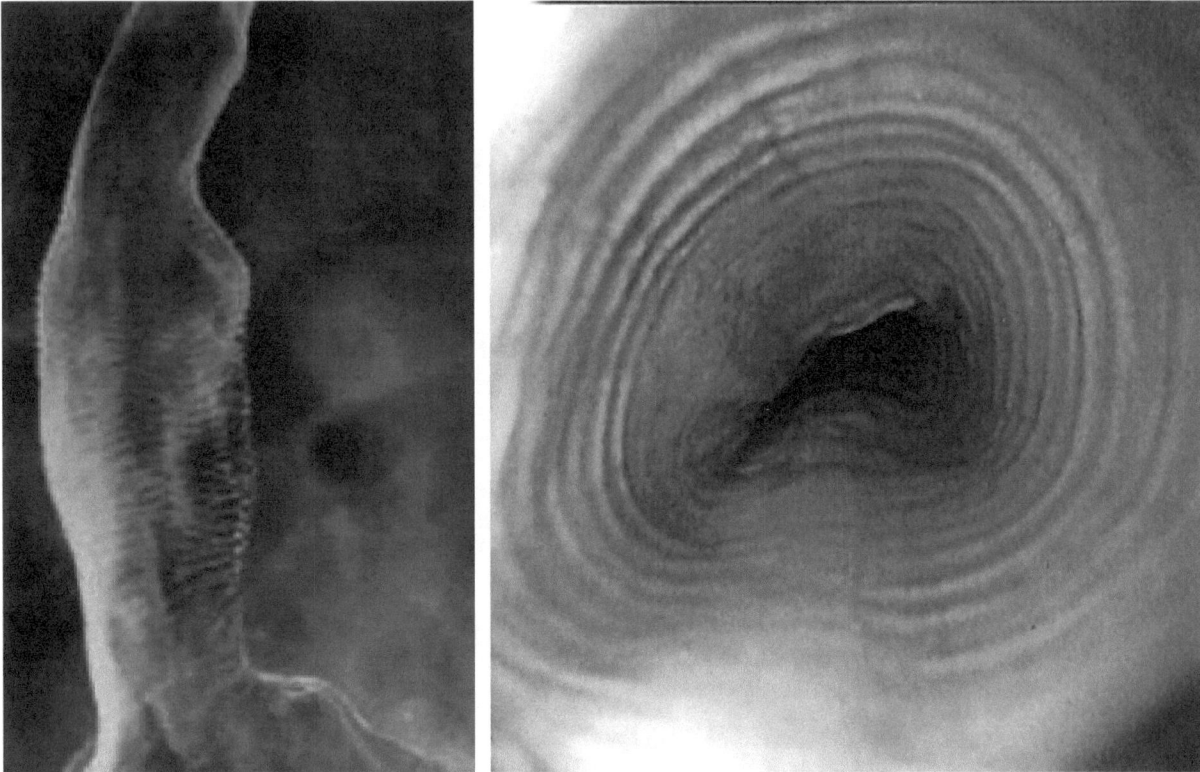

Fun Fact: most common benign tumor of esophagus is leiomyoma.

STOMACH

Benign Gastric Ulcer: most often happens along the lesser curvature of the stomach particularly in the middle body. The majority of ulcers found in the fundus are malignant. Most benign ulcers project outside the lumen and radiating folds are seen extending towards the ulcer crater (all the way to the edge).

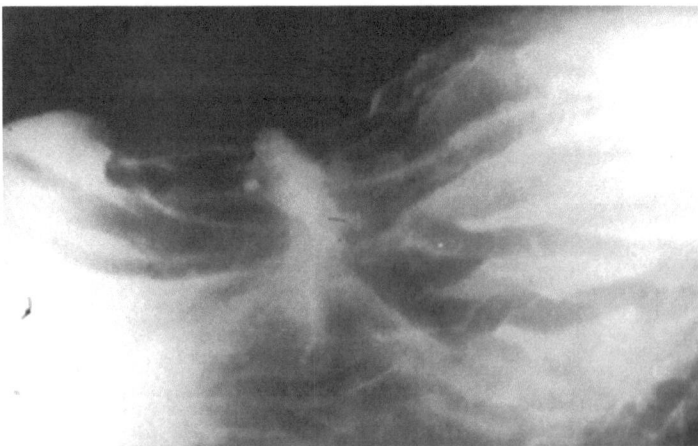

Gastric CA: refers to a primary malignancy arising from the gastric epithelium. It is associated with *H. pylori*. AdenoCA is by far the most common subtype (> 95%). Linitis plastic can happen and the stomach becomes small and contracted. On fluoro the stomach will be non-distensible.

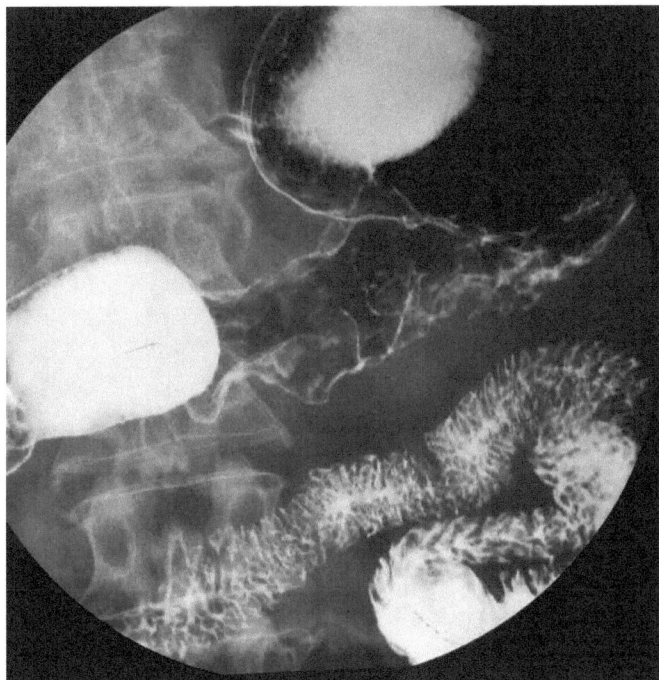

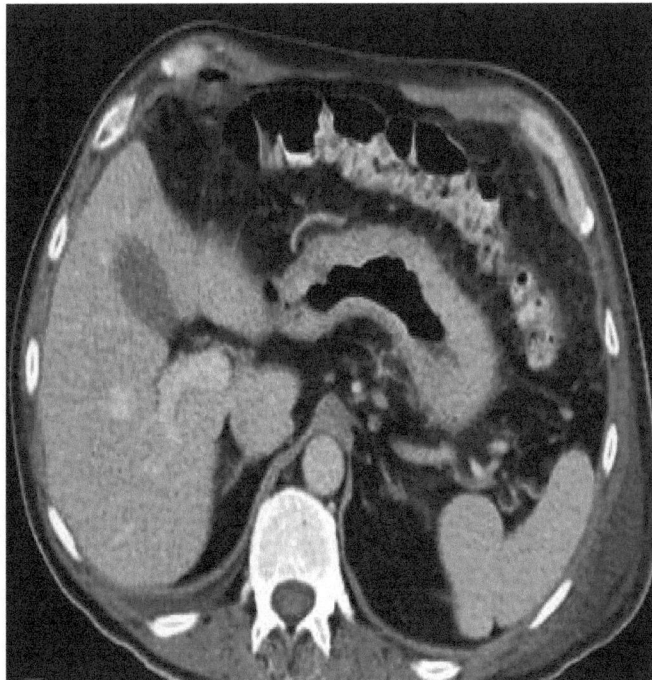

Menetrier Disease: is a rare idiopathic hypertrophic gastropathy. Characteristic of the disease is gastric mucosal hypertrophy, which causes the rugae to resemble convolutions in the brain. Thickening is most prominent in the gastric fundal region.

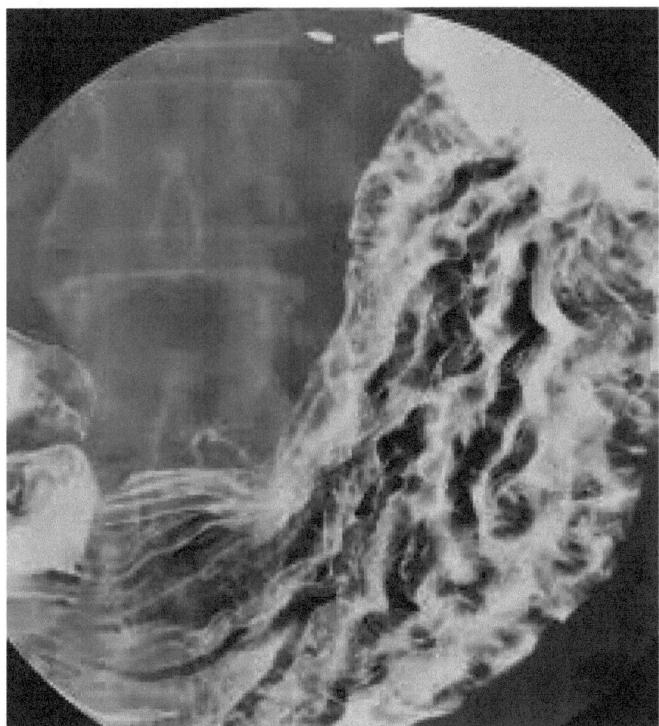

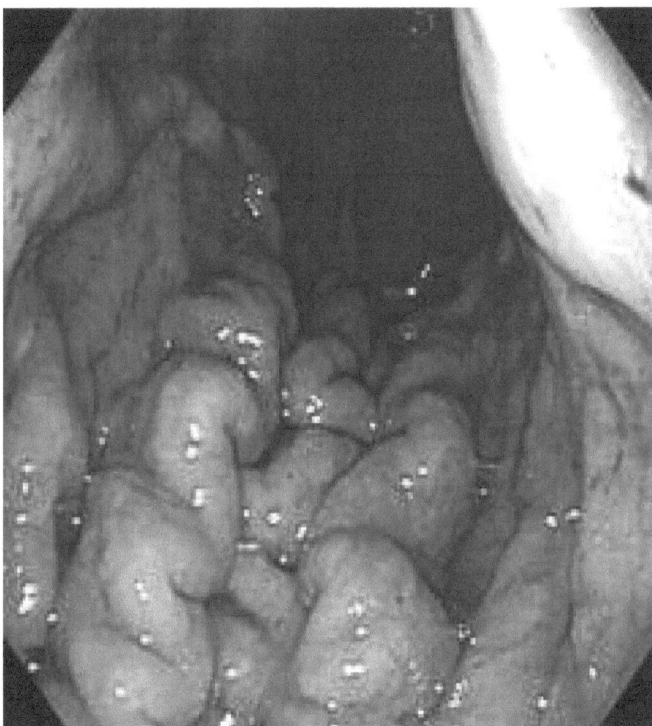

Pancreatic Rest: usually located on the greater curvature of the distal antrum. This is ectopic pancreatic tissue with its own duct (central umbilication).

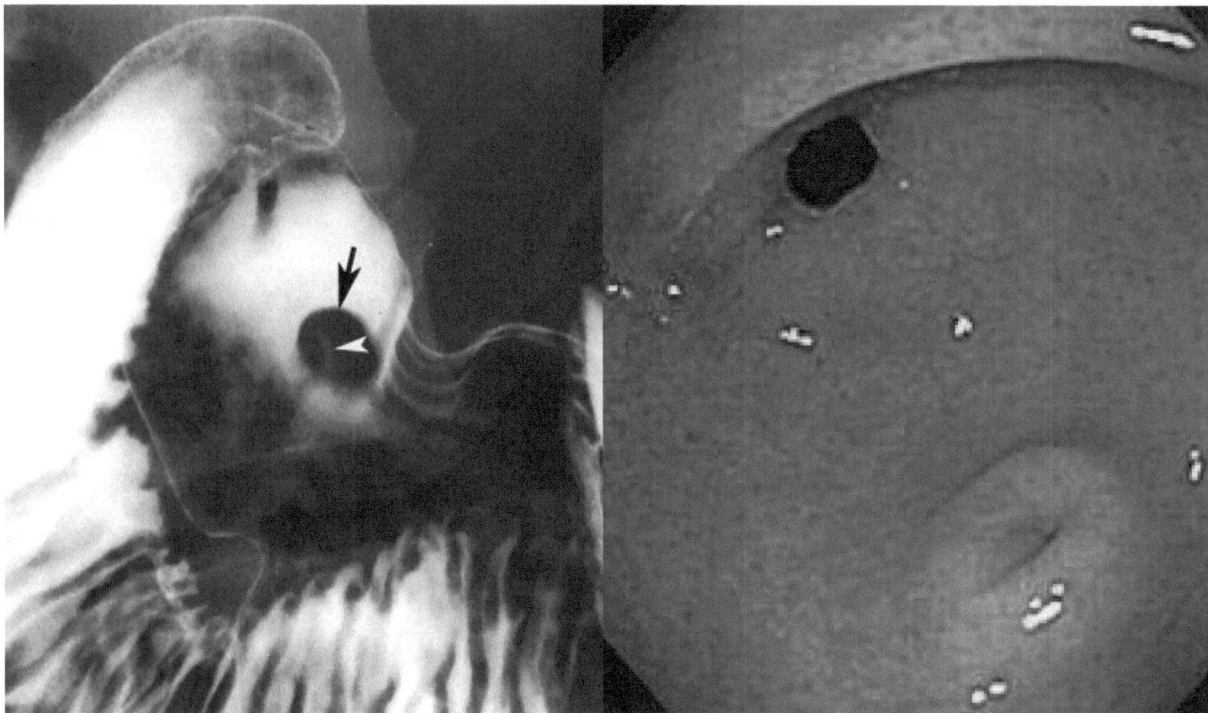

Gastric Volvulus: most result due to a large hiatal hernia and there are two kinds: organoaxial and mesenteroaxial. *Organoaxial* occurs when rotation of the stomach is around its long axis the antrum and greater curvature rotate superiorly and occupy a position above the fundus. *Mesenteroaxial* is when the stomach rotates from right to left about the axis of the gastroheptaic ligament. The antrum resides to the left of the cardia.

Type	Appearance	Description	Remarks
Organoaxial		Twist occurs along a line connecting the cardia and the pylorus along the luminal (long) axis of the stomach	• Most common type • Usually associated with diaphragmatic • Vascular compromise more common
Mesenteroaxial		Twist occurs around a plane perpendicular to the luminal (long) axis of the stomach from lesser to greater curvature	• Chronic symptoms more common • Diaphragmatic defects less common

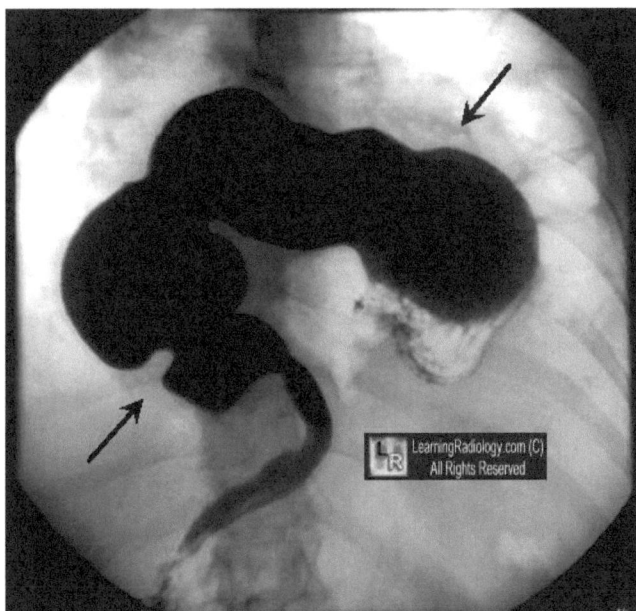

Fun Fact: leiomyoma is the most common benign tumor of the stomach and can be found anywhere in the stomach, but a leiomyosarcoma tends to be more proximal, enhances heterogeneously and can cause hemorrhage.

SMALL BOWEL

Perforated Duodenal Ulcer: use a water soluble UGI if suspecting this. Surgeons will ask to do this study after they repair a perforation to look for residual leak or suture dehiscence. Air in the RUQ is the key.

Small Bowel Diverticula: multiple outpouchings on the mesenteric surface. Complications can be due to diverticulitis, bleeding, and perforation. Can be associated with Vit B12 malabsorption caused by bacterial overgrowth.

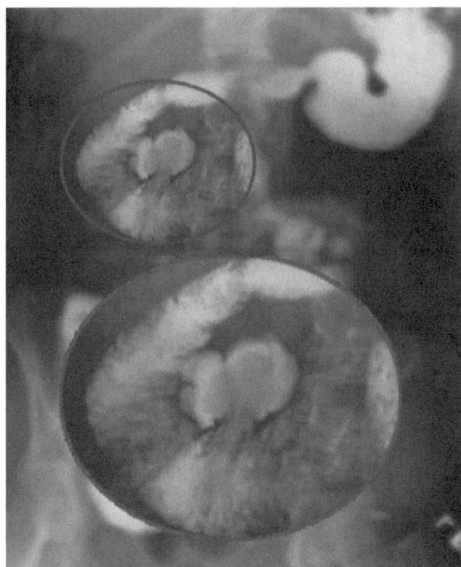

Brunner's Gland Hyperplasia: is an overgrowth of Brunner glands in the duodenum likely due to hyperacidity, this begins at the pylorus and extends into the proximal portions of the duodenum. These hyperplastic cells tend to be upto 1-cm, when > 1-cm it's called a Brunner gland adenoma. If it is a distal duodenal lesion – worry more about villous adenoma, which have an association with CA if enlarged.

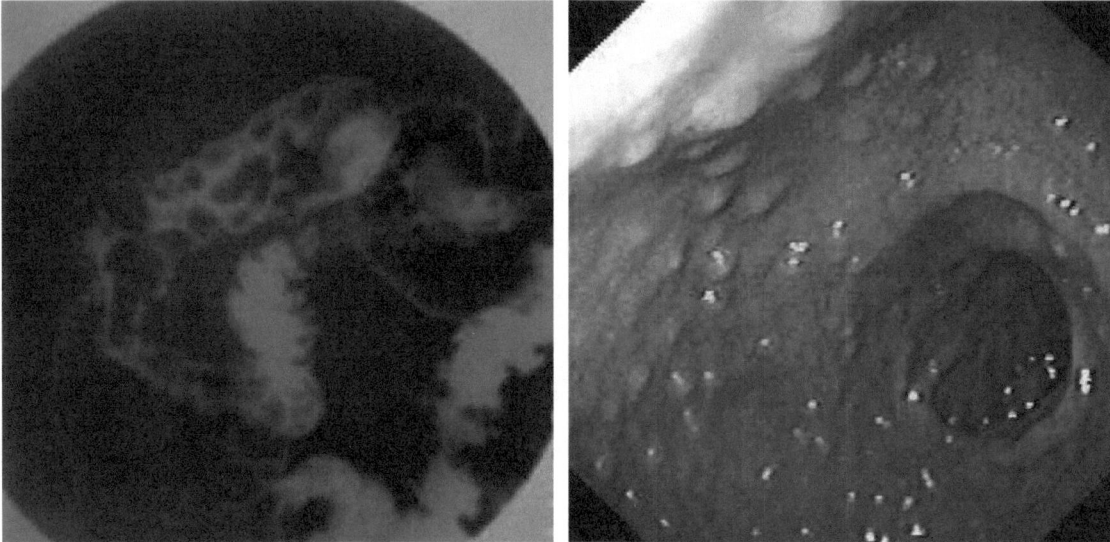

Scleroderma of the duodenum (2nd most common GI site) causes obstructive symptoms and has a very classic appearance on fluoro. Gastric and proximal duodenum dilated with signs of delayed gastric emptying. Can mimic SMA syndrome. Overall increased number of folds per inch.

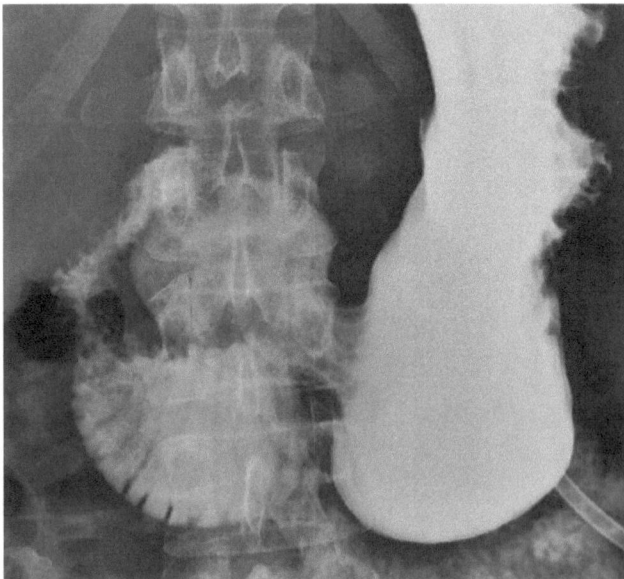

Celiac Disease: "ileojejunal reversal." A condition of GI malabsorption that is due to bad response to gluten – consider this in cases of Fe^{3+} deficiency anemia of uncertain cause. There is an increased risk of SB lymphoma (T-Cell) in long-standing disease. Overall decreased number of folds per inch.

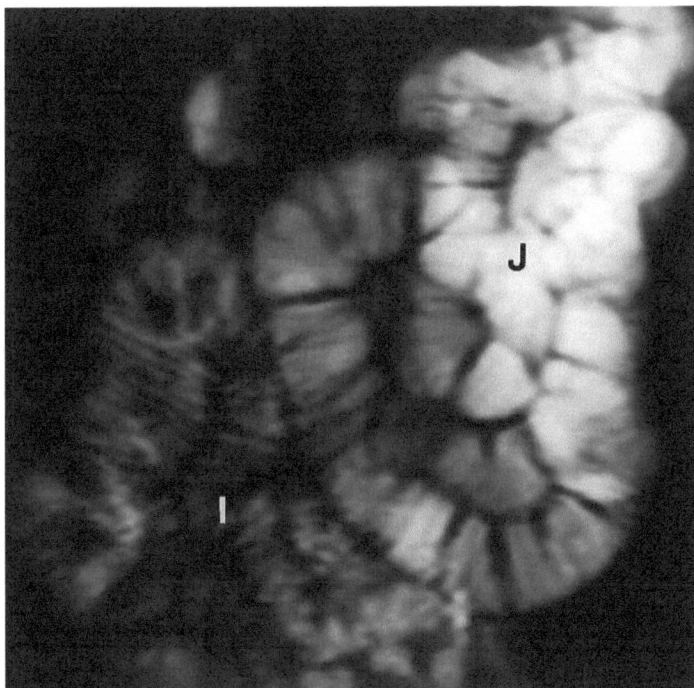

Crohn's Disease: is an inflammatory transmural disease process that has skip lesions from mouth to butt. Most often hits the TI and causes fistulas and strictures. If affecting the stomach, it'll be distal and cause erosions and stricture.

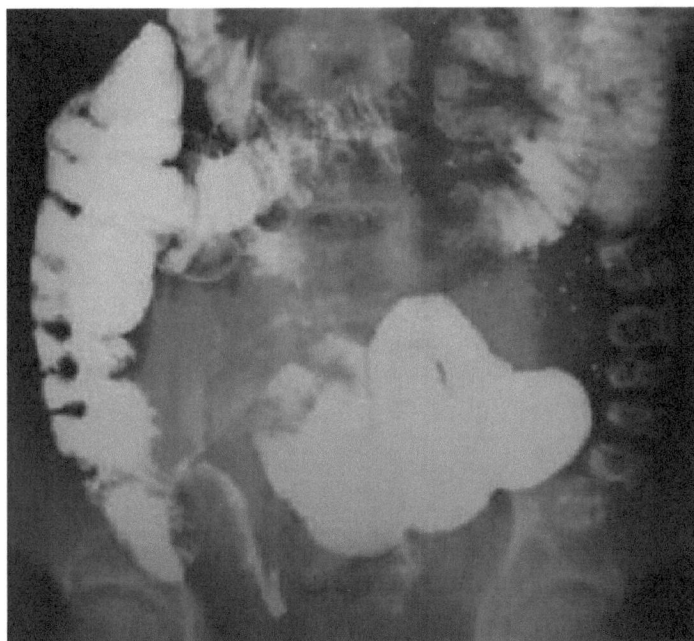

Backwash Ileitis: is extension of ulcerative colitis into the ileum due to failure of the ileocecal valve. It causes granular appearing mucosa with ulcerations and dilation of the ileum. Remember that Crohn's will cause narrowing, as will TB and *Yersinia*.

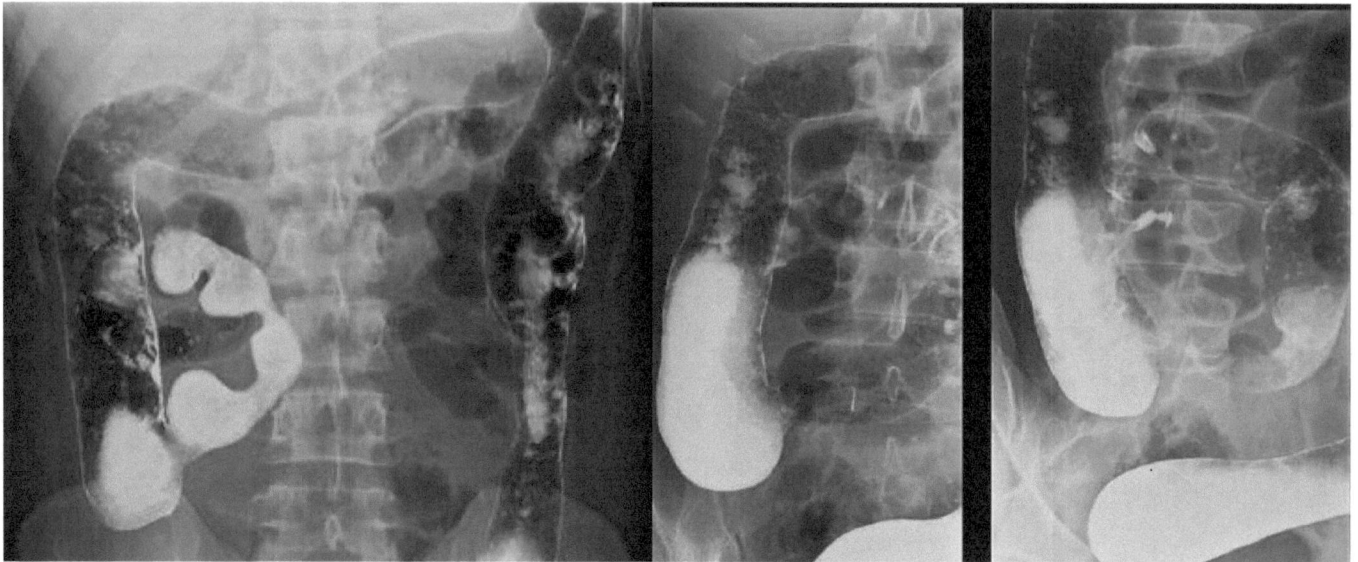

Small Bowel Lymphoma: can occur almost anywhere in GI tract (most often in stomach), it causes wall thickening and bowel dilation. Seen in people with AIDS and associated with EBV. Can be a focal mass or diffuse nodules (see image on next page).

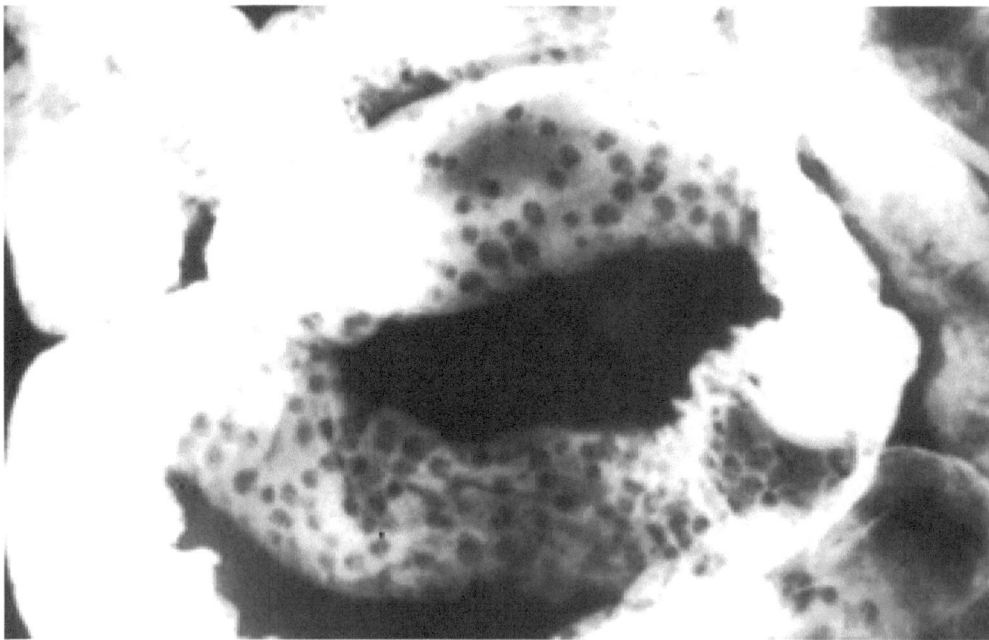

Small Bowel Lipoma: this is the second most common benign tumor of the SB (leiomyoma is #1 – tends to be in the jejunum and bleed), lipomas tend to be in the ileum can have a pedicle and cause intussusception.

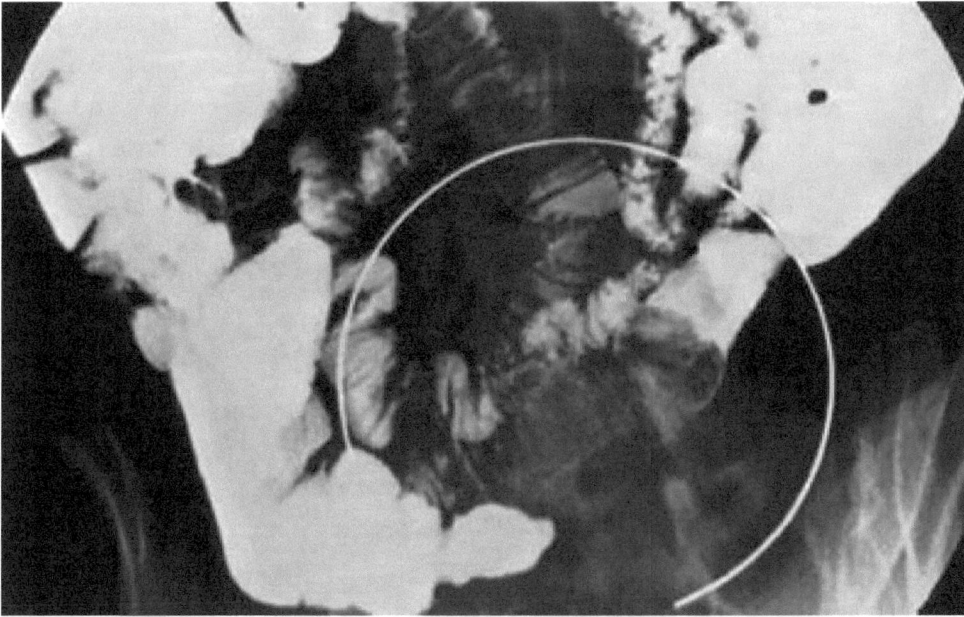

Whipple's Disease: think of this in middle-aged men with malabsorption and arthralgias. Caused by whipple's bacilli infection.

Peutz-Jeghers Syndrome: autosomal dominant polyposis syndrome characterized by multiple hamartomatous polyps involving the small intestine, colon, stomach, and mucocutaneous pigmentation of the mouth and fingers. There is an increased risk of intussusception and GI tract adenoCA (polyps themselves are NOT premalignant).

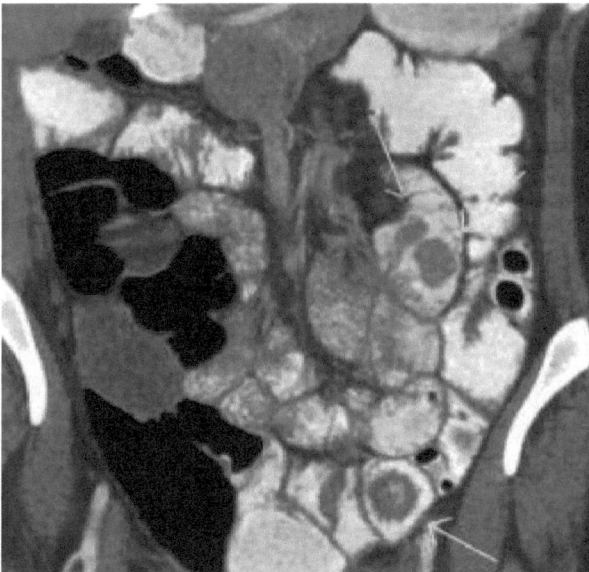

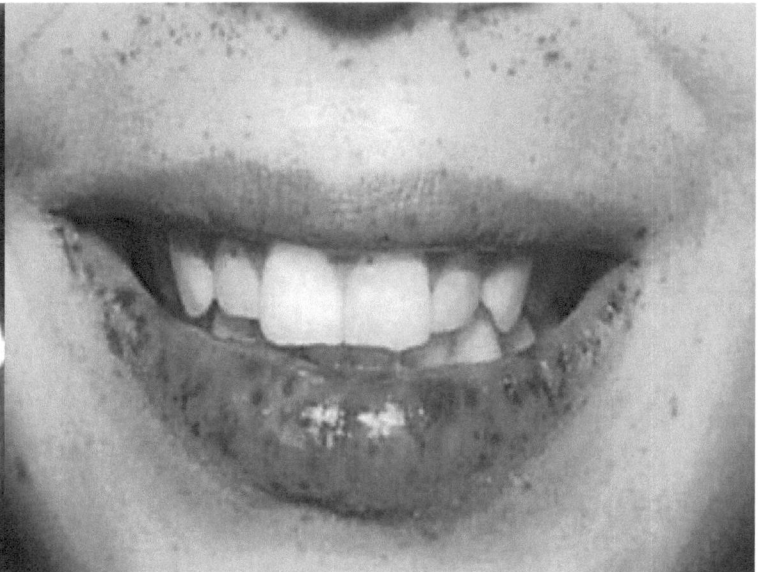

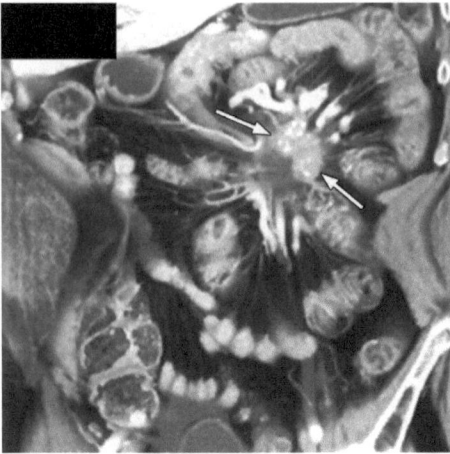

Carcinoid Tumor: can arise almost anywhere, when they arise in the small bowel, they prefer the ileum. They cause a lot of desmoplastic response and secrete 5-HIAA. Carcinoid syndrome occurs when liver metastases secrete hormones that cause flushing and vasodilation. With time right-sided endocardial fibrosis and valve prolapse occur.

COLON

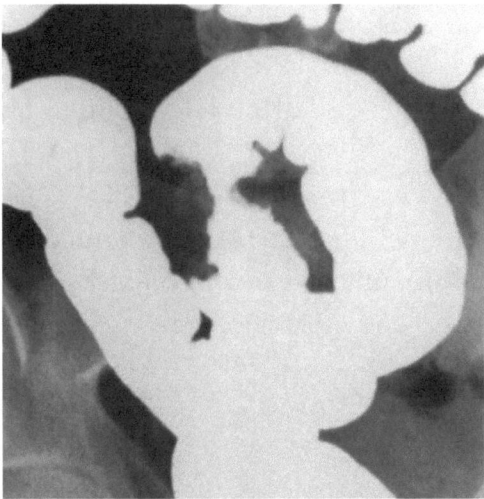

Colon CA: is the most common malignancy of the GI tract. 98% are adenoCA and arise from polyps that undergo malignant degeneration. Look for an apple core lesion.

Angiodyspalsia: Don't forget this is as a cause of lower GI bleeding in older adults, found in the right colon and is seen as a tangle of vessels near the cecum on angiogram. There is a loose association with aortic stenosis. The number one cause of bleeding is diverticular!

Familial Polyposis Syndrome: autosomal dominant condition characterized by adenomatous polyposis involving the colon >> stomach > small bowel. Predisposed to colon CA (#1 CA in these patients), periampullary CA (#2 CA in these patients)

- **Gardner's Syndrome** – polyps, osteomas and papillary thyroid CA
- **Turcot's Syndrome** – polyps and CNS tumors (GBM and medulloblastomas)

Neutropenic Colitis (typhlitis): seen in immunosuppressed individuals as infection of the cecum and ascending colon. Treated aggressively with antibiotics.

Benign Pneumatosis: this is kind of interesting because we will see intramural air in a patient not complaining of abdominal pain. Usually pneumatosis makes can tighten the Radiologists sphincter, but it can be due to steroids, asthma, COPD emphysema, and recent endoscopy and surgery.

COLON EMERGENCIES:

Cecal Volvulus: this is a surgical emergency because the cecum twists on its vascular pedicle causing a closed loop obstruction. Cecum displaces into the LUQ and appears bean shaped.

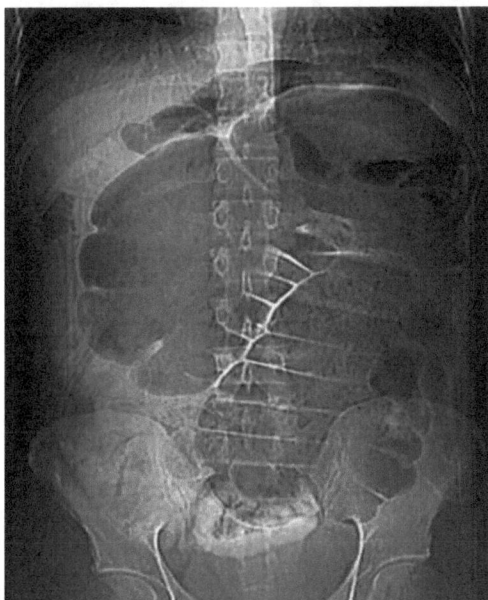

Sigmoid Volvulus: more common than a cecal volvulus. Happens in the elderly using laxatives. Sigmoid twists up into the RUQ with convergence of the sigmoid ends in the LLQ (to the left of S1). If not strangulated, tube deflation will work, if strangulated, surgery is needed.

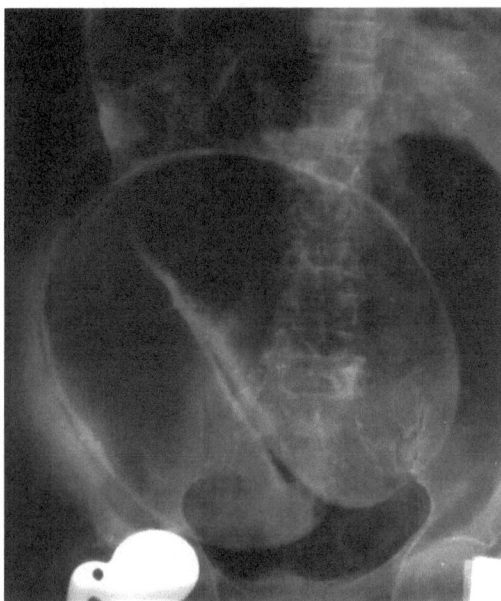

Toxic Megacolon: associated with ulcerative colitis, Crohn's, ischemia, and pseudomembranous colitis (*C. dificile*). Perforation is the most feared complication.

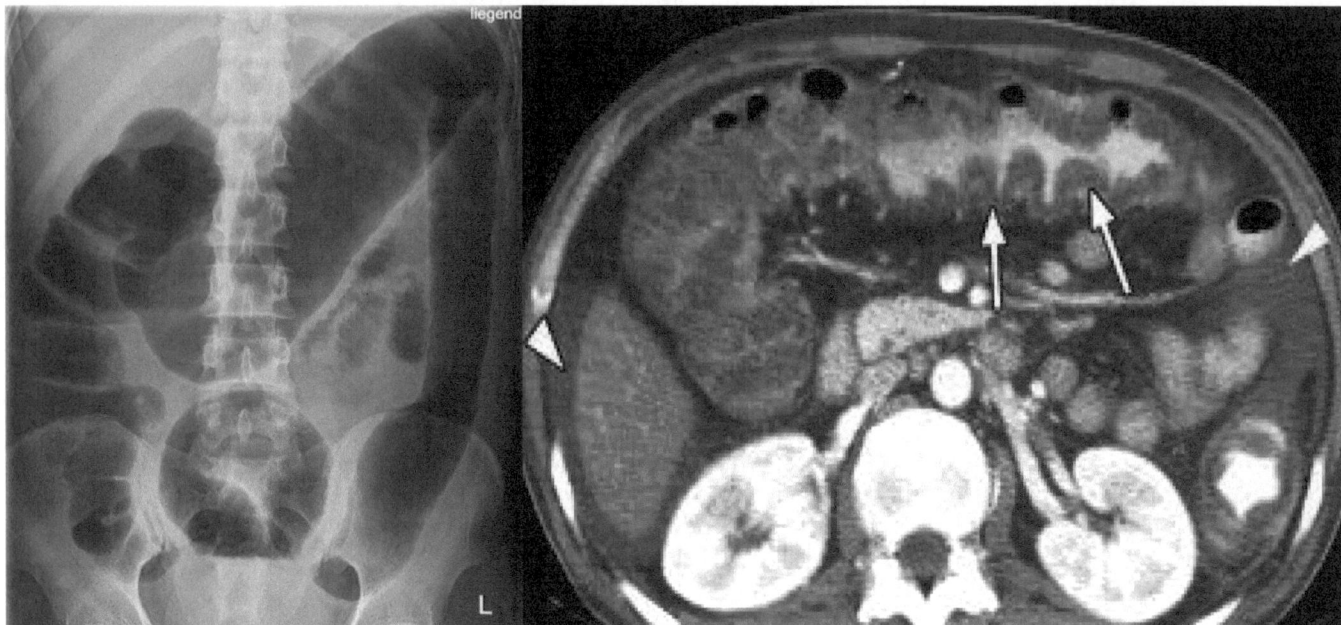

LIVER: going to focus on MRI appearance of liver masses in this section, however before we go into that, it's important to know liver segmental anatomy

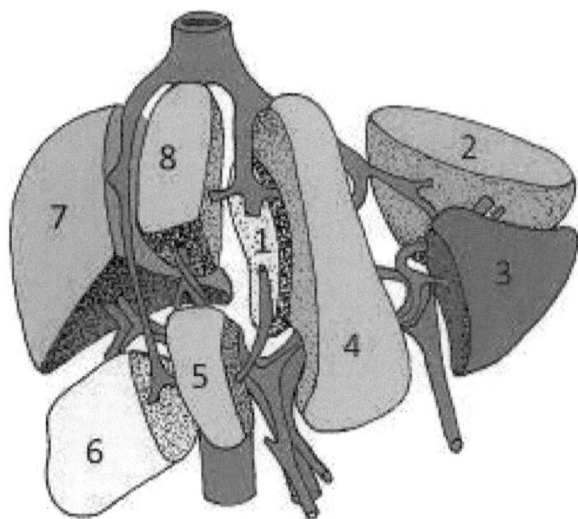

Caudate lobe is segment 1 and is located posteriorly. It is different from the other lobes because it directly connects to the IVC and tends to hypertrophy in cirrhosis while the rest of the liver is shrinking

Cysts: are benign lesions that are well demarcated and hypodense with water attenuation. No contrast enhancement.

Hemangioma: It is the most common benign liver tumor. Peripheral, nodular, interrupted enhancing pattern; can be giant. Homogeneous enhancement is atypical. These lesions should hold on to contrast and be brighter than the liver on delayed images.

MR: T1 hypointense relative to liver, T2 intensely bright, T1+gad shows peripheral enhancement

- PITFALL: Hemangioendothelioma has peripheral, coalescing lesions in a young kid with capsular retraction.

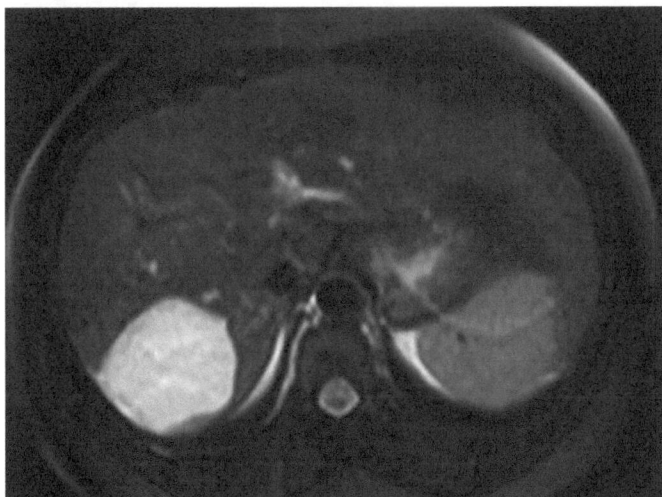

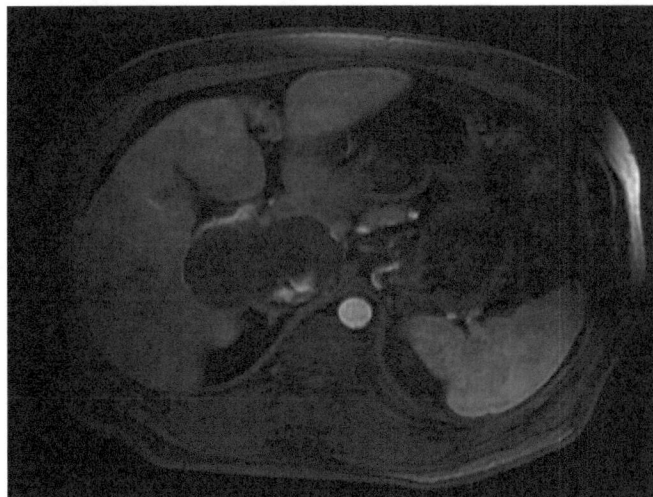

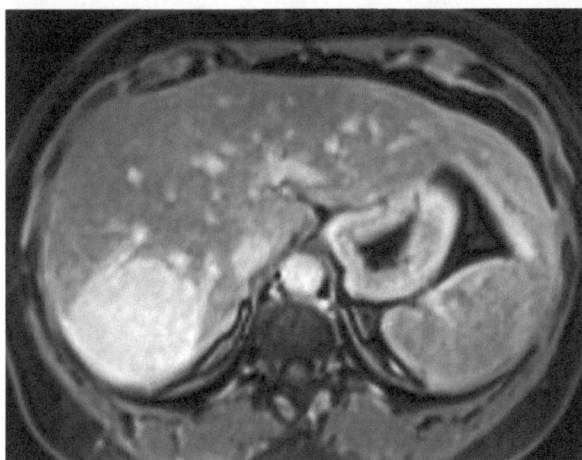

T2 (upper left), T1 + CE early (upper right), T1 + CE late (bottom)

FNH: incidental finding in young females. Referred to as "stealth lesions". If a patient has cirrhosis and you see something like this, go for HCC first, not FNH.

MR: T1/T2 similar signal to background liver. Central T2 bright scar. Homogeneous arterial enhancement of lesion, scar enhances on delayed images.

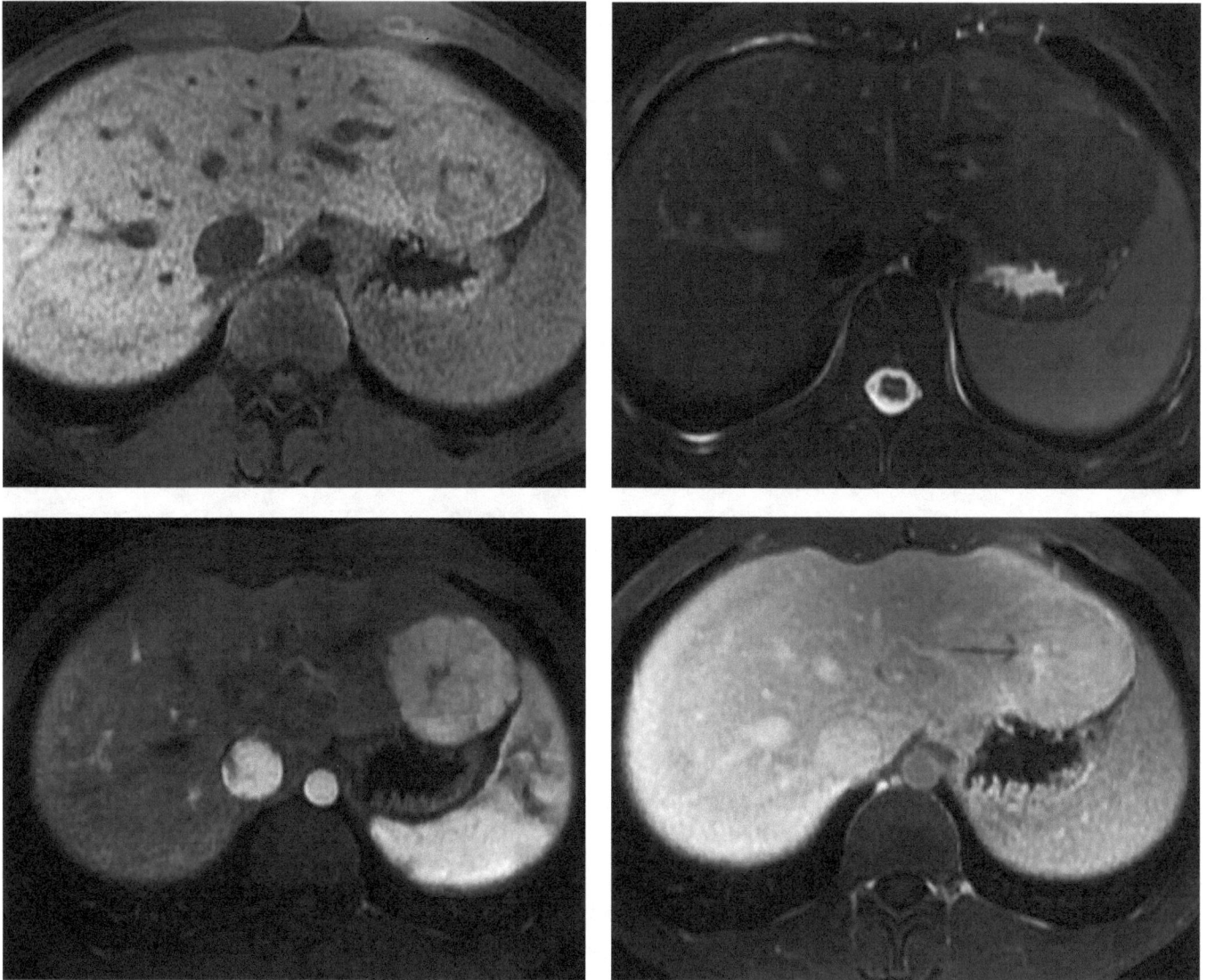

T1 (top left), T2 (top right), T1+CE early (bottom left), T1+CE late (bottom right)

Adenoma: young female on OCP or a muscular dude on 'roids, also if multiple (>10) then think about glycogen storage disease – Von Girerke's. Usually an incidental finding, but can have hemorrhage and fat content. This is a pre-malignant lesion. Use Eovist to help you out, because adenoma doesn't enhance on delays but FNH will. Adenoma does not have transport protein to take up Eovist.

MR: T1 variable (hyper to hypo intense), T2 mildly hyperintense, In/Out will cause some signal drop out because they can have fat, T1+CE shows early enhancement with isointense to liver on delayed, hypointense to liver on Eovist.

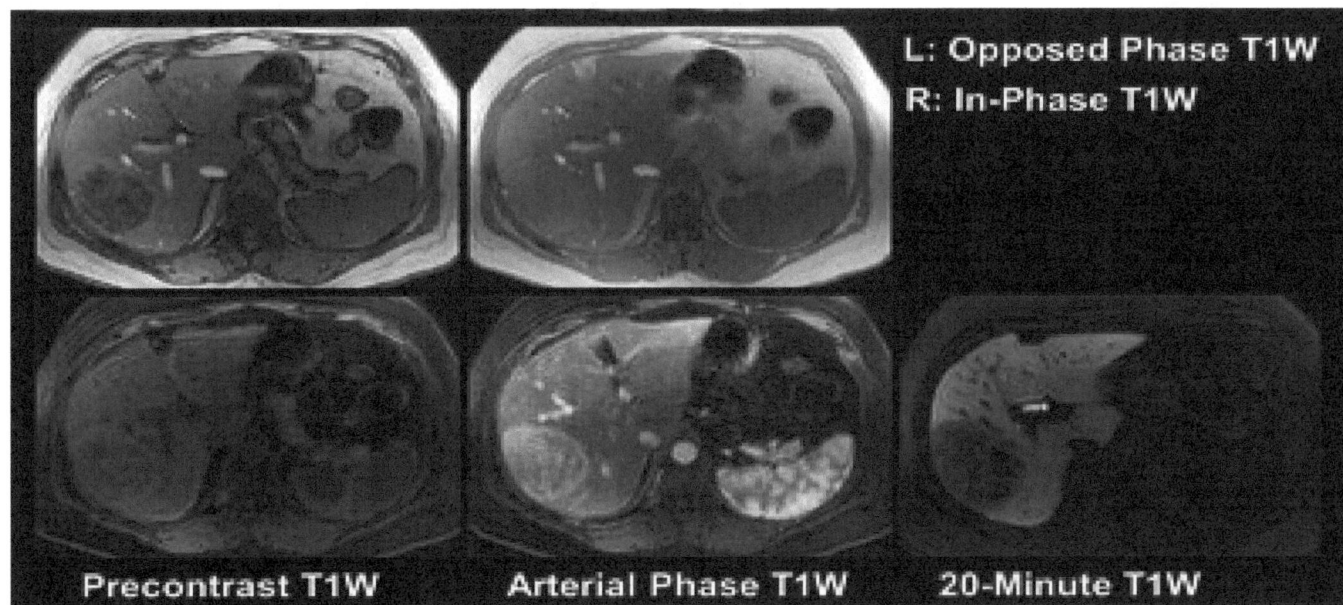

FOCAL MALIGNANT LESIONS:

Metastases: all tumors have a modified perfusion compared to the liver because of angiogenesis and hepatic artery recruitment. Fast growing masses will have cystic changes due to central necrosis. Look for multiple lesions. Calcifications are seen in: serous ovarian CA, mucin producing colon CA.

MR: T1 hypointense, T2 hyperintense, T1+CE can have lesional or peri-lesional enhancement. Small lesions enhance diffusely, larger lesions have rim enhancement with **wash-out.**

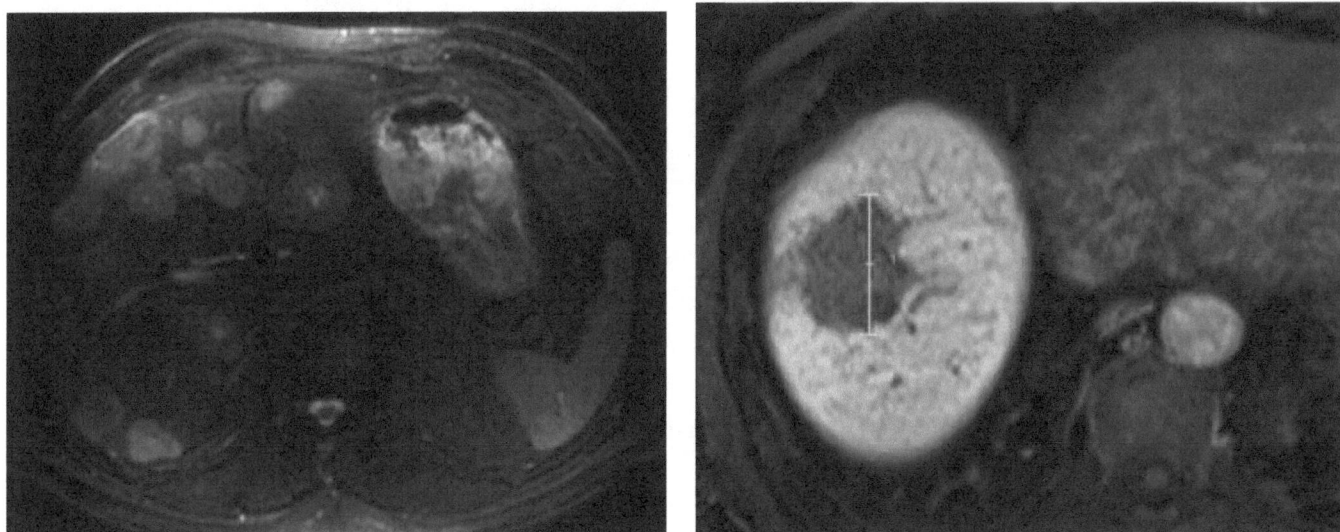

Multiple T2 bright lesions (left), Delayed image showing washout of lesion (right)

Hypervascular Mets – neuroendocrine tumors (islet cell, carcinoid, pheochromocytoma), thyroid, renal cell CA, and sarcoma

HCC: 5th most common cancer in the world and is associated with Hep B, Hep C, and EtOHism. Think about this in patients with cirrhosis and elevated AFP. Lesions are more hypervascular when > 2cm if < 2cm could be a dysplastic nodule or portocaval shunt, follow-up in 3 months to check for growth. Spreads to regional lymph nodes, look for venous invasion and extrahepatic disease because this rules out transplant as treatment option.

MR: T1 variable intensity, T2 typically hyperintense, T1+CE is usually avid early enhancement with **washout** becoming hypointense to the liver parenchyma

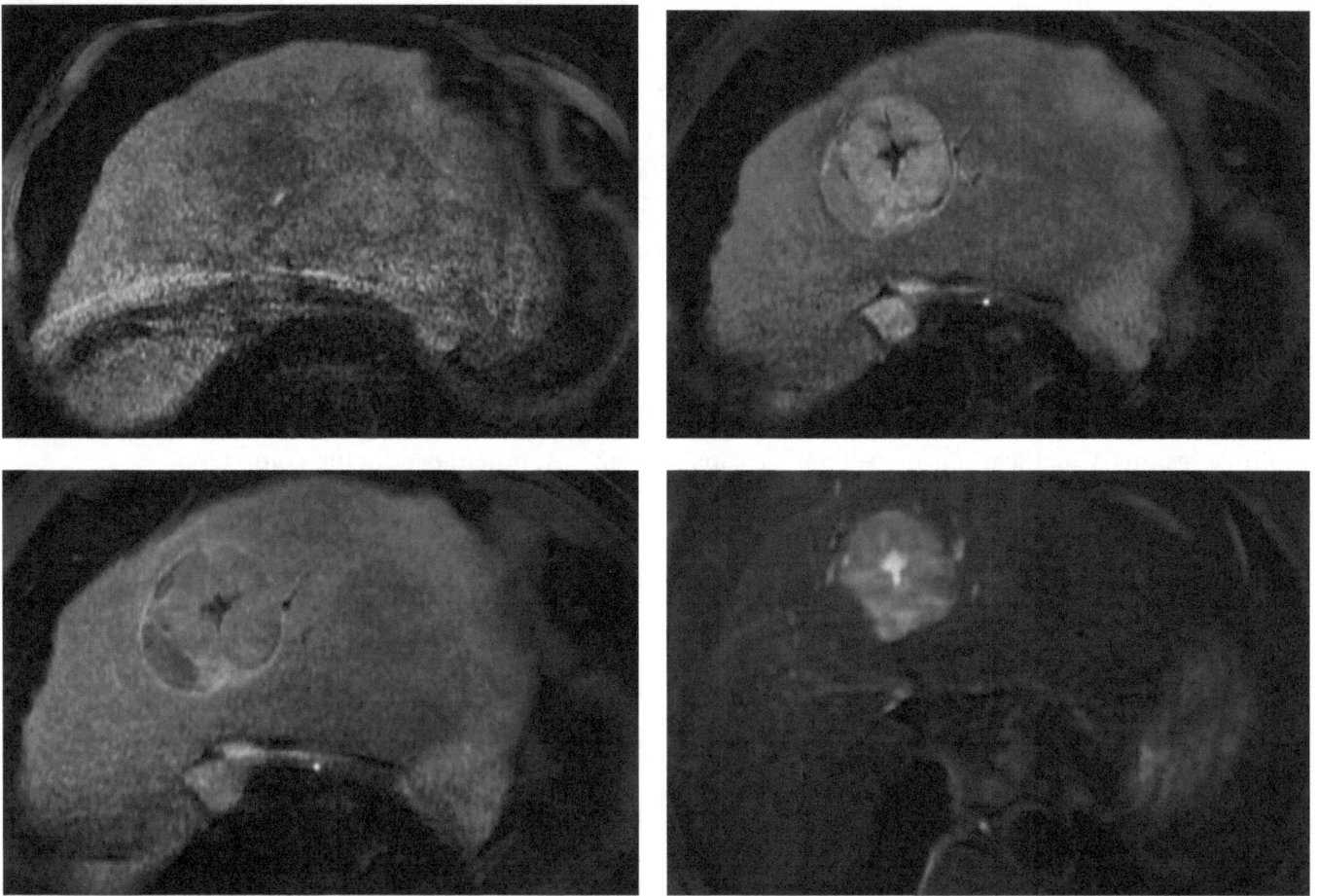

T1 hypointense (top left), T1+CE early enhancement (top right), T1+CE delayed starting to wash out peripherally (bottom left), T2 hyperintense

Cholangiocarcinoma: 2nd commonest primary liver malignancy. It is an infiltrating mass forming lesion that causes scarring of the bile ducts and liver capsule retraction. It is associated with PSC, Caroli's disease, and choledochal cysts

MRI: start of with peripheral enhancement that spreads centrally. Bile ducts distal to mass are dilated.

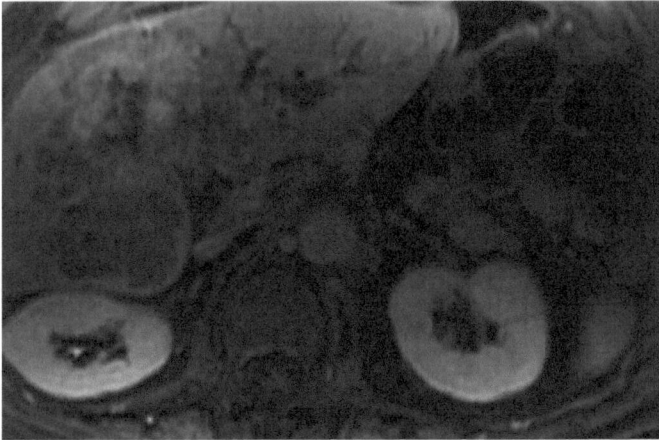

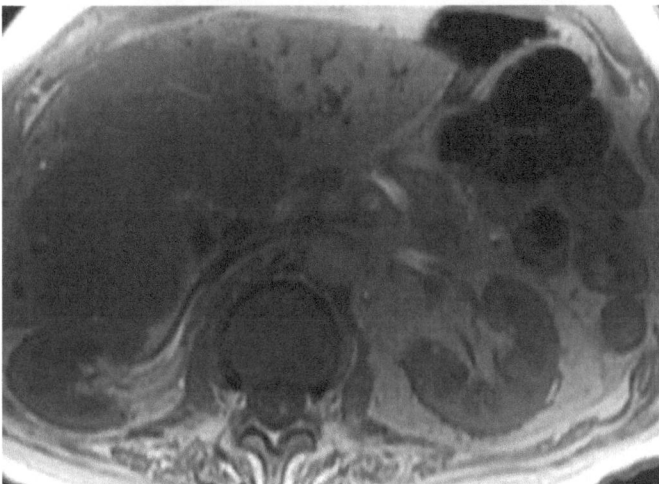

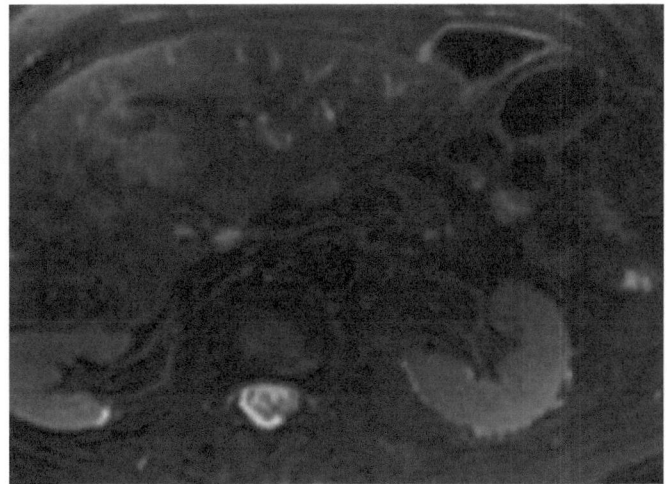

T1 hypointense (top left), T2 variable, but bright (top right), T1+CE heterogeneous enhancement (bottom left)

DIFFUSE LESIONS:

Cirrhosis: associated with HepC and EtOH abuse. Nodular appearing liver with portal HTN. The nodularity is the body's response to chronic injury (regeneration and fibrosis).

- **Regenerating nodules** are caused by chronic inflammation (T1 low T2 bright), **they enhance like the liver**
- **Dysplastic nodules** are associated with HCC and a growing dysplastic nodule is CA (T1 bright T2 low +/- CE, does not wash out)

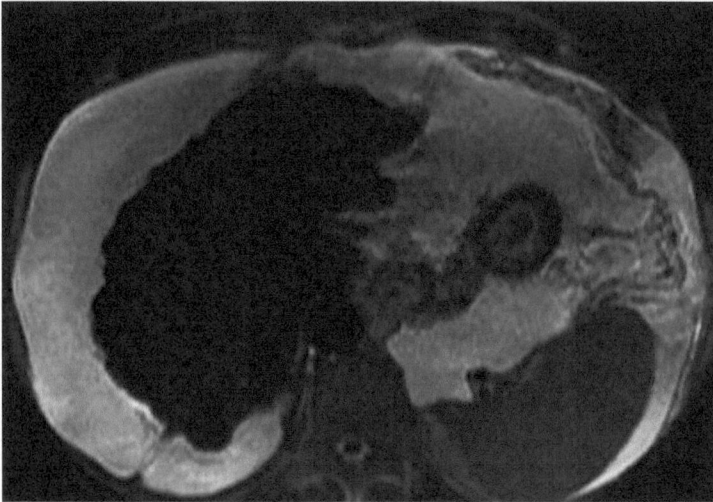

Fatty Liver: this is easy to diagnose, just use In/Out of phase imaging

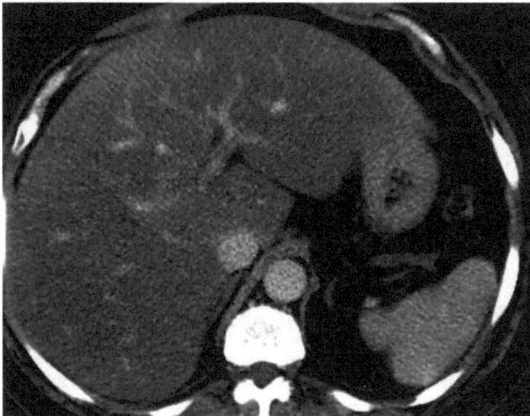

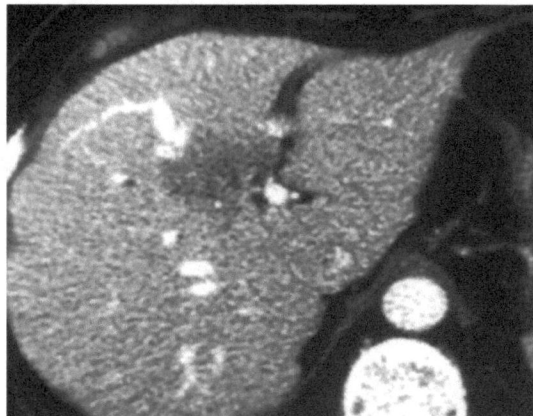

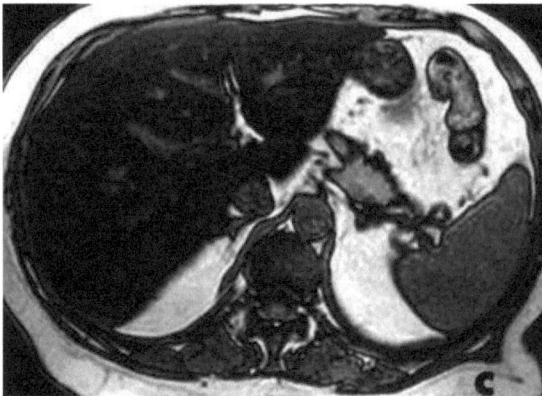

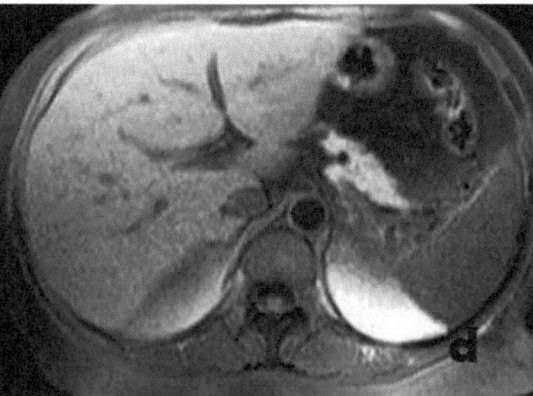

Diffuse fatty liver (top left), focal fat (top right), Opposed phase (bottom)

Hemochromatosis: autosomal recessive disease due to abnormal Fe^{3+} absorption from the GI tract. The reticuloendothelial system (RES) cannot store all of the Fe^{3+} so it gets deposited in liver parenchyma, pancreas, myocardium, and joints. Hepatomegaly, arthralgias, and heart failure – due to deposition of Fe^{3+}

MR: Super dark on T2, super-paramagnetic effects
CT: HU of liver increases (similar to amiodarone therapy)

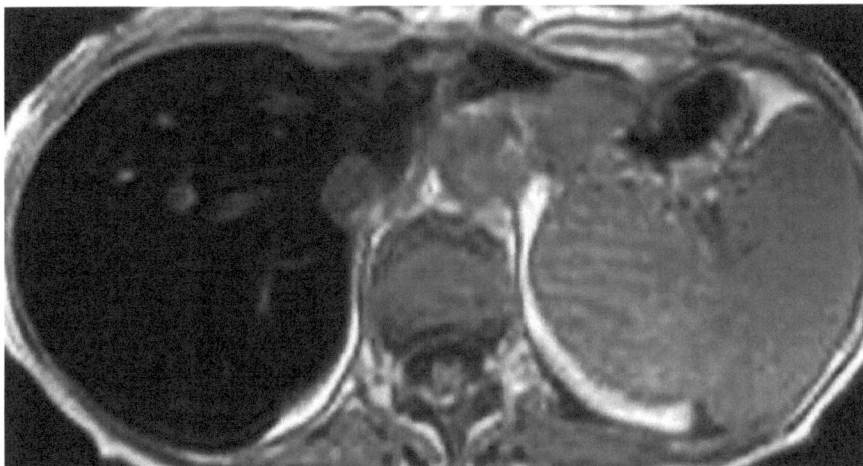

Hemosiderosis: due to repeat transfusions with Fe3+ in RES **without hepatomegaly**. Causes dark liver, dark spleen, dark marrow.

Budd-Chiari: hepatic vein thrombosis with patient's complaining of tender hepatomegaly, ascites and jaundice.

I   – IVC +/- secondary hepatic vein occlusion
II   – HV +/- secondary IVC occlusion
III – small veins of liver

The obstructed flow causes congested liver with reversal of flow. Caudate lobe enlargement with delayed enhancement and overall heterogeneity of the liver.

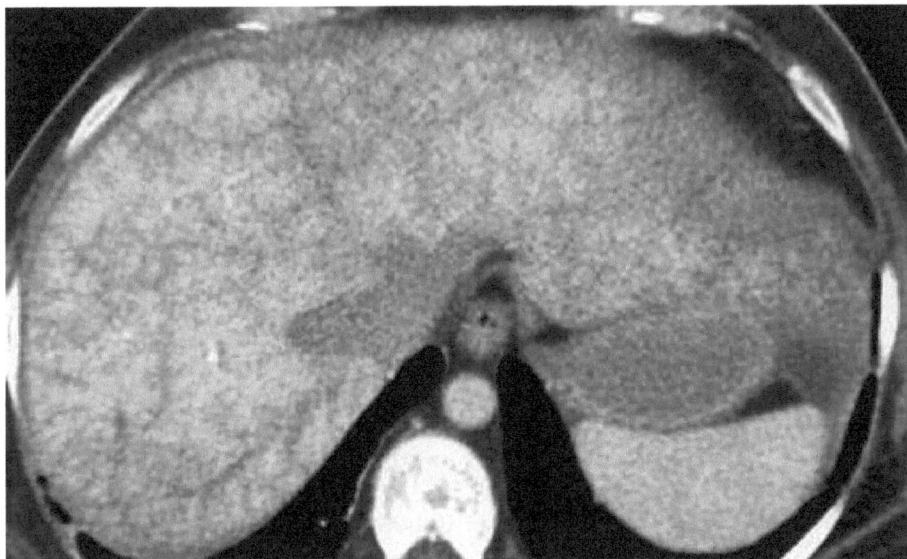

PV Thrombosis: causes include tumor, pancreatitis, cholangitis, etc. The chronic occlusion leads to collateral formation.

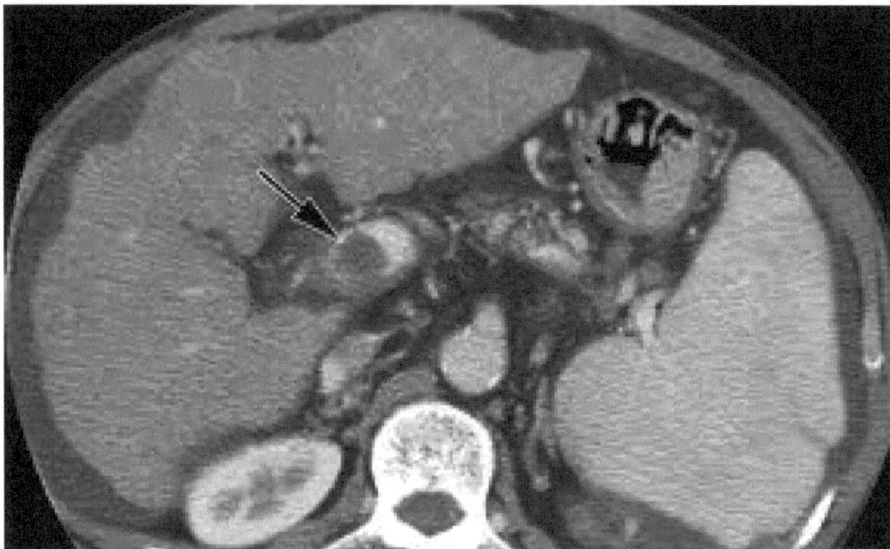

BILIARY TREE: There is an important fact to remember here, the **right posterior hepatic duct** can be variable in position and this variant is important for surgery because it may be accidentally ligated if the surgeon isn't made aware of it.

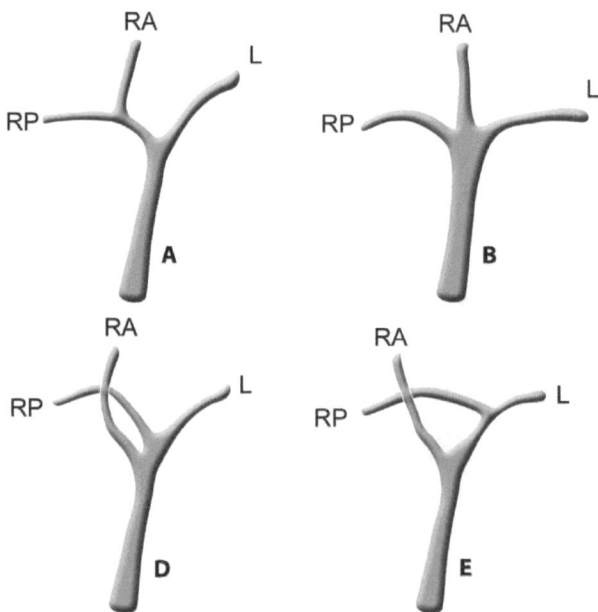

Some variants

Choledocholithiasis: look for filling defects in dependent locations, can be hard to see on CT (look for a subtle meniscus in the CBD around a soft tissue density to help ID a non calcified stone).

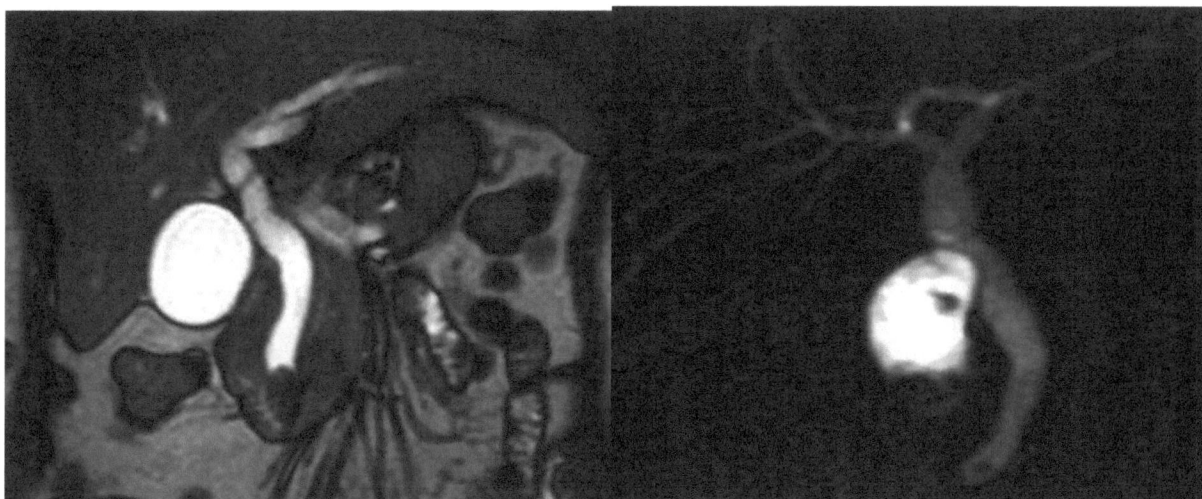

Cholecystitis: can be acute or chronic, calculous or acalculous (look for a GB > 5cm in transverse dimension in a febrile patient). Acalculous cholecystitis happen to sick patients, so drain this with a cholecystostomy tube.

Air in the GB wall is **emphysematous cholecystitis** seen in diabetics, caused by *C. perfringens*.

Gallstone Ileus: is when a large stone erodes through the GB wall and into the duodenum, it transits distally and gets stuck at ileocecal valve causing upstream obstruction.

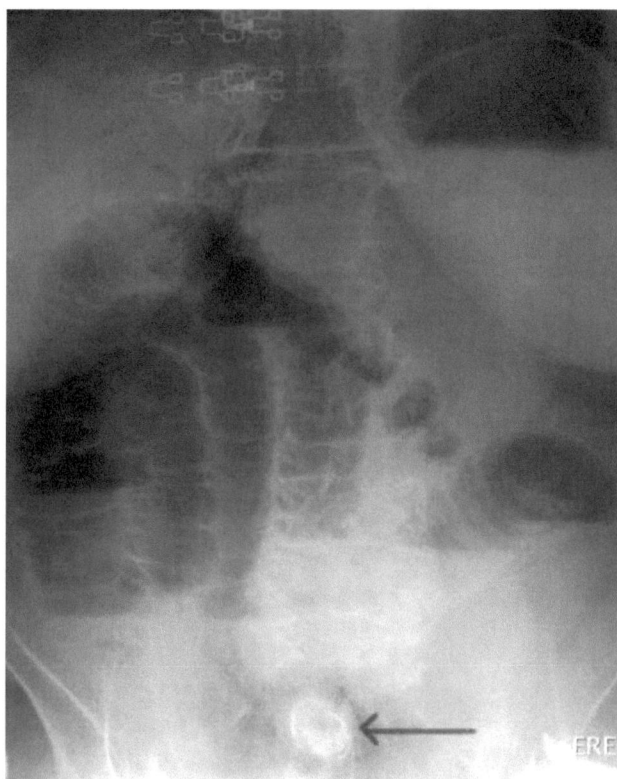

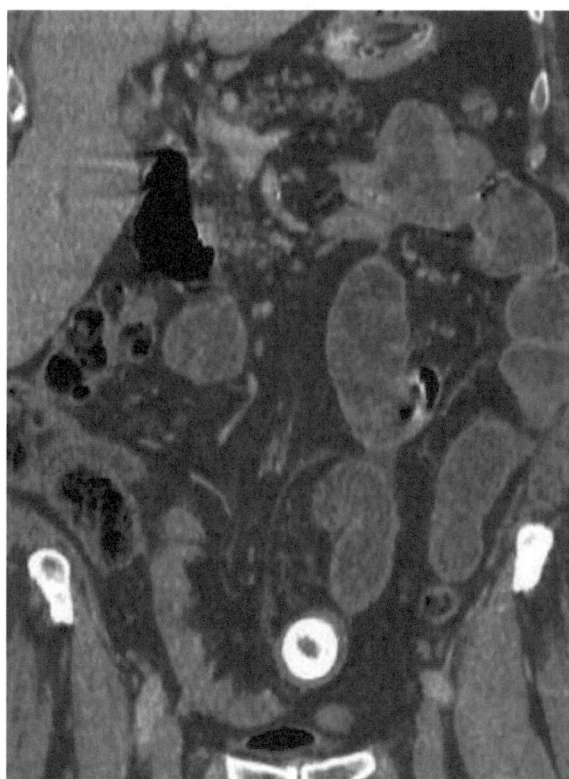

Porcelain GB: wall calcification, not as highly associated with malignancy as previously thought.

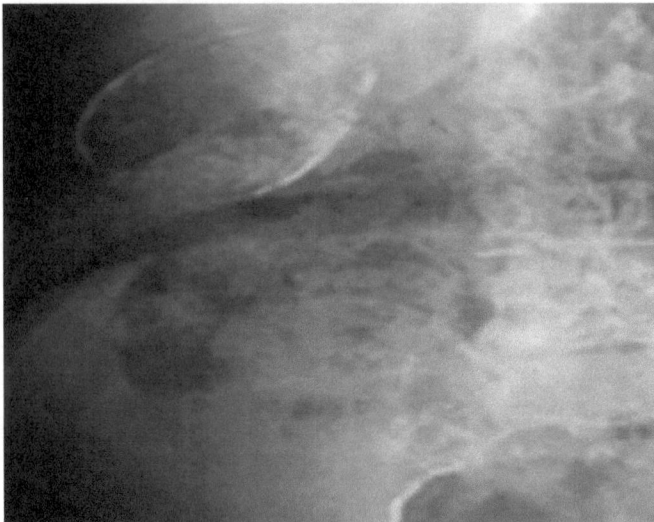

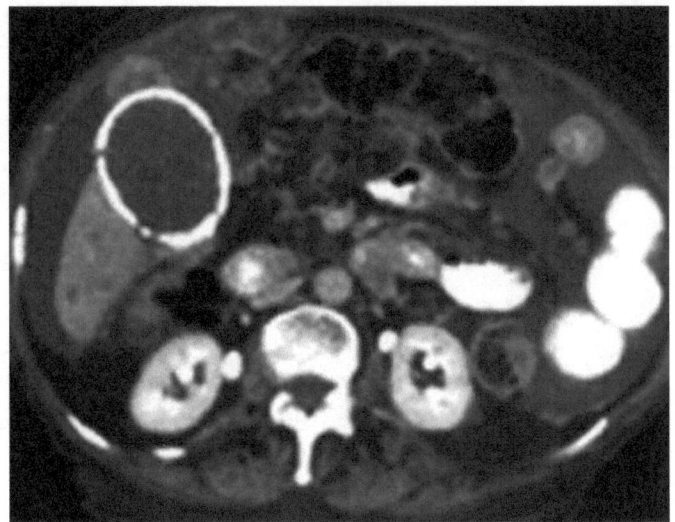

Mirizzi Syndrome: caused by a gallstone impacted in the cystic duct with severe local inflammation and obstruction of the common hepatic duct.

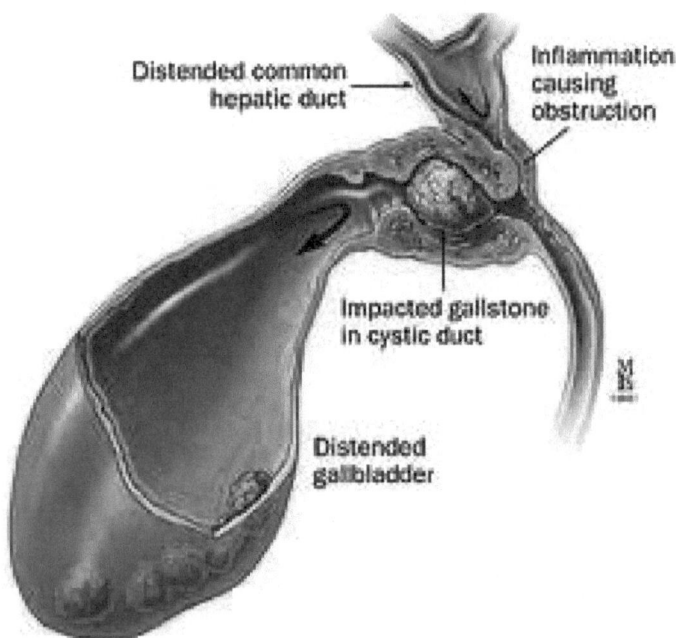

DUCTS

Pseudostricture: where the right hepatic artery crosses the common duct on MRCP

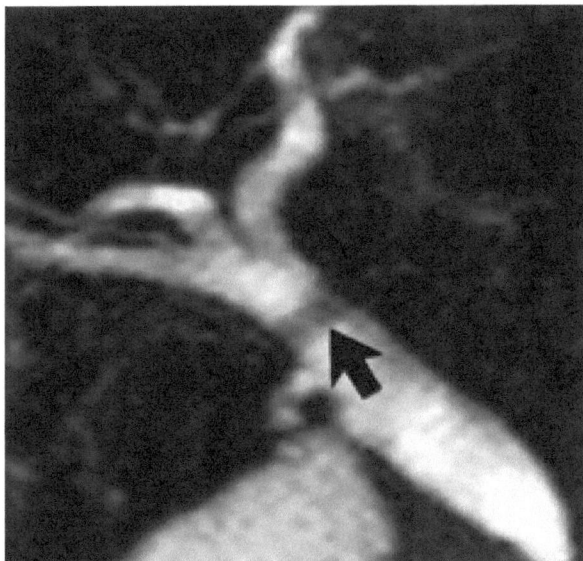

Primary Sclerosing Cholangitis: a disease of the intra-hepatic ducts, string of beads appearance, males > females, and a high association with IBD (especially ulcerative colitis)

Unlike primary biliary cirrhosis (females), the antibody titers are absent or low. Cholangiocarcinoma develops in 15% of these patients.

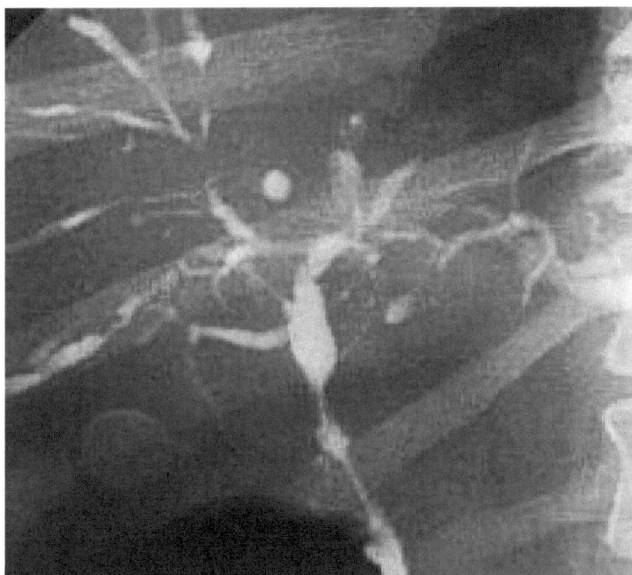

AIDS Cholangitis: refers to cholangitis in AIDS patients as a result of immunosuppression. Causative organisms: CMV and HSV and affects patients with CD4 < 135

Recurrent Pyogenic Cholangitis: is associated with gram-negative infection and liver flukes. Causes multiple soft IHD stones, look for centrally dilated ducts that taper near the periphery. Increased risk in the Asian population.

Ascending Cholangitis: this is a gram-negative bacterial infection associated with stones, stents, tumor, and pancreatitis. Patients present with pain, fever, and jaundice – no IHD stones

Choledochal Cysts: congenital cystic dilations of the biliary tree with a strong female predilection. Has an association with increased stone formation and cholangioCA. Cysts can rupture and lead to bile peritonitis (more frequently seen in neonates). Any CBD > 1 cm in a child is a choledochal cyst.

Surgical excision is cure of this, but the entire cyst has to be removed in order to prevent cholangioCA

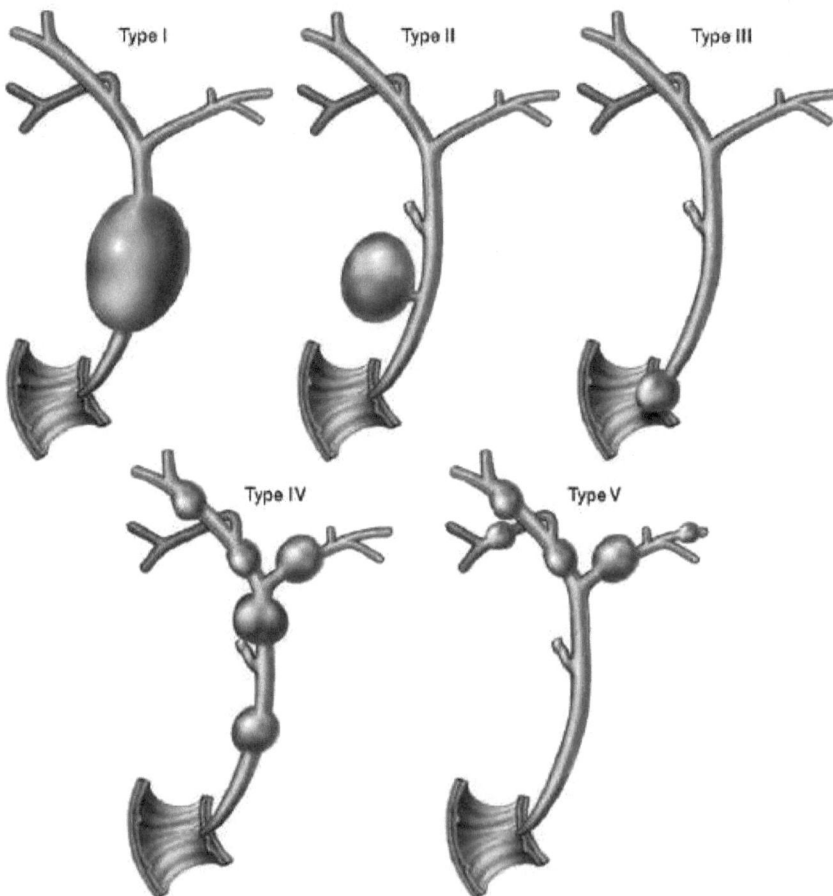

Type IV is split into A (intra and extra-hepatic ducts) and B (extra-hepatic ducts only). Type V is Caroli's disease (intra-hepatic only + fibrosis of liver)

MASSES & MALIGNANCY:

Adenomyomatosis: fundal thickening of the GB associated with stones (hyperplastic cholesterolosis). Look for cystic dilated spaces in the wall – benign finding with no follow-up needed

Cholesterol causes "ring-down" on US and on MRI look for "string-of-pearls" appearance of the wall

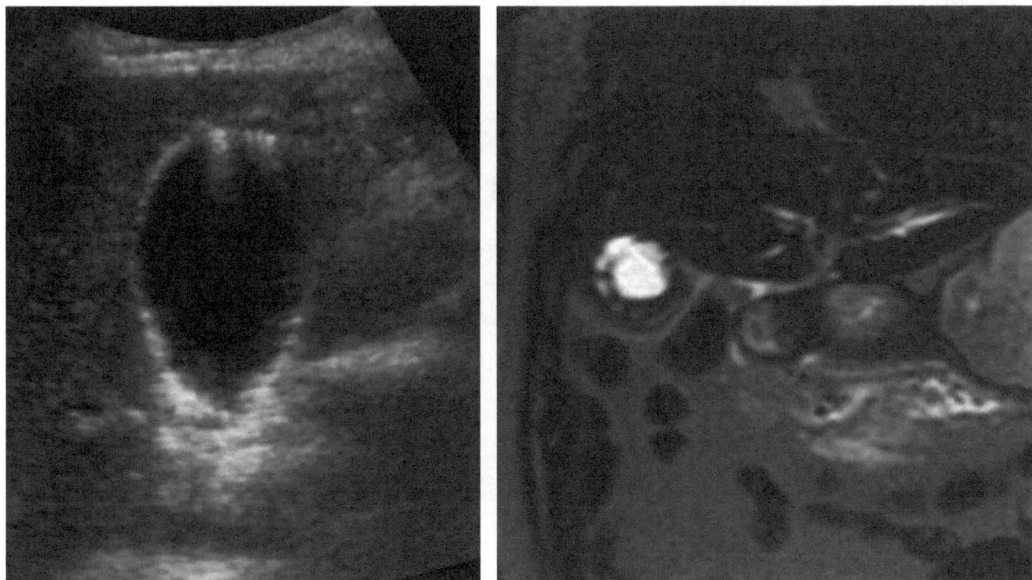

Polyp: an elevated lesion of the mucosal surface of the GB, which can be benign or malignant. 95% are related to benign conditions: cholesterol, adenoma, inflammation, adenomyomatosis and 5% are malignant.

Polyp < 5-mm are often benign and need no follow-up
Polyps 5-10-mm need follow-up to ensure no interval growth (variable 3-6 months) Polyps > 10-mm should be excised

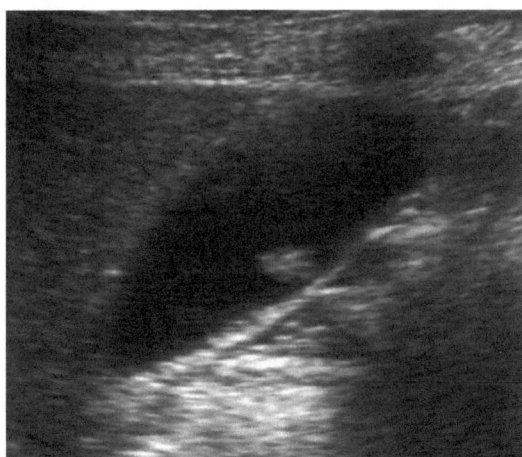

Hyperechoic non-shadowing lesion on US

Gallbladder CA: unfortunately this is usually an asymptomatic lesion until it's too late and the mass has already spread and invaded adjacent liver. AdenoCA is the most common subtype.

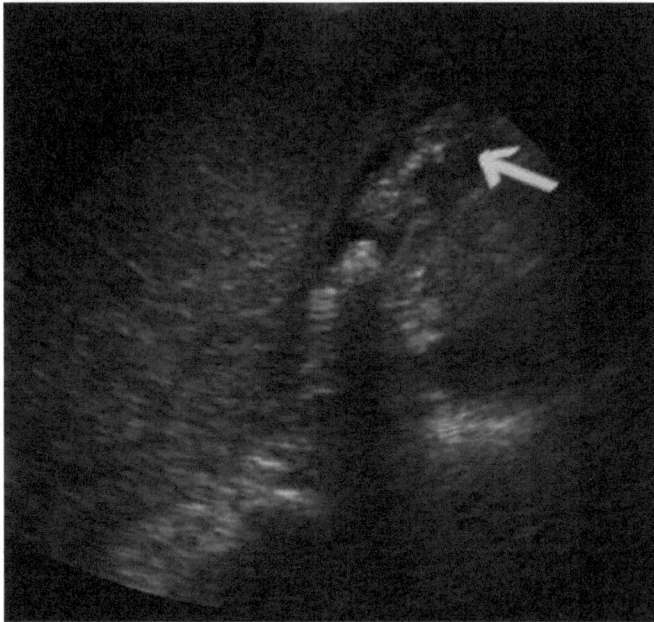

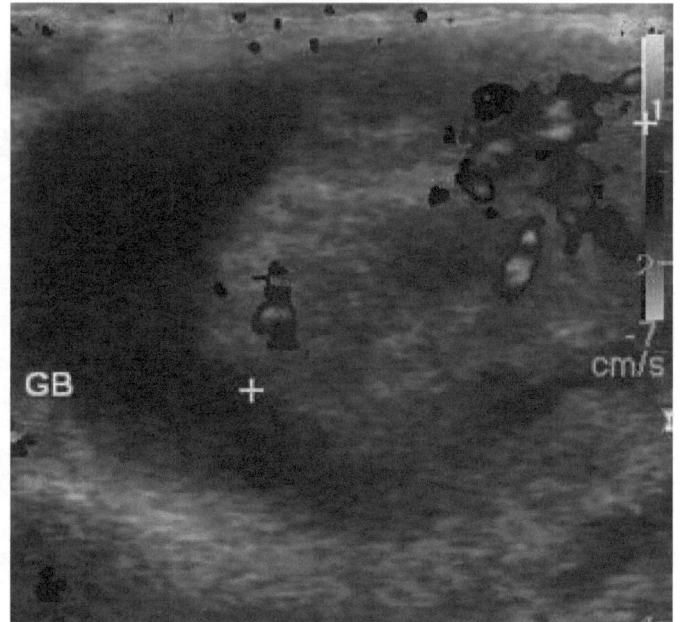

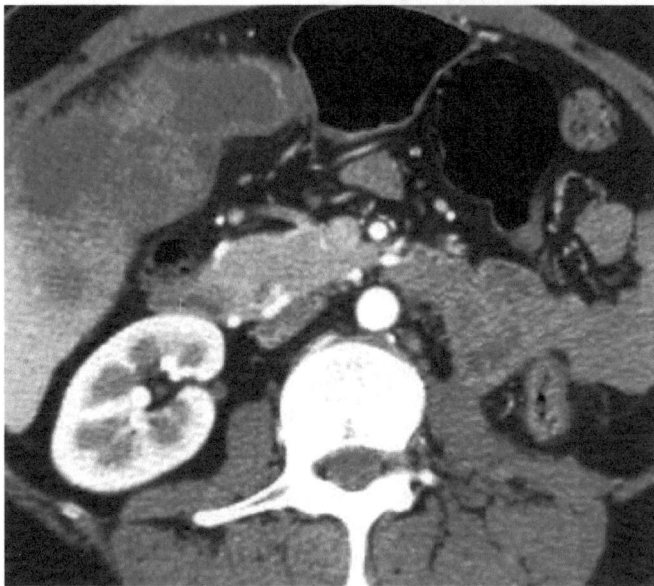

Fungating mass with internal blood flow

Klatskin Tumor: is the name for a hilar cholangioCA that causes IH biliary duct dilation.

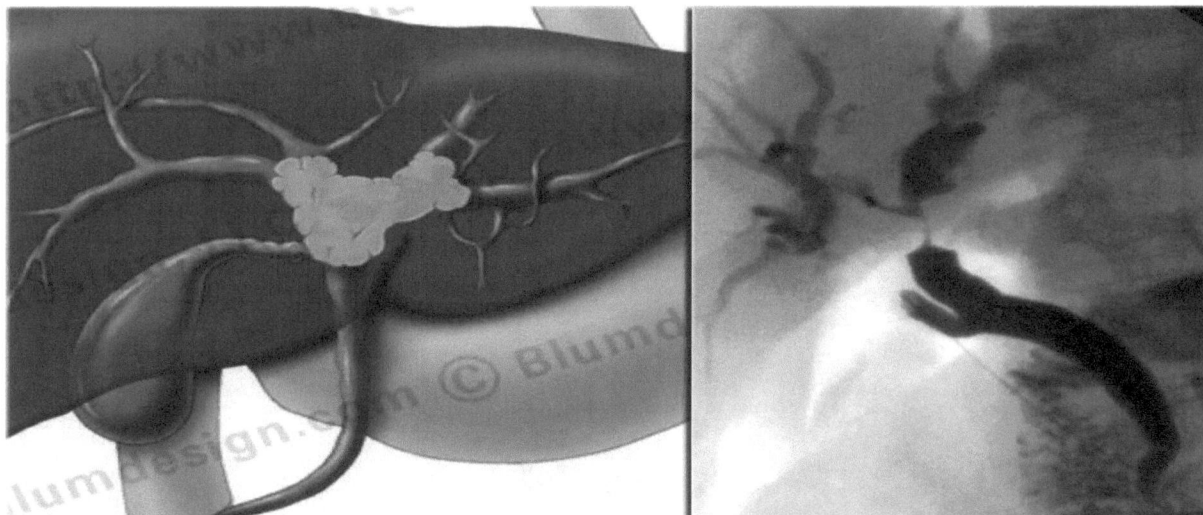

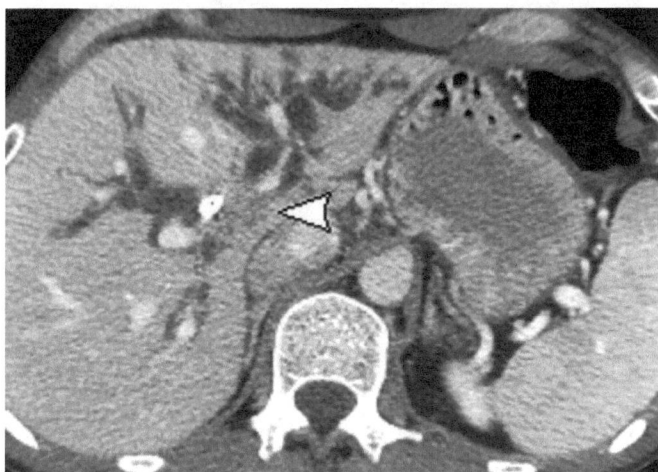

PANCREAS:

Pancreatic duct and variations are important to recognize because they can be associated with pathlogy:

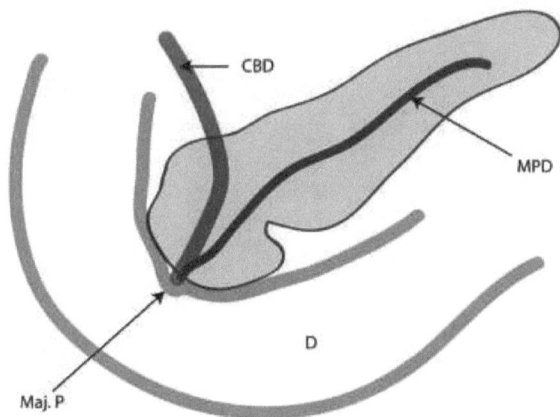

Pancreas Divisum: the most common variation of duct formation (4-10% of the population). Most patients with this are asymptomatic but it can be associated with pancreatitis.

Look for absent ventral duct with dorsal duct draining everything into minor paplla or inadequate connection between dorsal duct and short blunted ventral duct. **Crossing of CBD and PD is a key finding!**

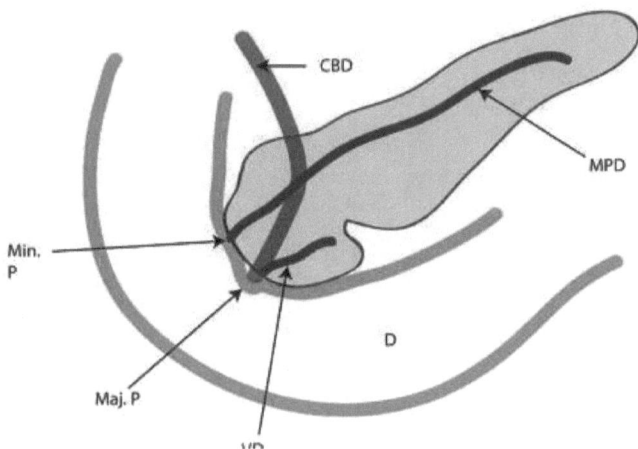

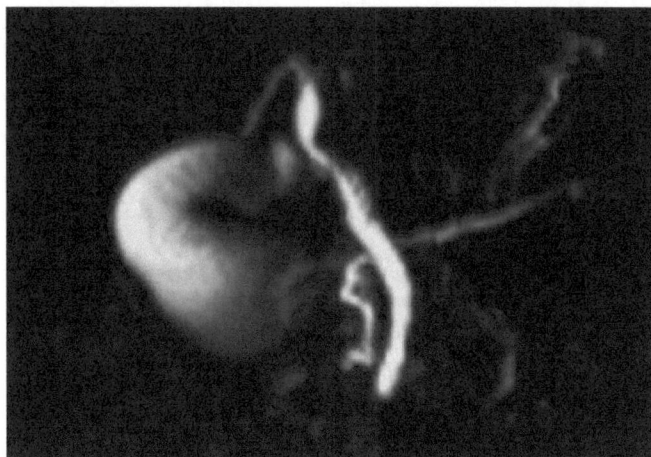

Annular Pancreas: rare morphological anomaly that can cause duodenal obstruction. It develops due to a failure of the ventral bud to rotate with the duodenum causing it to encase the bowel loop at its 2nd portion.

Acute Pancreatitis: edema, fluid, stranding in acute pancreatitis with pseudocyst being the most common complication. Pseudocyst should never have enhancing components, if it does, think cystic neoplasms. Most often caused by EtOH (men) and gallstones (women).

Other complications can be pseudoaneurysms (GDA and splenic arteries), venous thrombosis, pancreatic necrosis and abscess (most serious – life threatening). If abscess and necrosis occur, then surgical debridement is needed "necosectomy".

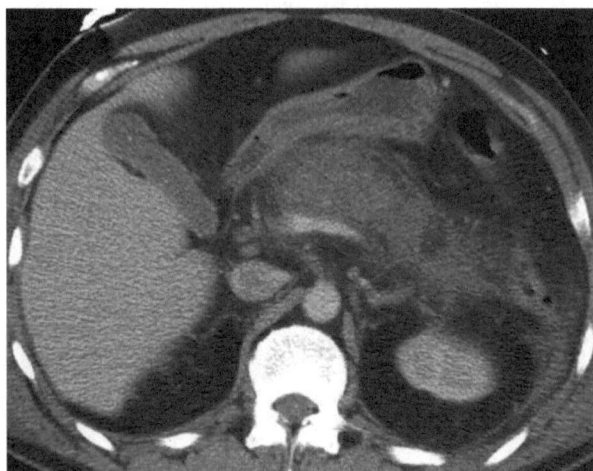

Acute Pancreatitis

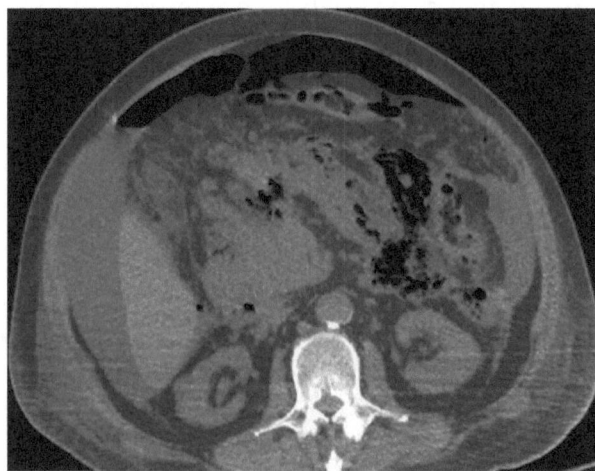

Pancreatic Necrosis

Chronic Pancreatitis: look for a dilated duct with Ca2+ in the parenchyma with atrophy and fatty infiltration.

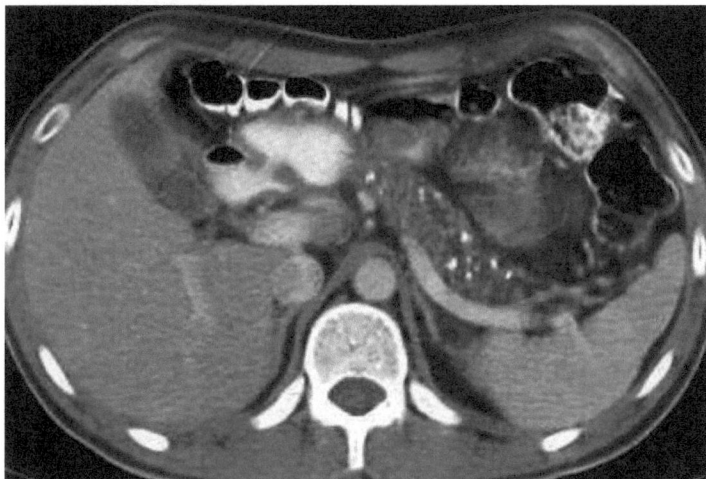

Autoimmune Pancreatitis: due to some systemic autoimmune disease and the pancreas becomes diffusely enlarged with loss of lobular contour. CBD becomes thick and the condition responds to steroids. Look for elevated levels of IgG4.

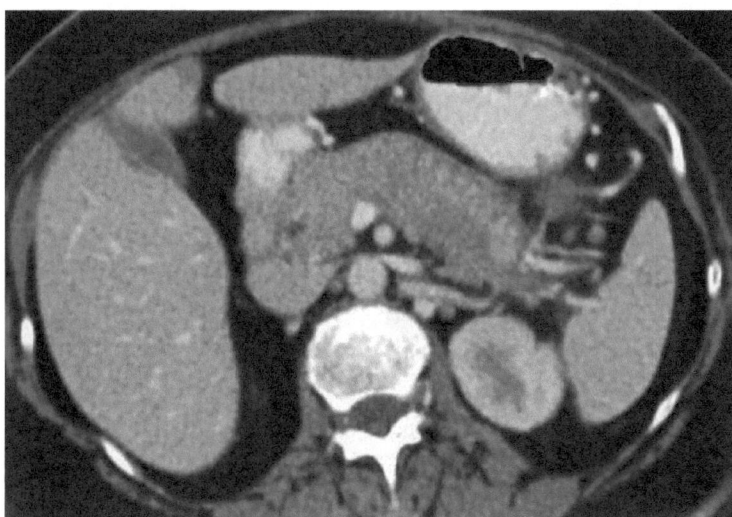

CANCER:

Adenocarcinoma: hypovascular mass causing dilated ducts (CBD and PD), venous invasion, and arterial encasement. Uncinate process tumor is a poorer prognosis because it presents later and has early SMA/SMV involvement. Non-resectable tumors are large, involve vessels, or have distant mets. Double-duct sign.

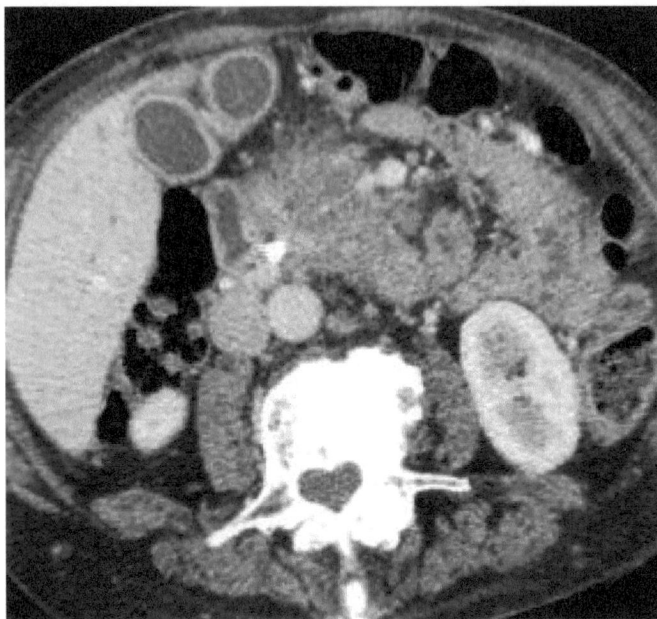

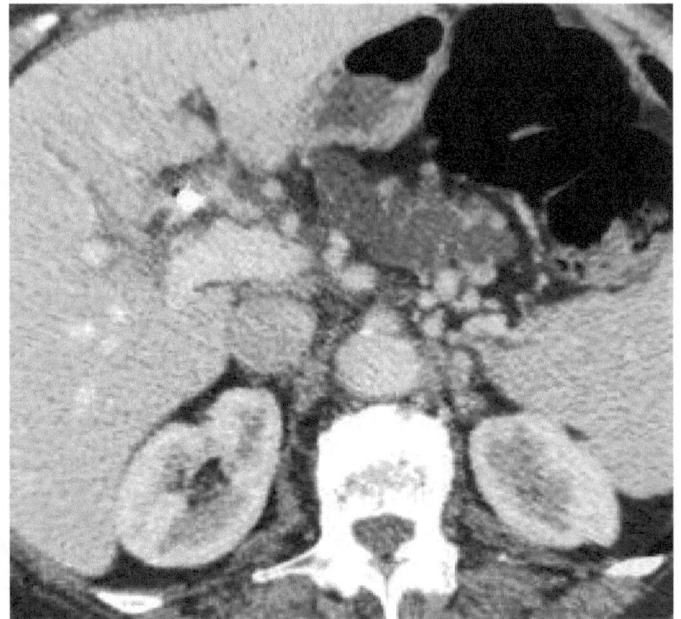

Cystic Benign Masses	Malignant Cystic Masses
Pseudocyst	Mucinous Tumor
Serous Cystadenoma	IPMN
	Cystic Metastases

Serous Cystadenoma: female > males (> 60 years of age). Cluster of small cysts with increased incidence in VHL. The septa enhance and may have a central scar and calcifications.

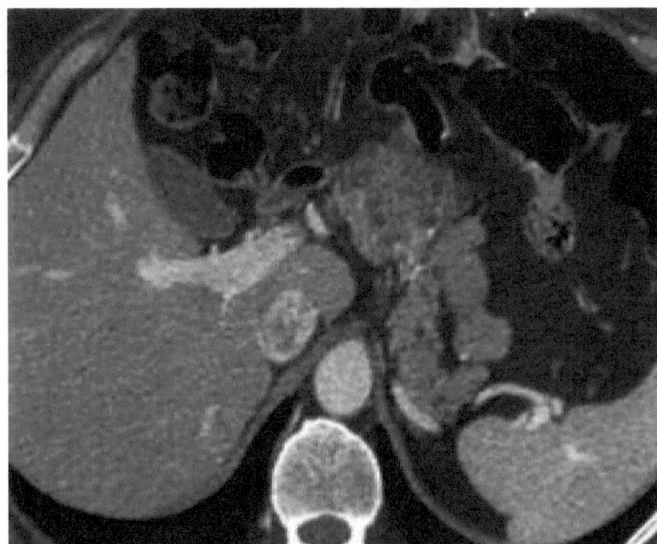

Microcystic

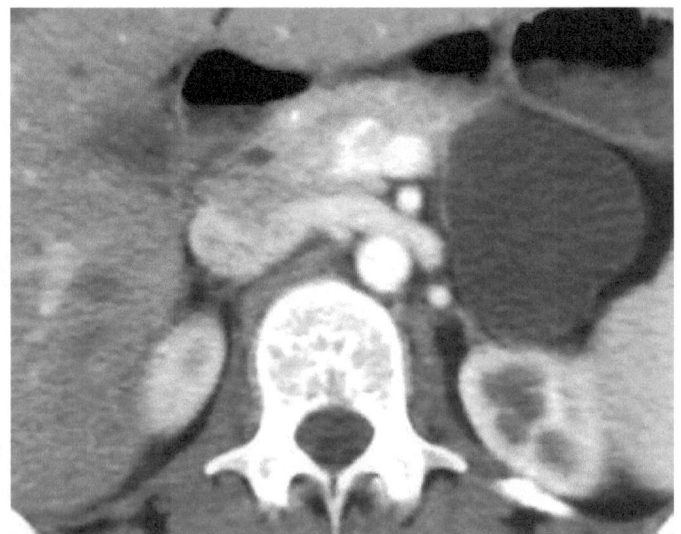

Macrocystic

This is an observable lesion unless it causes symptoms (due to compression from increased size).

Mucinous Cystadenocarcinoma: is a more malignant counterpart of the mucinous cystadenoma. Occurs almost exclusively in females and has numerous large cysts with an average diameter of 10-12 mm. Surgical treatment is the standard mode of treatment. Tail > body.

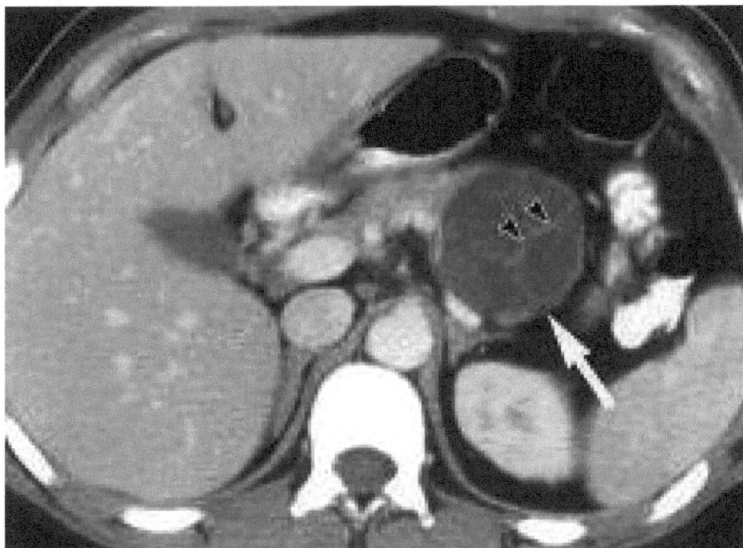

IPMN: mucinous tumors of the pancreas that cause ductal dilation (main and/or side branch), causing an absurd amount of mucin production. Usually indolent, but malignant degeneration does occur: duct dilated > 10-mm, thick septa, enhancing nodules, and Ca2+

Asymptomatic < 3-cm	Asymptomatic > 3-cm
Can be followed to assess for change	Surgical resection of aspiration

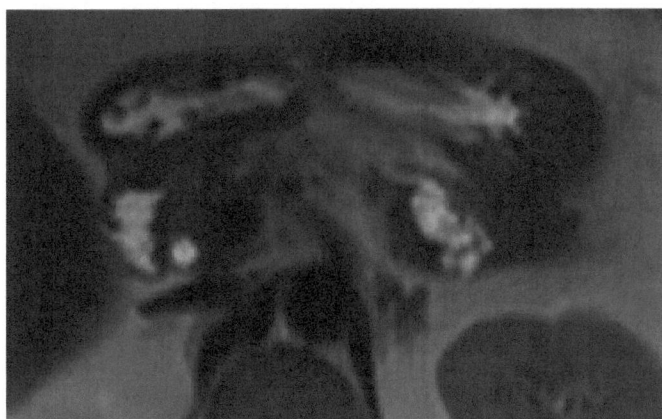

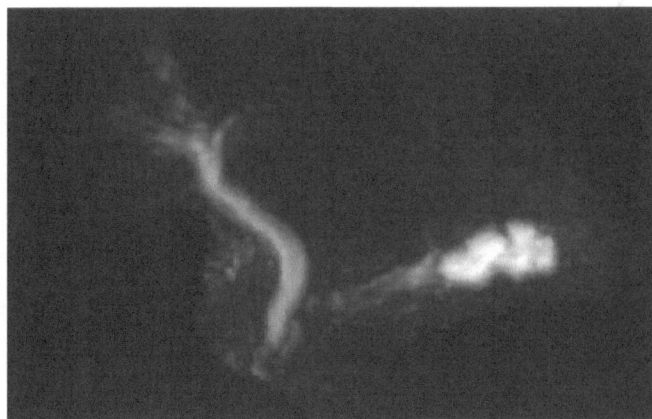

Neuroendocrine Tumors: discrete hypervascular masses seen best in the early arterial phase, do not cause obstruction, present with characteristic symptoms

I.   Insulinoma – most common subtype and most often benign, presents with hypoglycemia
II. Gastrinoma – most malignant and associated with ZE Syndrome

III. VIPoma – profuse diarrhea and flushing
IV. Glucagonoma – necrolytic migratory rash and diarrhea
V. Non-Functional – often large at time of presentation because no clinical syndrome associated with these

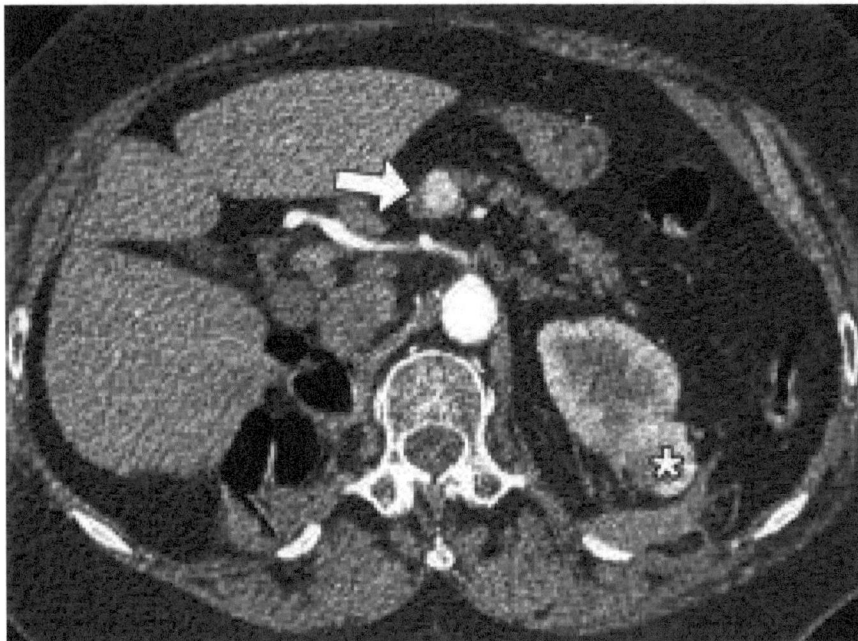

Hypervascular metastases will be multifocal and most often associated with RCC!

SPEN: rare tumors that are seen in young females. They present as large well demarcated encapsulated masses with heterogeneous enhancement that present more often due to compressive symptoms because of big size. 15% are malignant and resection is treatment of choice.

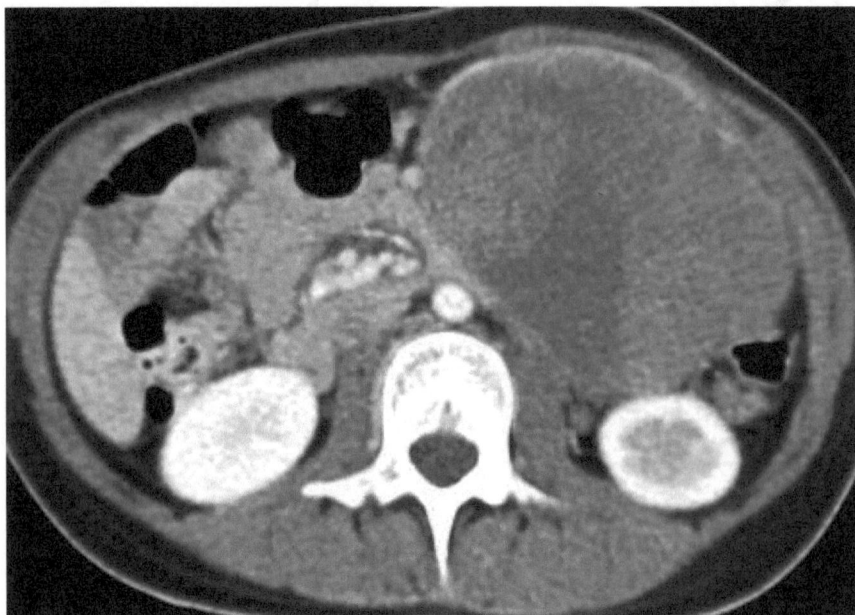

RANDOM OTHER STUFF:

Pelvic Lipomatosis: represents excess deposition of fat in the pelvis due to overgrowth of adipose leading to compression of pelvic organs. Patients usually present with features of compression of GU, vascular, or lower GI organs – dysuria, hematuria, urgency, etc. On IVP look for a **pear-shaped bladder** with dilated ureters. Most common cause of "pear-shaped" bladder is trauma and pelvic hematoma.

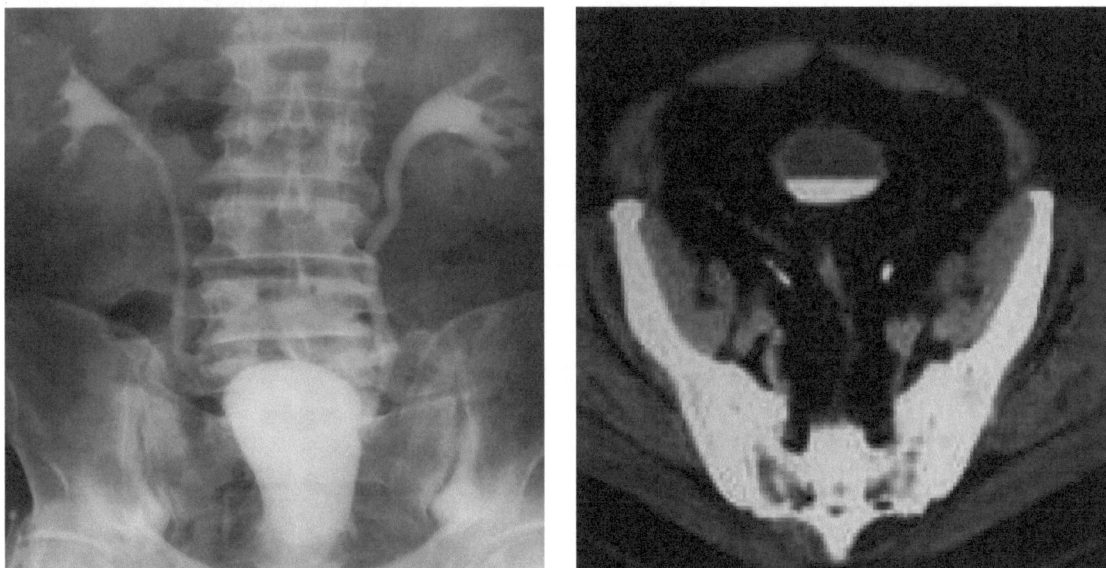

Spigelian Hernia: defect in the linea semilunaris occurring in the right or left lower quadrants. Characteristic location is lateral to rectus muscles and inferior to the umbilicus.

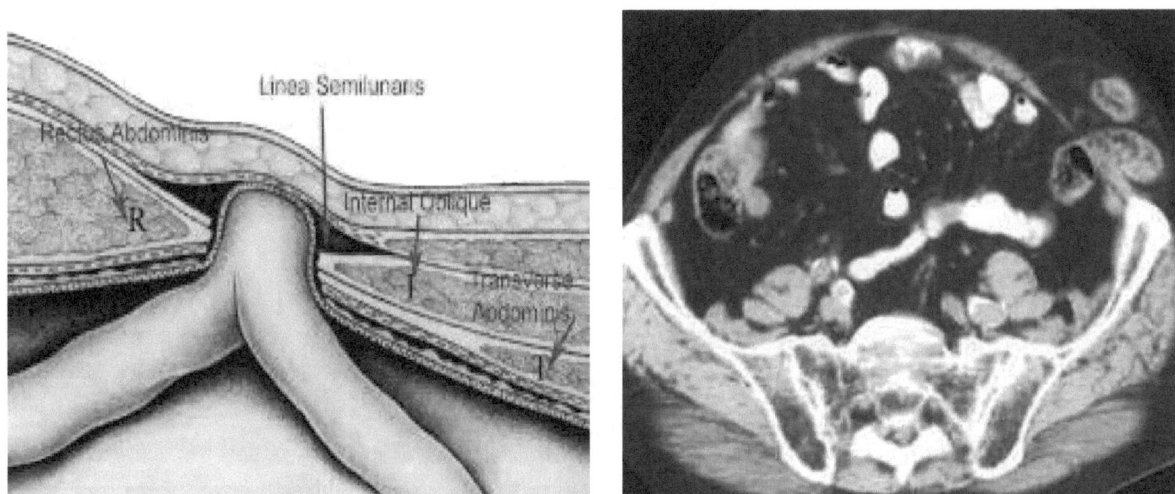

Internal Hernia: most common type is a left paraduodenal hernia. Right paraduodenal through the fossa of Waldeyer and left paraduodenal is through the fossa of Landzert. Can become obstructive requiring surgery to decompress and prevent ischemic injury.

Genitourinary

Bosniak Criteria: is a CT descriptor, do not use this on US

<u>Benign</u>

I.   A benign simple cyst
II. Mildly complex cyst with thin septa or eccentric calcification, hyperdense cyst < 3cm

IIF. The "f" is for follow-up needed. This is a cyst with thick septa, nodular calcs, or a cyst that is hyperdense and > 3cm in size

<u>Malignant</u>

III. Irregular walls/septa, thick calcs, **no enhancement**
IV. **Enhancing** nodules or walls (cystic renal cell)

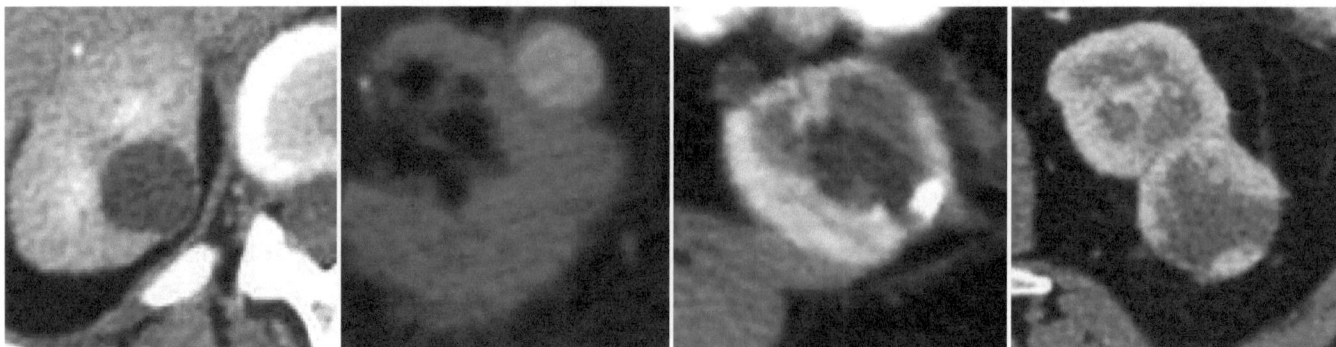

| I | II | III | IV |

ADPCKD: kidneys are normal at birth but over time the kidneys become very enlarged and develop multiple cysts of varying sizes, some with hemorrhage (responsible for hematuria), progresses to ESRD. Cysts in liver > pancreas. Remember the association with **berry aneurysms.** No increased risk of CA.

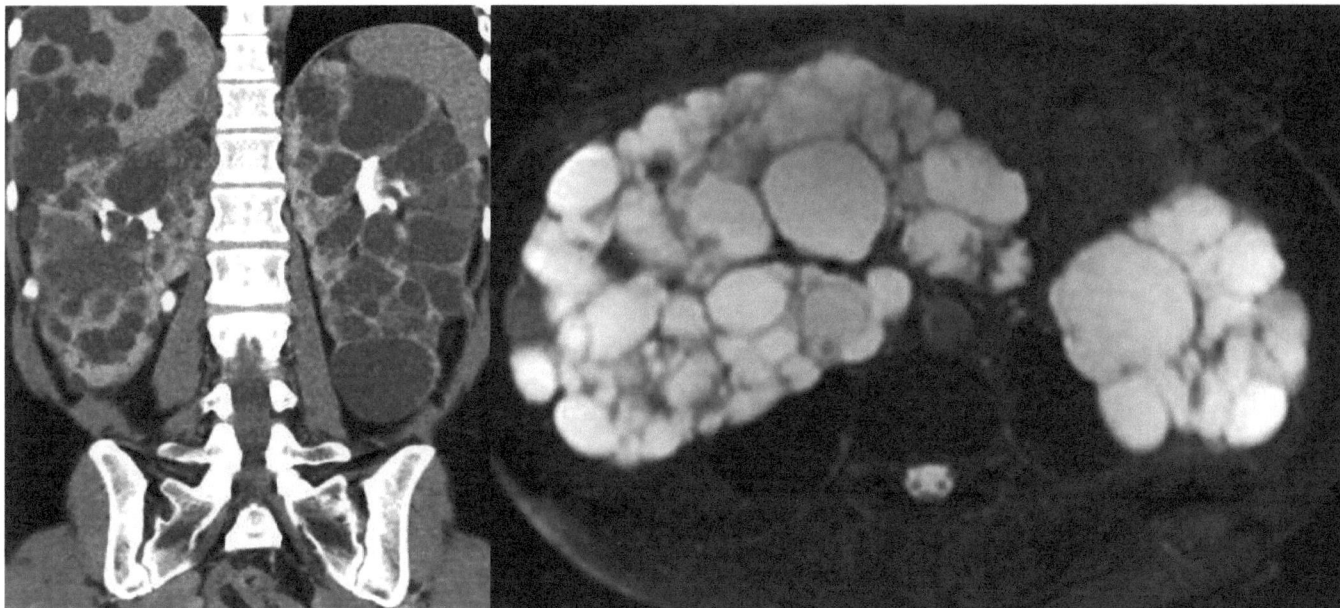

Acquired Cystic Disease: this happens in patients with ESRD on dialysis. The kidneys become small and enhance poorly. There are cysts of varying sizes and there is an association with **clear cell RCC.**

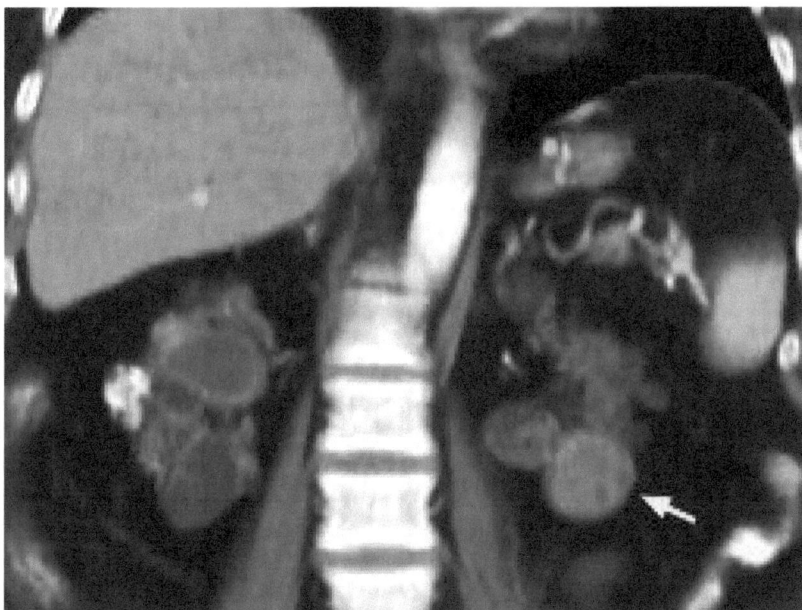

Arrow points to RCC.

Multilocular Cystic Nephroma: is a cystic renal tumor with a bimodal age distribution (young males and older females). It presents as a cystic mass invading the renal hilum – benign tumor with multiple septations. Resected because it cannot be differentiated from RCC by imaging.

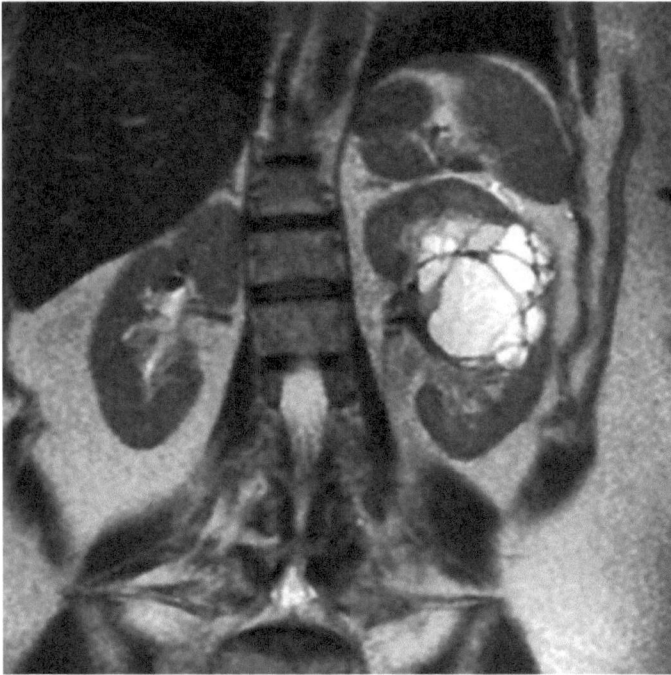

SOLID RENAL MASSES:

1. Macroscopic fat – makes the lesion benign (AML)
2. Enhancing lesion without fat – malignancy until proven otherwise!

Renal Cell CA: most common renal malignancy with a variety of appearances. Basically if it looks suspicious (enhancement, nodules, irregularity, growing), just call it an RCC and let the surgeons take it out. Has association with VHL – tends to be bilateral.

Staging:

I.   Confined to capsule
II.   Extra-renal but confined by Gerota's fascia

1-A. Vascular invasion (renal veins, IVC)
1-B. Local nodal spread
1-C. Vascular invasion and local node spread

1-A. Adjacent organ invasion
1-B. Distant mets

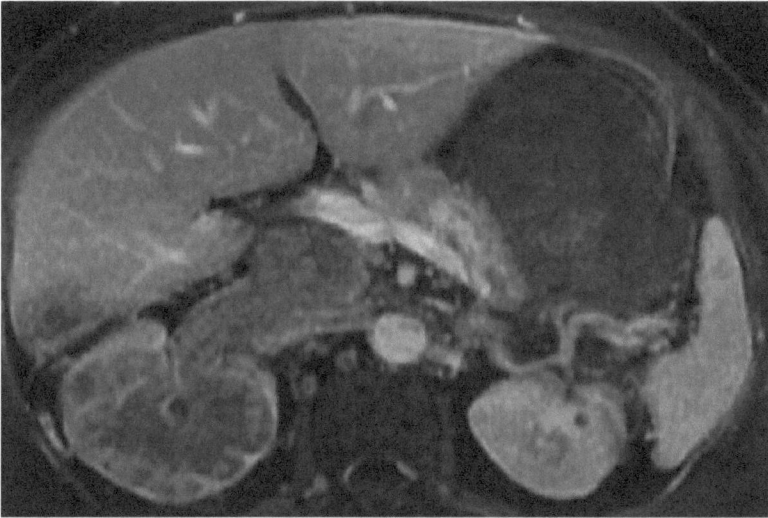

Renal vein and IVC invasion – stage III-A

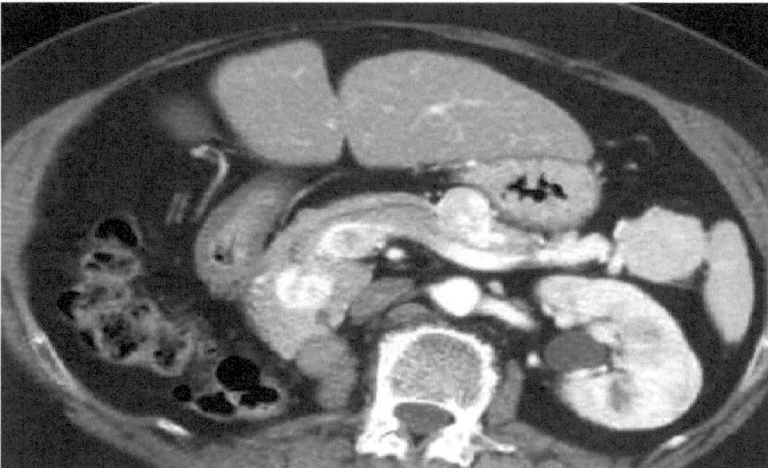

Hypervascular mets to pancreas and mesentery – stage IV-B

VHL: autosomal dominant inheritance, defect on chromosome three associated with bilateral RCC, pheochromocytomas, islet cell tumors, pancreas serous cystadenomas, hemangioblastomas, epididymal cystadenomas, retinal angiomas.

TCC: presents as a filling defect in the collecting system, concurrent CA rate is almost 40%, can also be circumferential wall thickening of ureter. Associated with cigarettes, cyclophosphamide, and phenyl compounds. Hematuria is the most common symptom.

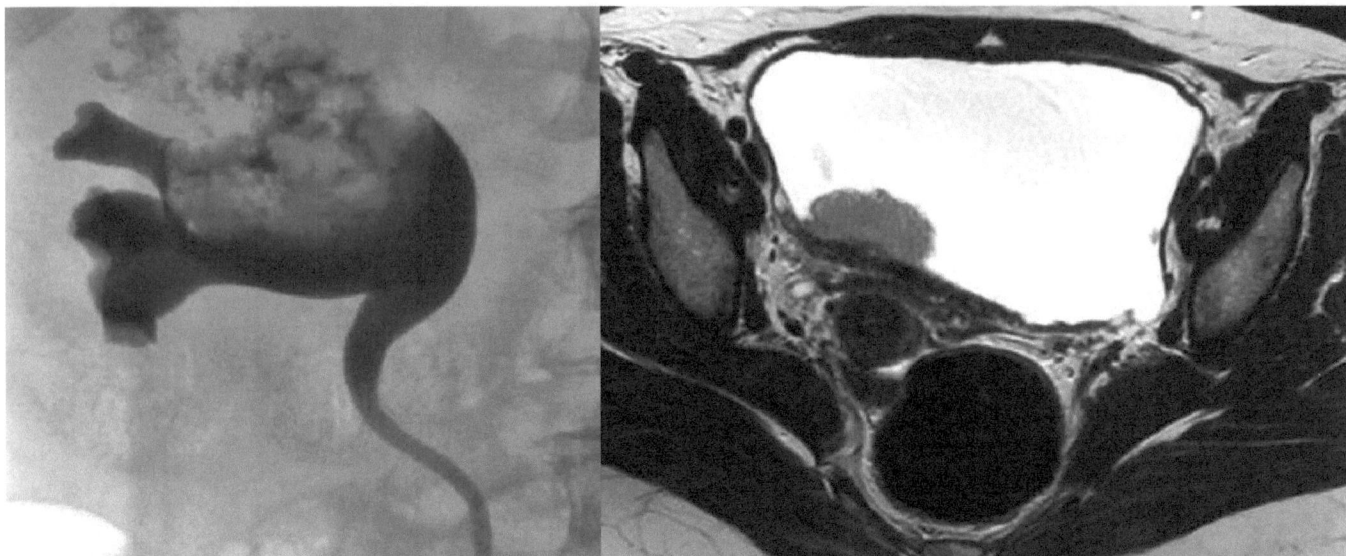

Also look for "goblet sign" – this is TCC of the ureter

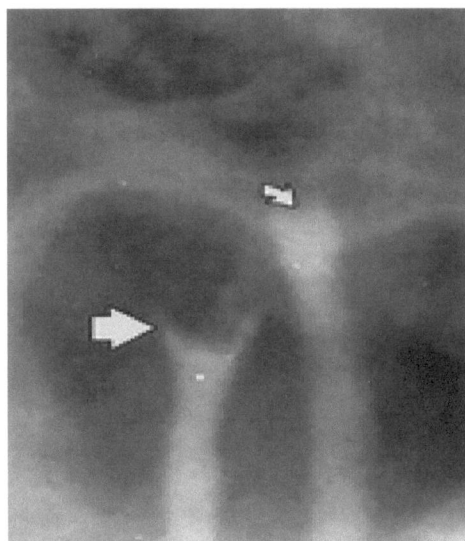

AML: macroscopic fat containing lesion – benign. This can bleed if it gets bigger than 4-cm, in which case we embolize. This is easy to ID and should not be called a malignancy.

Lymphoma: most commonly with non-Hodgkin disease and presents as unilateral or bilateral renal enlargement with diffuse hypodensity or multiple hypodense masses. Look for LAD in the RP as well.

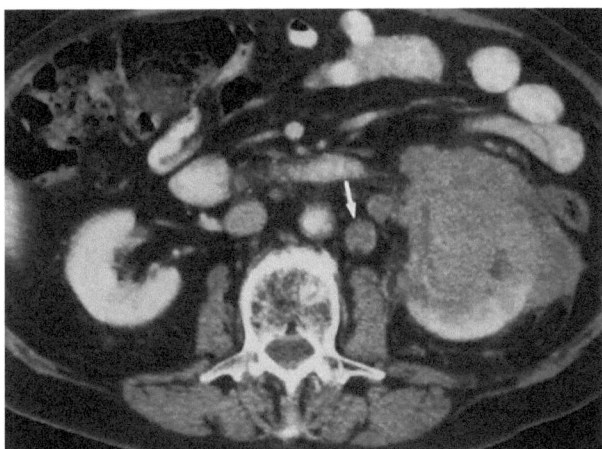

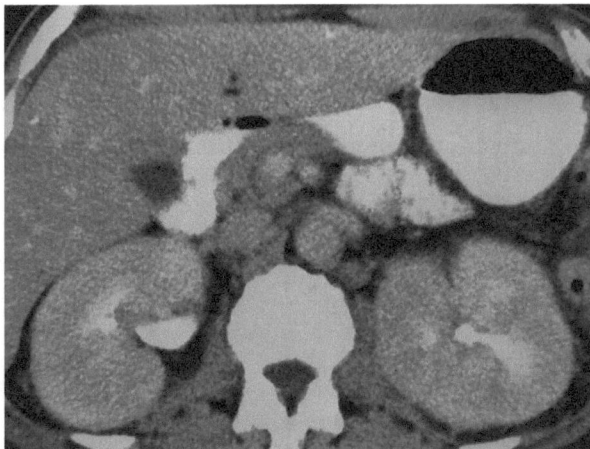

Oncocytoma: benign tumor that is radiologically indistinguishable from RCC so it has to be excised. 13% of the time it is bilateral, look for a sharply demarcated lesion with a central scar, "spoke-wheel" pattern on angiography (can be seen with RCC).

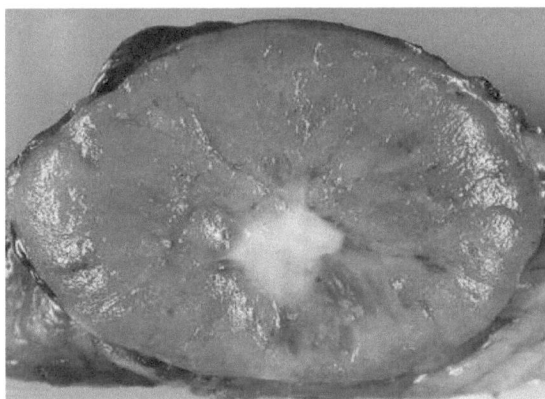

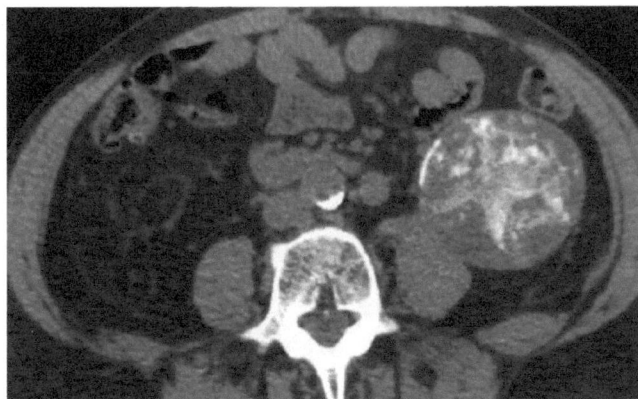

Page Kidney: refers to the phenomenon of HTN that develops following long-standing compression of renal parenchyma by a sub-capsular renal collection (hematoma, seroma, urinoma). Parenchymal compression leads to vessel compression and activation of the renin-angiotensin system.

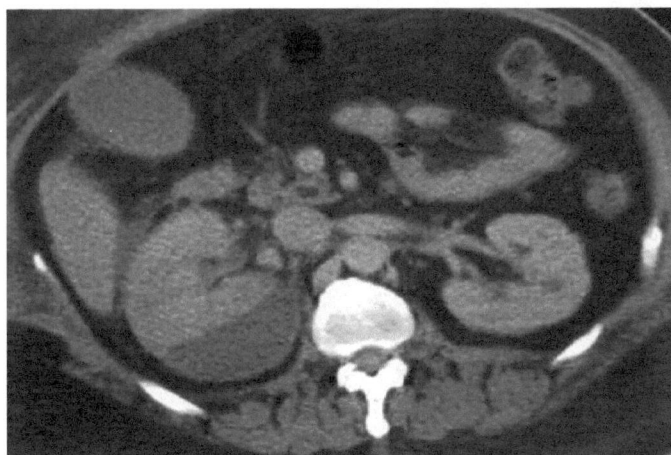

ADRENALS

Adenoma: the most common adrenal mass lesion, benign with HU density < 10 on NCCT, > 50% washout with dynamic imaging, or fat signal loss on In/Out phase MRI. **Do not call a lesion adenoma if greater than 4 cm**. When adenoma is hyperfunctioning the patient has Cushing's.

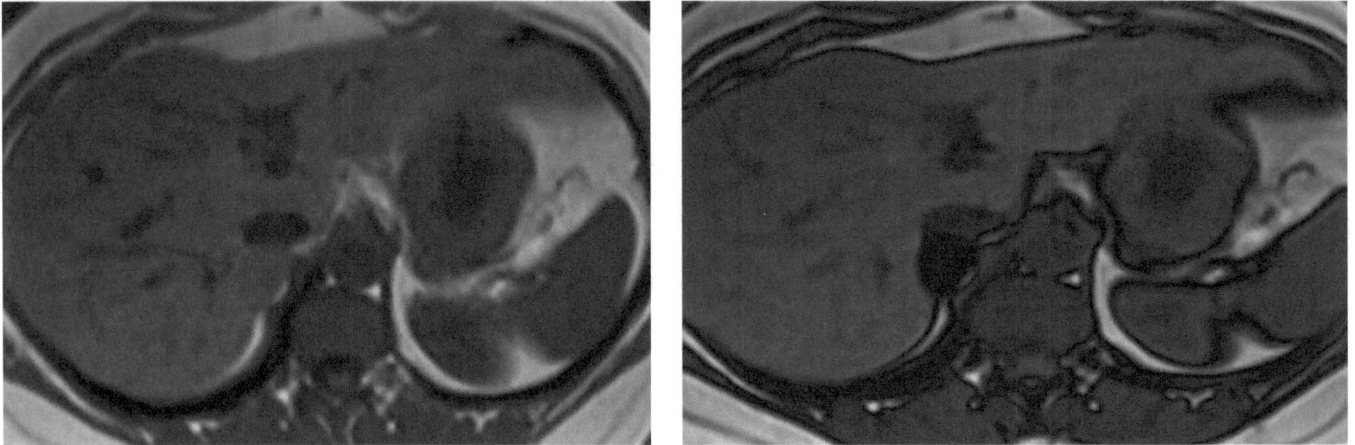

Myelolipoma: fat-containing benign lesion that can hemorrhage when it gets bigger than 4-cm.

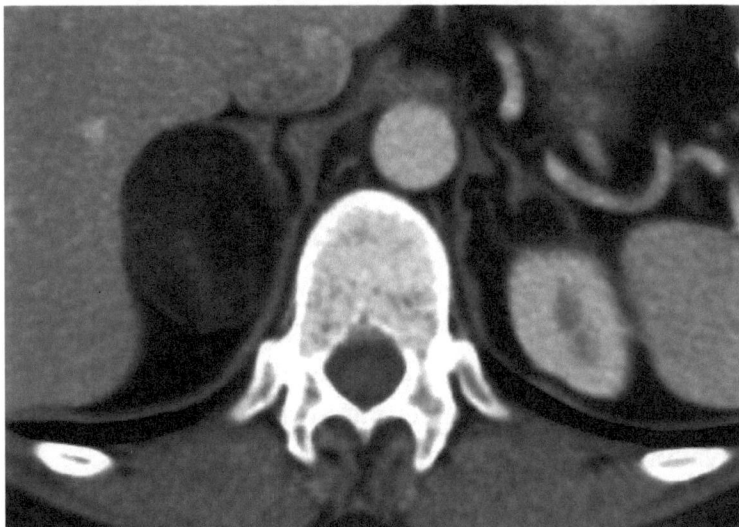

Pheochromocytoma: uncommon tumor that follows the '10% rule' – extra-adrenal, bilateral, familial. Can be seen in MEN II and VHL. Causes uncontrolled HTN with patients sometimes having HTNsive crisis. This is a paraganglioma, so avidly enhances. If it's not in the adrenal gland, go inferiorly and look for it near the Organ of Zuckerkandal (at aortic bifurcation). I-123 MIBG avid.

CT: large enhancing mass with areas of necrosis
MRI: T2 bright 'light bulb' lesion, with heterogeneous enhancement

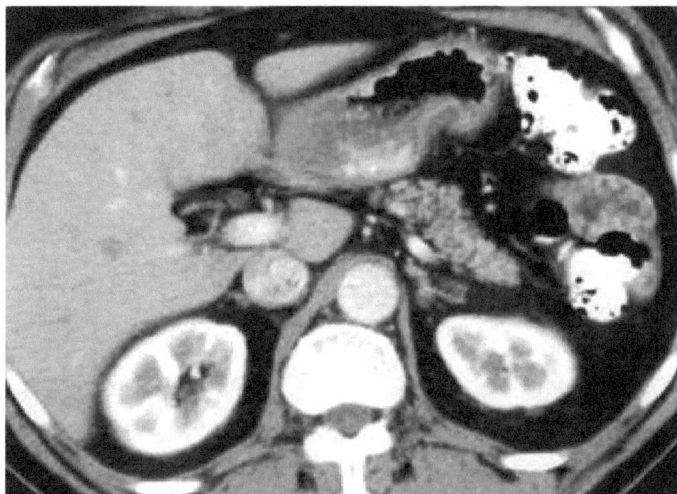

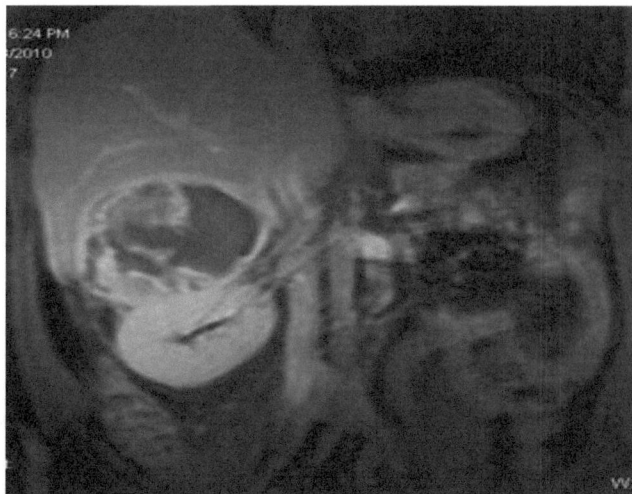

Adrenal Carcinoma: highly malignant but rare lesion that can be hormonally active or inactive. Aggressive lesion that tends to invade vessels and adjacent structures. It has heterogeneous enhancement due to necrosis and tends to be > than 6 cm.

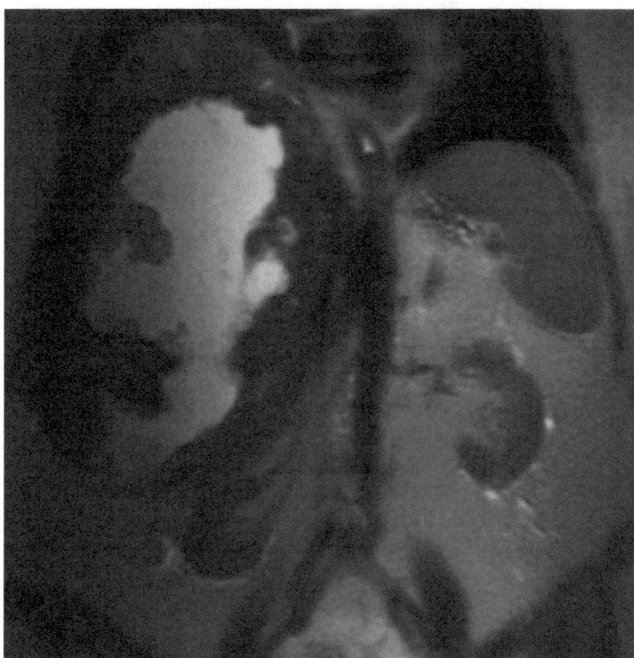

Larger necrotic mass is displacing the right kidney inferiorly

Metastases: this is the most common adrenal malignancy. Hypervascular irregular mass in a patient with known primary. Be wary of collision tumors.

Adrenal cyst: rare lesion, but like a cyst anywhere in the body, it is a simple lesion with HU < 10 and no enhancement

Waterhouse-Friderichsen Syndrome: cause of non-traumatic adrenal hemorrhage due to meningococcal sepsis. Need clinical history to make this diagnosis. Remember adrenals can bleed in patients with elevated INR, babies with ischemia, and in trauma.

RENAL DISEASES

Crossed Fused Ectopia: one or both kidneys on the wrong side of the abdomen with the ureter crossing back across the midline to insert at normal position in trigone of bladder. The ectopic kidney suffers from reflux.

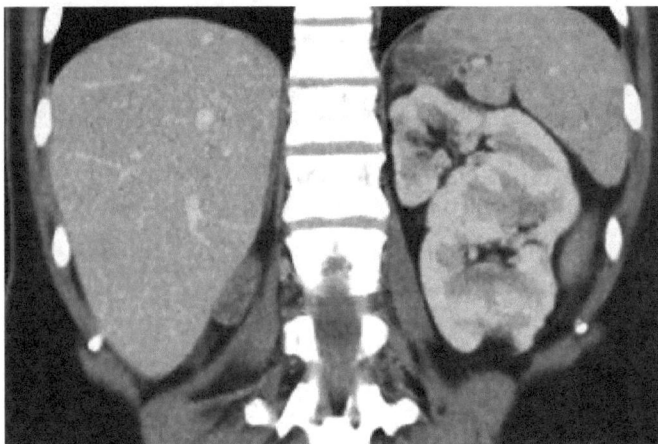

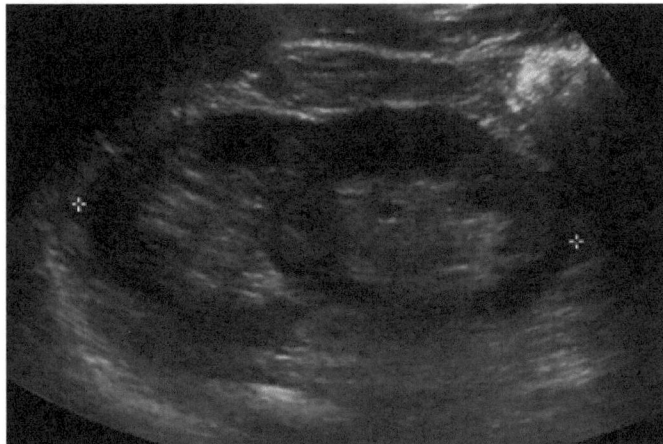

Horseshoe Kidney: This is the most common fusion anomaly of the kidneys. Fusion of lower renal poles with arrested cranial migration at the level of the IMA. More susceptible to trauma, stones, and infections.

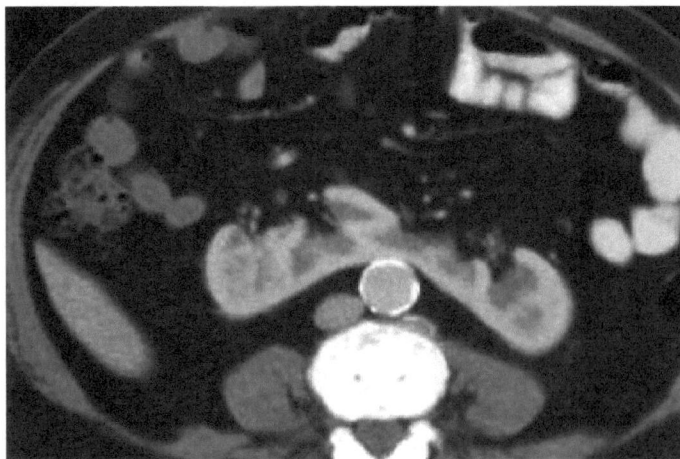

FUN FACTS:

With any congenital anomaly of the kidneys always image the pelvis to look for Mullerian Duct Anomalies (covered in the next section).

Renal Enlargement has a variety of causes: cystic disease, lymphoma, leukemia, amyloid, HIV nephropathy, infection, RV thrombosis, etc.

Lithium toxicity causes multiple bilateral microcysts.

Pyelonephritis: edematous hypodense kidney with surrounding stranding and overall diminished perfusion. Look for the classic 'striated nephrogram' and urothelial enhancement. Be careful and make sure to look for abscess. Most common offending organism is *E. coli*.

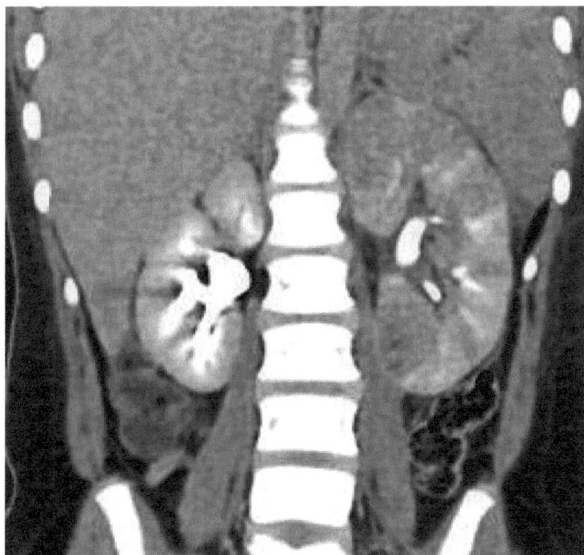

Xanthogranulomatous Pyelo: chronic infection resulting in a non-functioning kidney with very specific radiographic features. Look for a **staghorn** calculus and hydronephrosis. Infectious changes can be marked, extending out of the kidney into the RP and even through the musculature of the flank.

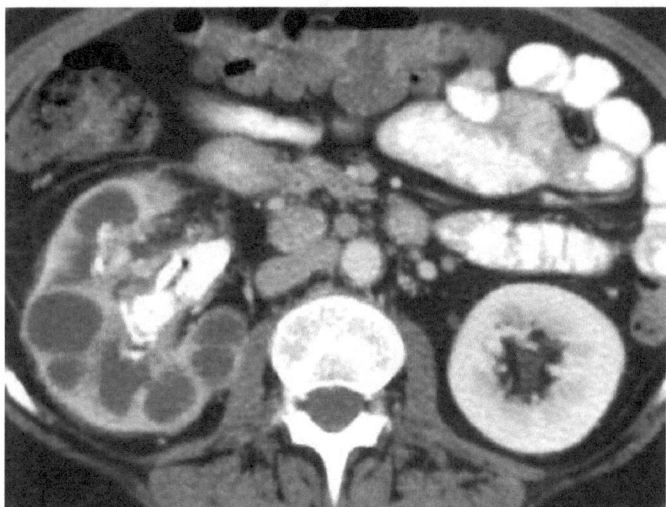

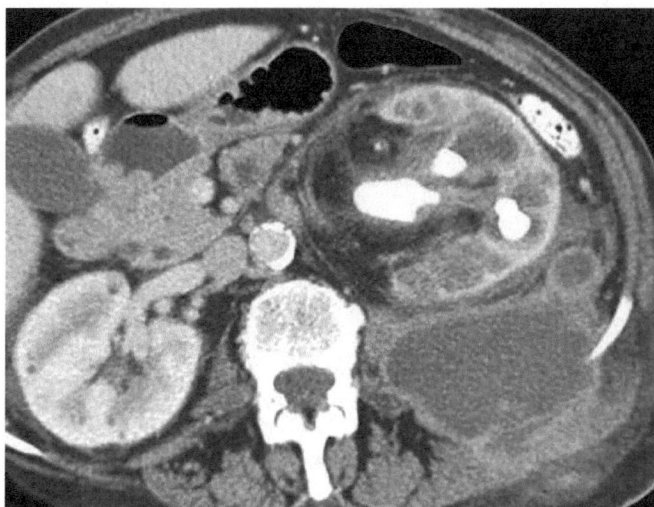

Fungus Ball: seen in **neutropenic** patients as a mass in the collecting system, since it's a filling defect, the differential is broad, use the clinical history to help guide you this way.

Renal Infarct: wedge shaped peripheral hypodense defect. Look for a cause for the infarct (embolic, atherosclerosis, vasculitis, dissection). Look for the rim sign (cortex stays perfused very peripherally) because capsular artery maintains perfusion.

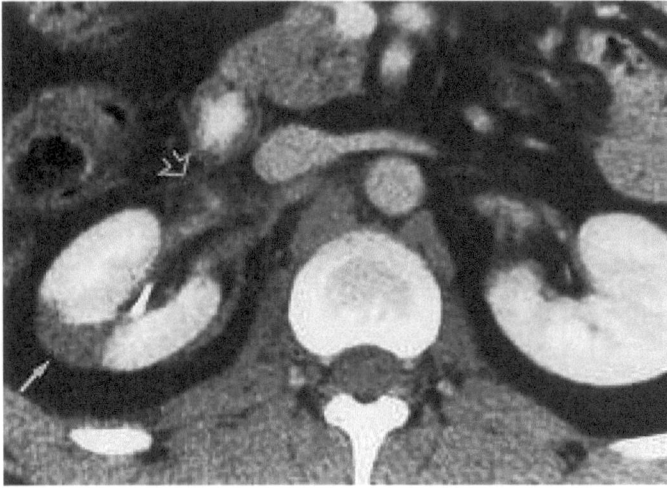

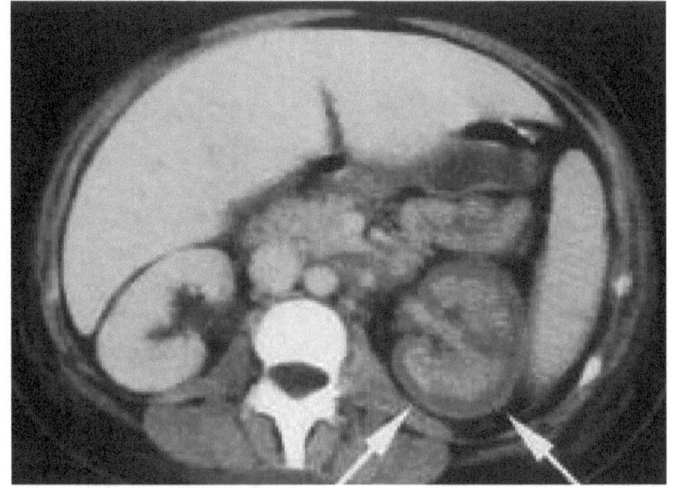

Renal TB: accounts for almost 20% of extra-pulmonary TB and results in shrunken kidneys with **coarse calcifications** and big dilated calyces "cotton ball calyces" and papillary necrosis.

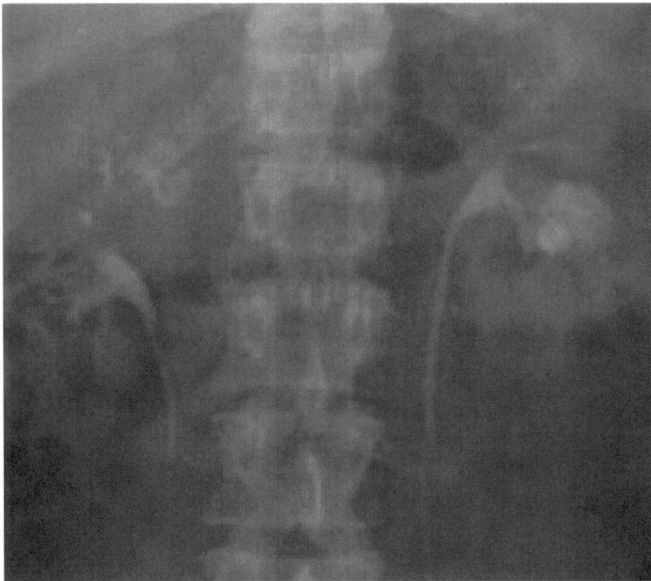

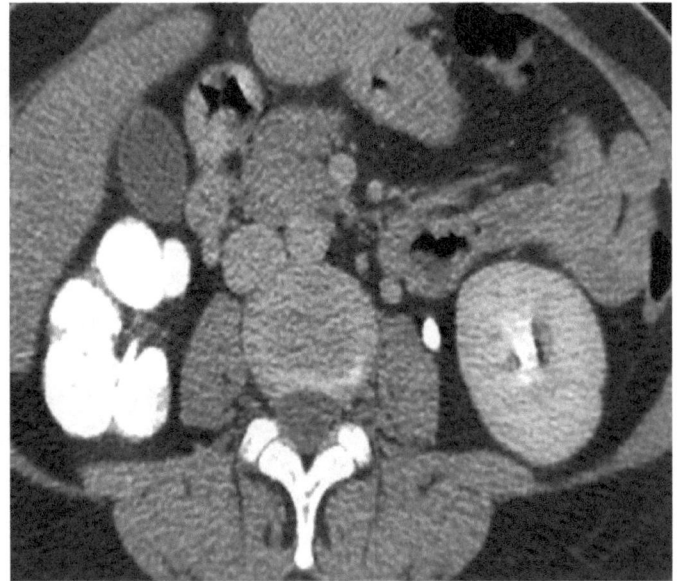

Medullary Nephrocalcinosis: deposition of calcium salts into the medulla of the kidney. Many causes: hyperparathyroidism, medullary sponge kidney (most likely if the other kidney is normal), RTA, milk-alkali syndrome to name a few. Predisposes to urolithiasis.

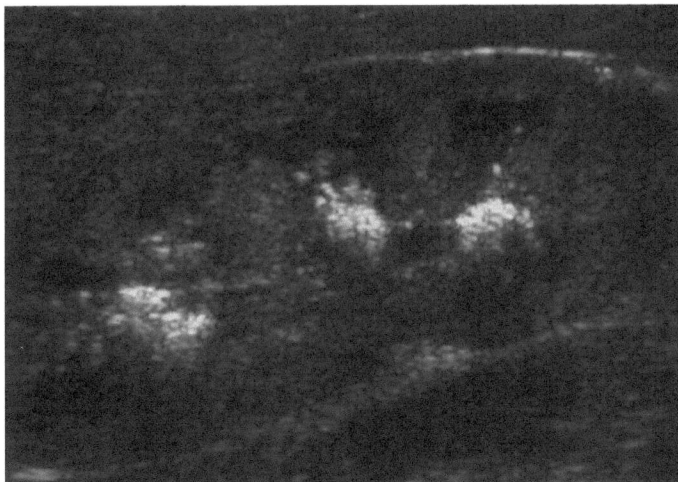

Cortical Nephrocalcinosis: less common than medullary but also has a whole host of causes: chronic glomerulonephritis, HIV, and ischemia. On CECT there will be a thin rim of non-enhancing cortex.

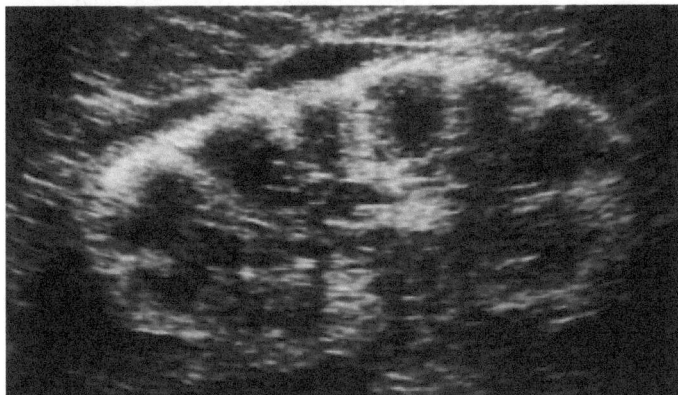

Papillary Necrosis: is ischemia of the renal papillae leading to necrosis. It has a very typical look 'golf ball on a tee' and results in loss of renal function.

Pyelonephritis	Cirrhosis
Obstruction	Analgesics (#1 cause)
Sickle Cell	Renal vein thrombus
Tuberculosis	Diabetes (#2 cause)

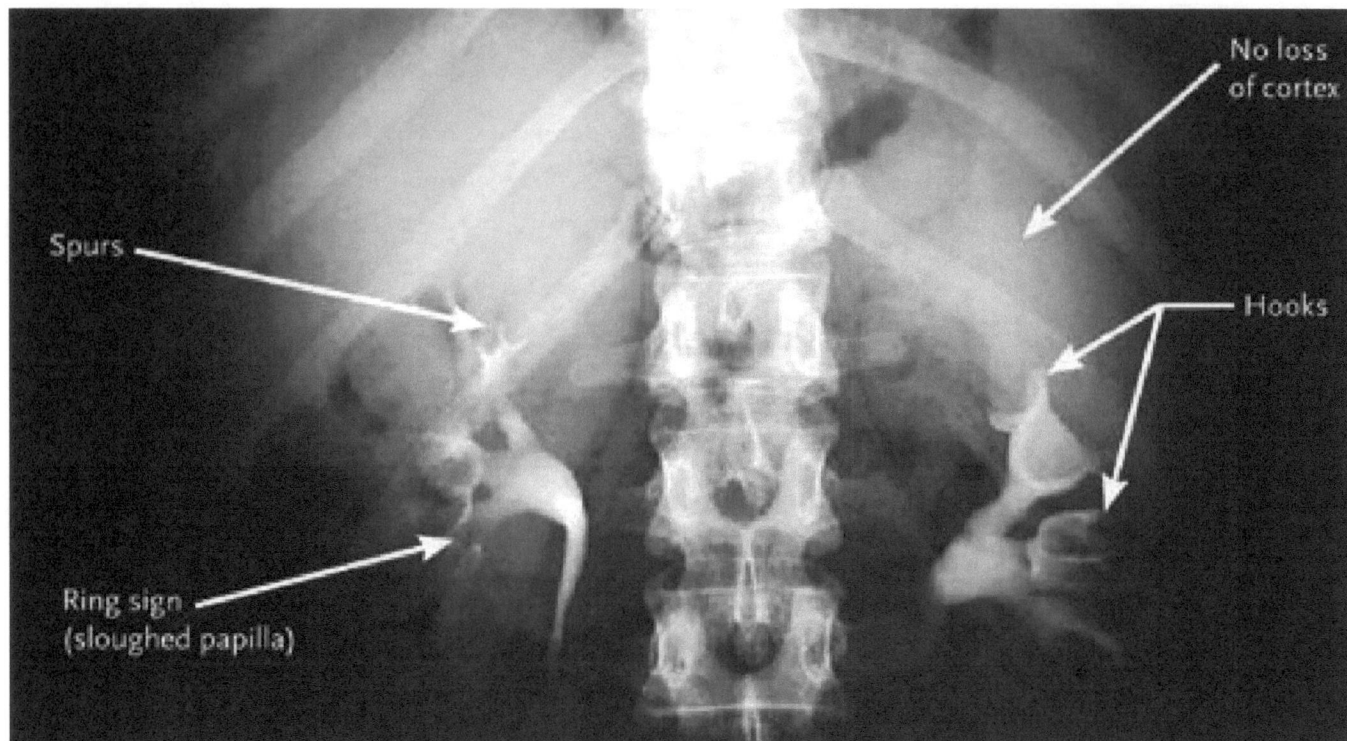

When thinking about a **Delayed Nephrogram** it is a two-fold process, one there is a delay in enhancement and then the contrast stays longer than it should. Think about: RV thrombus, obstruction, RAS, hypotension, ATN, myeloma

Renal Ptosis: this is a hypermobile kidney that can slump on its suspensory ligaments causing UPJ obstruction. Do not confuse this with duplication of the collecting system (will discuss this in pediatric GU chapter).

Megaureter: ureter dilates more as we progress distally and narrows to a birds beak configuration prior to UVJ (aperistaltic segment). Most common type is non-refluxing, non-obstructed.

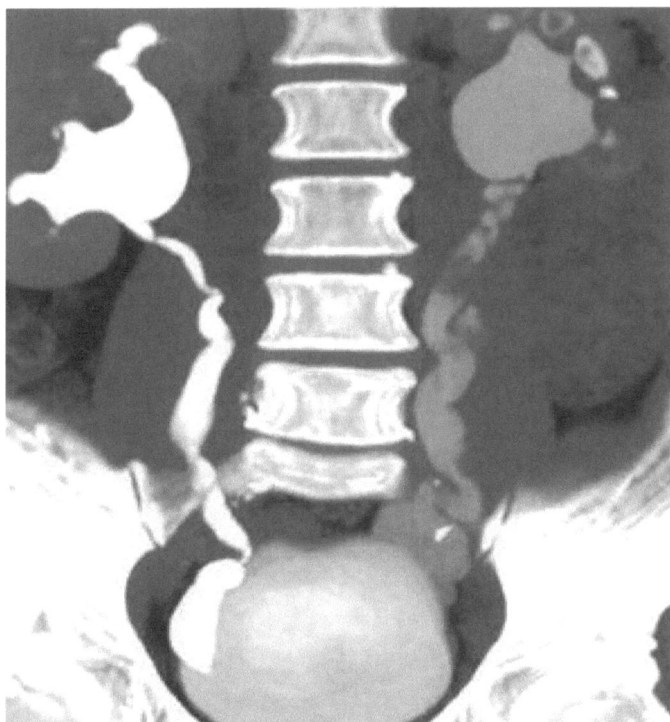

Megacalycosis: congenital condition more likely to affect males. This is too many dilated calyces in a big kidney. If unilateral it can be associated with **ipsilateral megaureter** and **contralateral UPJ obstruction**.

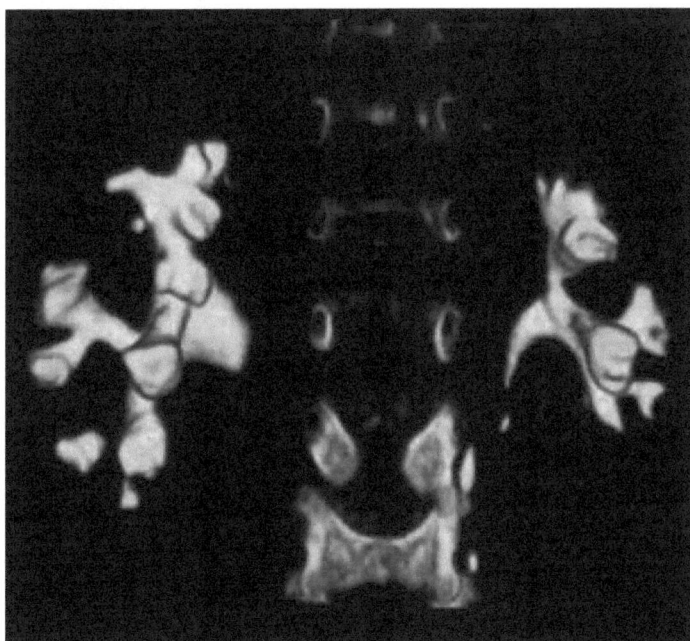

Posterior view recons show an enlarged L-kidney and supernumerary dilated calyces

BLADDER, PROSTATE & URETHRA
Bladder filling defect:

Hematoma	Non-enhancing mobile mass
Calculus	Hyperdense, mobile calcified mass
TCC	Enhancing soft tissue mass adherent to the wall or asymmetric wall thickening, look for other sites of GU TCC
Leiomyoma	Smooth contour tumor with fat density – rapid increase in size is a leiomyosarcoma
Pheochromocytoma	Classic history is passing out while peeing, highly vascular tumor

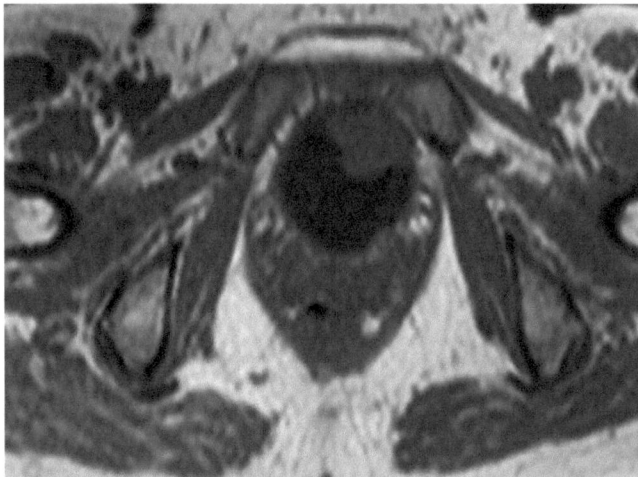

Leiomyoma T1

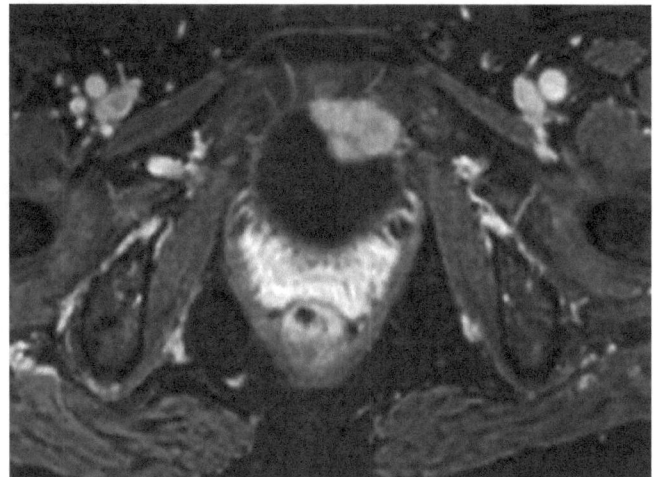

Leiomyoma T1+Gad

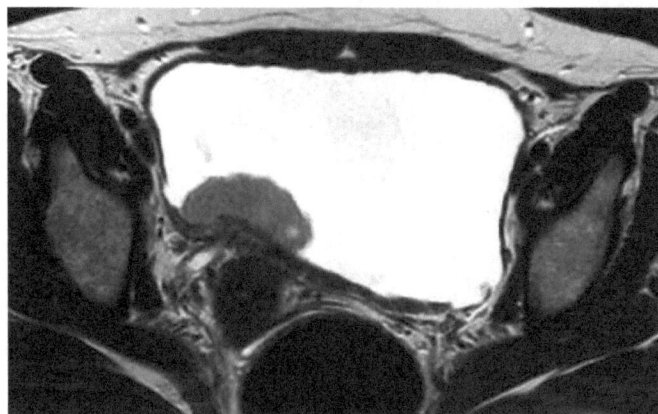

Bladder TCC

Risk factors for bladder cancer:

TCC – smoking and alanine dye
AdenoCA – congenital defects (urachal remnant)
Squamous Cell CA – stones, schistosomiasis

Bladder Schistosomiasis: *Schistosoma hematobium* causes a granulomatous reaction in the bladder with wall calcifications and fibrosis. I thought I had this after swimming in a waterfall in Hawaii with warning signs…

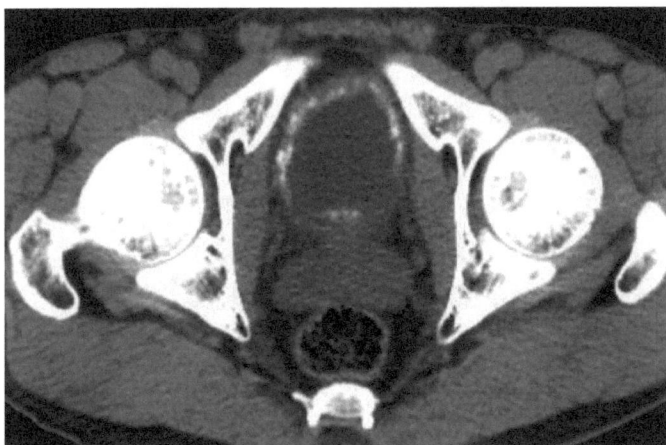
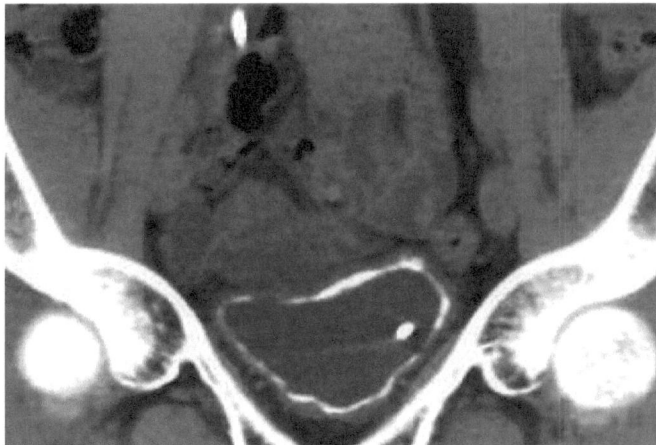

Neurogenic Bladder: comes in two varieties, spastic (small pine-cone shaped with trabecular wall) or atonic (large smooth walled). When you see a spastic neurogenic bladder, look at the spine for congenital defects. Atonic bladders can be seen in people with really horrible spine degenerative changes.

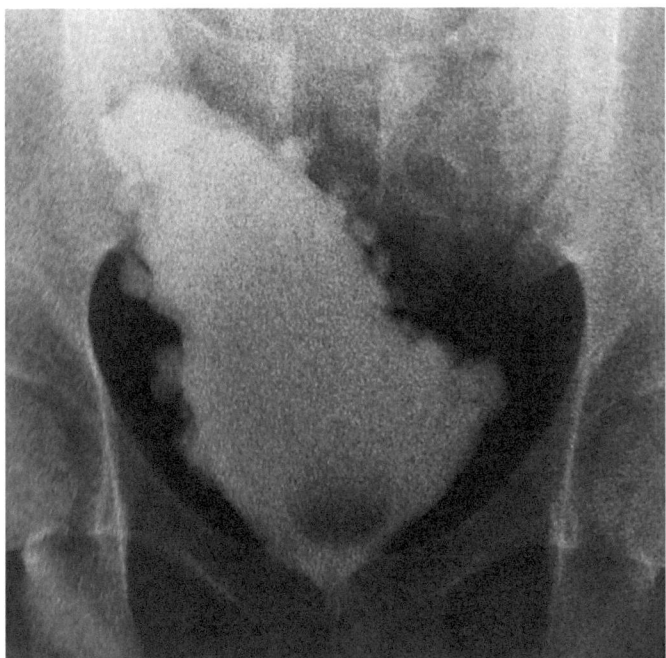
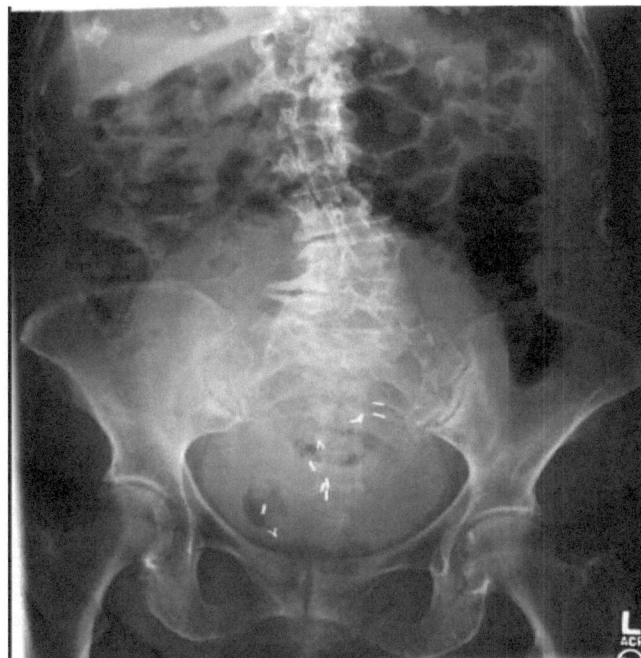

Spastic   Atonic

Emphysematous Cystitis: seen in diabetic patients with poor control and in patients with urinary stasis. *Proteus* species are responsible for this. Not a surgical emergency, can treat by lowering blood sugar and giving antibiotics as well as bladder drainage.

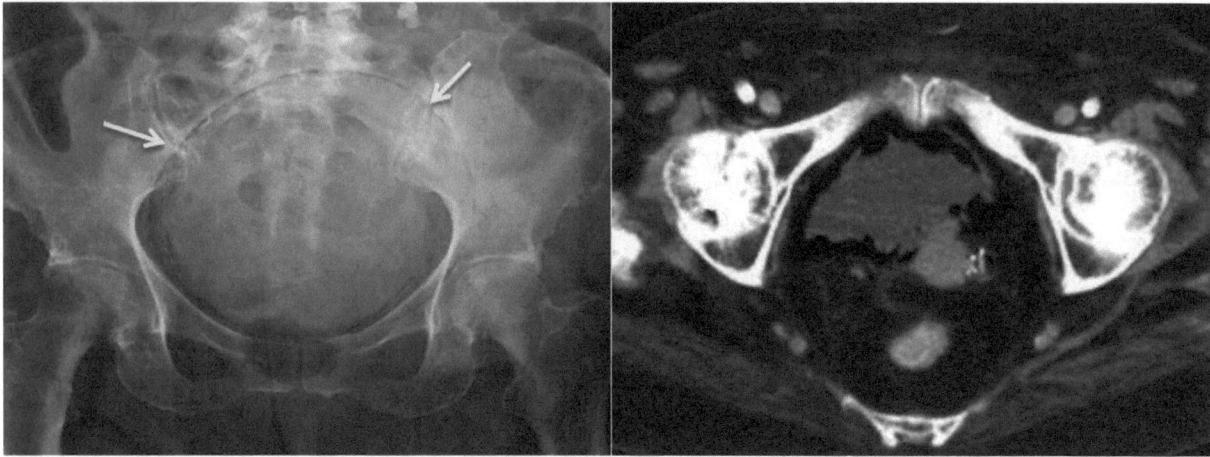

Bladder Diverticula: predispose patient to urinary stasis, which causes stone formation and infection. The chronic irritation can lead to TCC formation. Cancer forming in a tic has a worse prognosis because it can have earlier transmural spread.

Bladder Injury: seen after significant pelvic trauma and can be sub-divided as follows

1. Extra-peritoneal – most common with a flame-shaped appearance to extravsated contrast collecting in the perivesicle, anterior prevesicle (Retzius), and retrorectal spaces.
2. Intra-peritoneal – this happens when there is a direct blow to a distended bladder with a cloud-like appearance to extravasated contrast. This will track along bowel loops and in the paracolic gutters.

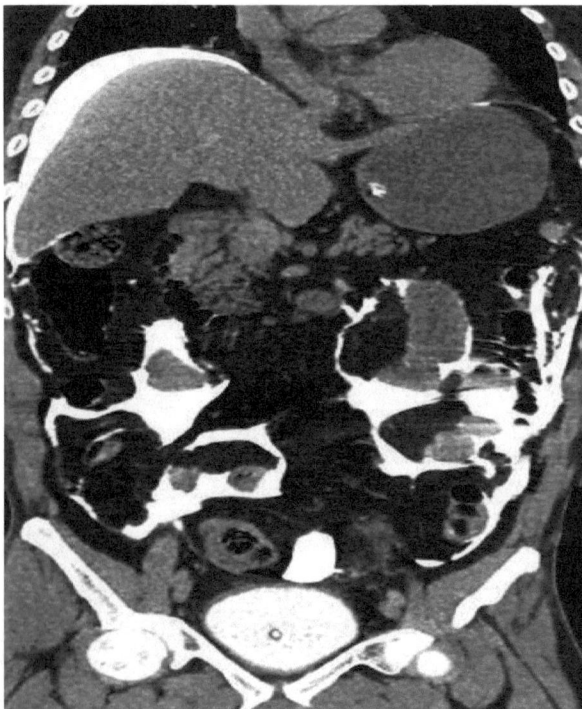

Intra-peritoneal   Extra-peritoneal

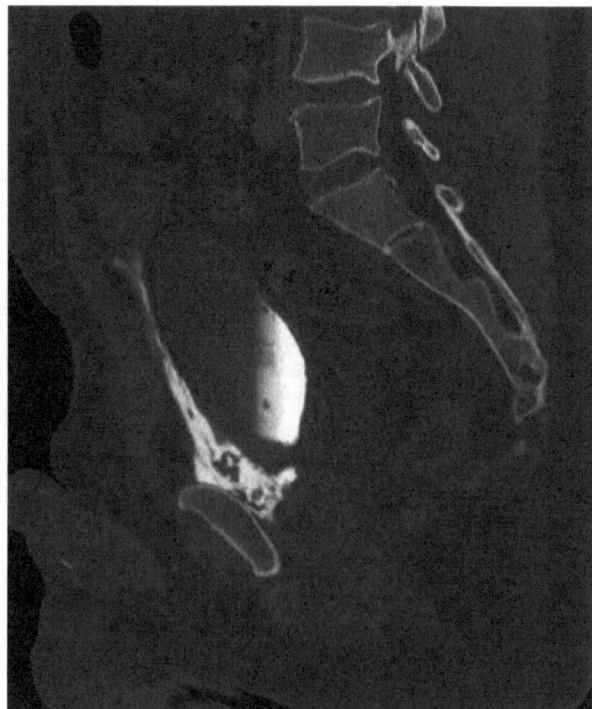

PROSTATE: Zonal anatomy is important to understand as it helps guide your differential diagnosis.

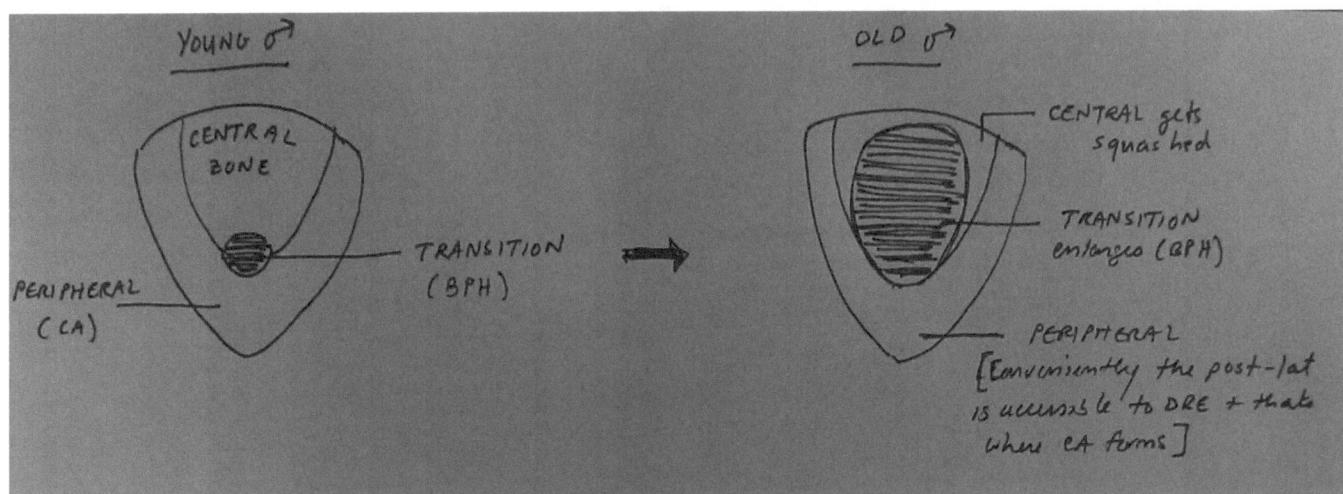

BPH: as demonstrated above, the transitional zone enlarges as we age and causes obstruction by squashing the prostatic urethra. MRI shows a bubbly appearing prostate on T2 imaging.

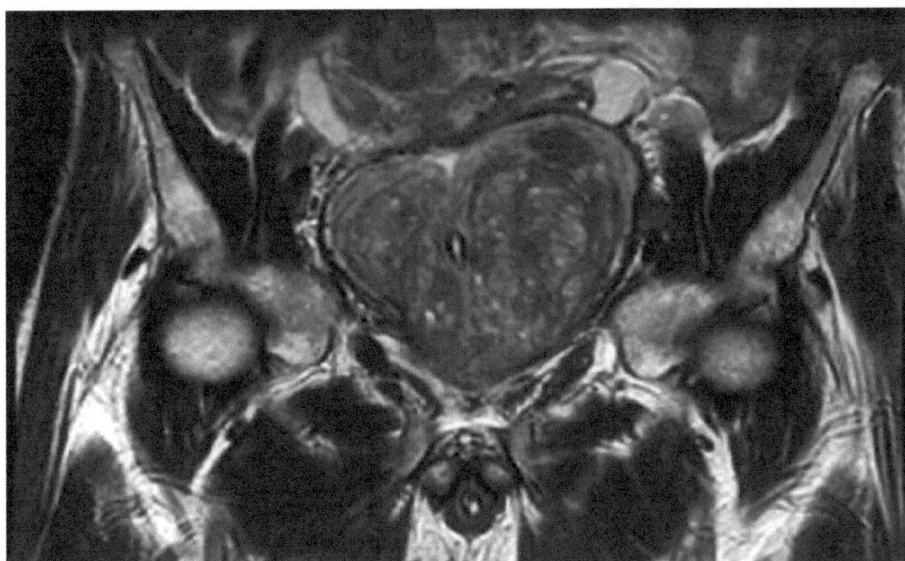

Prostate CA: is going to occur in the peripheral zone, the key is to describe organ bound disease versus local invasion of neurovascular bundle and pelvic nodes. The tumor will be T2 hypointense (because fibrous nature). Look for a bulging capsule and obliteration of the rectoprostatic angle.

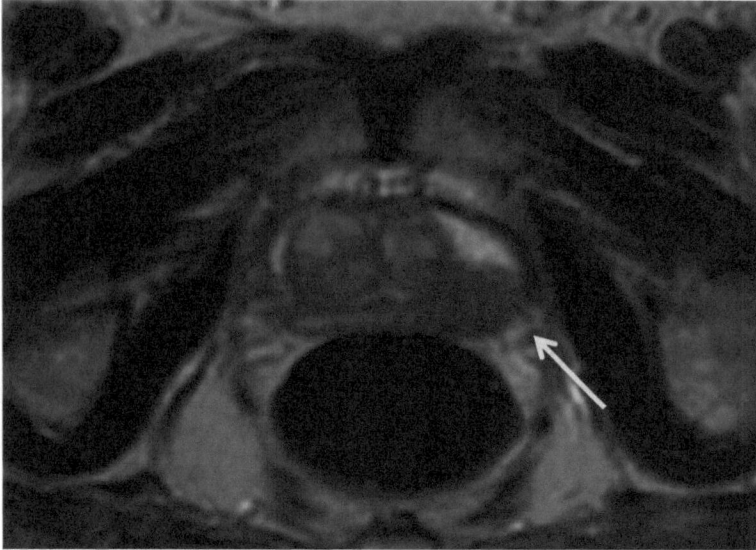

There is a T2 hypointense mass in the left posterior peripheral zone cause a bulge in the capsule and impression on the left rectoprostatic angle (triangle of fat between prostate and rectum)

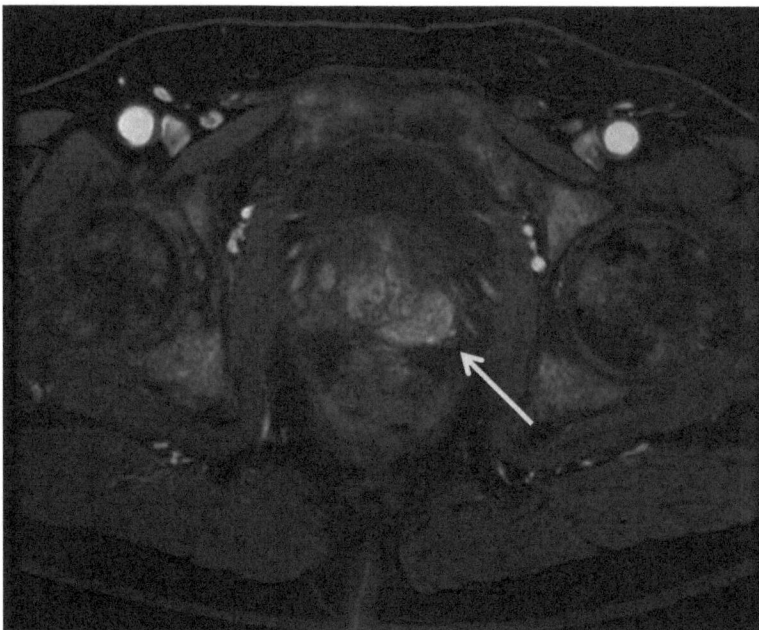

T1+Gad shows enhancement of left prostate cancer with narrowing of the rectoprostatic

Remember to look for lymph nodes and bony pelvic mets, especially if you have enhanced images.

Important Staging: Stage T2 is still confined to the prostate and the surgeons can do a radical prostatectomy. Stage T3 is locally invasive and the treatment is palliative XRT and hormonal therapy.

URETHRA: Normal anatomy is important to understand how trauma is classified

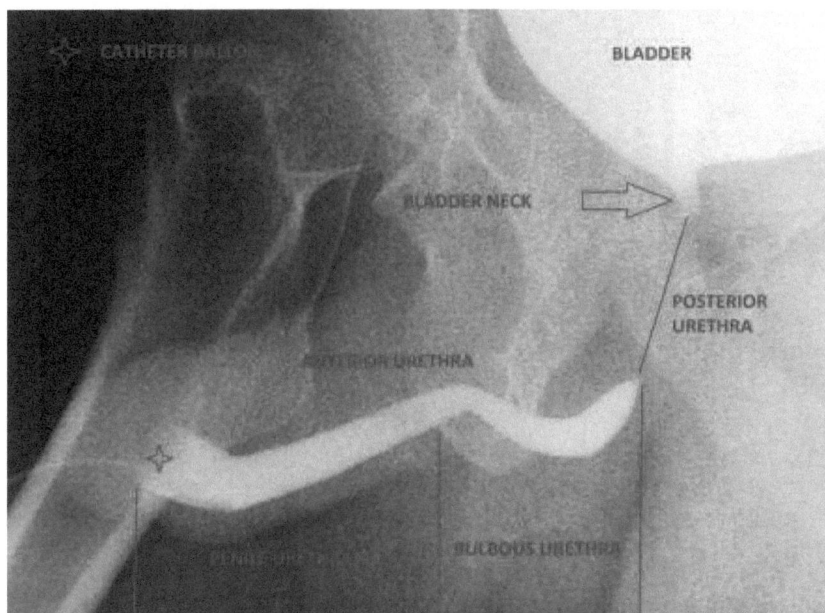

Trauma: most injury is due to blunt trauma to the pelvis resulting in fractures, especially involving the anterior arch. Posterior urethral injury more likely with pelvic fractures while anterior injury is due to a straddle type mechanism where the pelvis isn't fractured.

Type I – urethra stretched but not torn
Type II – membranous urethra is torn above the urogenital diaphragm
Type III – membranous and bulbar urethral injury with urogenital diaphragm injury
Type IV – bladder neck and proximal urethral injury
Type V – anterior urethra injury only

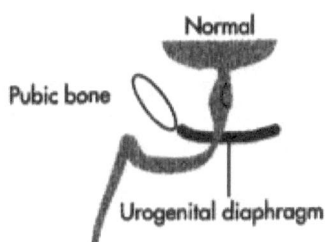

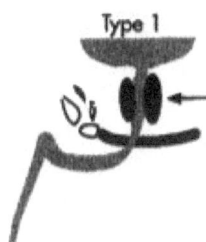

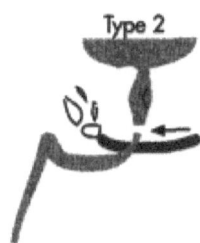

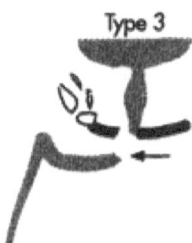

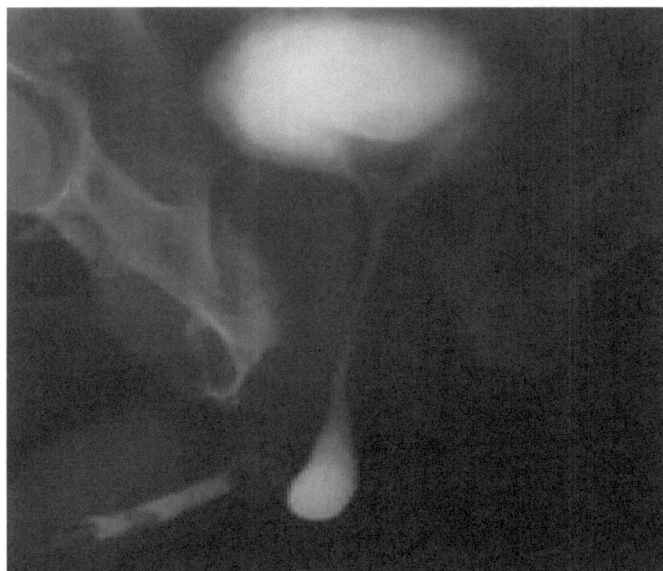

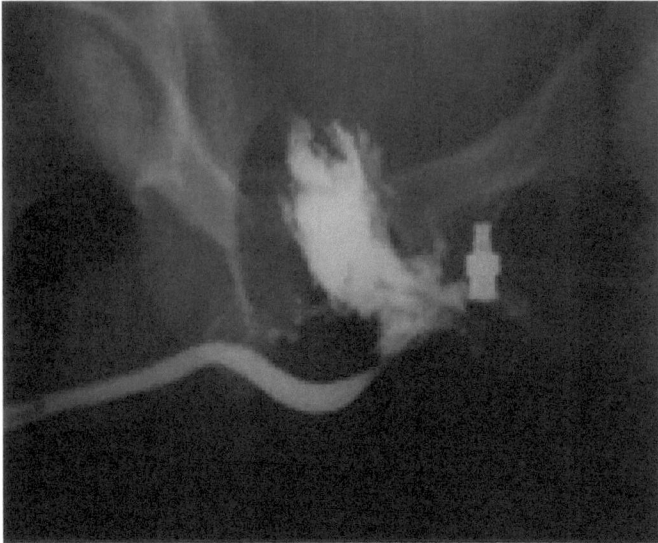

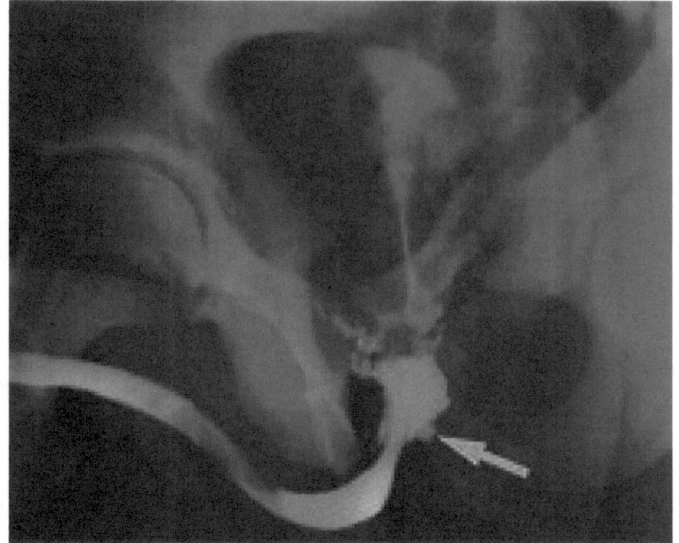

Top right – Type I injury with stretching of the urethra but no extravasation
Bottom left – Type II with extravsation from posterior urethra above bulbous part
Bottom right – Type III injury through urogenital diaphragm involving the bulbous portion

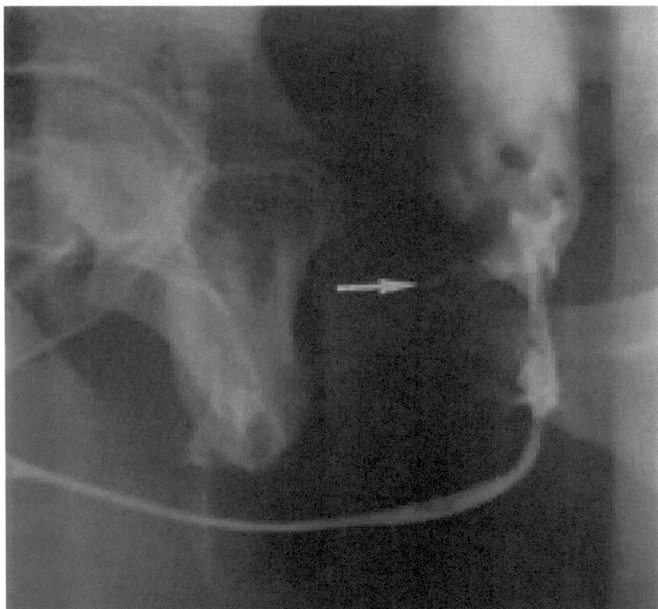

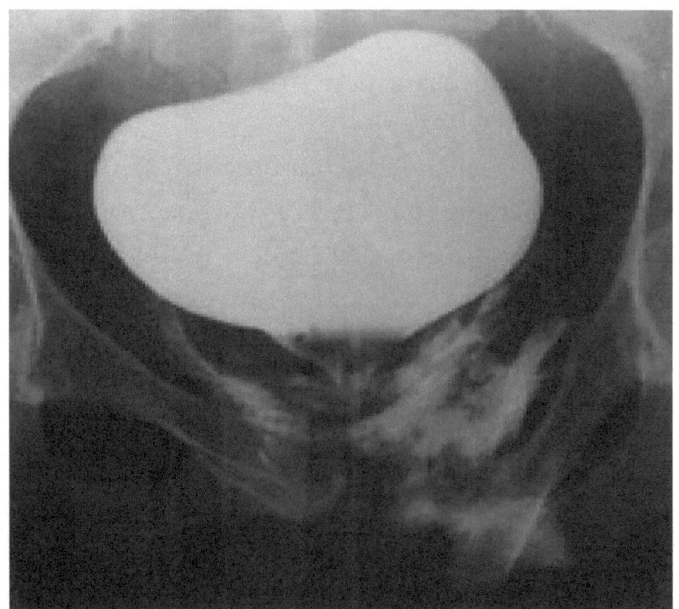

Left – Type IV injury with proximal injury and extra-peritoneal extravasation

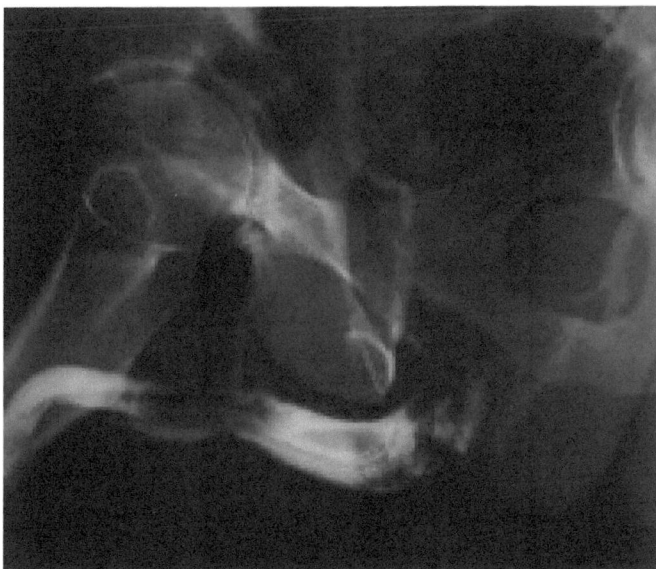

Right – Type IV injury with bladder neck injury and contrast extravasation Type V injury, involving only the anterior urethra

Mutlifocal penile uretha strictures

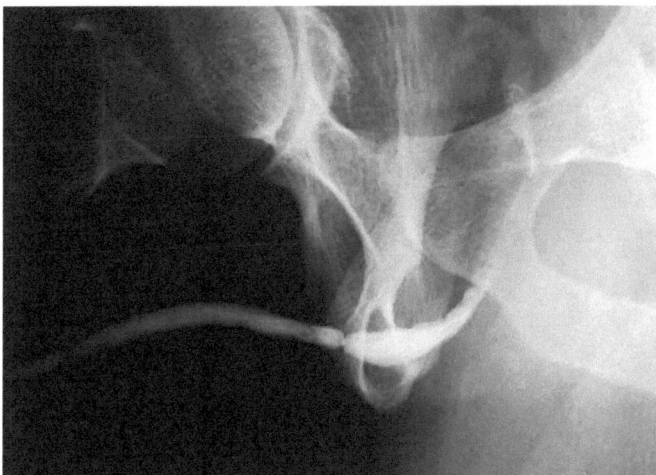

Strictures: usually due to trauma or infection. The length of the stricture dictates treatment, if > 1.5 cm it cannot be resected and re-anastamosed. To fully evaluate do a VCUG and RUG.

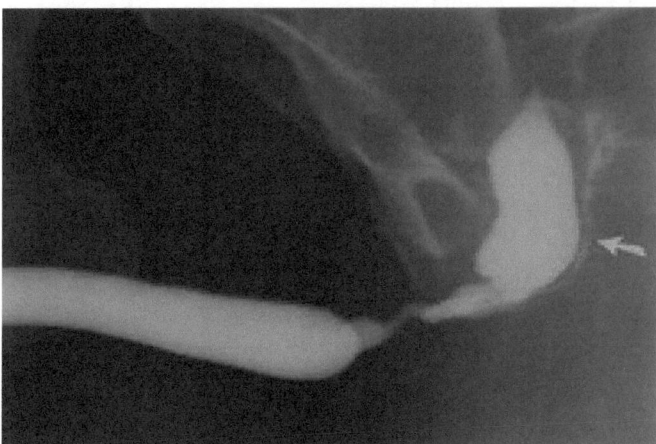

Arrow points to glands of Cowper filling because of back pressure from stricture

Urethral Diverticulum: mostly in females and they complain of non-specific symptoms. It's usually a posterior fluid-filled structure that can have stasis of urine causing stones, infection, or TCC.

Gonococcal Urethritis: post-inflammatory strictures and filling of Glands of Littre causes a shaggy appearance to the urethra.

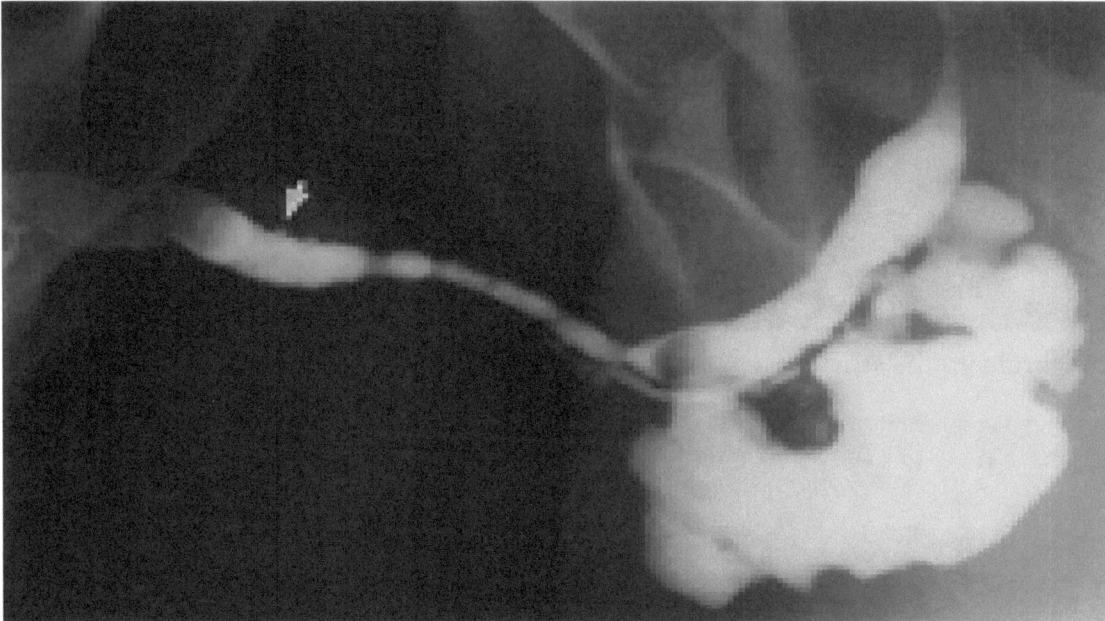

Arrow points to small outpouchings of contrast pooling in glands of Littre – this tells you that this is gonococcal urethritis

BENIGN GYNECOLOGICAL DISEASES

Mullerian Duct Anomalies: 1-3% of the population is affected and these are associated with reproductive dysfunction. Also, patients with MDA have GU anomalies (renal agenesis).

Normal Mullerian ducts are paired structures that look like bananas. They have three phases of fusion; a defect in any of these three steps causes abnormalities.

I   – organogenesis – defect here leads to hypoplasia/agenesis or unicornuate uterus
II   – lateral fusion – defect here causes bicornuate or didelphys
III – septal resorption – defect here causes septate uterus
   • arcuate uterus is considered a normal variant by many
   • septate is the most common variant

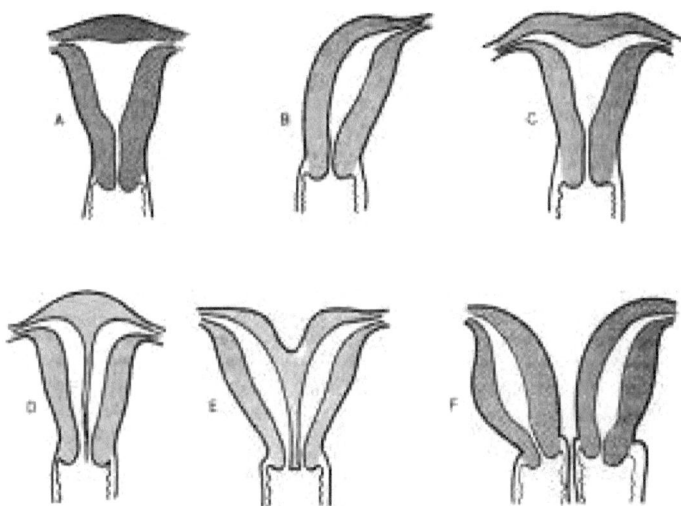

A – Normal (convex fundal contour)

B – Unicornuate

C – Arcuate – convex or flat fundal contour

D – **Septate – most common variant** E – Bicornuate unicollis (1 cervix) bicollis (2 cervices)

F – Didelphys (2 cervices and 2 vaginas)

Women whose mothers used DES have 'T-shaped' uteri and are at increased risk of cervical and vaginal malignancy.

Leiomyomas: most common benign tumor of the uterus and symptoms relate to size and location. Welldemarcated **T2 hypointense lesion** with homogeneous enhancement unless there is internal degeneration (high T2, non-enhancing).

Transmural is the number one location (in the muscle substance)

Submucosal is right next to the endometrium and can protrude into the endometrial canal, can be pedunculated

Subserosal if pedunculated they can rotate on axis and torse causing pain

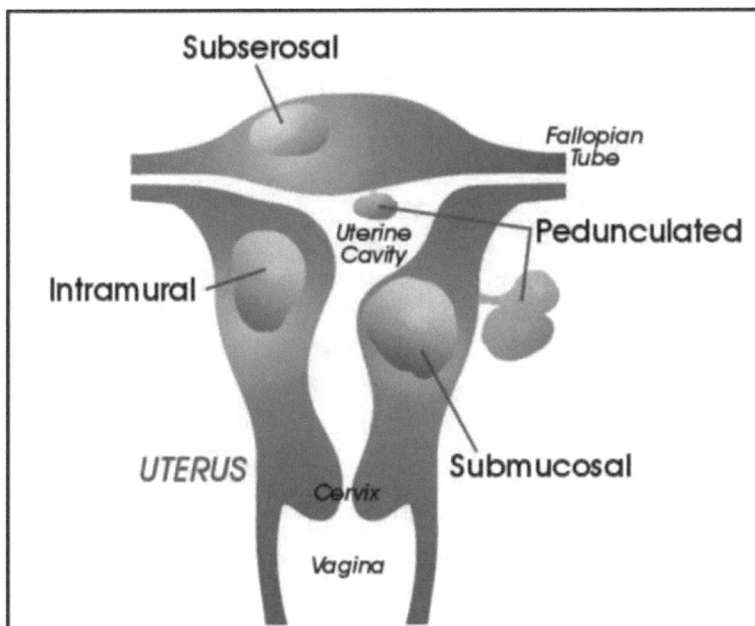

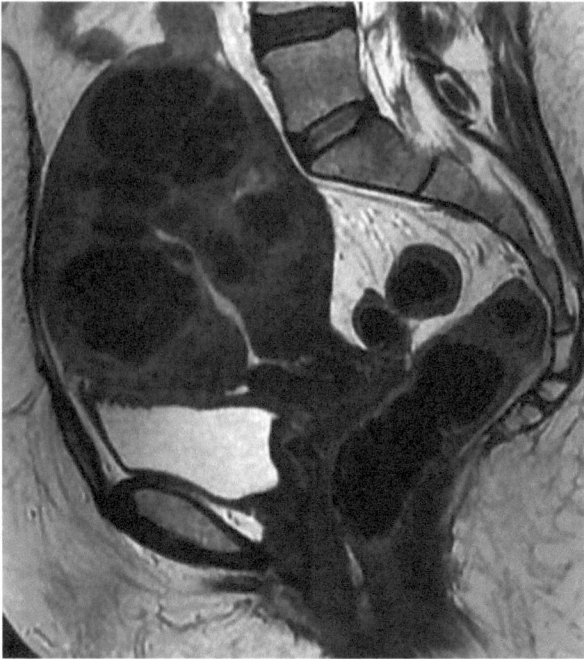

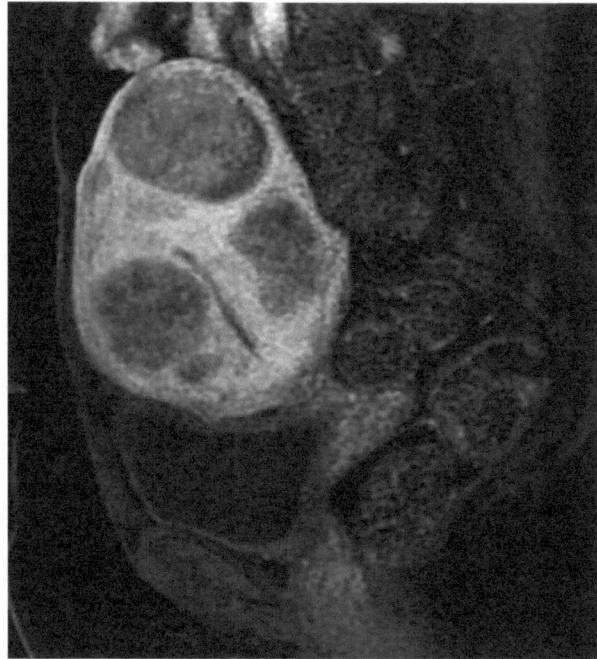

Multiple leiomyomas: left image T2, right image T1+gad

Adenomyosis: ectopic endometrial tissue in the myometrium can be focal or diffuse. Borders are ill defined and has a "starry sky" appearance on T2 MRI. The bright spots are glandular deposits. This disease is characterized by an abnormally large junctional zone > 12-mm

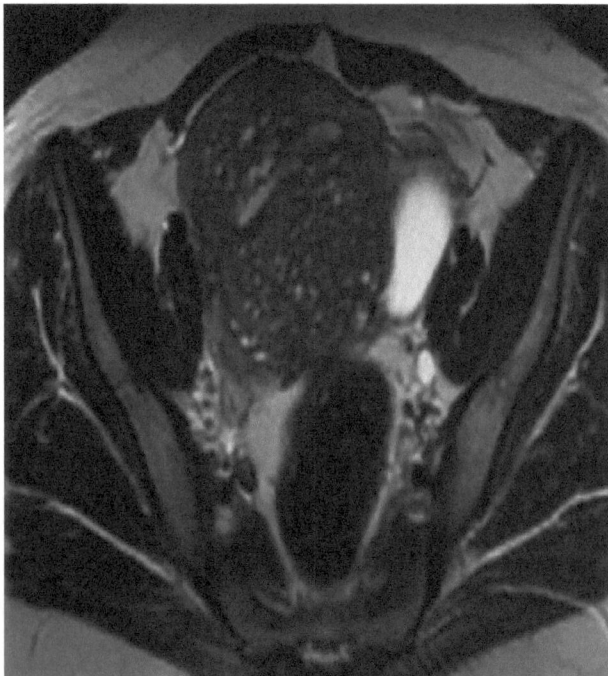

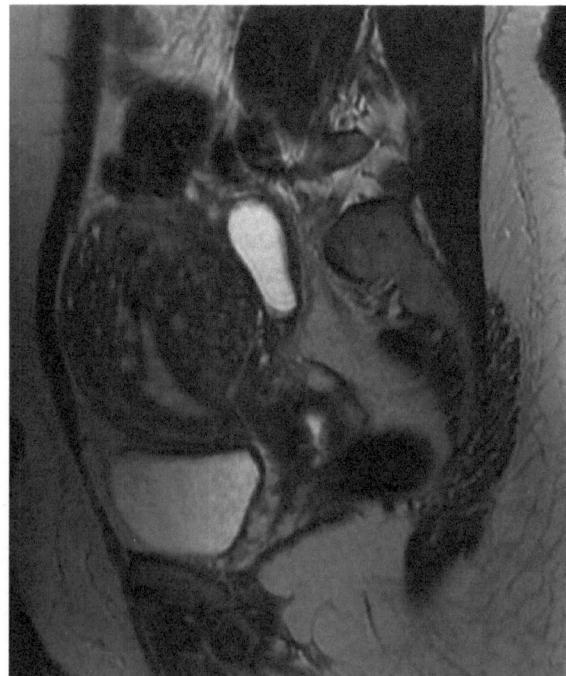

Endometriosis: is ectopic endometrial tissue outside of the uterus with most implants on the surface of the ovaries, uterine ligaments, and pouch of Douglas. Causes dysmenorrhea, dyspareunia, and **infertility**. These can have malignant transformation – look for solid components. They can be anywhere; catemenial pneumothorax is endometrioma in pleura.

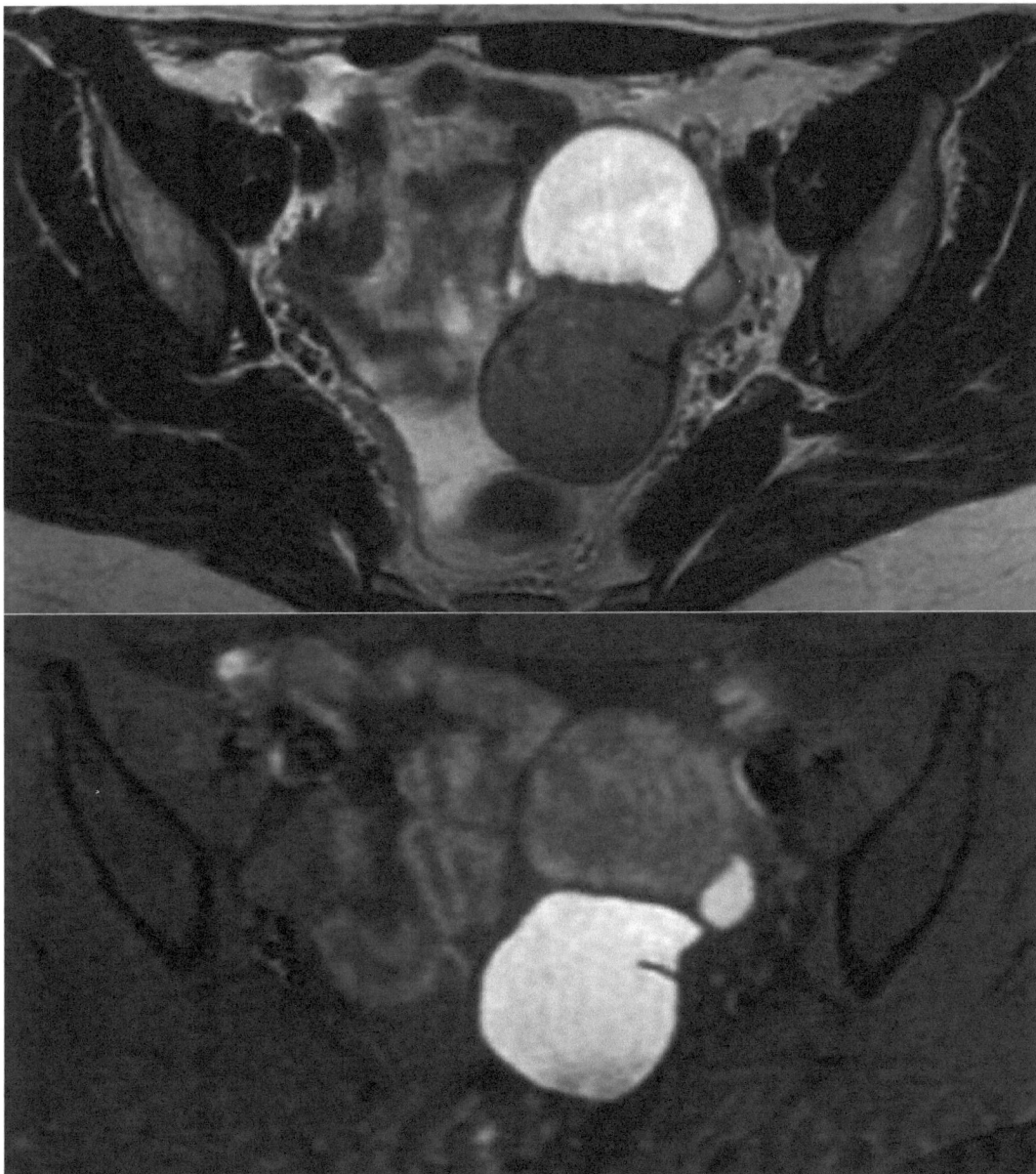

The classic MRI appearance is of a T1 bright lesion (blood products) with T2 'shading'

T1 – top image
T2 – bottom image

Peritoneal Inclusion Cyst: walled off ovulatory fluid in premenopausal women with a history of surgery, trauma, PID, or endometriosis. The appearance is of a normal ovary sitting in a loculated fluid collection.

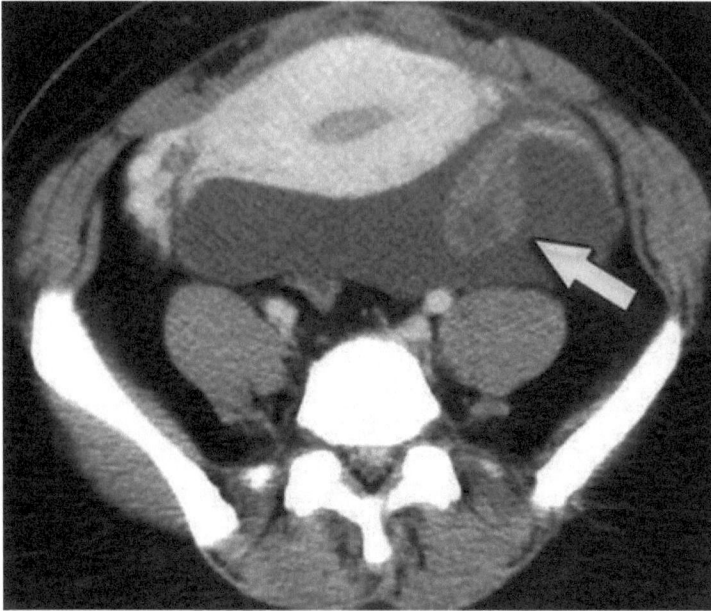

HSG: this procedure should be performed during the **proliferative stage** (follicular days 6-14) of the cycle when the endometrium is at its thinnest. Make sure the patient is not pregnant. Commonly used to evaluate for causes of infertility.

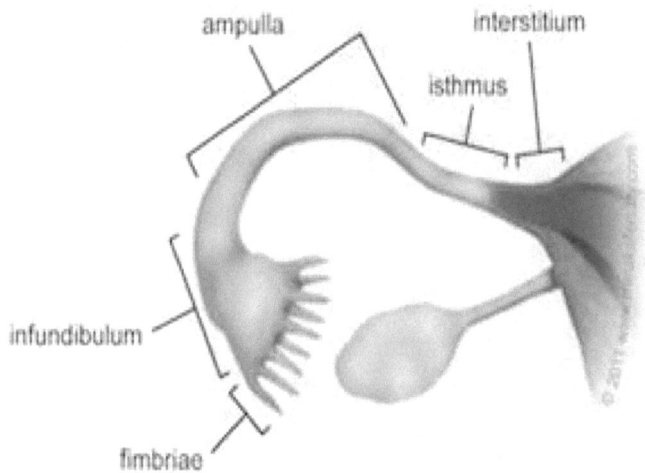

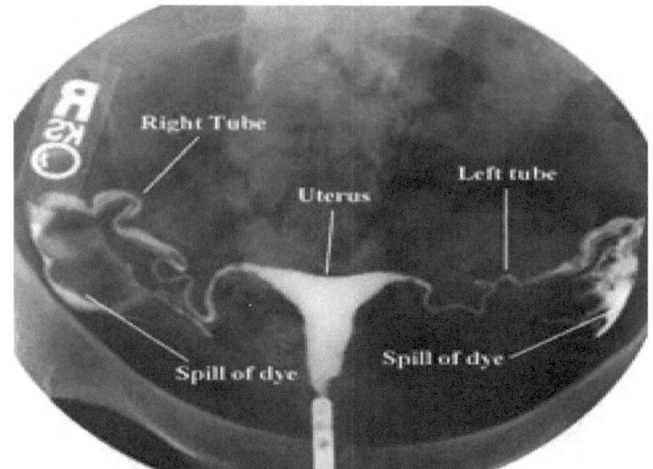

Salpingitis Isthmica Nodosa: is an inflammatory and post-infectious disease of the fallopian tubes that is characterized by **multiple diverticula**. It may be associated with tubal obstruction and is best characterized with HSG. This increases the risk of a tubal ectopic.

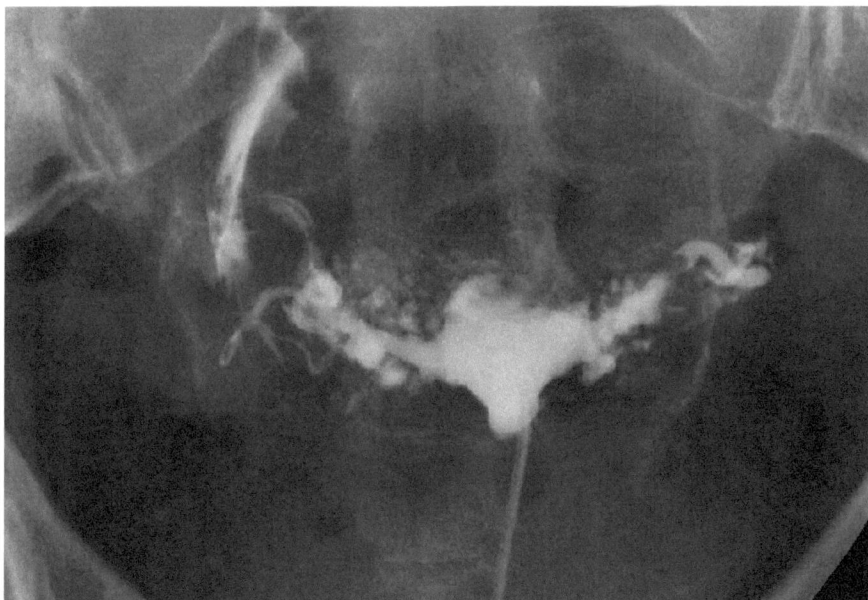

Asherman Syndrome: a condition where there are intra-uterine adhesions from injury to the endometrium, associated with infertility and pregnancy loss. Look for linear filling defects with inability to distend the endometrial cavity.

Other detectable conditions: MDA, submucosal fibroids, malignancy, adhesions, tubal polyps, hydrosalpinx

GYN MALIGNANCIES

Ovarian Malignancy: the majority of ovarian tumors are adenocarcinomas and they spread by direct extension, peritoneal seeding, and via RP LAD.

Malignant characteristics are: solid components, enhancing nodules, thick septa, necrosis, and peritoneal deposits.

Staging of malignancy should be thought about as intra-pelvic vs. extra-pelvic disease:

I   – confined to one or both ovaries
II   – one or both ovaries with pelvic extension can be treated with TAHBSO
III   – disease extends into the abdomen, omental caking anterior to transverse colon, nodules (earliest will be in the paracolic gutters)
IV   – distant metastases

Epithelial Tumors (60-70%)	
Serous Cystadenoma (most)	Benign tumor filled with watery fluid
Serous CystadenoCA	Largest portion of malignant ovarian CA, 6th decade of life, elevated CA-125, **frequently bilateral** mixed cystic solid lesions

Mucinous Cystadenoma	Larger than serous tumors, secrete mucin, and contain septations (rare to be unilocular)
Mucinous CystadenoCA	Malignant tumor with multilocular appearance with some nodular soft tissue density. Rupture can lead to pseudomyxoma peritonei – less likely to be bilateral than serous tumors

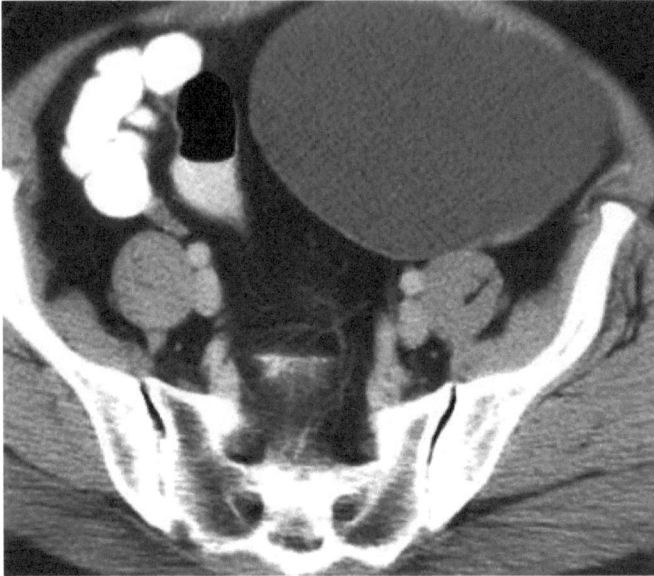

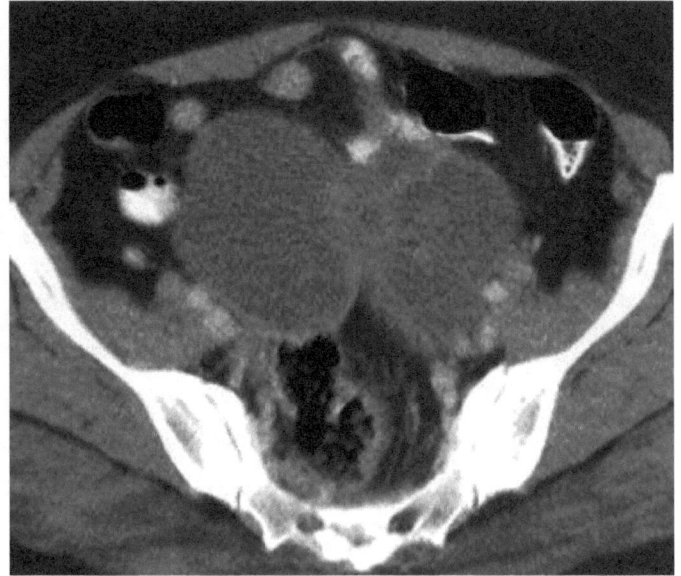

Left image – unilocular serous cystadenoma
Right image – bilateral serous cystadenoCA with enhancing nodules and thick septa

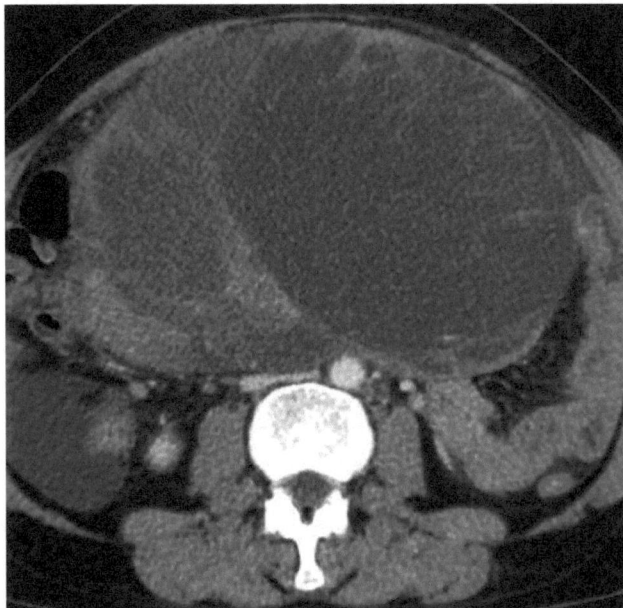

Mucinous cystadenoCA displaying typical properties of very large size, multi-locular, thick septa and enhancing nodules

Germ Cell Tumors: commonest is the **ovarian mature teratoma** (dermoid); contain mature elements of fat, calcium, and hair. Typically asymptomatic incidental finding, but can predispose to torsion. Look for macroscopic fat and calcium to clinch this diagnosis.

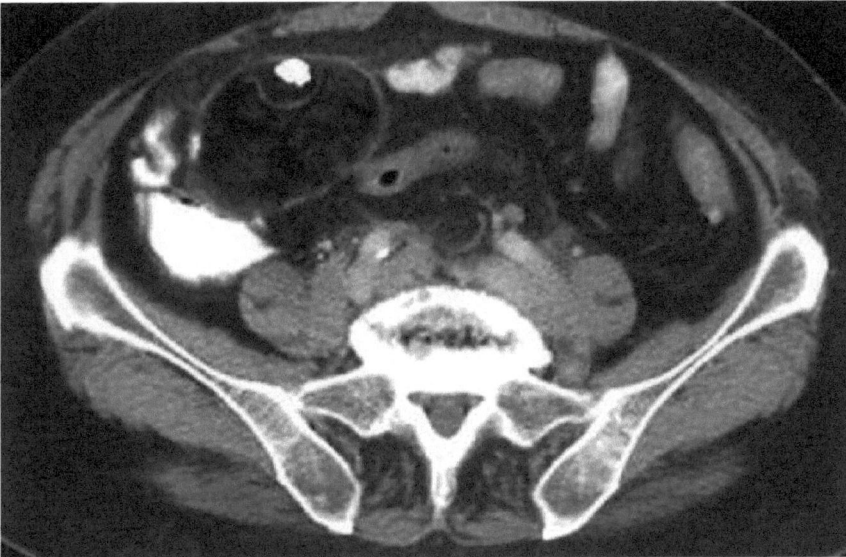

Sex Cord – Stromal Tumors: these are the rarest forms of ovarian tumors. Keep a couple in mind because they have classic presentations for testing purposes:

1. Fibroma-thecoma – benign fibrous tumor associated with Meig's Syndrome (ascites and right sided pleural effusion)
2. Granulosa cell – originate from the ovarian stroma and secrete estrogen (66% in post-menopausal women) and lead to endometrial hyperplasia or carcinoma. In younger girls it can cause precocious puberty.

Next we will look at endometrial and cervical cancers. To be able to find these things on MRI you have to know the normal appearance, so lets start with a normal sagittal T2 MRI. It shows a hyperintense endometrium surrounded by a thick black junctional zone (incidental leiomyoma). The cervix is the lower 1/3rd of the uterus and should be jet black on T2 imaging because of its fibrous build. On this sagittal image you can also see the anterior and posterior vaginal fornices (inferior to the 'C' – the hyperintense slits curving upwards).

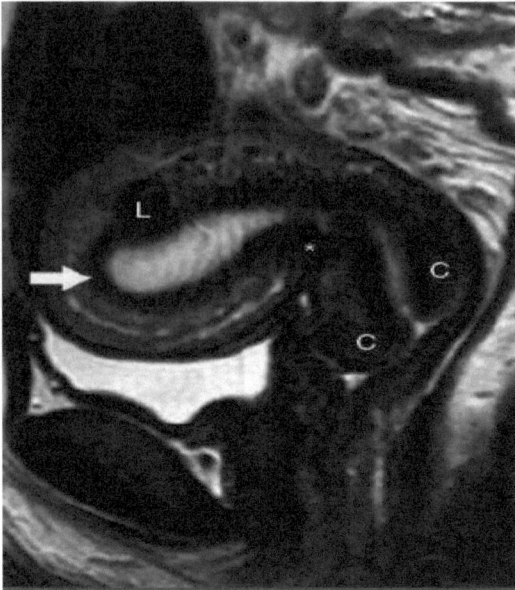

Endometrial Cancer: this is the commonest GYN malignancy and the warning sign is post-menopausal bleeding. A woman not on Tamoxifen has an endometrial thickness cutoff value of 5-mm, biopsy that thing if it's thicker! On Tamoxifen, can push that limit to 8-mm.

The majority is adenoCA and it spreads by direct extension and to the paraaortic and RP lymph nodes as well as peritoneal seeding. Use the sagittal T2 image on MRI to look for this. Normal endometrium is T2 bright and the cancer disrupts this pattern and has variable enhancement.

Stage 0 – carcinoma in situ
Stage 1 – limited to the body of the uterus with up to ½ the myometrial thickness invaded
Stage 2 – cervical stromal involvement
Stage 3 – local spread (uterine serosa, adenexa, vagina)
Stage 4 – distant metastases

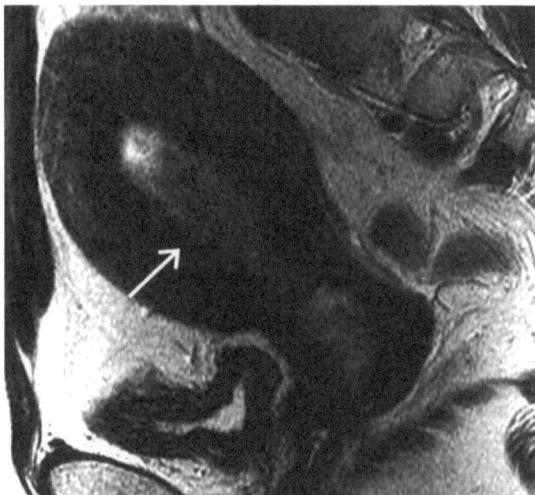

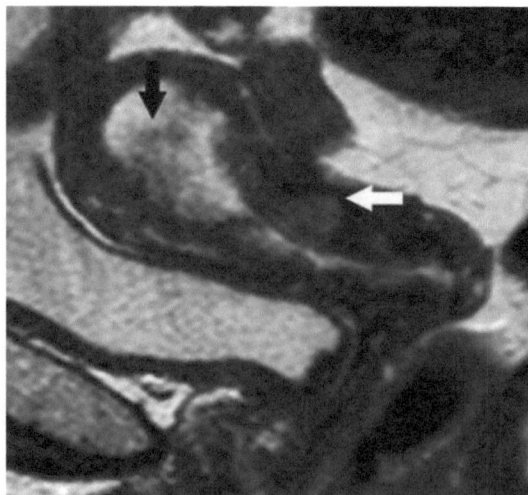

Cervical Cancer: patients present with intermenstrual, post-coital bleeding. HPV is a risk factor and squamous cell cancer is the biggest culprit. On MRI the two key things are 1) axial view to look for parametrial invasion (through stroma) and 2) look for intermediate signal intensity in the normally dark cervix on sagittal T2.

The most important thing to remember here is **stage IIb** as this indicates parametrial invasion and therefore, the treatment changes from surgery to XRT

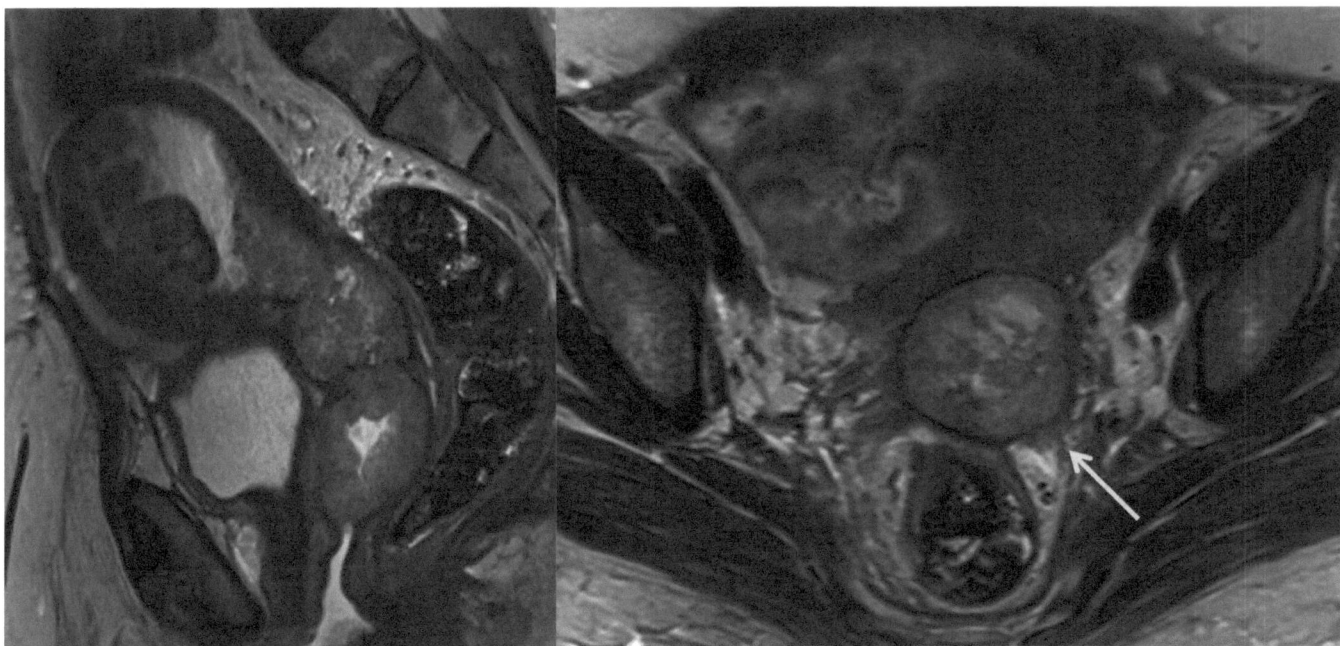

Contrast this uterus and cervix to the normal above. There is soft tissue filling the endometrial cavity and there is intermediate increased signal in the cervix replacing the normal stroma. The axial view shows that the tumor is not contained by the thick dark stromal band (left posterior) so it is stage IIB and therefore surgery is not an option.

Mammography

The breast is divided into three zones:

- Pre-mammary – from subcutaneous tissue to anterior mammary fascia
- Mammary – between anterior and posterior mammary fascias
- Retro-mammary zones – posterior mammary fascia to chest wall

BI-RADS:

0 – incomplete evaluation
1 – negative
2 – benign
3 – probably benign – f/u 6, 12, 18 months (2% risk of CA)
4 – suspicious (30% risk of CA)
5 – highly suggestive of malignance (95% risk of CA)
6 – known malignancy

BIRADS II lesions
Calcified fibroadenomas
Multiple secretory calcifications
Oil cysts
Galactoceles
Mixed density hamartomas
Simple breast cyst

BIRADS Lingo: when in doubt always go with the more suspicious descriptor.

Mass – 3D structure demonstrating convex borders evident on 2 views

Asymmetry – lacks convex borders

Global asymmetry – large volume of glandular tissue occupying > 1 quadrant in a breast compared to the other breast

Focal asymmetry – seen on 2 views

Developing asymmetry – any change to a focal asymmetry, this is BIRADS IV until proven otherwise

Density Descriptors
Almost entirely fat
Scattered fibroglandular densities
Heterogeneously Dense
Extremely dense

Shape
Round
Oval
Irregular
Lobular

Margins
Circumscribed < 25% obscured
Microlobulated
Angular
Indistinct
Spiculated

BENIGN MASSES:

Oil Cyst: a benign lesion where an area of fat necrosis becomes walled off by fibrous tissue. If multiple, bilateral, and in the dermis – steatocystoma multiplex

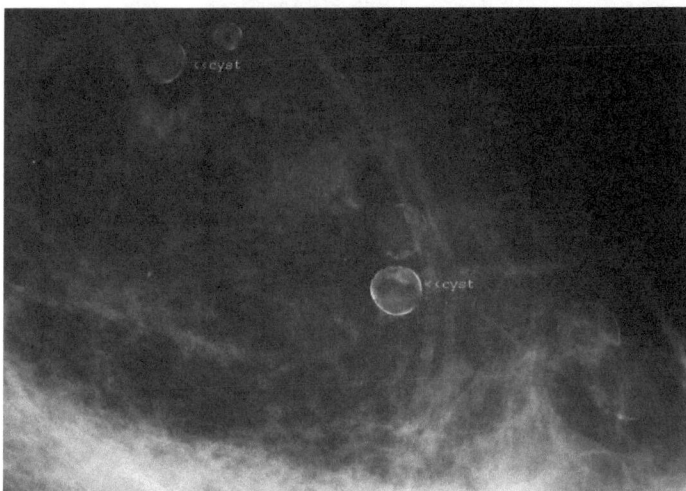

Lipoma: can be a painless palpable mass or discovered incidentally. Radiolucent mass on mammogram and rounded iso-to-hyper-echoic lesion on US.

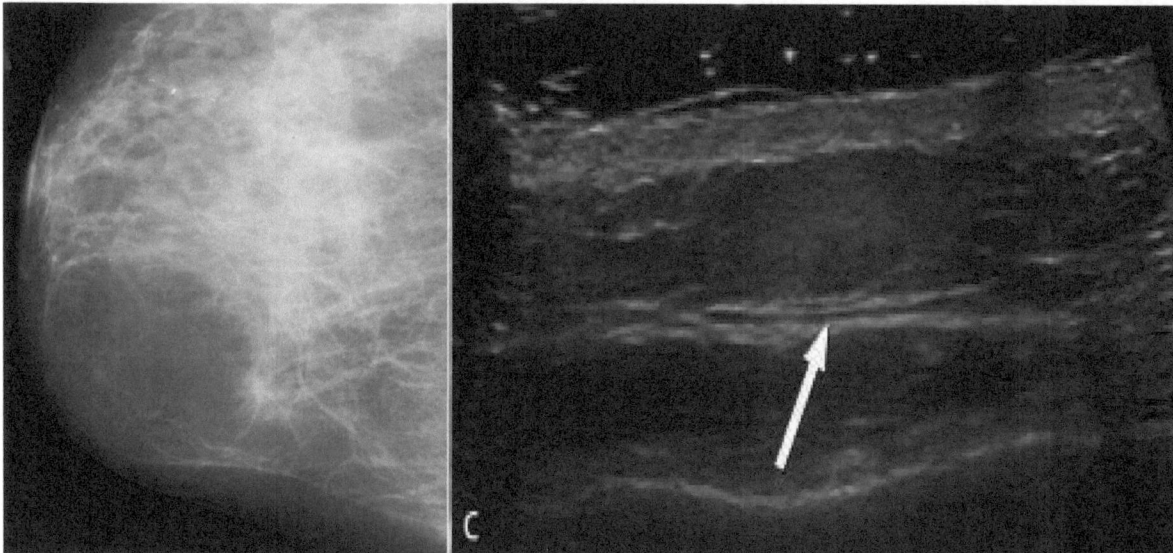

Galactocele: benign lesion that occurs in young women during lactation. Patients present with a painless palpable lump occurring over weeks to months. Essentially it is a retention cyst due to lactiferous duct occlusion.

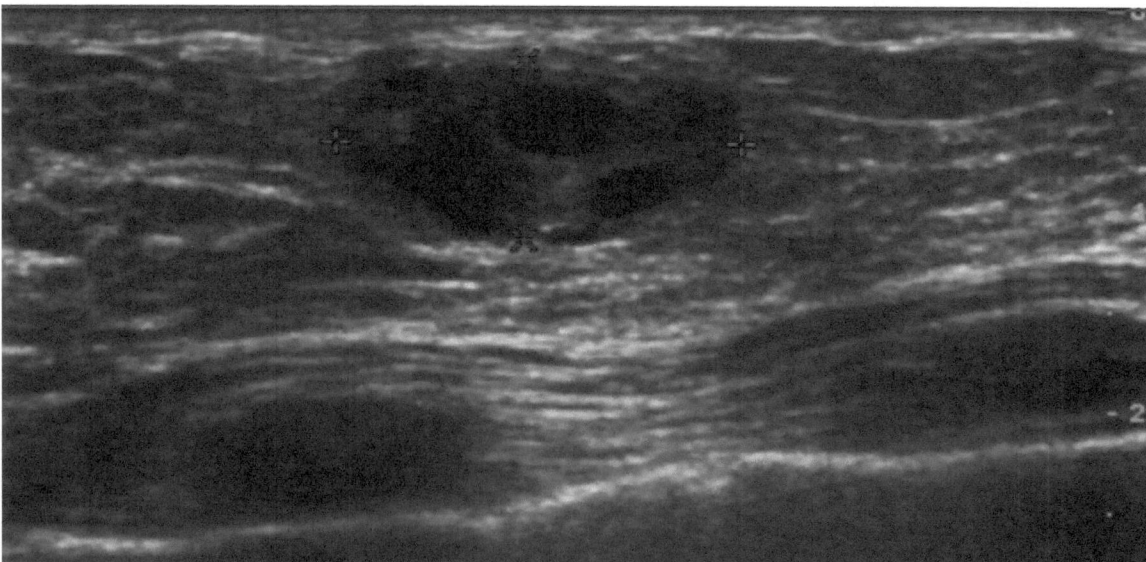

Hamartoma: are also called fibroadenolipomas and are a benign lesion. Can present as a soft lump or unilateral breast enlargement. It is composed of fibrous, glandular, and fatty tissues – all normal breast elements. Look for a pseudocapsule.

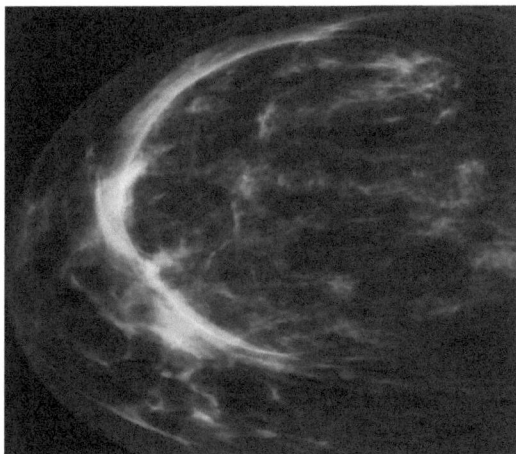

Lymph Node: can be solitary or multiple. Have to be sure that it is a benign lymph node to call it that. Look for the hypoechoic cortex and hyperechoic fatty core.

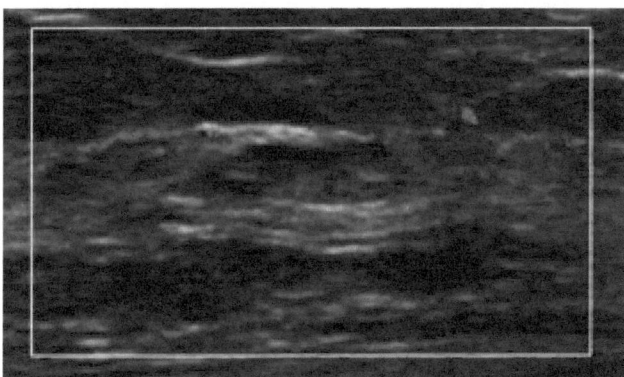

Lactating Adenoma: is one of the most common peripartum period masses. Present as a painless mass late in pregnancy or in the post-partum period. They are palpable, mobile lesions that undergo rapid growth. They resolve with the cessation of lactation.

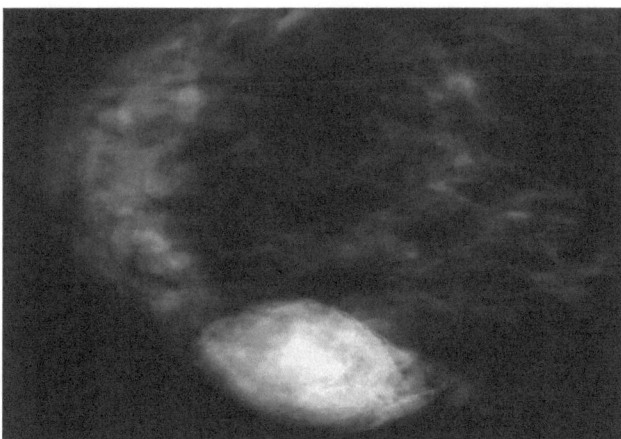

Sternalis Muscle: normal variant of chest wall musculature. Has a typical look and is typically unilateral.

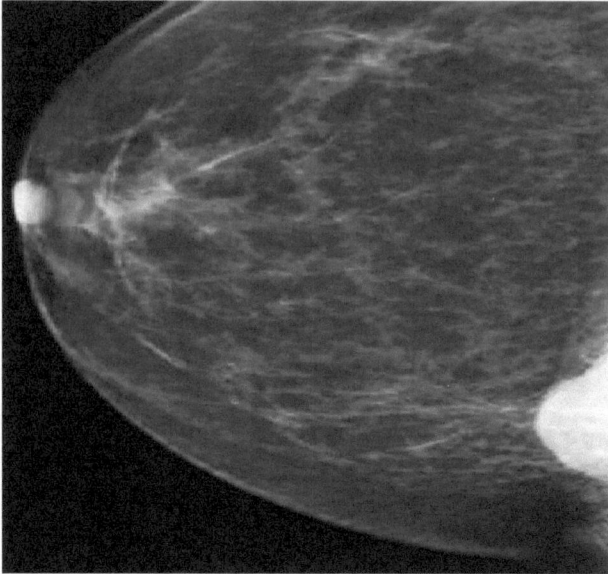

Radial Scar: also called complex sclerosing adenosis. It is an idiopathic process. Usually not palpable and clinical exam is often normal. There should never be any skin thickening or nipple retraction. It's called a "black star" because center is lucent and dense lines radiate out from it.

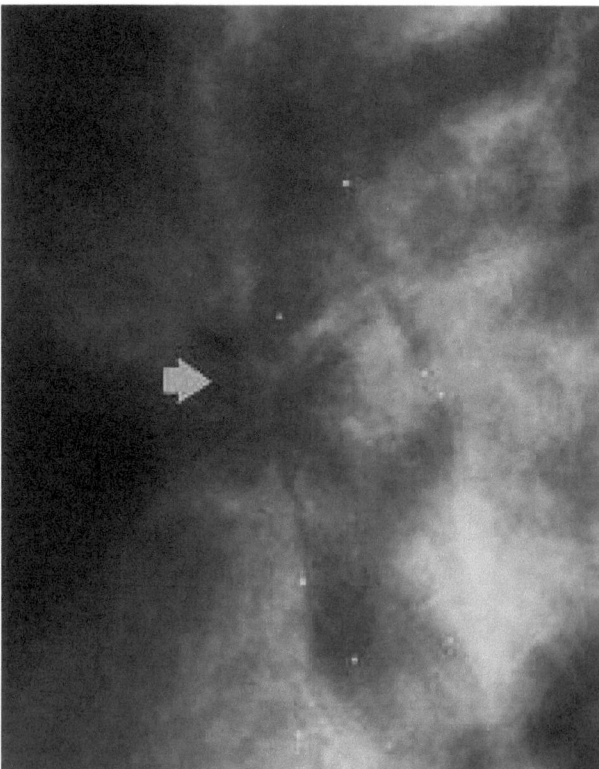

Diabetic Mastopathy: occurs in younger patients with DM1. It is a palpable mass that just 'shows up' one day and is an ill-defined hypoechoic mass on US. Needs biopsy to exclude malignancy. Otherwise, it is a selflimited entity that doesn't require treatment.

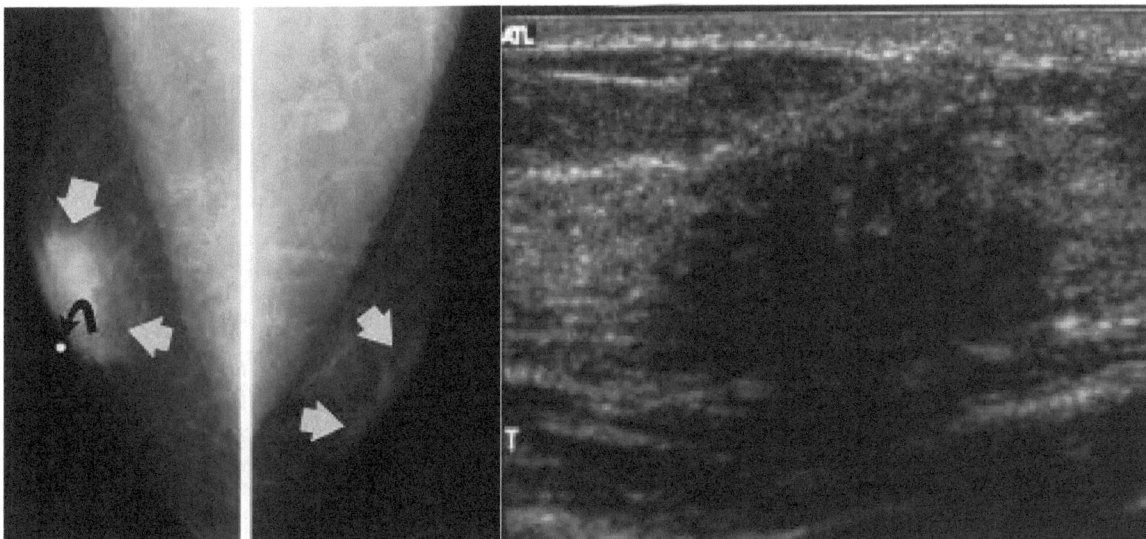

Gynecomastia: benign excess of male breast tissue. Not a risk factor for developing male breast cancer. Flame shaped uni- or bilateral lesions starting at the areola and extending posteriorly. The excess tissue just blends in with the normal fat.

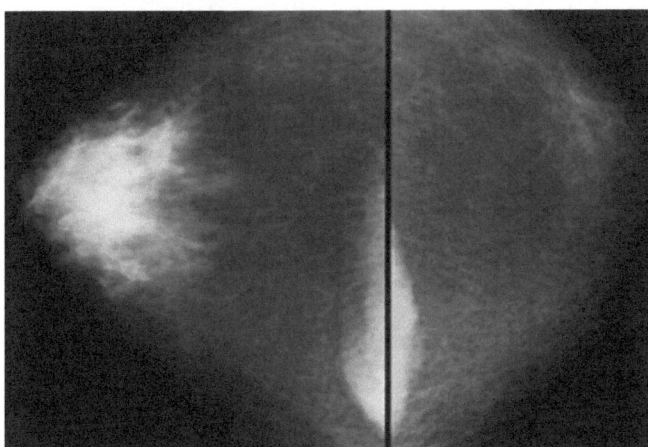

Fibroadenoma: number one mass in a young femal (<30). Well defined hypo-echoic mass on US. If the patient is on cyclosporine, they can get cyclosporine induced fibroadenomas.

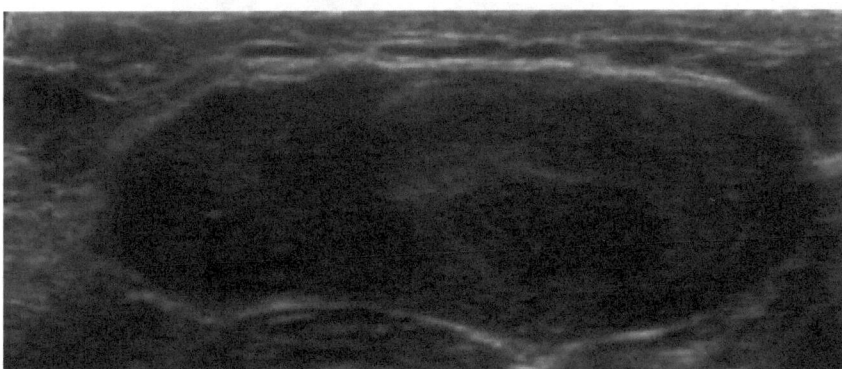

PASH: is a benign hormonally responsive process seen in premenopausal women that clinically gets called fibroadenoma. Biopsy is used to prove it, then we can recommend routine follow-up.

On mammo, it will be a circumscribed or partly circumscribed mass lacking calcification. On US, it is a hypoechoic mass with similar imaging characteristics to fibroadenoma.

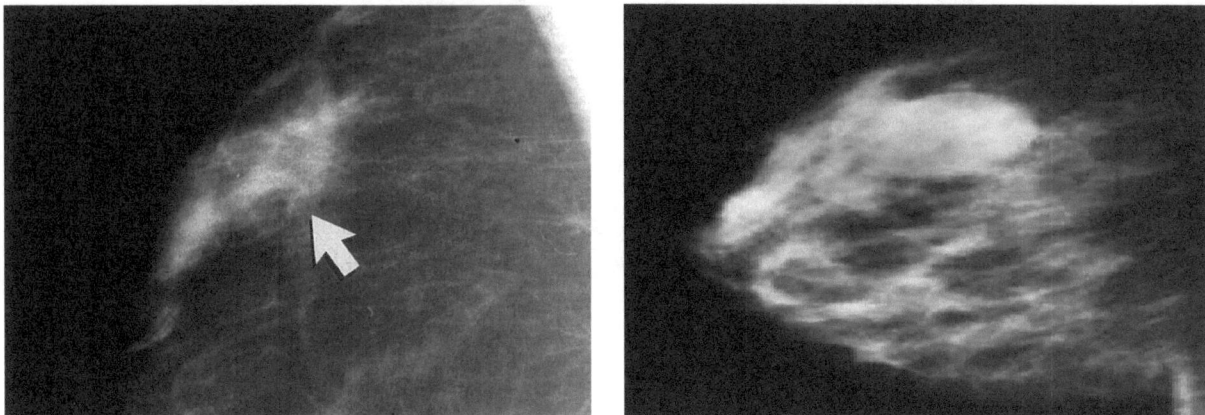

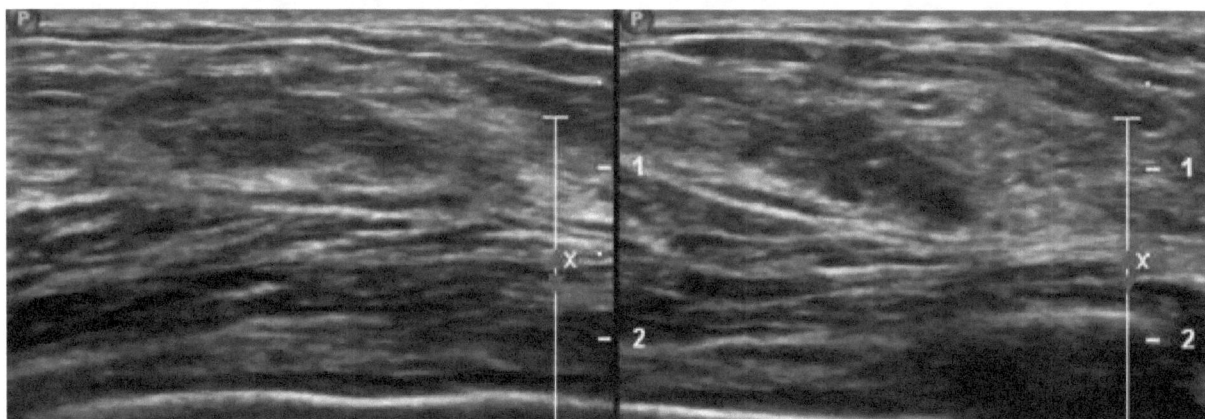

Intraductal Papilloma: benign lesion which is the most common intraductal mass of the breast. Patients report bloody nipple discharge. Solitary papilloma has no increased risk of malignancy, but if any atypia is present, excise the whole thing.

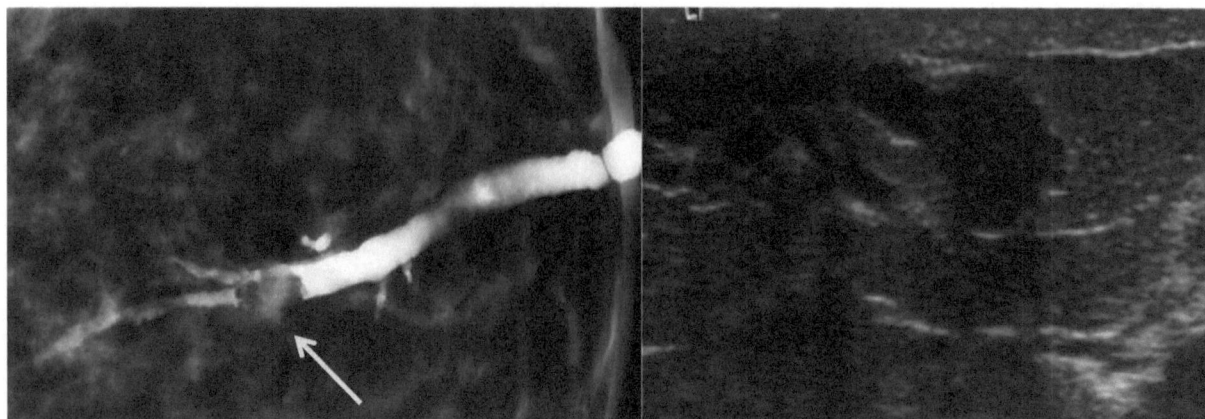

MALIGNANT LESIONS: mammographic appearance of malignant lesions includes ill-defined or spiculated margins, something that has been growing over time, new or suspicious calcifications. On US, there are soft tissue nodules with vascularity and posterior shadowing.

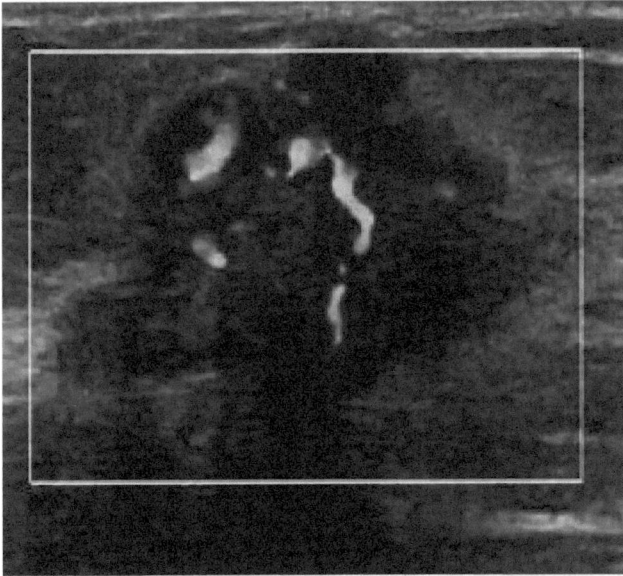

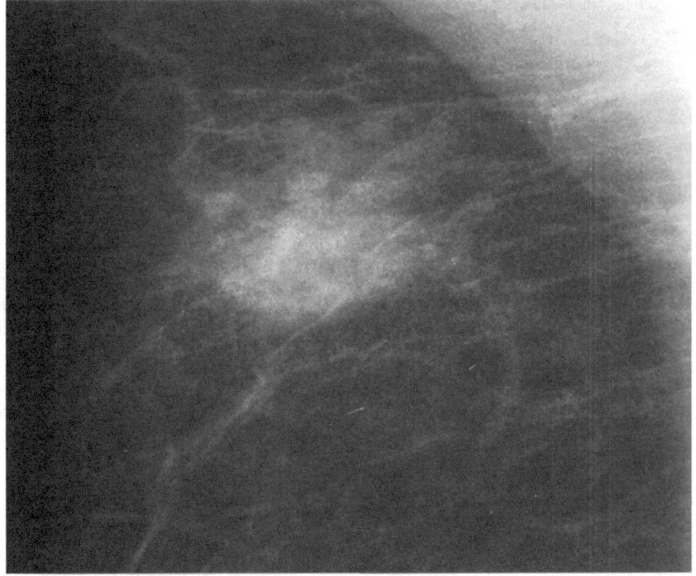

Invasive Lobular CA: doesn't incite a lot of desmoplastic reaction so it can present later. Doesn't have calcifications and has a high incidence of being multicentric or bilateral.

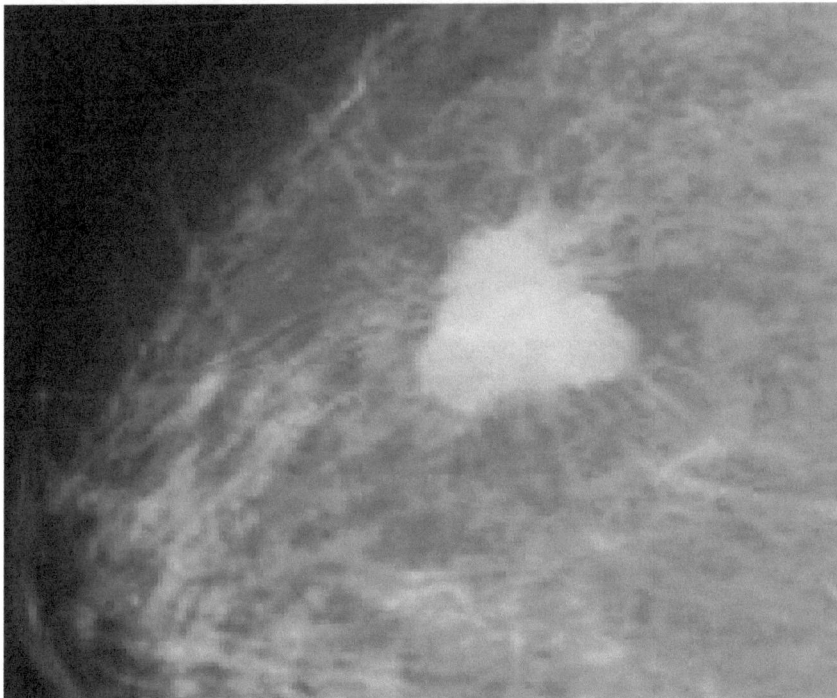

Ductal Carcinoma in Situ: is cancer of the ducts without infiltration of the basement membrane. It accounts for 25% of breast cancer detected at screening mammography. The most common mammographic finding is microcalcifications and may also present as a mass with architectural distortion. MRI is more sensitive than mammogram and shows non-mass like segmental enhancement. Cannot use conventional MRI kinetics to predict malignancy because this has a plateau curve instead of rapid washout.

– 40% non-comedo: small cell, less aggressive
– 60% comedo: large cell, more aggressive
– 11% will have invasive component at time of biopsy

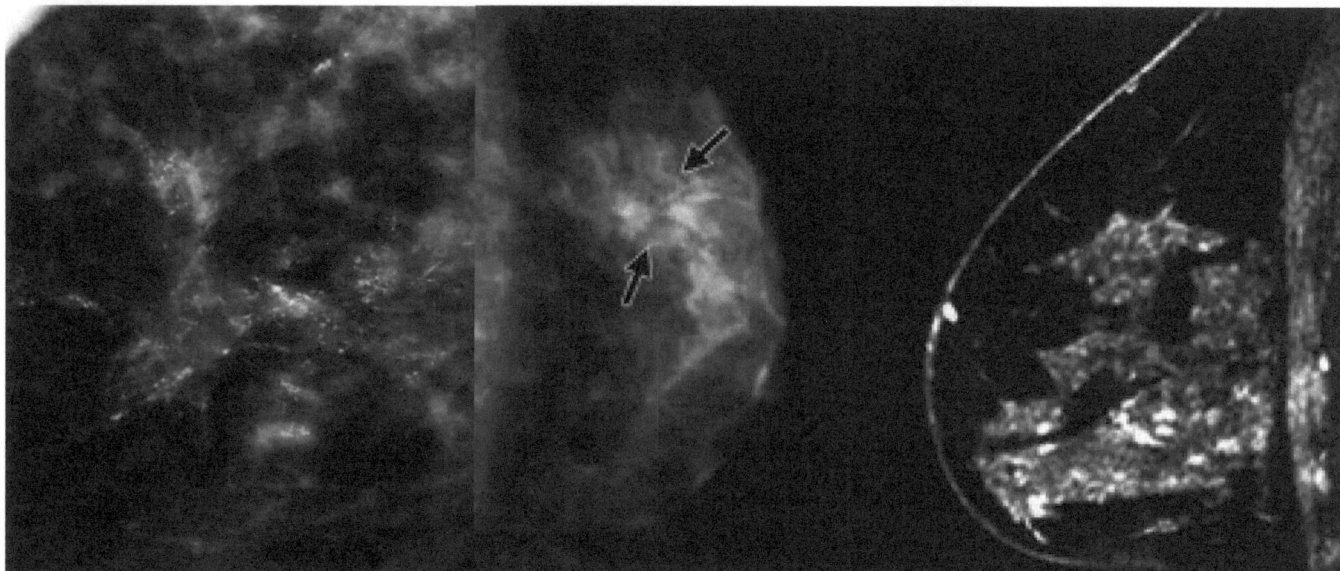

Left – microcalcifications, Middle – architectural distortion, Right – segmental enhancement

Tubular Carcinoma: is a sub-type of invasive ductal carcinoma, they account for 1% of breast CA. There are usually found incidentally because the majority are not palpable. Often it is a small spiculated lesion with or without calcifications. Spicules are longer than the central mass.

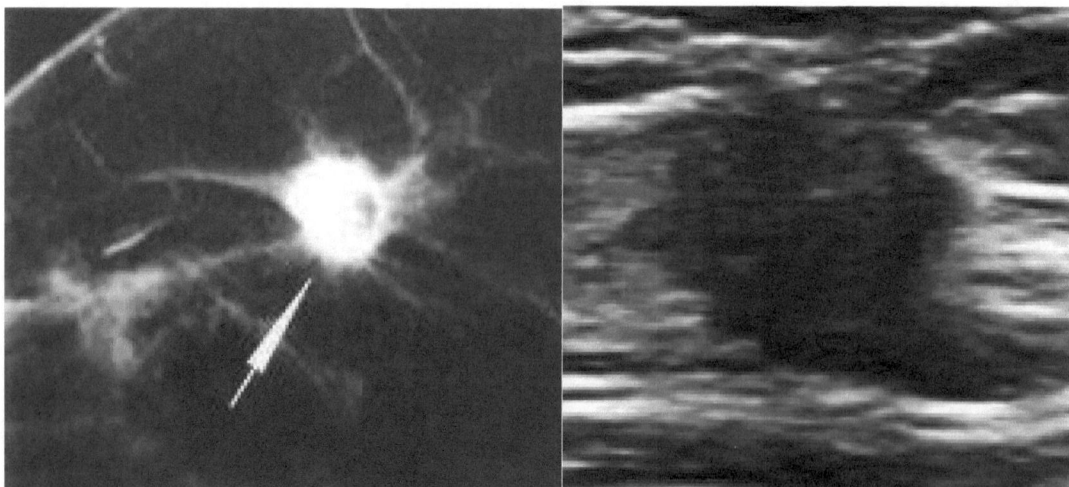

Phyllodes: large, fast growing mass that can have malignant degeneration. These clinically manifest as a firm or hard round tumor, large in size, with rapid growth. Wide local excision is used for malignant lesions.

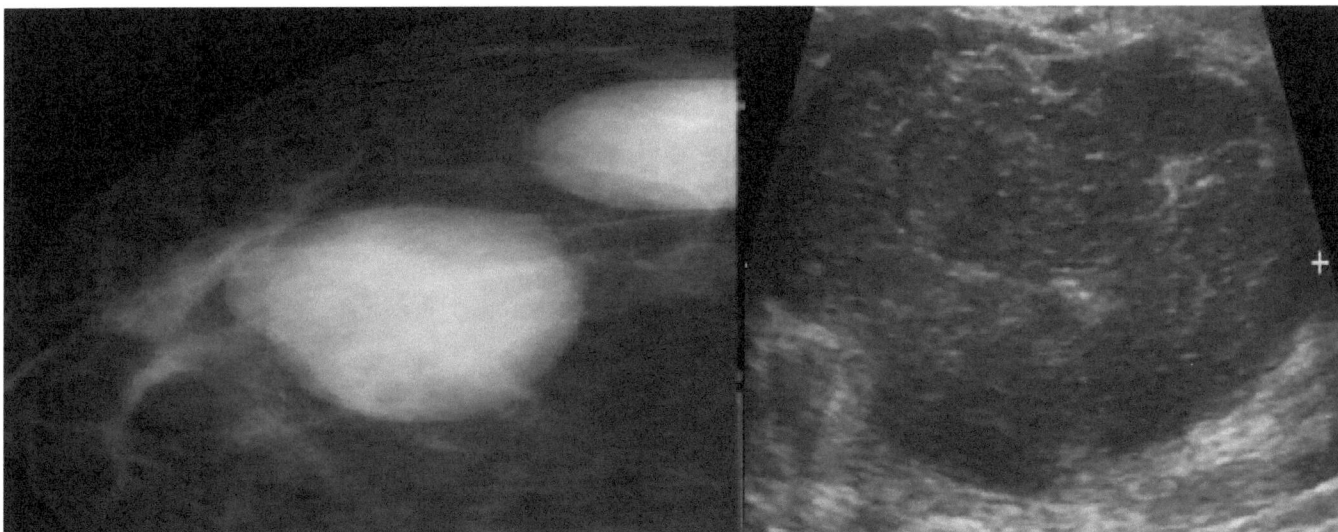

Paget's Disease of the Breast: malignant adenocarcinoma cells extending into the nipple surface through the terminal lactiferous ducts. 90% of the time there is an underlying malignancy of the breast (DCIS). A wedge biopsy of the nipple is necessary to make the diagnosis. Lesion can be confined to the epidermis.

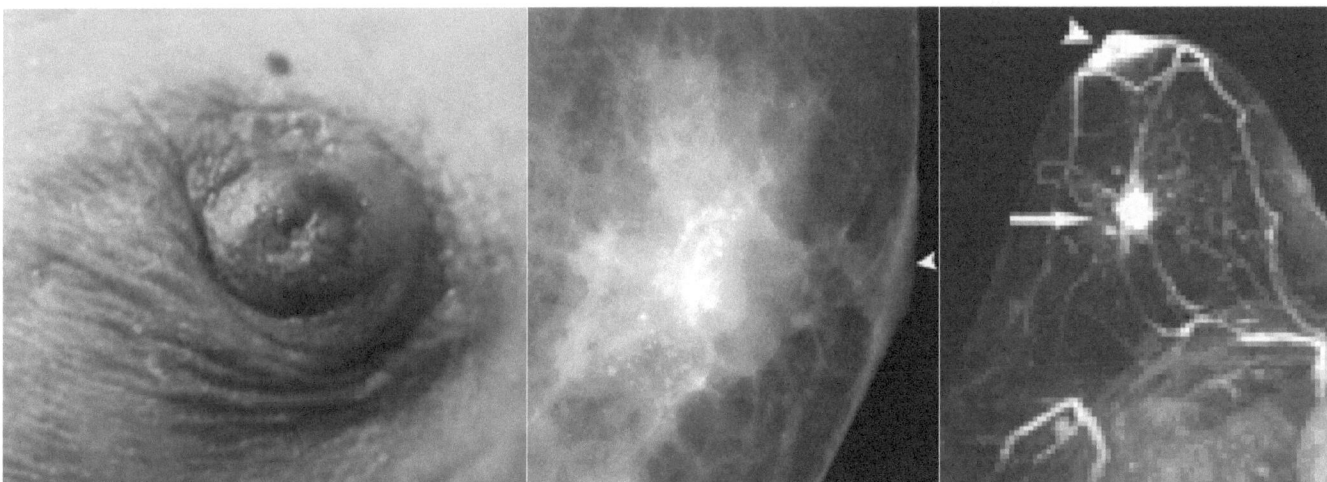

Left – skin thickening and redness of the nipple; Middle – areolar skin thickening and ductal calcifications; Right – MRI showing enhancing nipple and enhancing invasive ductal cancer

Invasive Ductal Cancer: is the most common invasive malignant breast cancer accounting for almost 80% of carcinomas. This is a very cellular tumor and as such presents as a solid mass. Presents as an irregular mass on mammogram, the high cellularity causes it to be T2 hypointense, it demonstrates avid enhancement.

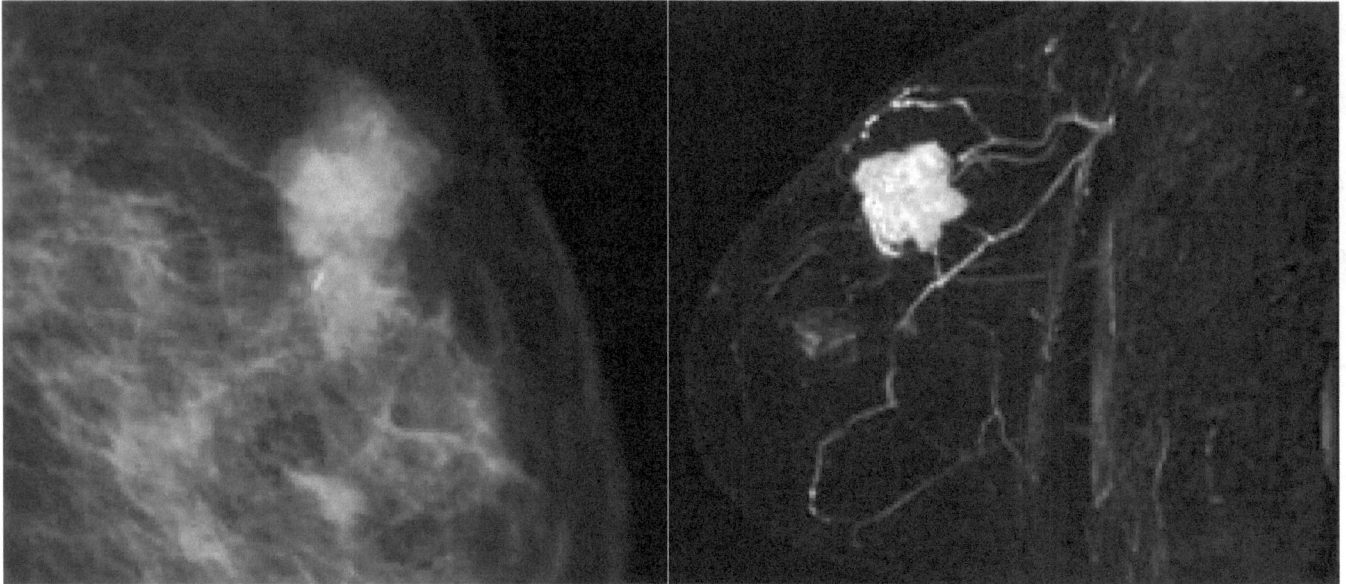

ULTRASOUND: the best position for US is arm abducted and hand behind head

- 10 MHz or higher frequency is mandatory
- For depth, center the lesion and be able to see the chest wall
- Color Doppler box should be as small as possible to cover size of target

Describe shape, orientation (parallel vs anti-parallel), and margins

Indications for US:

- Young patient with palpable mass
- Additional evaluation needed for mammographic finding

Cyst: benign lesion, round, anechoic, sharp posterior wall, acoustic enhancement, and no blood flow

Complicated cyst: have internal echoes due to debris; can have ring down, but no internal flow

Complex mass: papillary neoplasms until proven otherwise, this is a cyst with a thick septa, mural nodule, eccentric wall thickening

Sebacious cyst (epidermal inclusion cyst): look for a tract to the skin

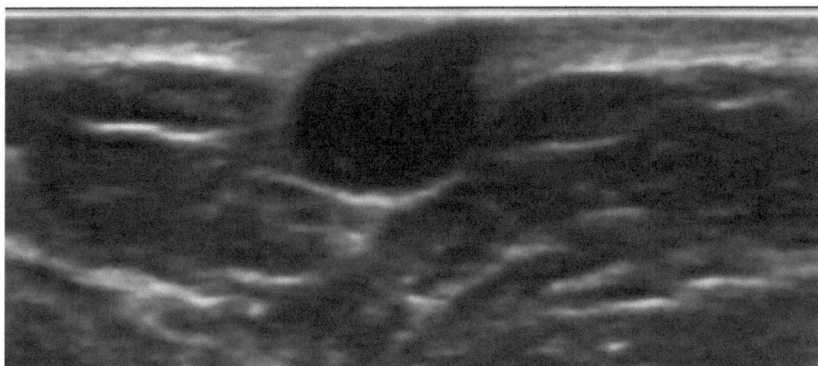

Implant: looking for rupture

1. Step ladder sign – intracapsular rupture
2. Snowstorm – extra-capsular rupture

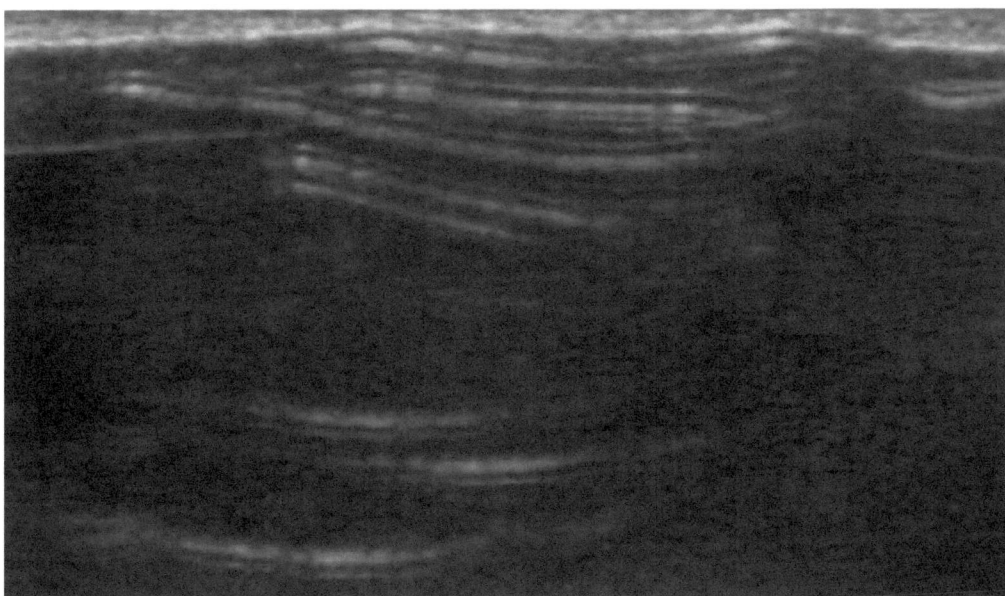

Stepladder Sign – intracapsular rupture

<u>**BREAST MRI**</u>: never done alone, it is an adjunct to mammogram

Indications:

1. Evaluate extent of known disease
2. Axillary LAD with unknown primary
3. One time screening of contralateral breast in patient with new CA
4. High risk screening in young patient
5. Evaluating treatment response

Technique: exam is done prone with breast hanging through a dedicated breast coil. Hormonal fluctuations cause increased background enhancement. Therefore, the MRI should be done during days 3-14.

In MRI like in mammogram, we have to describe the background tissue, in this case enhancement:

None/minimal: < 25%
Mild: 25-50%
Moderate: 50-75%
Marked: > 75%

DCIS shows clumped non-mass like enhancement extending towards nipple.

KINETIC CURVES:

Type I – progressive enhancement pattern. Shows a continuous increase in signal throughout time, usually considered benign.

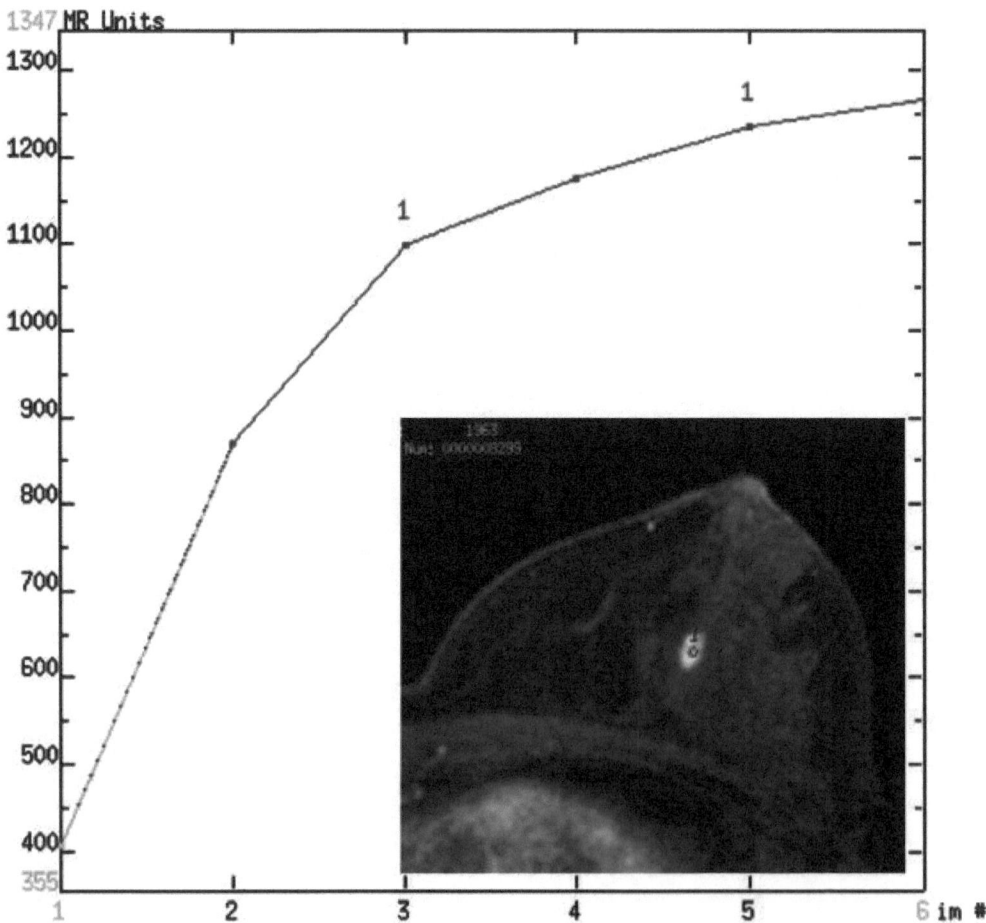

Type II – plateau pattern, initial uptake followed by the plateau phase, considered concerning for malignancy

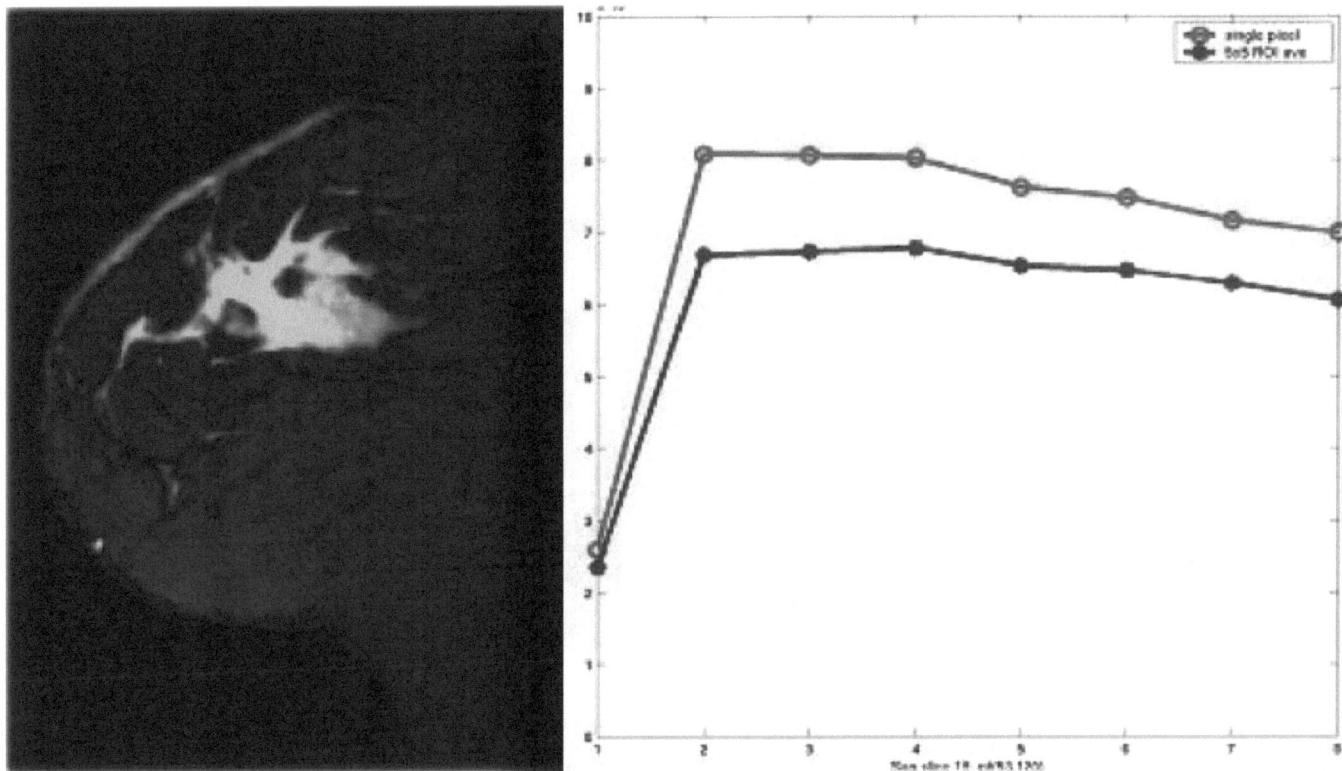

Type III – rapid enhancement with washout, highly concerning for malignancy

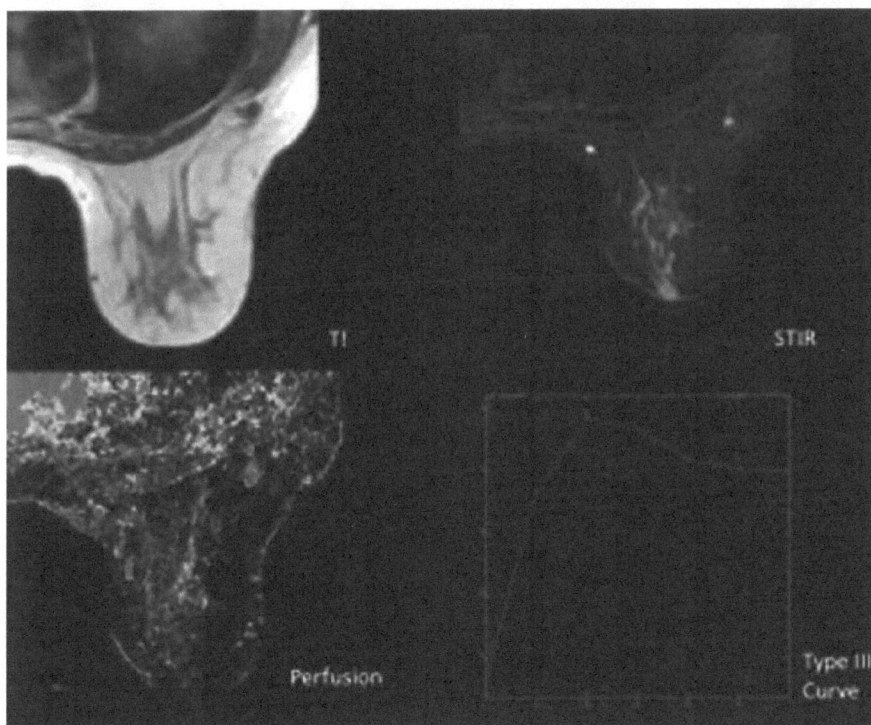

IMPLANT EVALUATION: can be placed in front of or behind the pectoralis muscles.

MRI is done to evaluate the integrity of the implant. Normally the body walls off the implant with a fibrous capsule.

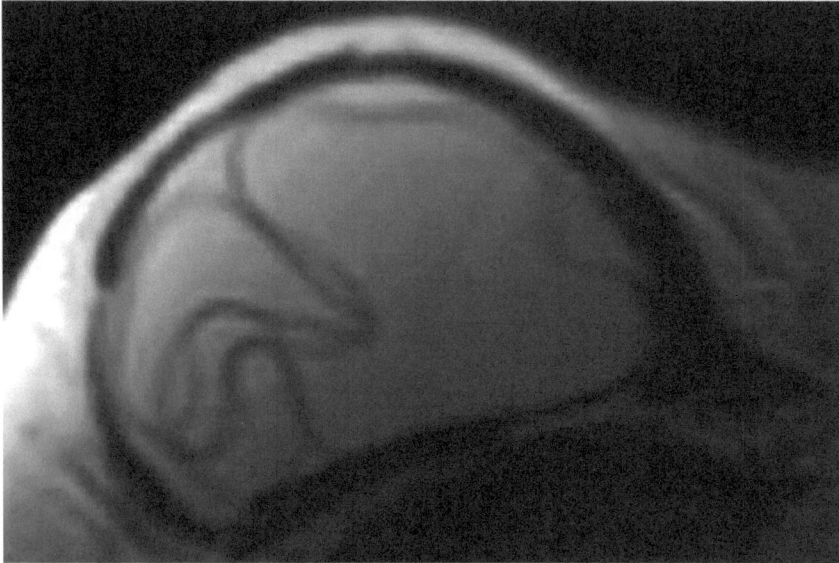

Intra-capsular rupture – "linguine sign"

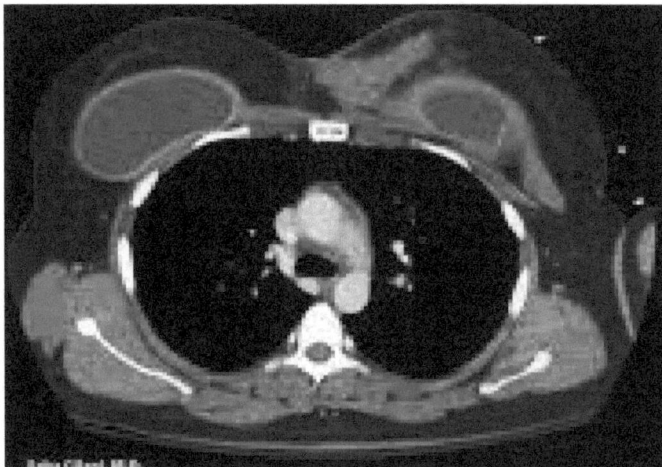

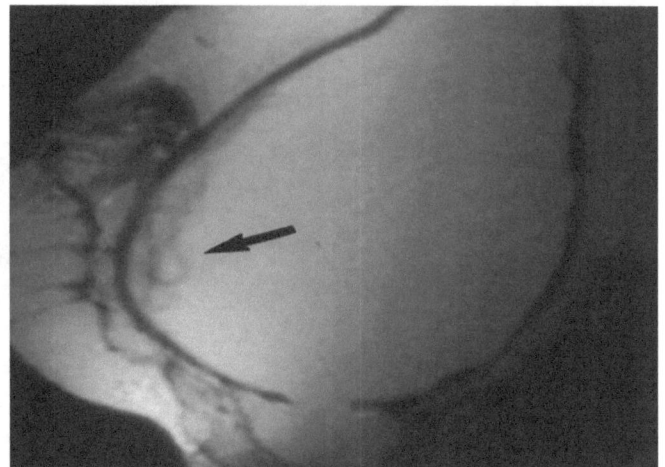

Extra-capsular rupture and focal bulge and defect at inferior aspect

CALCIFICATIONS: need to be analyzed by morphology and distribution

Benign Calcifications	
Vascular	Tram-track calcs surrounding soft tissue of the vessel
Skin	Tightly clustered with lucent centers, typical location is the inframammary fold
Radiolucent center	Oil cyst
Dytrophic	Coarse, thick – due to trauma or prior surgery
Sutural	Looks man-made
Popcorn	Large, thick – fibroadenoma
Secretory	Large bilateral rod-like – plasma cell mastitis
Injection	Silicone or paraffin injection
Milk of calcium	Change shape with differing positions, on lateral view, meniscus

	Distribution
Diffuse/scattered	Randomly distributed but all calcs look the same
Regional	Large volume with calcs > 2cc of tissue
Grouped/ clustered	5 or more in one cc of tissue
Linear	Suggests deposits in a duct – suspicious
Segmental	Deposits along a duct – v. suspicious

	Morphology – decide only on MAG view
Round	Small, round, or punctate – usually benign unless they change or are new
Amorphous	Small with hazy boundaries, difficult to characterize
Coarse Heterogeneous	Big irregular calcs, intermediate concern b/c cant tell if they are early benign process or malignancy
Fine Pleomorphic	Small, irregular – high probability of malignancy
Fine Linear/ Branching	Thin curvilinear, filling the ducts - CA

Benign calcifications:

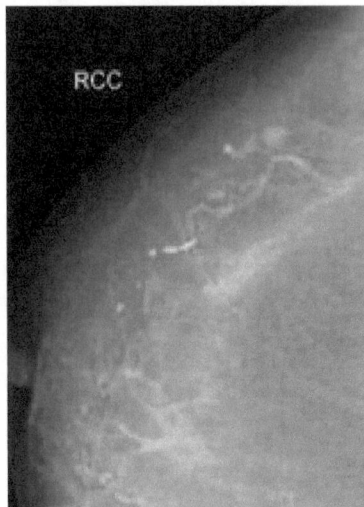

Vascular

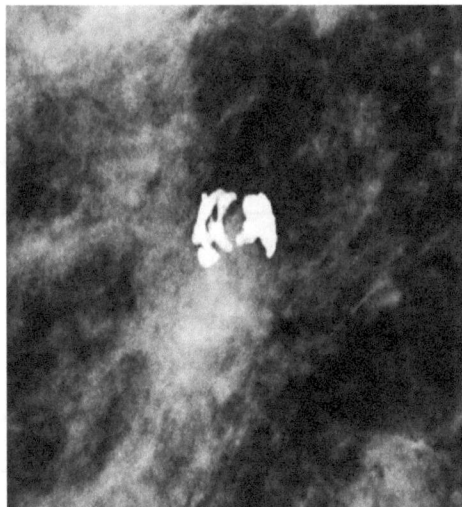

Coarse

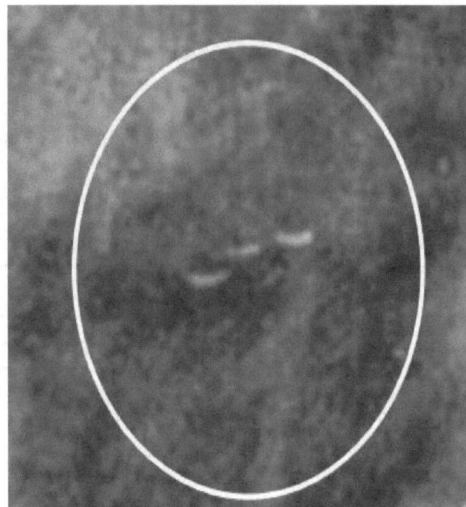

Milk of CA

Malignant calcifications:

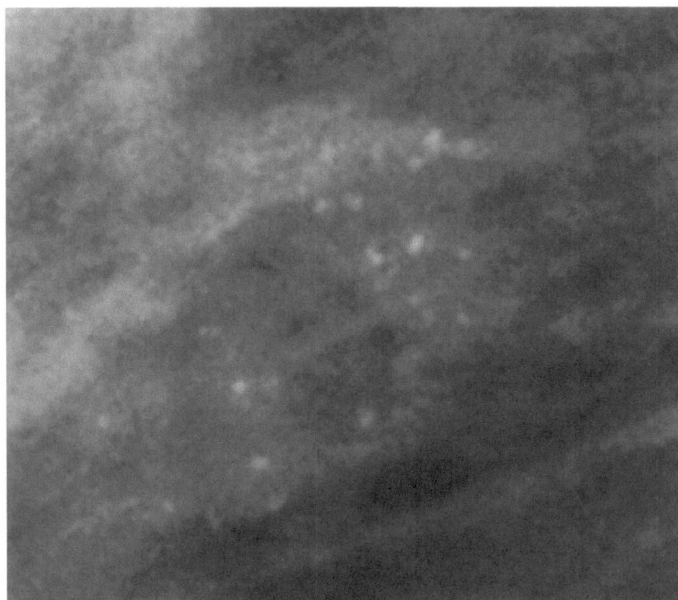

Pleomorphic

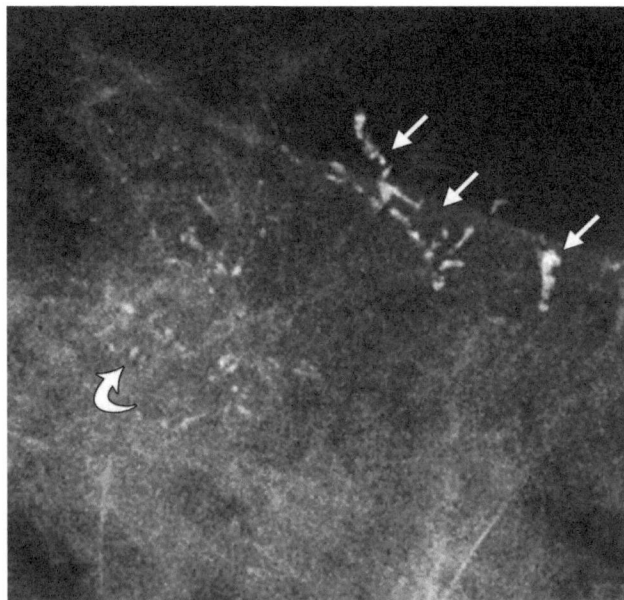

Linear Branching

FUN FACTS:

1. There is a 1 in 8 lifetime chance of getting breast CA
2. Dense breasts have a higher risk of breast CA than fatty breasts
3. The most common cause of symmetrically increasing density involving the glandular tissue, not the skin is exogenous HRT
4. The standard MLO view can miss structures in the **medial** breast
5. Mammo screens need to be cleaned once a week
6. Bucky should be cleaned after every use
7. Bilateral breast masses are a benign finding, unless changing.
8. Digital Mammographys is good for (DMIST trial)
   - Dense breasts
   - Females < 50 years old
   - Women not yet in menopause
9. Fibroadenoma calcs start outside and go in
10. Breast to breast metastases are the number one source of mets followed by melanoma.
11. Metallic densities in lymph nodes can be from prior gold therapy for RA

Musculoskeletal

TRAUMA

<u>Wrist</u>: when evaluating the wrist, remember to look at the arcs of Gilula on the AP

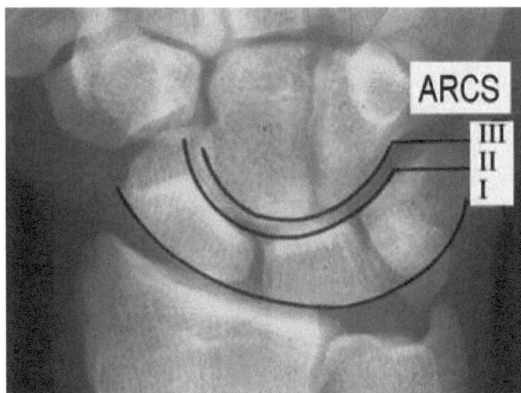

If these don't look perfect, something is wrong, especially in the post– traumatic patient. Look carefully at the lateral view for dislocations.

The AP view is also used to look at the S–L ligament distance (normally < 2mm); if widened, it's torn

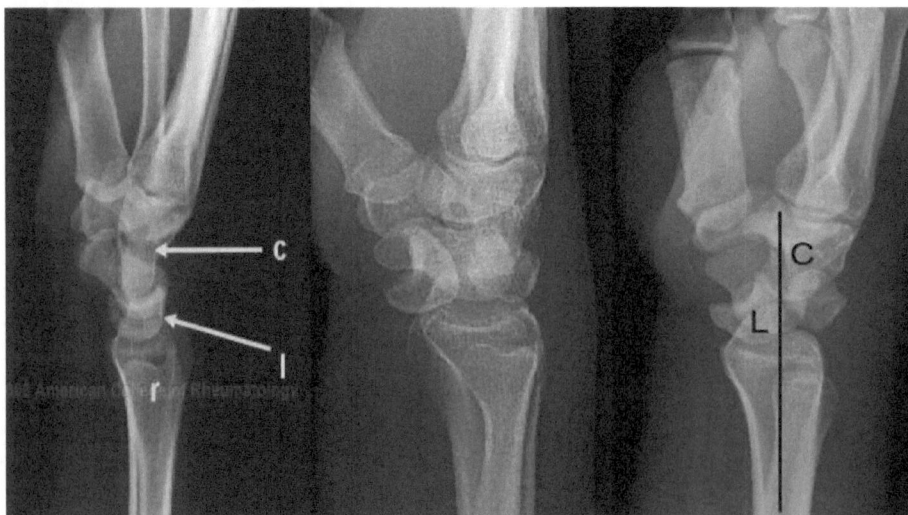

The lateral view should demonstrate the capitate, lunate, and radius to lie on top of each other in a straight line – any deviation is a dislocation.

Lunate dislocation – lunate slips out and capitate and radius maintain alignment

Peri-lunate dislocation –lunate and radius stay put but the capitate slips out of the lunates cup

Triquetrial fracture can be seen as a subtle avulsion and soft tissue swelling over the dorsum on the lateral view, don't miss it.

Fatigue fracture is abnormal stress on normal bone and an **insufficiency fracture** is normal stress on abnormal bone.

<u>Forearm & elbow</u>: pretty basic anatomy, looking for a few things here most of which have eponyms. Also keep in mind normal elbow alignment, fat pads, and lines

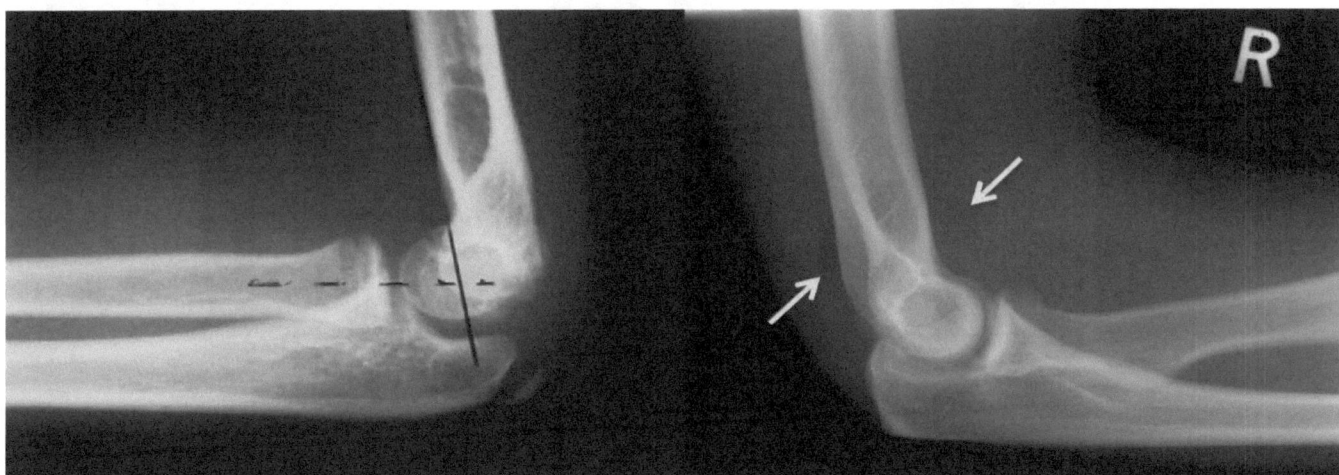

Normal radiocapitellar line should always go through the capitellum on all views unless dislocated. The anterior fat pad can be seen all the time, but when elevated 'sail sign' that's a problem. Posterior fat pad is never seen unless there is a joint effusion.

Colle's Fracture	Distal radius fracture as result of FOOSH, dorsal angulation of fragment (extra-articular)
Smith Fracture	Distal radius fracture with volar angulation of the distal fragment (extra-articular)
Monteggia	Fracture of the ulna shaft and dislocation of the radial head (image on left below)
Galeazzi	Fracture of the radius with dislocation of the radioulnar joint (image in the middle below)
Nightstick	Isolated injury of the ulna mid diaphysis from direct blow
Radial Head	Most common elbow fracture in an adult – can be subtle – get a radial head view if you have any doubts (image on right).

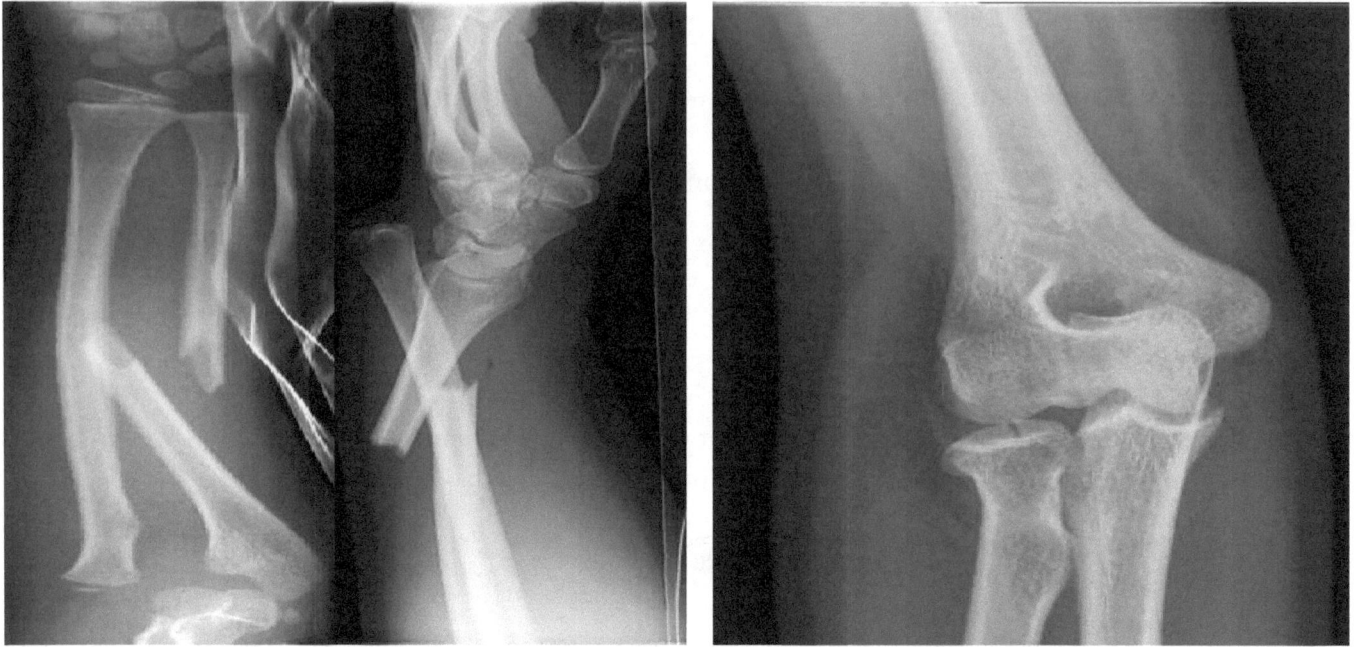

Pediatric Elbow: keep the ages of ossification centers in mind when evaluating the pediatric elbow

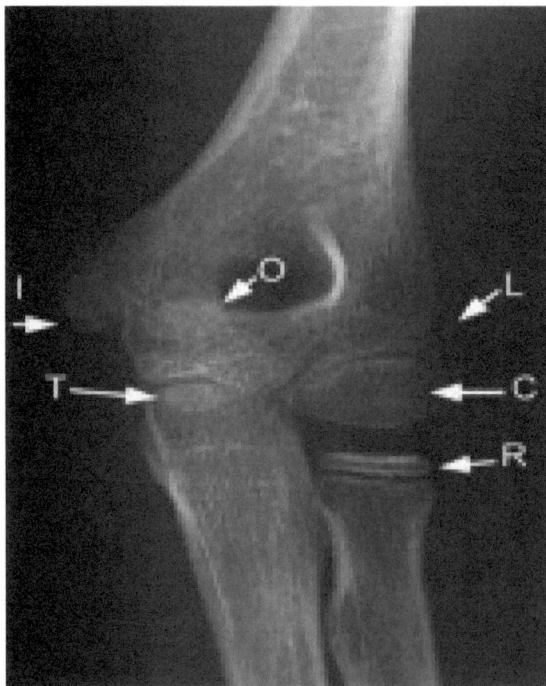

Capitellum	1
Radial Head	3
Internal Epicondyle	5
Trochlea	7
Olecrenon	9
External Epicondyle	11

Osteochonditis, Panner disease, and other pediatric injuries will be discussed in the pediatrics chapter.

Shoulder dislocation

Anterior	The most common type, results from forced abduction and external rotation. Associated with Hill–Sachs lesion (depression of posterolateral humeral head) and Bankart lesion (detached anterior inferior labrum)
Posterior	Humeral head is forced posteriorly in internal rotation – classic causes are seizures and electrocution. Associated with reverse Bankart (posterior inferior labrum detachment)
Inferior	Least common form, also called luxatio erecta because the arm appears to be permanently held in fixed abduction. Caused by a hyper abdution of arm.

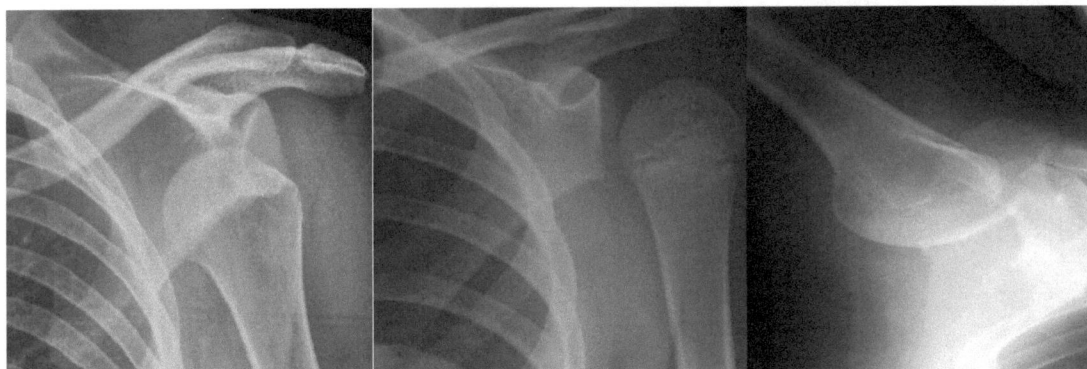

Left – anterior dislocation in classic position with humeral head projecting inferior and medial
Middle – posterior dislocation with widened GH distance
Right – inferior dislocation with arm fixed in abduction

AC Injury: common injury to the shoulder ranging from sprain to disruption. Graded from I – VI based on severity.

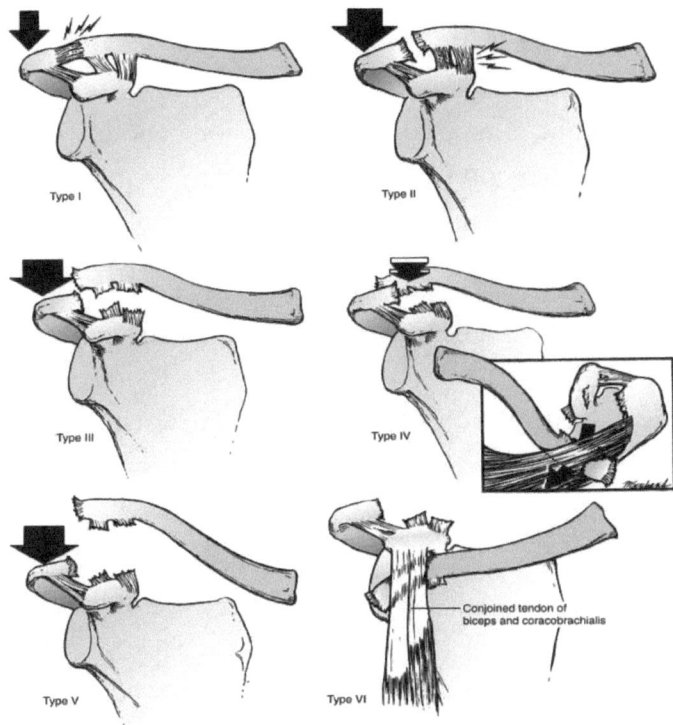

Grade I – AC sprain only no disruption

Grade II – AC ligament ruptured with widening of the AC distance > 6–7 mm

Grade III – AC and CC ligaments ruptured with clavicle elevated, CC distance > 13 mm

Grade IV – ligaments ruptured and clavicle displaced posteriorly into trapezius muscle

Grade V – ruptured ligaments with clavicle raised > 25 mm

Grade VI – totally jacked up with clavicle displaced inferiorly behind the coracobrachialis muscle

Lower Extremity: Base of the 5th metatarsal has two key injuries that you need to be able to distinguish

Apophyseal Avulsion	Horizontally oriented fracture below the metaphysis treated with walking cast, allowed to bear weight – avulsion due to peroneus brevis
Jones Fracture	Fracture at the metadiaohyseal junction, cannot bear weight, has high incidence of non–union

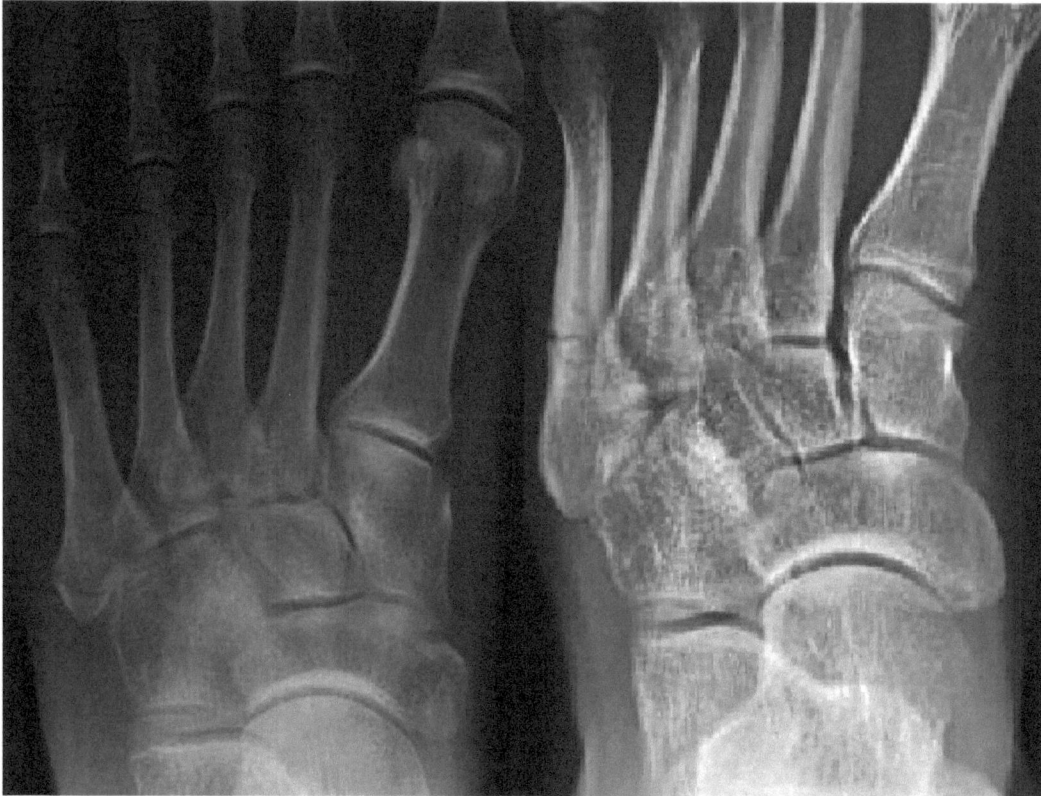

Lisfranc Injury: most common dislocation involving the foot, it is a do not miss lesion. The Lisfranc ligament attaches the medial cuneiform to the 2nd metatarsal base on the plantar surface.

There are two types of dislocation: homolateral and divergent

- Homolateral: lateral displacement of the 1st – 5th metatarsals OR the 1st stays in normal position while 2nd – 5th dislocate laterally (image on left)
- Divergent: lateral dislocation of 2nd – 5th with medial dislocation of the 1st metatarsal (image on right)

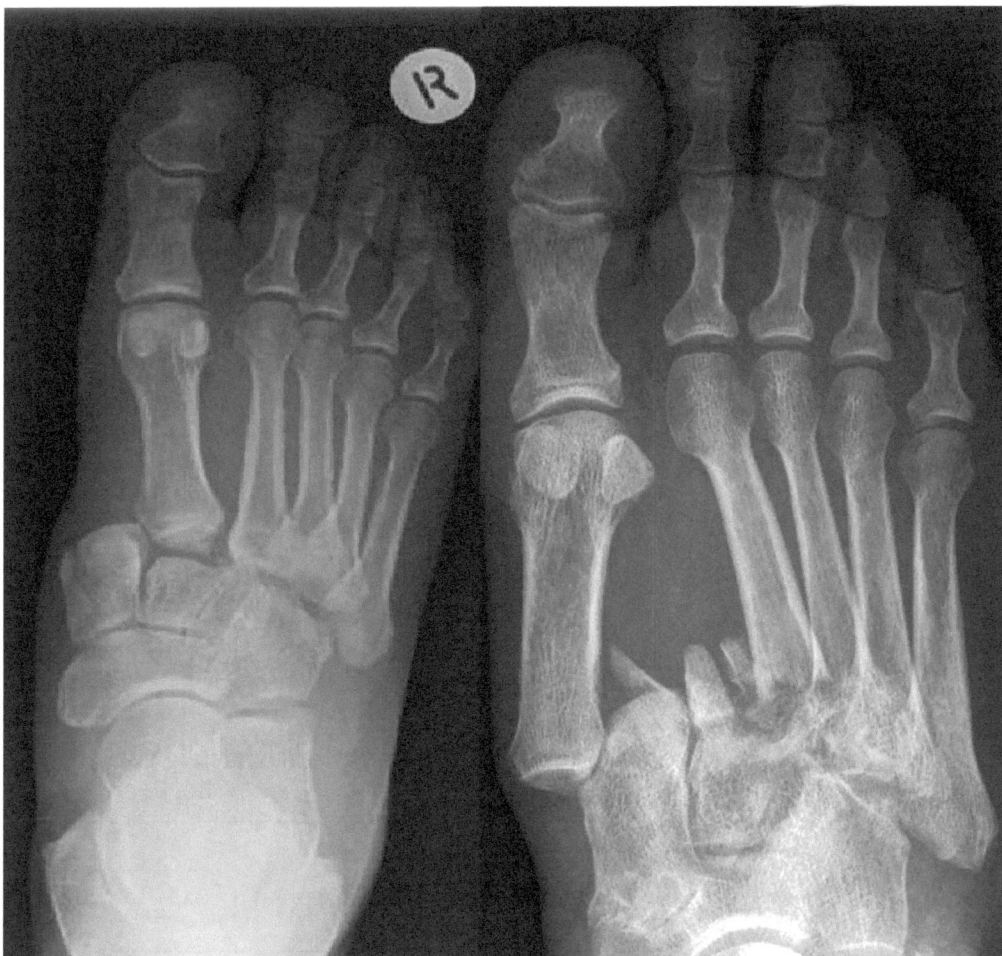

Calcaneus: if Bohler's angle is reduced < 20 degrees there is a calcaneal fracture, most often of the posterior facet

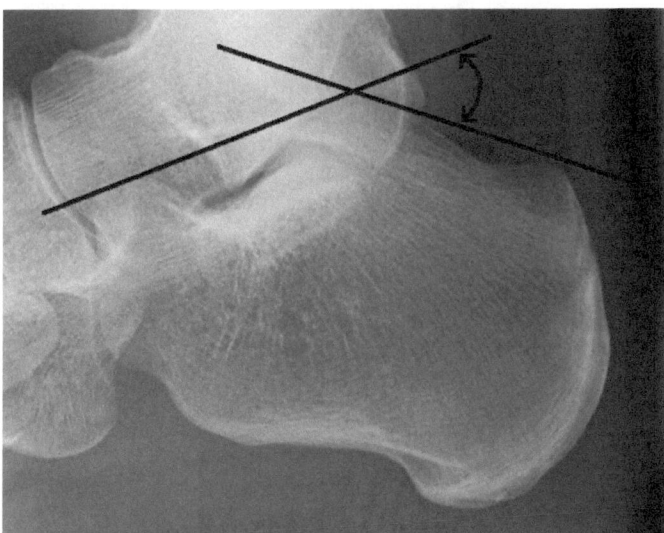

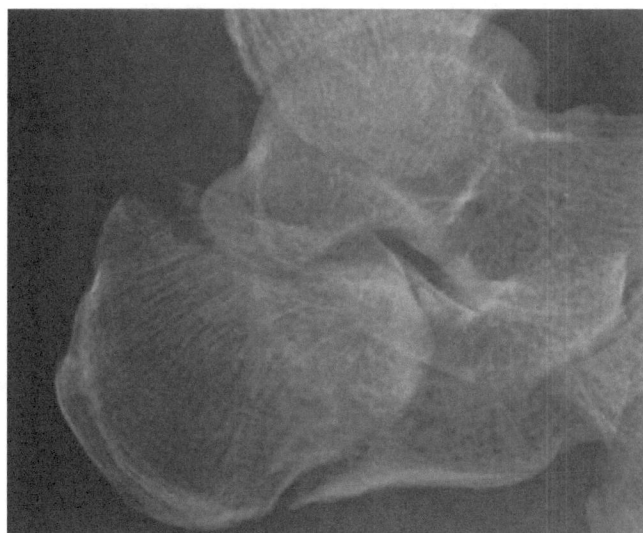

Calcaneal Tuberosity Avulsion: strongly associated with DM and can be spontaneous. Also seen in patients with osteoporosis and hyperparathyroidism.

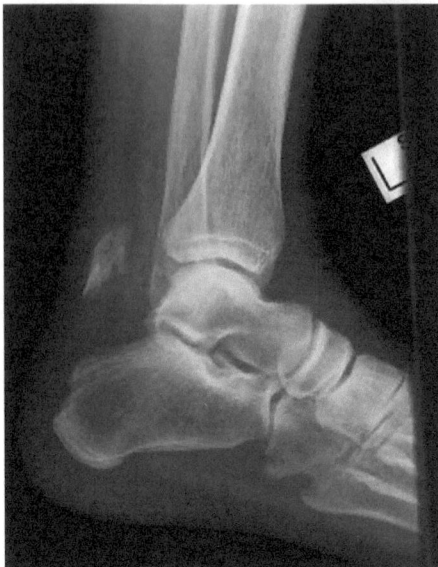

Weber Fractures: the most common mechanism of injury to the ankle is inversion external rotation

Weber A	Below the level of the tibial plafond – syndesmosis is intact
Weber B	Begins at the level of the tibial plafond extending superiorly – syndesmosis can be partially torn but no widening noted – variable stability
Weber C	Above the tibial plafond – syndesmosis is torn and the injury is unstable needing ORIF

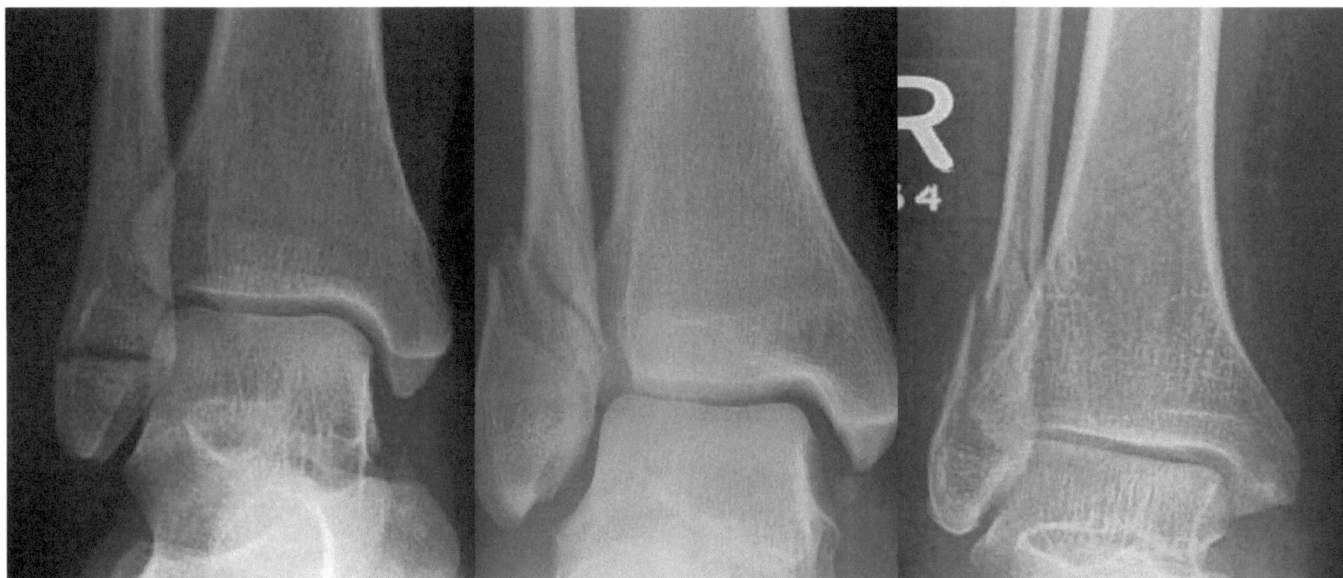

Maisonneuve Fracture: unstable injury with the medial malleolus fractured and force of injury going up and out through the syndesmosis into the proximal fibula. Deltoid ligaments are frequently disrupted.

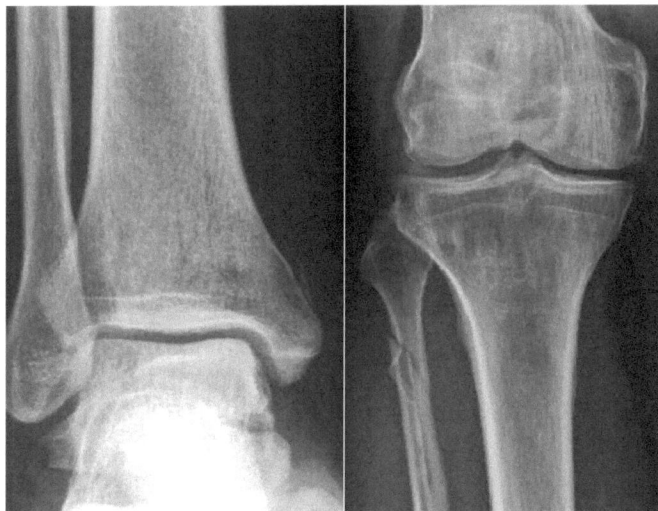

Schatzker Injury: tibial plateau fracture, sometimes the only clue is a fat–blood level in the knee joint on a lateral film.

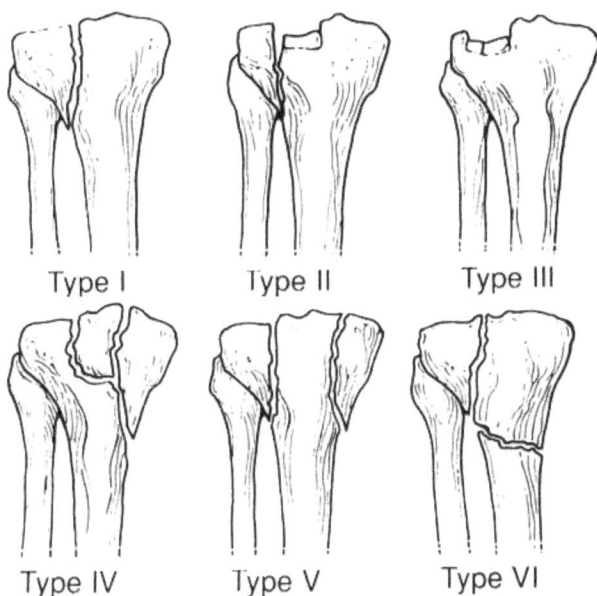

Type I – lateral split only

Type II – lateral split with depression

Type III – lateral depression only

Type IV – medial split

Type V – bicondylar split

Type VI – metadiaphysis extension of fracture

Segond Fracture	Avulsion of the lateral tibial plateau with associated **ACL tear**
Reverse Segond	Avulsion of the medial tibial plateau with associated **PCL tear**

SI Joint	Anterior 1/3rd is true synovial joint, posterior 2/3rd ligamentous bridge
Lateral Compression	Look for buckled arcuate lines
Vertical Shearing	Look for vertical distraction of the pubic symphysis - unstable

ARTHRITIS

Distribution	
Proximal	Rheumatoid arthritis, CPPD
Distal	Psoriasis, Reiters, Osteoarthritis

Osteoarthritis: primary vs secondary – but just by looking at the film, you cannot tell the two apart. Primary occurs almost exclusively in women. Subset called **erosive OA (only in the hands!)**. Secondary is due to overuse or trauma.

Hallmarks: sclerosis, osteophytes, and joint space narrowing – if you don't have osteophytes do not mention DJD

With erosive osteoarthritis the buzz word is "gull–wing" deformity

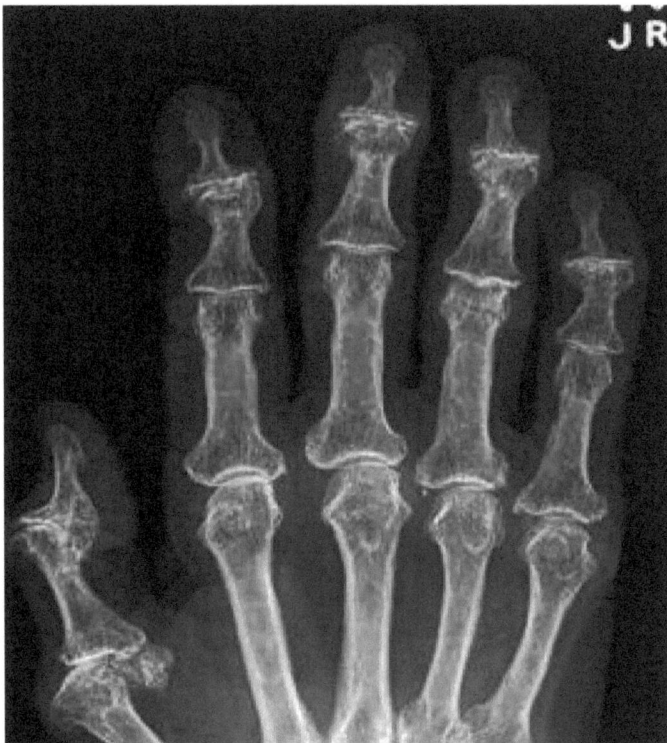

DISH: the only thing other than OA that causes osteophytes. The key here is 3–4 contiguous segments with large bulky anterior osteophytes in a spine with **normal disc spaces**. Look for associated PLL ossification. In C–spine the big anterior osteophytes will rarely cause dysphagia. The other thing to remember is that in the lumbar spine osteophytes may only be on the right side because the aortic pulsations prevent left–sided osteophytes from forming.

Rheumatoid Arthritis: proximal hands going out to MCPs. Look for soft tissue swelling, osteoporosis, joint space narrowing, and marginal erosions. This leads to secondary degenerative disease after a long time.

Radiographic findings display a "crowded carpus" with loss of joint space, there is **soft tissue swelling over ulnar styloid process with erosions** – this is a target area of RA (look here first for erosions). The 5th metatarsal head is a target area in the foot.

There will be joint fluid on MRI and the MRI will show signs of RA much earlier than plain film.

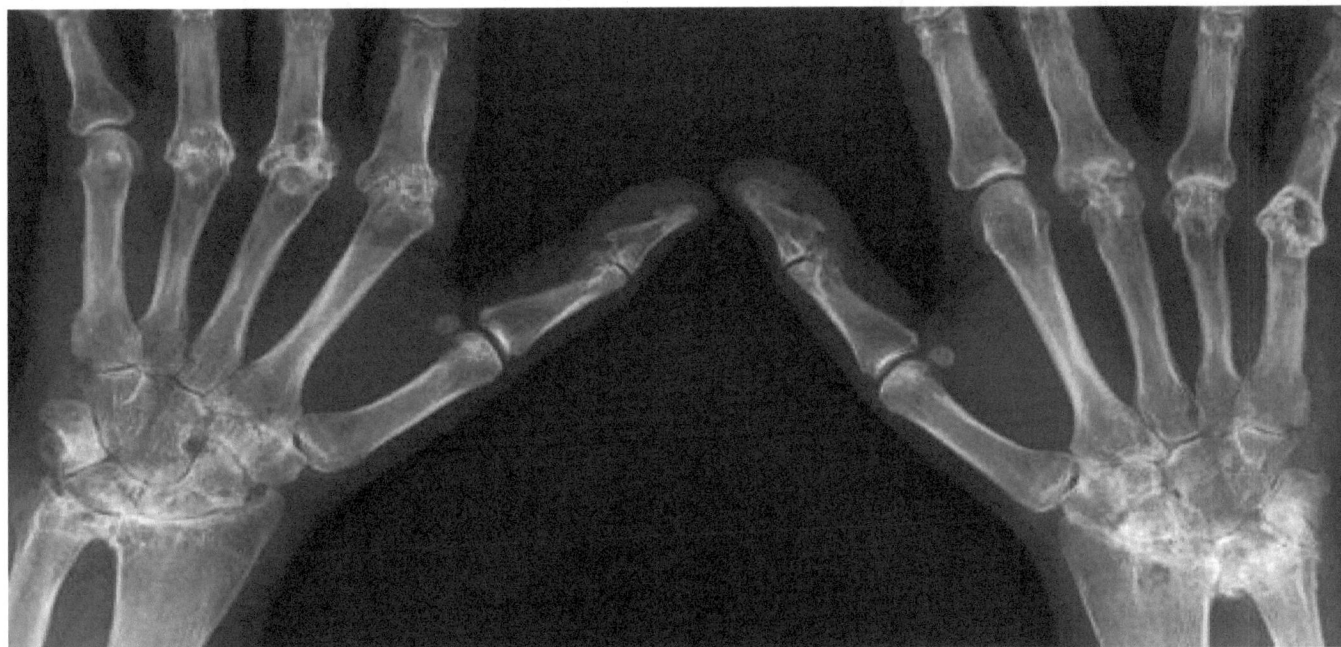

HLA-B27 Arthropathies
Ankylosing Spondylitis
Inflammatory Bowel Disease
Psoriasis
Reiters – not in females

With these look for paravertebral ossifications:

1. Osteophytes – laterally oriented and bulky
2. Syndesmophytes – vertically oriented
   - Bulky and asymmetric: Reiters or Psoriasis
   - Fine and symmetric: Ankylosing Spondylitis or IBD

Ankylosing Spondylitis and IBD: Bilateral SI joint involvement (100% of the time), bilateral symmetric syndesmophytes, **vertebral body squaring**, and high risk for spinal fracture – bamboo spine

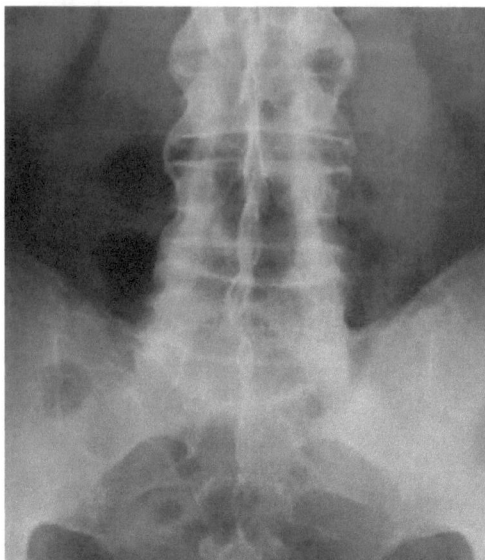

This spine can be fractured distally with minor proximal trauma. The spine is like a long glass pipette. Plain film is not enough for assessment in trauma, need CT and or MRI.

Reiters (reactive arthritis) and Psoriasis: **distal disease** with soft tissue swelling "sausage digit", proliferative fuzzy erosions, bulky asymmetric syndesmophytes, and ankylosis. If the ankylosis involves a joint other than SI, think psoriasis first. Unilateral sacroiliitis not bilateral.

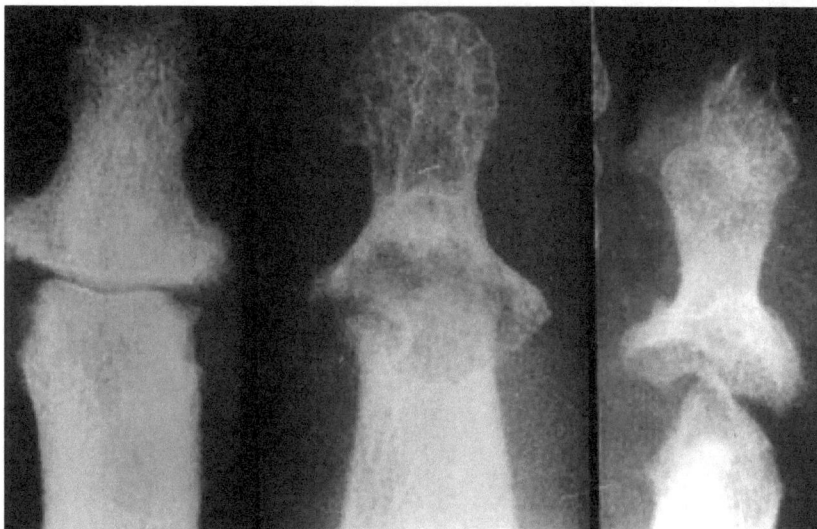

Fuzzy erosions, joint space loss and fusion, pencil in cup deformity

Reiter's and Psoriasis like the IP joints

These two diseases usually start off unilateral but can progress to bilateral. But ankylosing spondylitis and IBD do not start off unilateral.

Fun Fact: when you see SI joint changes, rule out infection 1st in younger patients and in older people think of gout as well.

Gout: normal mineralization, sharply marginated erosion often with sclerotic margins, soft tissue nodules, and a predilection for the 1st MTP. Pathology is monosodium urate crystal deposition in and around the joint.

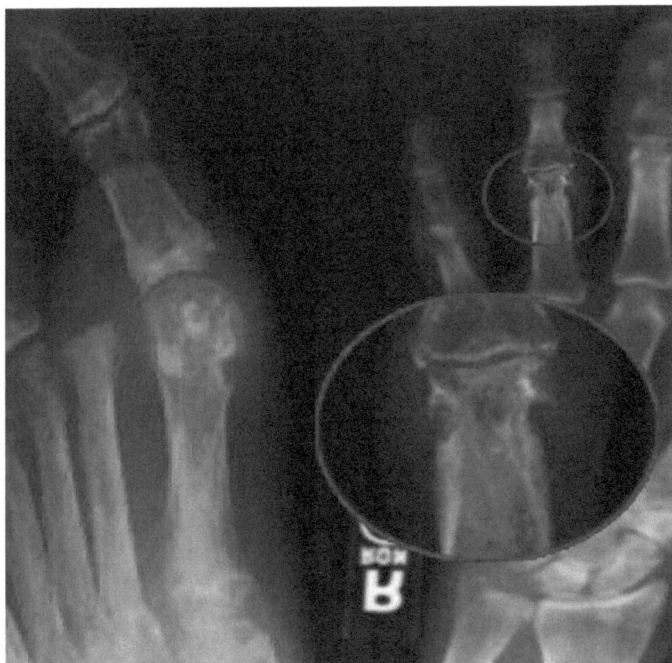

Podagra on the left with soft tissue swelling and punched out erosions

Gout in the hands demonstrating the classic 'rat bite' erosions in the juxta–articular region

Fun fact: olecranon bursitis – think RA or Gout

CPPD: pyrophosphate deposition in the fibrocartilage of the TFC, menisci, tri–radiate cartilage, or symphysis pubis. Pain, chondrocalcinosis, and arthropathy are the three classic features.

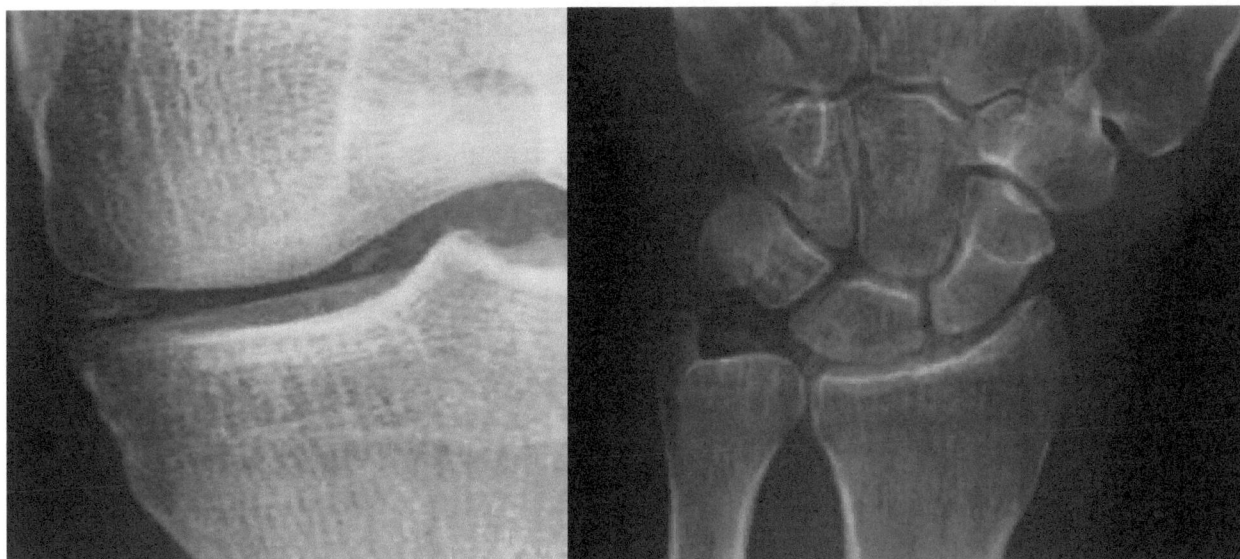

The other thing to look for is **isolated patella–femoral** degenerative change – unique to CPPD. Narrowing of MCPs and TFC chondrocalcinosis is classic for CPPD.

Hemochromatosis: causes repeated bleeding into the joints with pseudotumor and arthritis.

PVNS: is proliferation of the synovium that cause joint space loss and will be hypointense on T1, T2, and blooms. **Never calcifies!**

Neuropathic Joint: most often seen in diabetes, rapidly progressive joint space destruction. Remember the association with distal clavicle resorption and syringomyelia.

Osteochondromatosis: loose cartilageneous bodies in the joint that are nourished by the synovium, can grow in size over time

Primary – if all same size, needs complete synovectomy Secondary – different size, treat the underlying OA

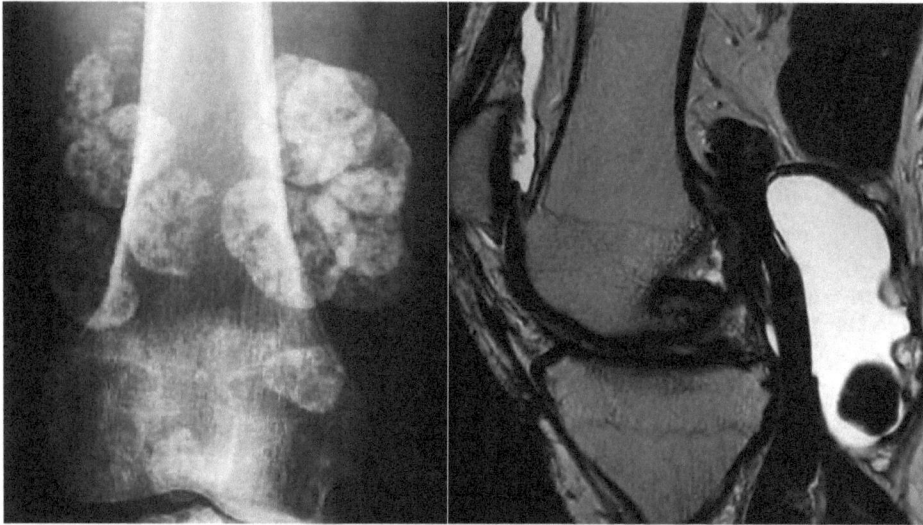

INFECTION

Acute Osteomyelitis: *S. aureus* is the most common pathogen and method of infection is direct inoculation or hematogeneous spread. Patient will have signs of infection, look for a skin ulcer. T1 low marrow intensity, T2 high signal from edema and reactive marrow changes, plus soft tissue edema and cellulitis, T1+gad shows contrast enhancement and abscess.

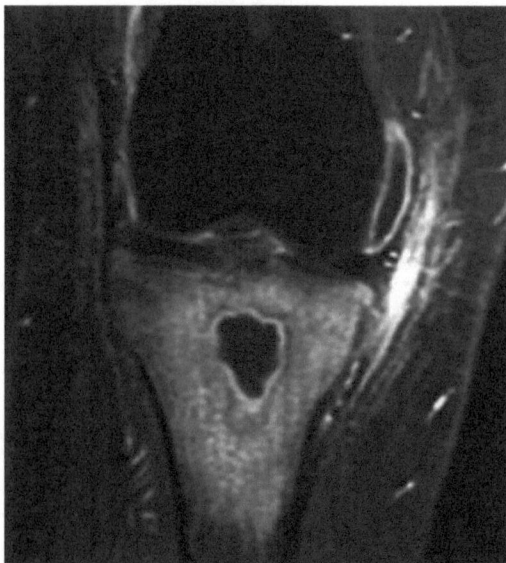

Brodie's Abscess: focus of chronic osteomyelitis with abscess. Can occur in any location at any age. Looks like the example of osteomyelitis above. In kids looks for a lucent, tortuous tract extending towards the physis – pathognomonic.

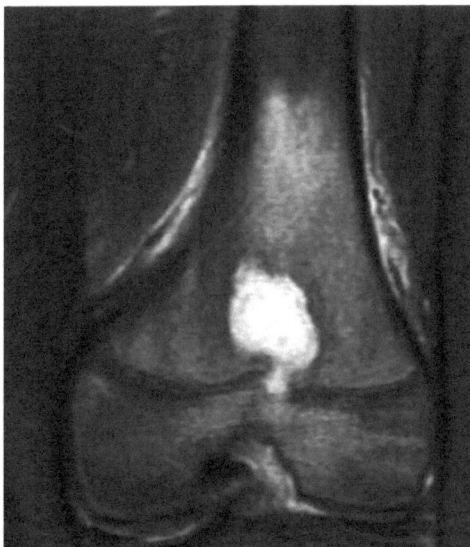

CRMO: will be multifocal and can simulate metastases on bone scan, but in younger patients with long term complaints. This is characterized by chronic pain and a low–grade fever, without bactermia. Treat with steroids and NSAIDS.

METABOLIC
The most common metabolic bone disease is osteoporosis – have to lose 30–50% bone mineral density before this is picked up on x–rays

Transient Osteoporosis of the Hip: diminished bone density of hip without joint changes. Bone marrow edema noted on MRI and the whole process resolves on its own. Also bone scan will be hot on the affected side.

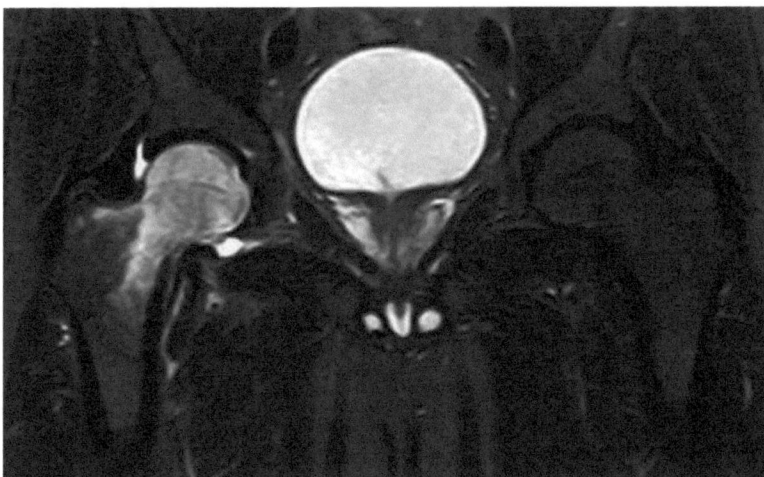

Rickets: osteomalacia in the pediatric population due to Vit D deficiency. Look for wide frayed metaphyses, loss of bone mineral density, and coarsened trabecular markings.

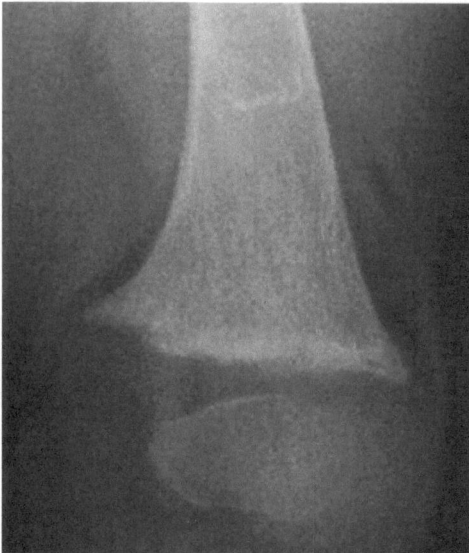

Scurvy: a vitamin C deficiency causes impaired wound healing, blood vessel integrity, and osteoid matrix formation. It is very common to have subperiosteal bleeding from vessel fragility.

Osteomalacia: caused by accumulation of excess uncalcified osteoid with bone softening. Due to a dietary deficiency of Vitamin D and lack of solar radiation. Look for looser's zones – sites of partial insufficiency fracture located on the **concave** side of the bone. Characteristically in the proximal femur, lateral scapula, and proximal tibia.

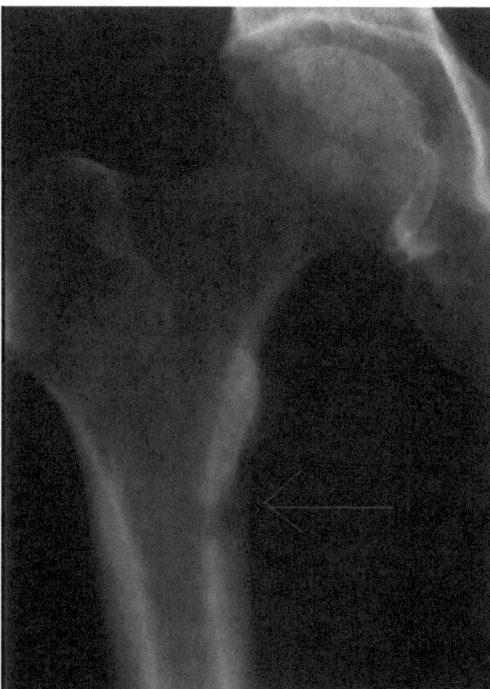

Hyperparathyroid	High Ca, Low Phosphate, High PTH – brown tumors and subperiosteal bone resorption. Bone resorption occurs at the phalanges and undersurface of clavicle – associated with MEN I and MEN IIa
Primary	Autonomic adenoma
Secondary	Hypocalcemia, hyperphosphatemia due to renal failure or GI malabsorption
Tertiary	Parathyroid gland hyperplasia due to secondary HPT

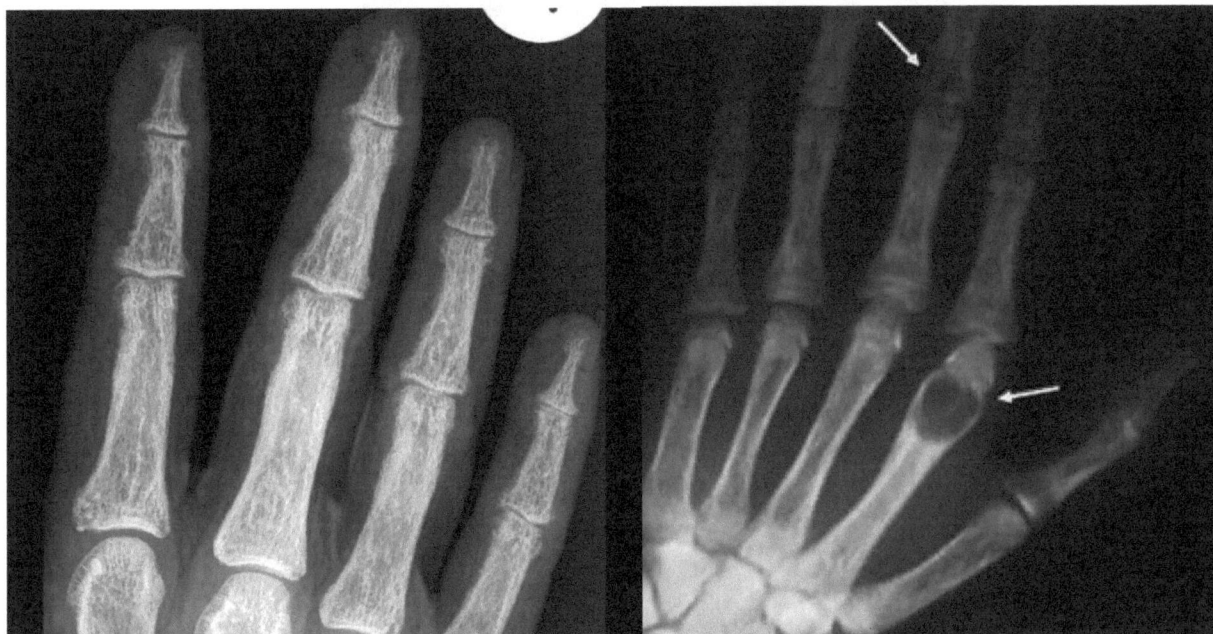

Subperiosteal bone resorption along the radial aspect of the middle phalanges is pathognomonic.

Renal Osteodystrophy: bone abnormalities in patients with chronic renal failure as a combination of secondary HPT and osteomalacia. Look for the rugger jersey spine, increased bone density, vascular and periarticular calcifications.

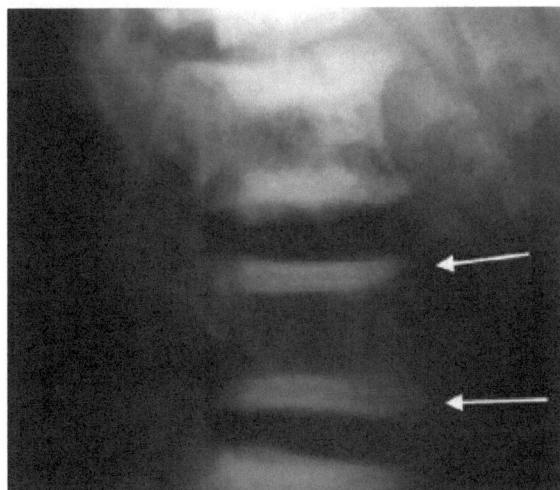

Hypoparathyroidism: triad of hypocalcemia, osteosclerosis, and soft tissue calcifications. Look for calcifications in the basal ganglia and brachydactyly.

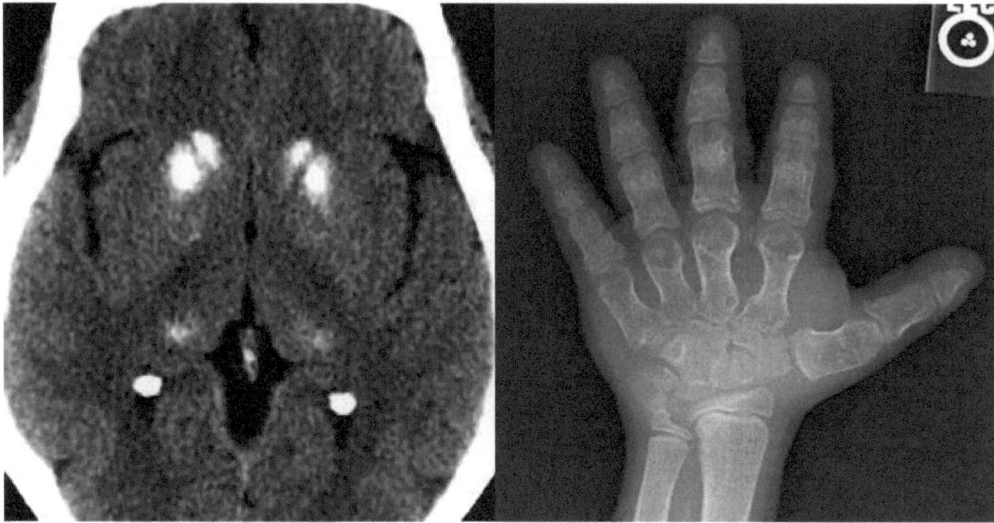

Acromegaly: excess growth hormone from pituitary adenoma causes bone growth and soft tissue swelling. Look for spade–like tufts, thick heel pads, large sella and frontal sinuses.

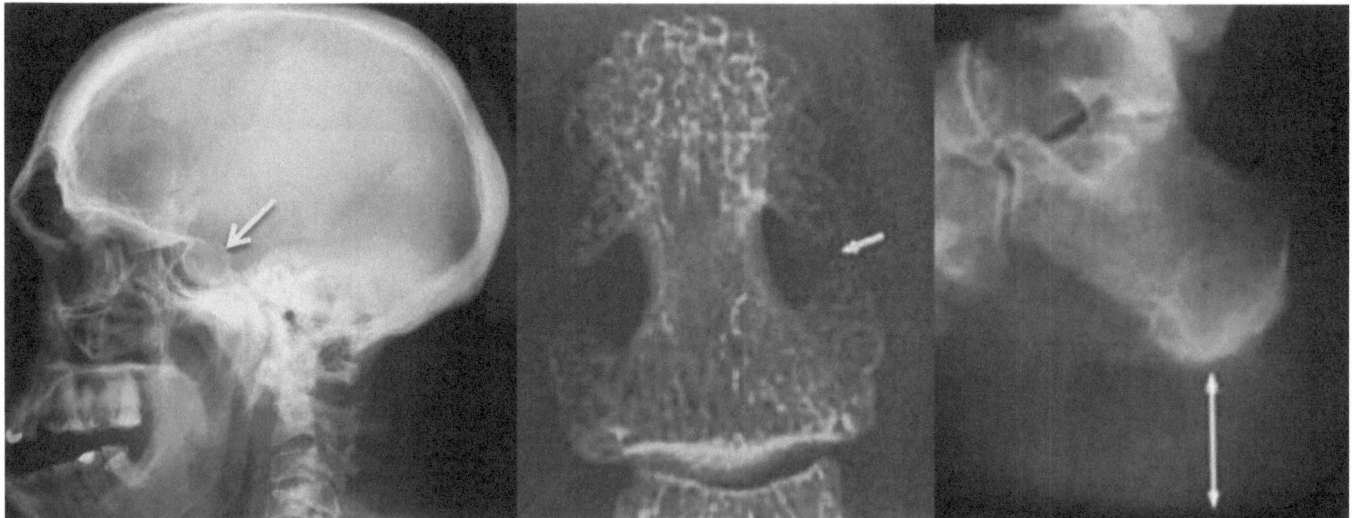

Osteopetrosis: is a bone disease caused by lack of absorption of the bone due to an underlying enzyme deficiency in osteoclasts. Look for really dense bones, bone–in–bone appearance of the spine, and obliteration of the diploic spaces in the skull.

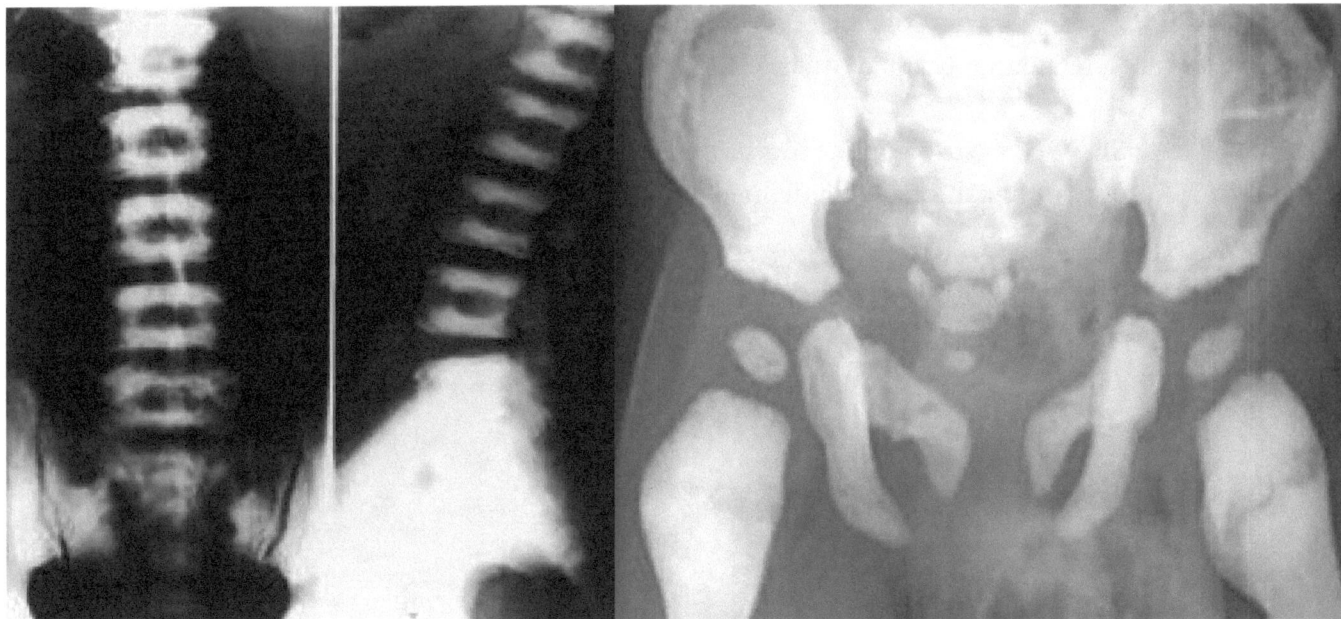

Ochronosis (Alkaptonuria): rare disease (Helm's has only seen one case – per his lecture), the characteristic findings are calcifications of the intervertebral discs. Look for chondrocalcinosis and joint space loss.

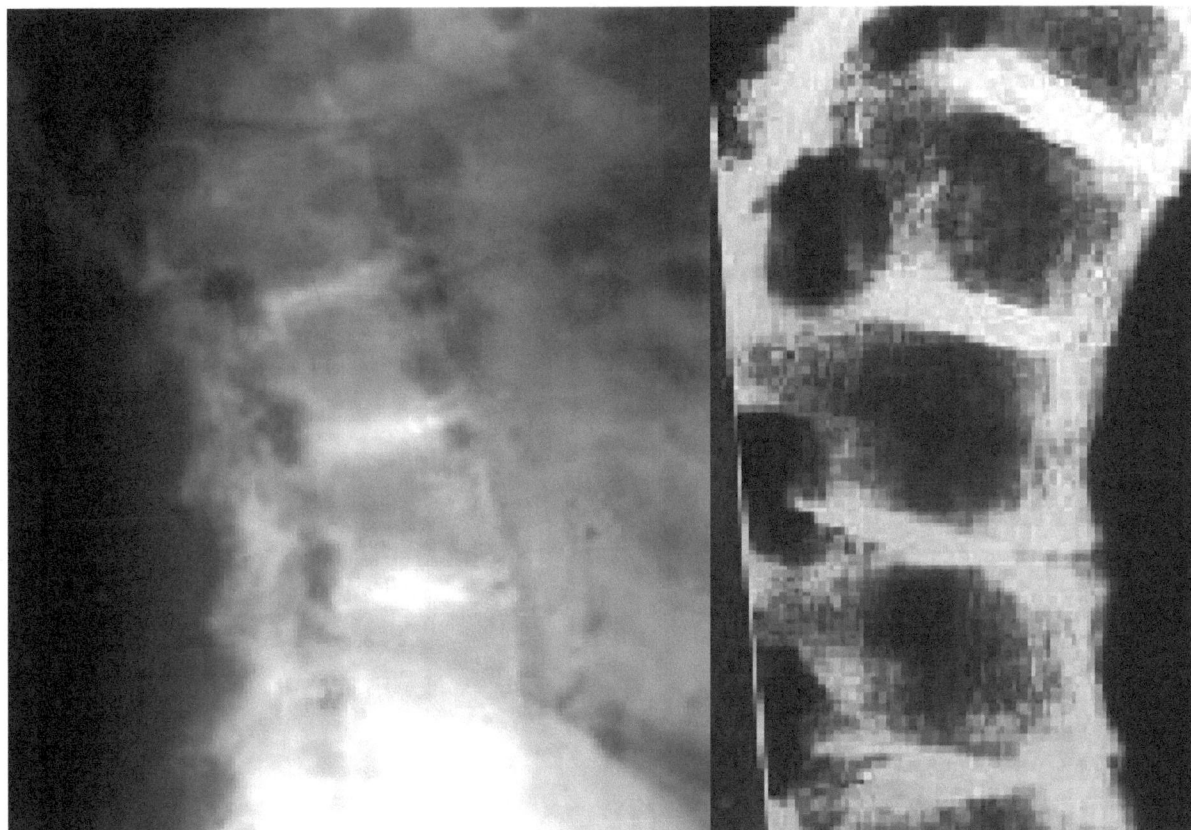

FEGNOMASHIC: this is a review of lytic bone lesions both benign and malignant. To figure out what the lesion is, there are a few things that have to be evaluated:

ZONE OF TRANSITION: narrow zone of transition is indicative of slow growth and tends to be a sign of benignity. Wide zones of transition are ill–defined borders indicating malignancy or infection.

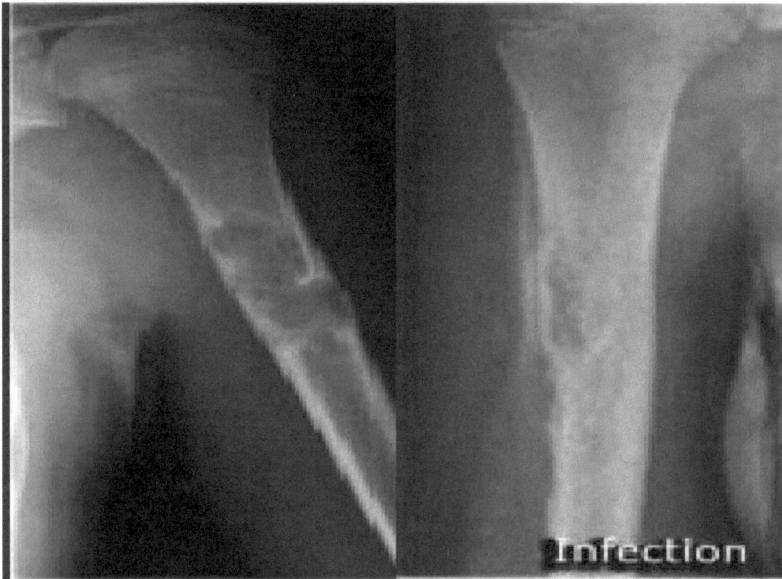

AGE: is an important way to narrow the differential diagnosis, Helms likes to use < 30 and > 30 as nice cutoffs; with patients > 40 having mets/myeloma/lymphoma thrown into almost every differential

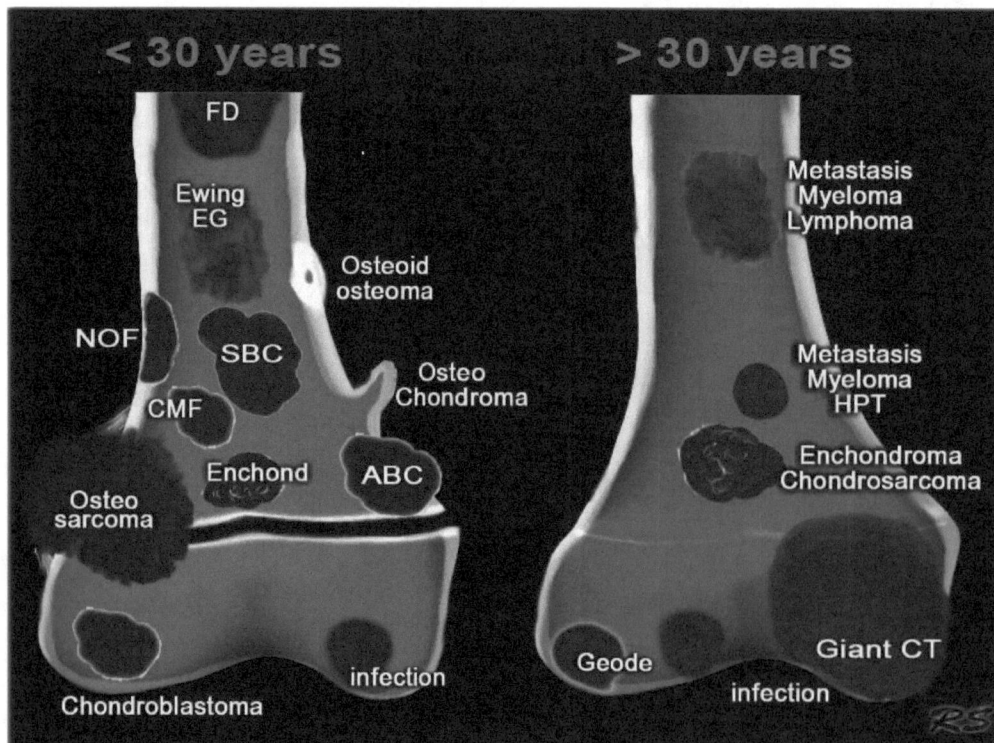

PERIOSTEAL REACTION: is a non–specific reaction and will occur anytime the periosteum is irritated (tumor, infection, or trauma). There are benign and aggressive patterns.

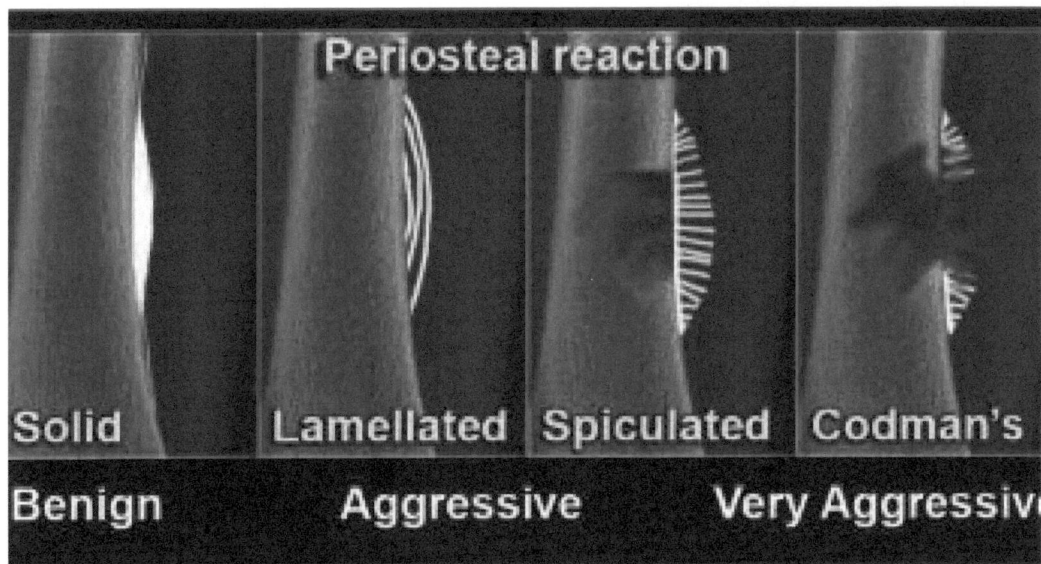

Fibrous Dysplasia: can look like anything, but it **never has periosteal reaction**. Prediliction for the pelvis, femur, ribs, skull; in fact this is the most common solitary lesion in a rib.

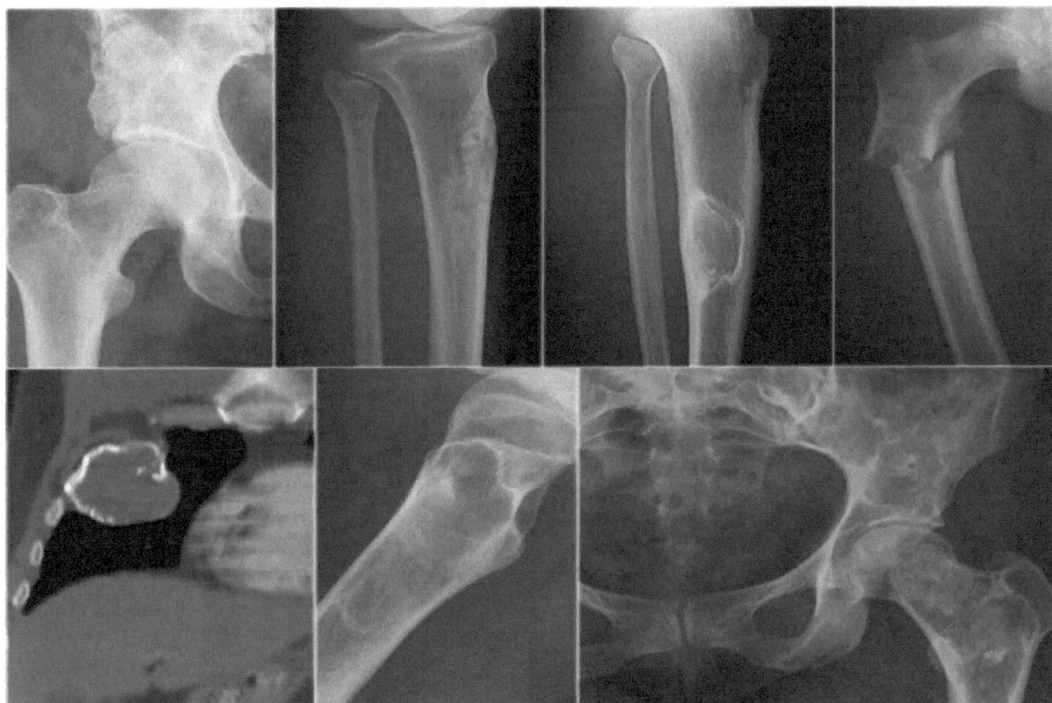

Adamantinoma: is a primary malignant bone tumor presenting in the 2nd–3rd decades and is locally aggressive. Almost exclusively occurs in the tibial diaphysis (anterior cortex). It has an expansile osteolytic appearance with areas of lysis and sclerosis. This lesion lacks periosteal reaction.

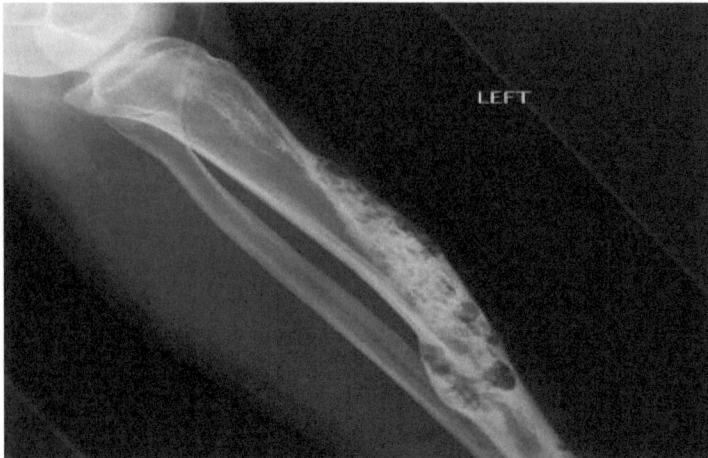

Enchondroma: most common benign cystic lesion of the phalanges, they have chondroid matrix (except in the phalanges), difficult to differentiate from a bone infarct. Enchondroma and chondrosarcoma look a lot alike, except chondrosarcoma has a soft tissue component and causes pain.

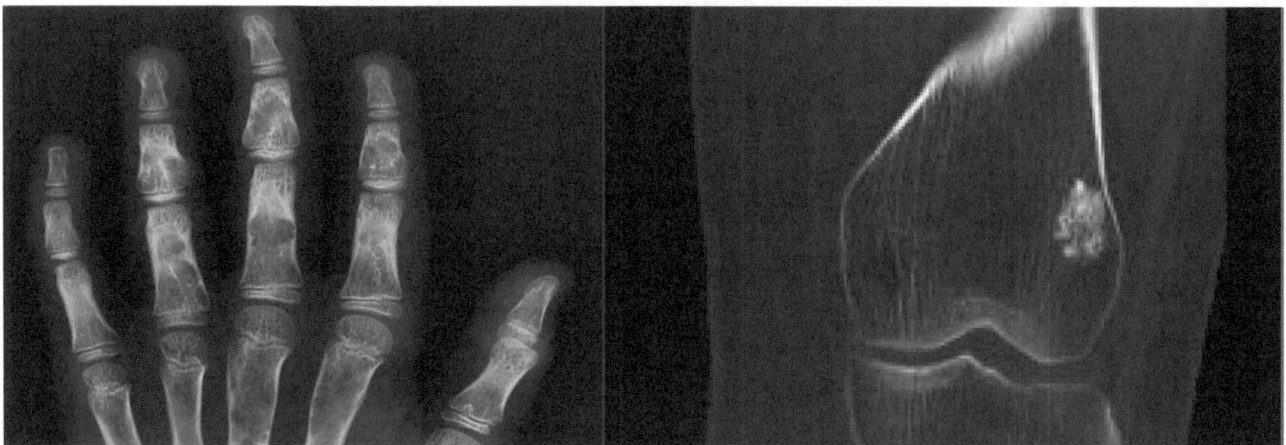

Ollier Disease: this is multiple enchondromas located in the metaphyseal region and has a very characteristic appearance. There is an increased risk of chondrosarcoma.

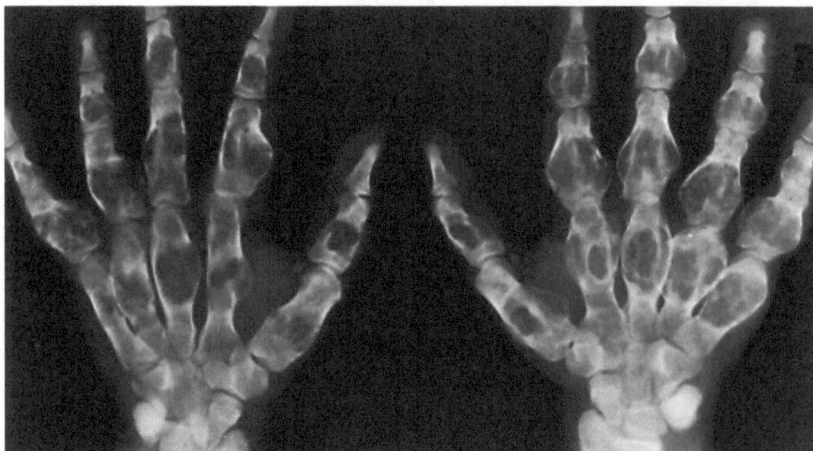

Fun Fact: if it looks like this but has soft tissue calcifications (hemangiomas), then it's Mafucci's Syndrome

Eosinophilic Granuloma: this is only in people under 30 years of age and it can look like anything. It occasionally has a bony sequestrum. Only three other things have a sequestrum: fibrosarcoma, osteomyelitis, and lymphoma.

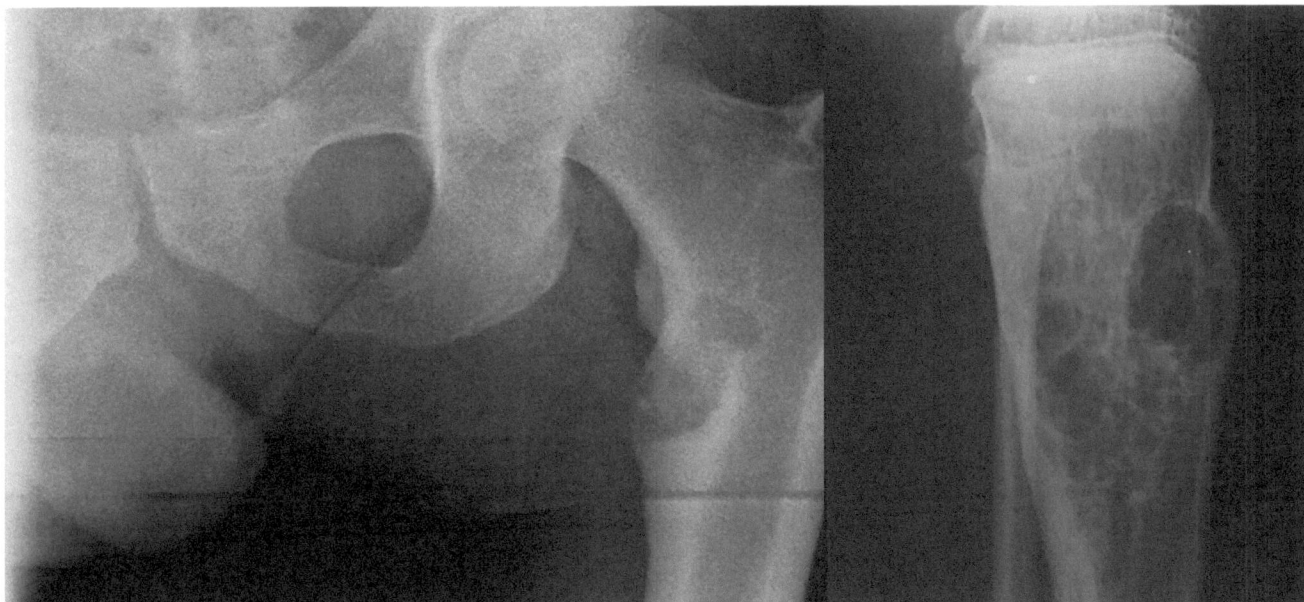

Giant Cell Tumor: most are benign but up to 15% can be malignant, if it does metastasize it likes to go to the lung. 4 criteria: only in patients with **closed epiphyses**, epiphyseal and abuts the articular surface, **eccentrically** located, sharp zone of transition that is NOT sclerotic. XRT can transform these into osteosarcoma or fibrosarcoma.

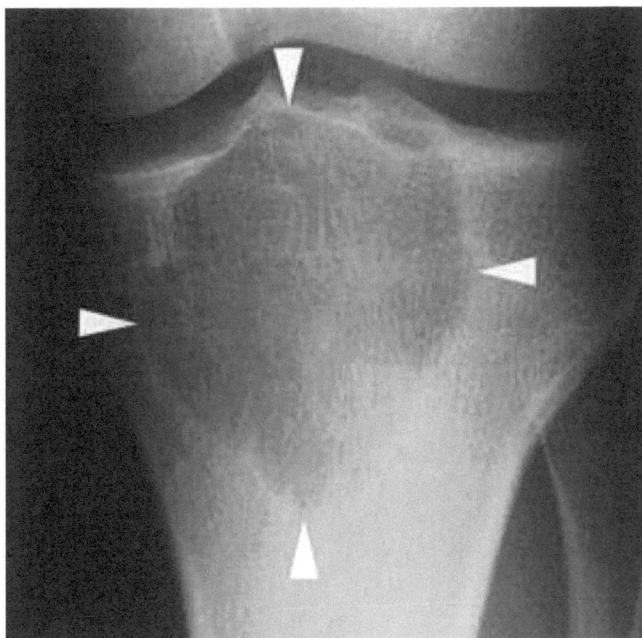

NOF: seen in kids and it usually regresses by the age of 30. It is a benign asymptomatic lesion occurring in the metaphysis of long bones. Has a thin sclerotic border with scalloping. Slightly expansile and as they heal, they become sclerotic.

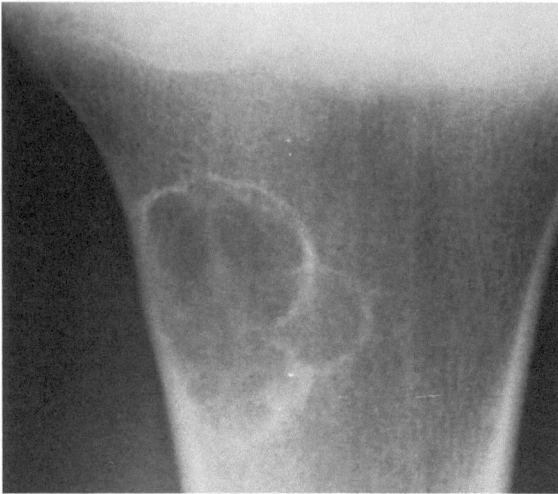

Osteoblastoma: expansile lesion with a "soap bubble appearance". One of the few things that likes the posterior elements of the spine and can cause painful scoliosis. This is an osteoid osteoma > 1.5–cm.

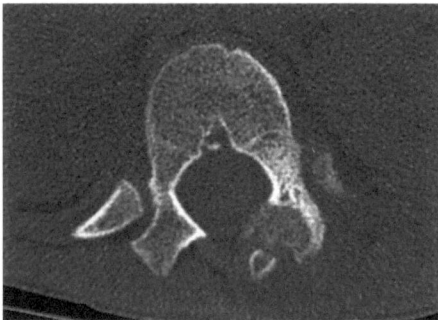

Metastatic Disease and Myeloma: consider this in anyone over the age of 40 with a lucent lesion of the bones. Can be solitary or multifocal. Lytic mets come from thyroid or renal cell CA.

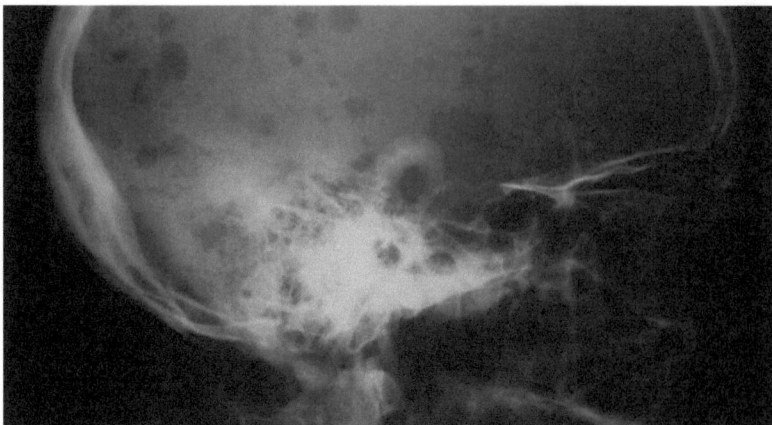

Aneurysmal Bone Cyst: always expansile, patients younger than 30 years old, MRI shows fluid–fluid levels, can be painful and can also be in the posterior elements.

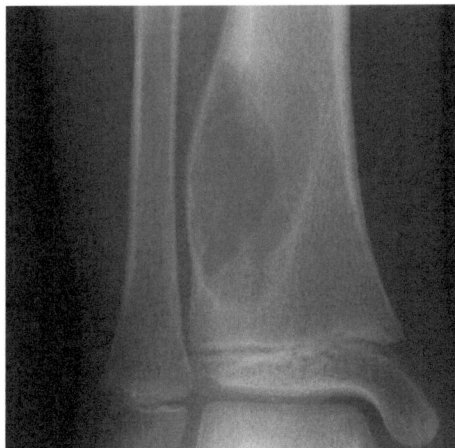

Solitary Bone Cyst: only lesion in FEGNOMASHIC that is always **centrally** located. Two thirds to three fourths are in the proximal humerus or femur. Asymptomatic unless a fracture occurs "fallen–fragment" sign. Patients younger than 30. Also commonly seen in the calcaneus where it has a triangular shape and located anteriorly–inferiorly.

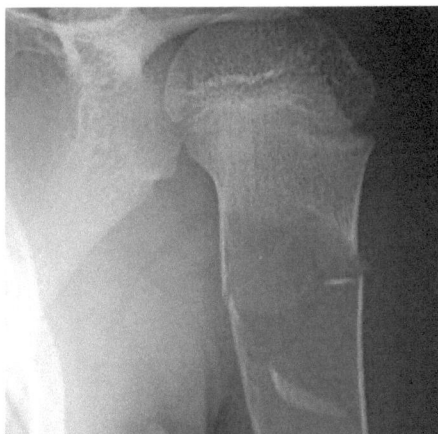

Fallen fragment in fractured UBC

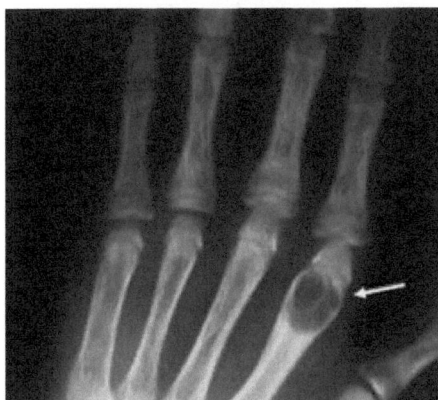

Hyperparathyroidism: causes brown tumors

Infection: can occur anywhere and in patients of any age, if there is a sequestrum then strongly consider osteomyelitis. Get MRI to confirm.

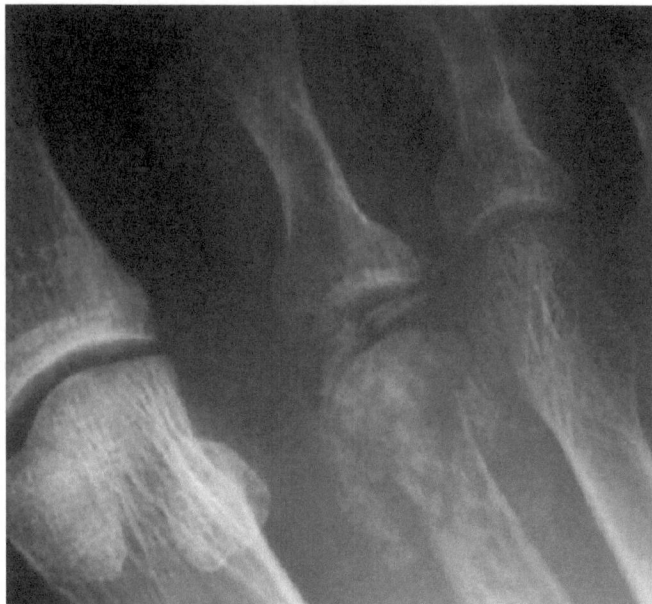

Chondroblastoma: only occurs in the **epiphyses** in patients < **30 years old**. The differential for a lytic lesion of the epiphyses in a patient younger than 30 is: infection (most common), chondroblastoma, and GCT.

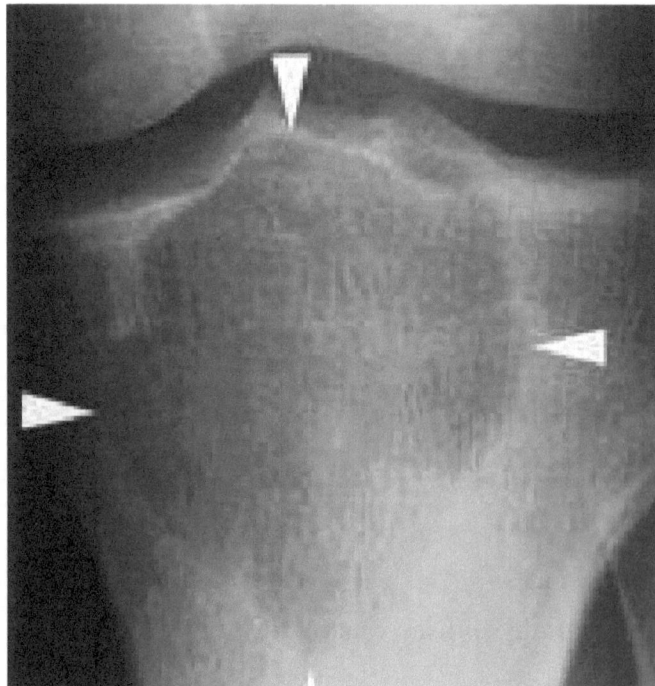

Lesion	
FD	No pain or periosteal reaction, single or multifocal (Mc-Cune Albright)
Enchondroma	Must have calcifications, except in the phalanges < 30 years old
GCT	Epiphyses must be closed
NOF	Asymptomatic lesion in < 30 year old
Osteoblastoma	Mentioned whenever an ABC is mentioned, "soap bubble"
Mets & Myeloma	In patients > 40 years old
ABC	Expansile in patients < 30 years old, likes posterior elements
Solitary Bone Cyst	Centrally located
HPT	Look for brown tumors
Infection	Anything goes
Chondroblastoma	Younger than 30 years old and epiphyseal with aggressive features of joint invasion and extension into the soft tissues – benign tumor

< 30 years	No Periosteal Reaction	Epiphyseal	Multiple
EG	Fibrous Dysplasia	Chondroblastoma	EG
ABC	Enchondroma	Infection	Enchondroma
NOF	NOF	GCT	Mets and Myeloma
Chondroblastoma	Bone Cyst	Geode	HPT
Bone Cyst			Infection

Fun Fact: Multiple Myeloma with sclerotic lesions is part of POEMS syndrome: polyneuropathy, organomegaly (hepatosplenomegaly), endocrine dysfunction, and M–protein and skin abnormalities.

COMMON TESTED MRI DIAGNOSES not to be a douche, but to figure these sets of images out, you have to know the basic MRI anatomy of these structures, I don't' have time to type out an anatomy chapter.

SLAP Tear: this is a tear of the superior glenoid labrum from anterior to posterior. In the figure below, the superior labrum is frayed and has fluid signal tracking under it indicating tear.

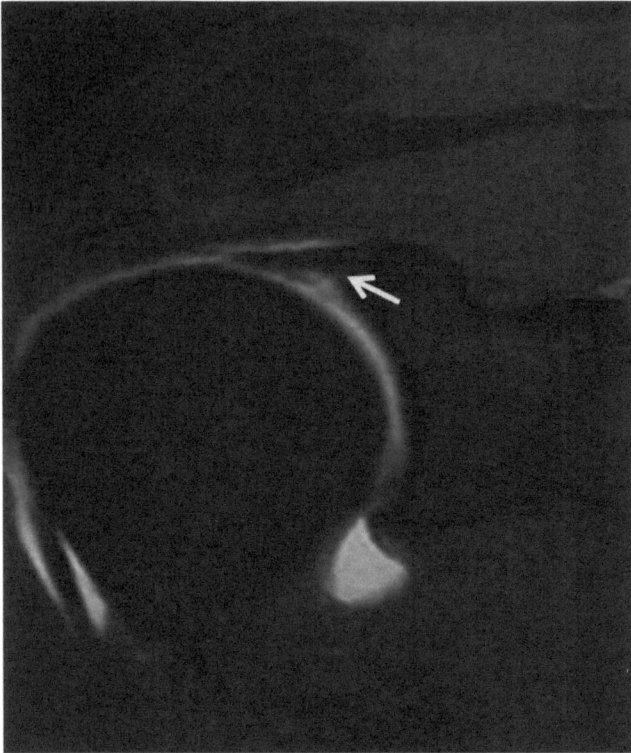

Perthes Lesion: anterior GH injury in which the anterior labrum is lifted from the edge of the glenoid along with a sleeve of the periosteium from the underlying bone. This is an **unstable lesion.**

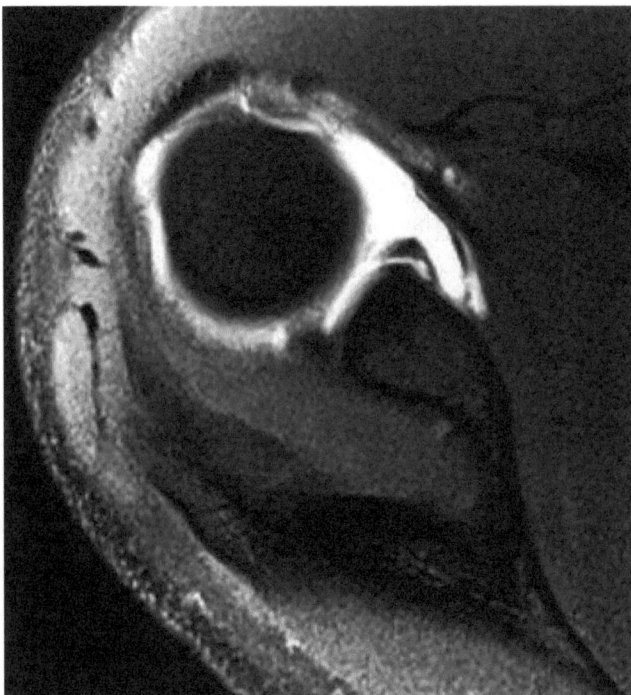

Buford Complex: congenital labral variant where the superior labrum is absent and the middle GH ligament is thickened. Look how there is a thick band anteriorly – that's the thickened MGHL.

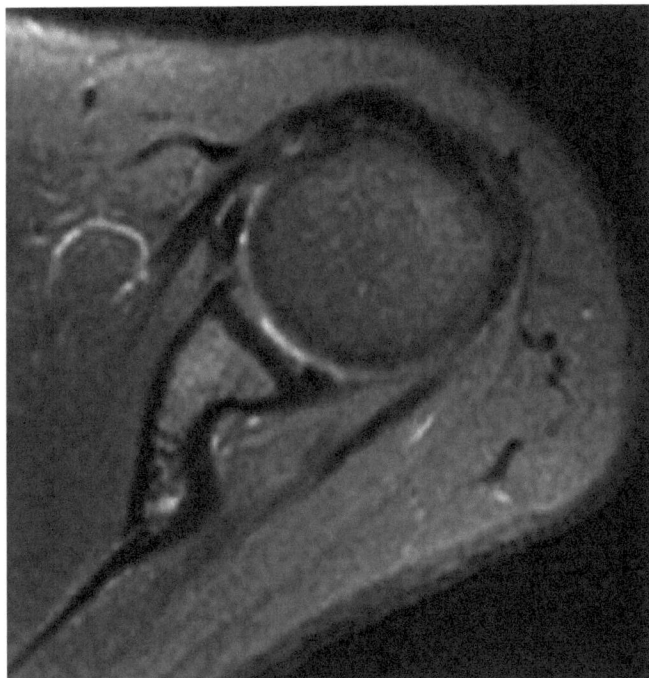

Parsonage Turner Syndrome: idiopathic neuropathy with wasting of the rotator cuff muscles. Presents with sudden onset pain and gradual weakness.

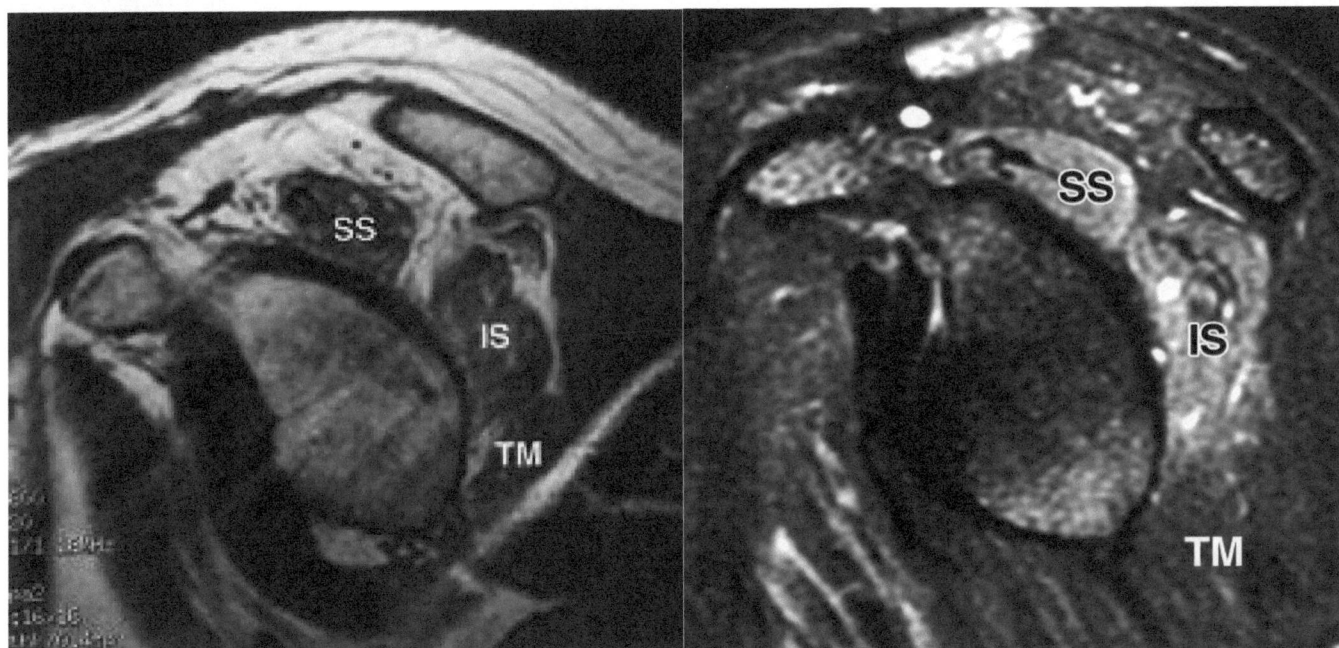

On sagittal T1 there is muscle atrophy in the supraspinatus, infraspinatus, and teres minor muscles with fatty striations being more prominent. On the STIR sequence there is muscle edema.

Supraspinatus Tear: This can be a partial thickeness or full thickness tear. Remember that if you see any fluid in the subacromial subdeltoid bursa, it is abnormal and either is due to DJD or a full thickness tear (especially if the fluid is injected gadolinium for an arthrogram).

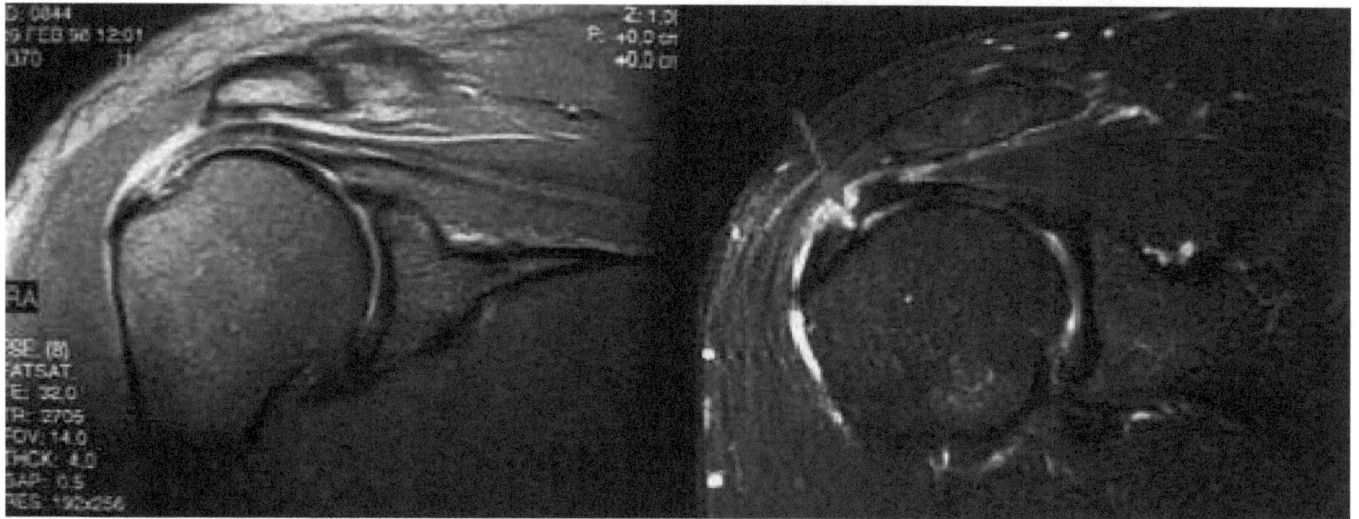

Subscapularis Tear: This is an important tear to remember because the normal attachment of the subscap muscle to the lesser tuberosity helps keep the biceps tendon in place. If this tears, the biceps tendon can sublux and it subluxes medially.

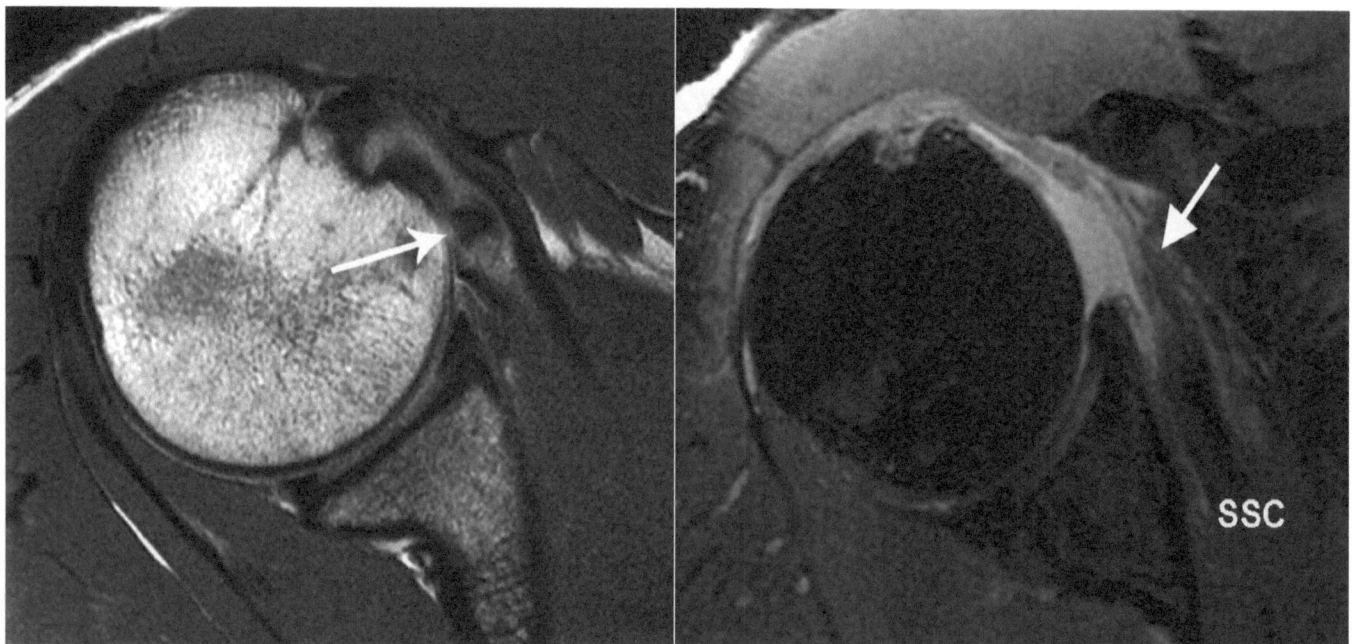

Fun Fact: With the tendon tears, remember to describe how much retraction there is.

Fun Fact: supraspinatus, infraspinatus, teres minor attach to the greater tuberosity while the subscapularis attaches to the lesser tuberosity. Biceps attaches to the supraglenoid tubercle.

Biceps Tear: most commonly involves the long head of the biceps, and when it happens the biceps balls up in the arm and looks like a softball. Look for edema in the biceps muscle and retraction of the tendon from its attachment site (radial tuberosity). Distal tear is seen in younger patients due to trauma and proximal tear is seen in older patients from degenerative changes.

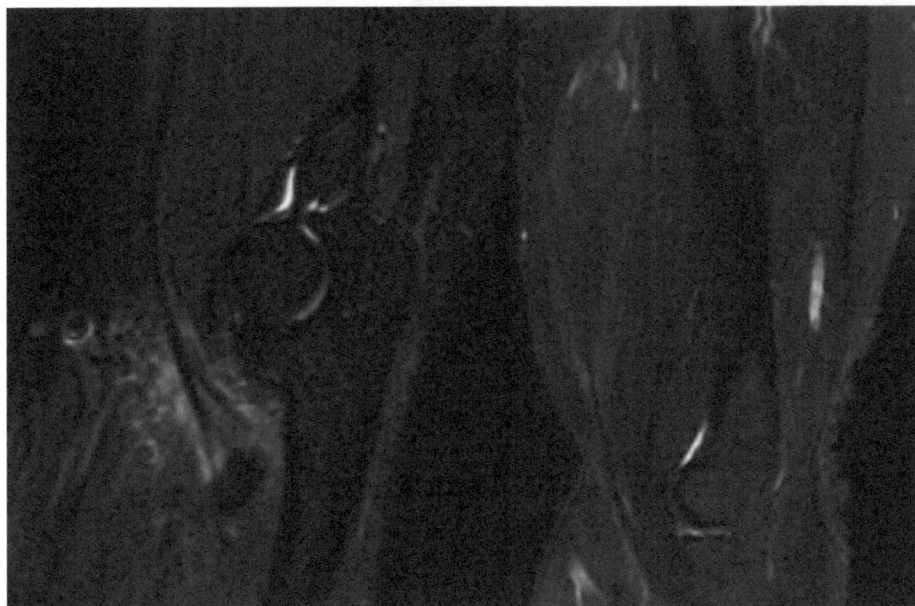

Triceps Tear: This is a posterior injury and like the biceps injury, look for tendon tear on a sagittal view and measure tendon retraction.

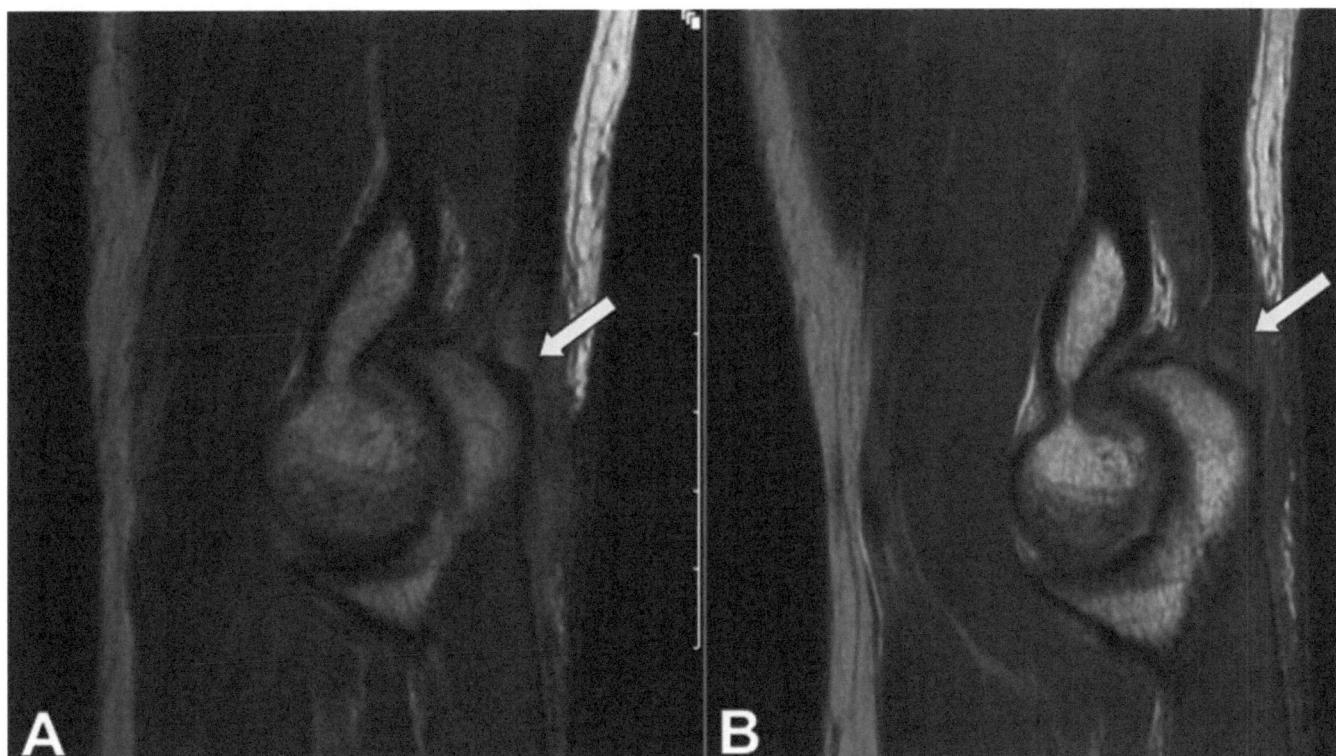

Cubital Tunnel Syndrome: ulner nerve neuropathy due to compression of the nerve as it passes beneath the cubital retinaculum resulting in impaired sensation in the 4th and 5th fingers. This is the second most common UE neuropathy.

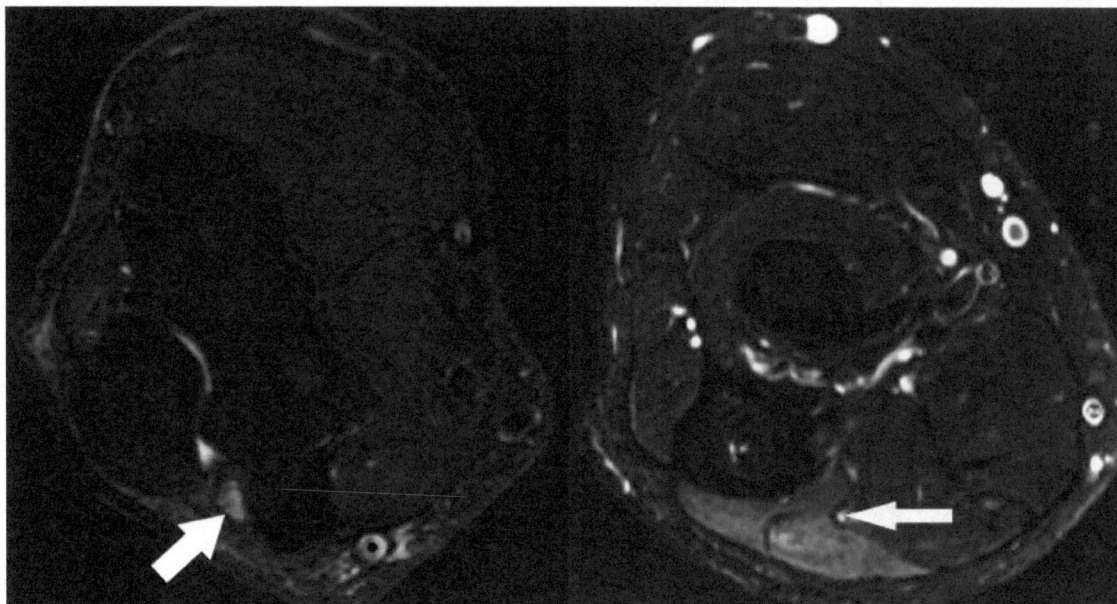

The image on the left shows increased signal and swelling of the ulnar nerve in the cubital tunnel. The nerve is most visible on imaging posterior to the medial epicondyle. The image on the right shows typical swelling and increased signal of the flexor carpi ulnaris (closer to the nerve, medial) and flexor digitorum profundus (lateral).

Ulnar Collateral Ligament Injury: this is seen commonly in throwing athletes due to tremendous force placed upon the elbow. If the valgus stress is too great, we injure the ulnar collateral ligament. This is more common of an injury than injury of the radial collateral ligaments.

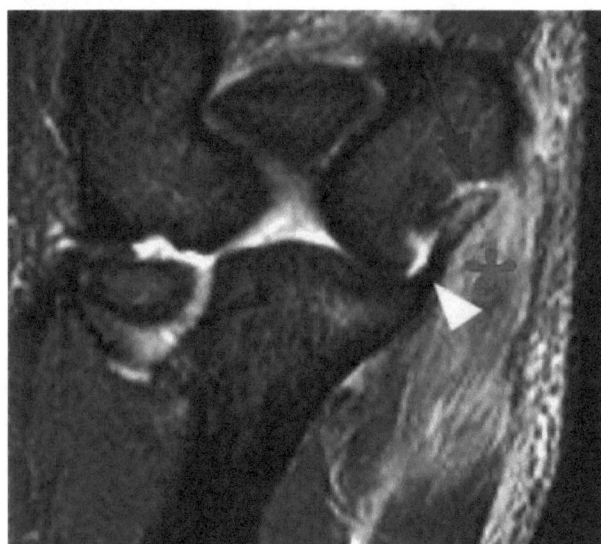

An abnormal gap is seen at the proximal attachment of the UCL (blue arrow). The distal attachment is intact (white arrowhead). There is edema in the pronator muscle (asterix).

Lateral Epicondylitis: refers to an overuse syndrome common in tennis players due to repeated rotatory motion in the forearm. On MRI look for thickening of the tendinous insertion and acute avulsive injuries. Extensor carpi radialis brevis is the most often injured.

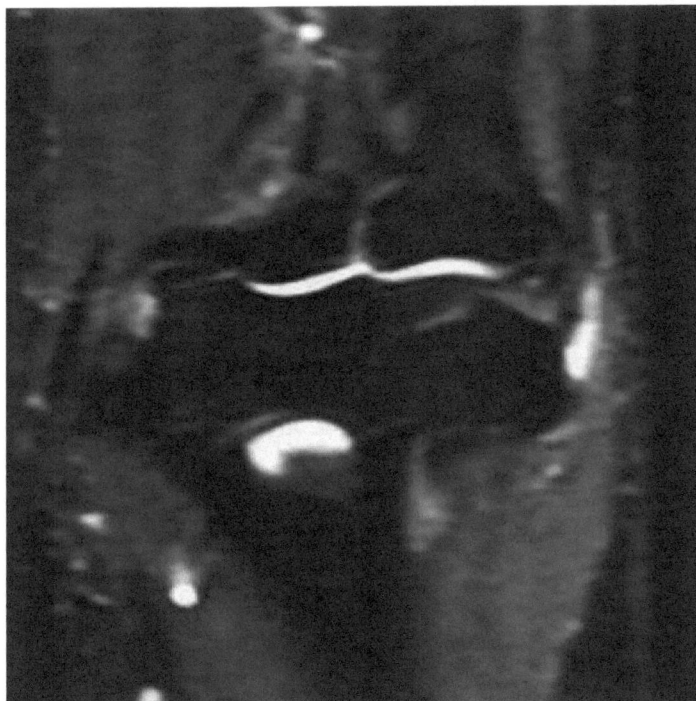

Medial Epicondylitis: also known as Golfer's elbow (and common in baseball pitchers), is an inflammatory condition involving the **elbow flexors.** This happens due to forceful flexion and valgus stress on the elbow.

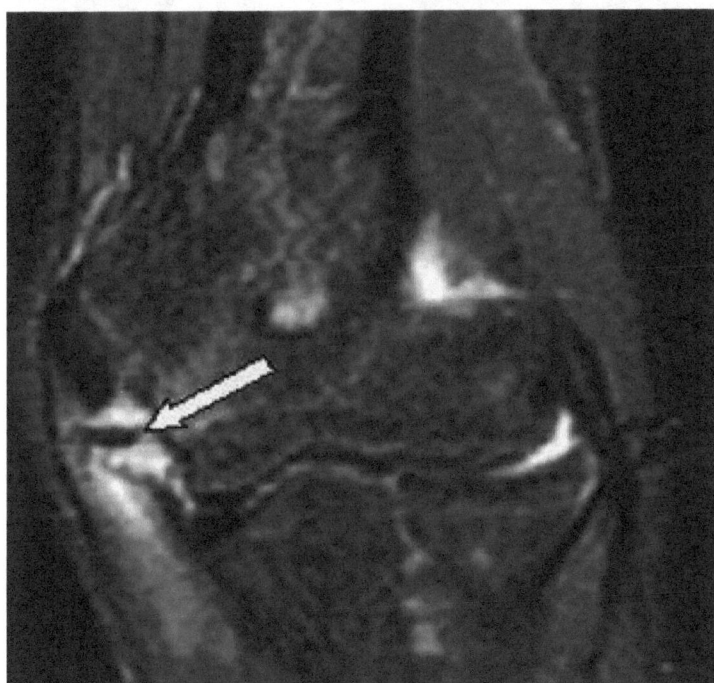

Carpal Tunnel Syndrome: typing this study guide is giving me carpal tunnel. This is a compression of the median nerve as it passes through the carpal tunnel (formed inferiorly by the flexor retinaculum extending between the hook of the hamate and tubercle of the trapezium and superiorly by the carpal row). The contents of the tunnel are the flexor tendons and the median nerve.

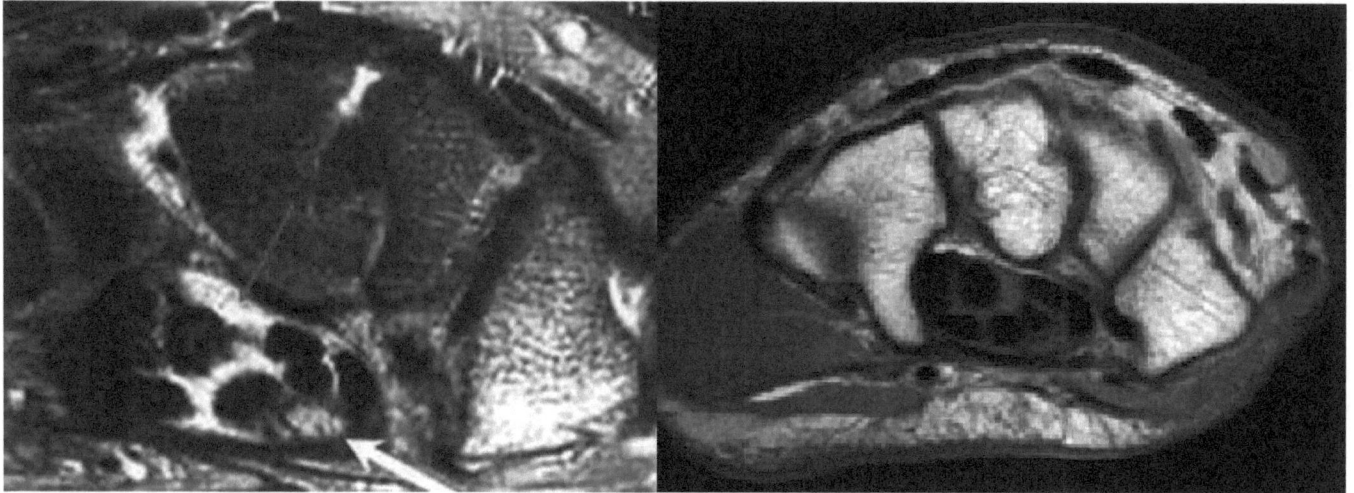

Left: the median nerve is swollen and enhances suggesting carpal tunnel syndrome (white arrow). Right: the median nerve is hypointense and does not enhance (normal)

De Quervain Tenosynovitis: painful syndrome affecting the first tendon compartment of the wrist which contains the APL and EPB tendons.

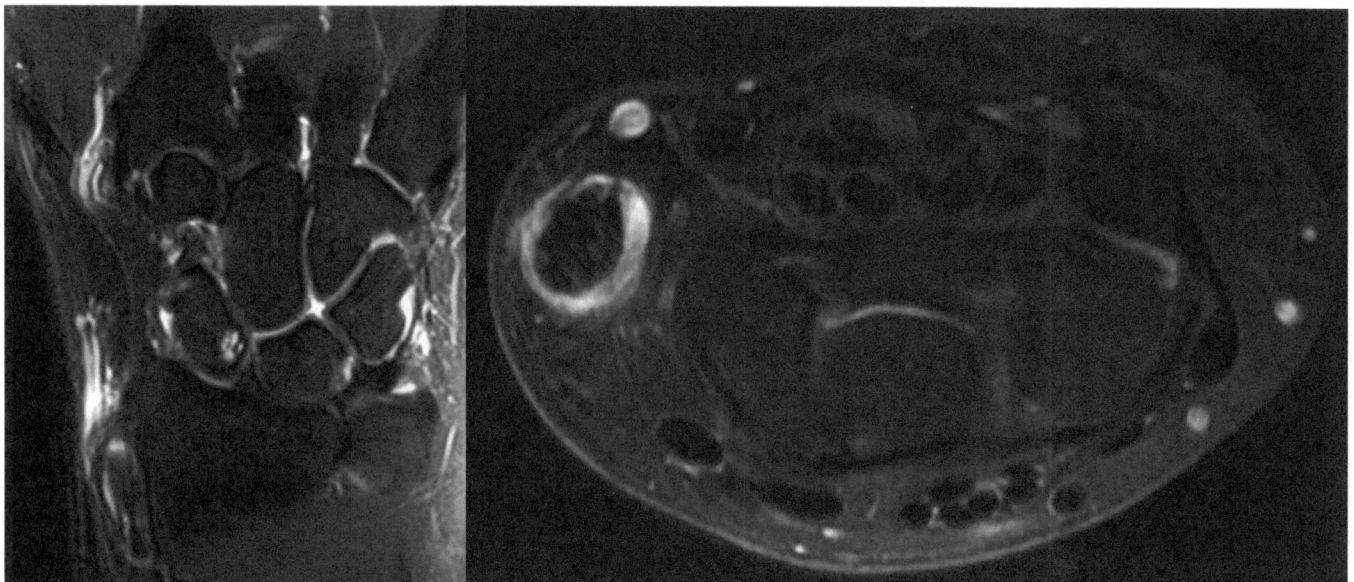

Guyon Canal Syndrome: entrapment neuropathy of the ulnar nerve as it passes through Guyan's canal. Guyon's canal contains the ulnar nerve, artery, and vein.

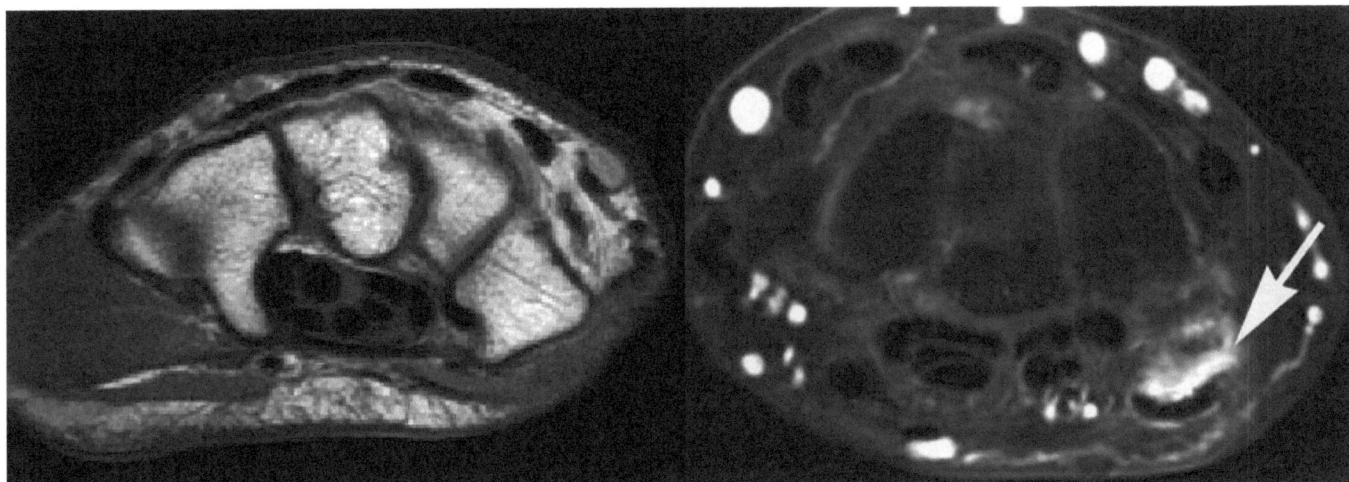

Normal Ulnar Nerve   Ulnar Nerve Inflammation

Gamekeeper's thumb: is when the UCL of the thumb is injured. If that's the only injury then immobilization and casting will be enough. However, if the torn end is dislocated dorsally above the adductor aponeurosis/ adductor pollicis muscle, that is characterized as a Stener lesion. This prevents healing and is an indication for surgical repair.

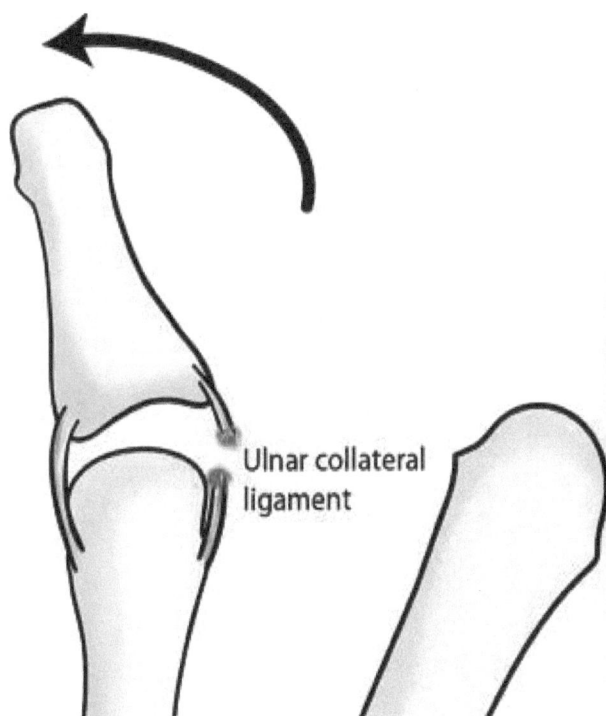

Ulnar collateral ligament

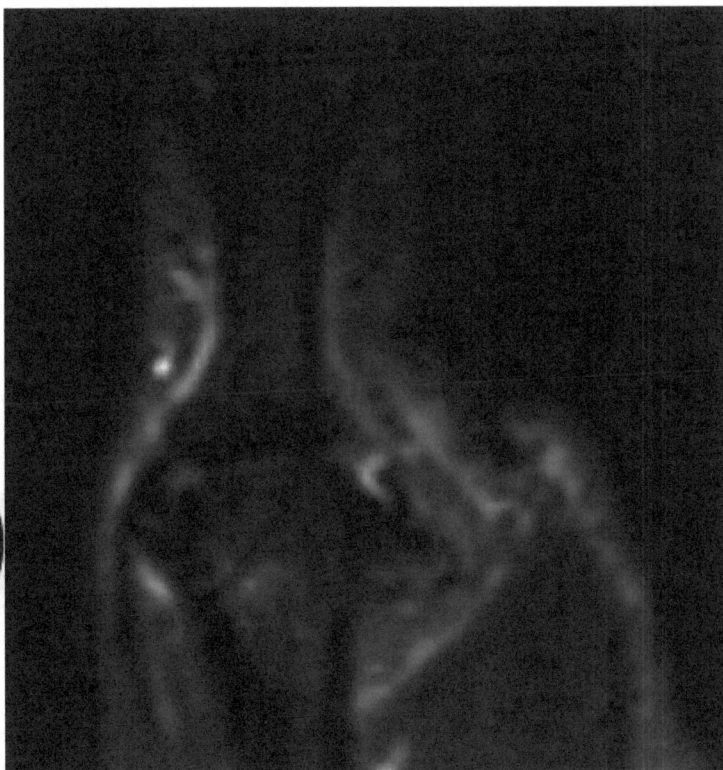

Soft tissue edema and discontinuity of the MCP UCL.

ACL Tear: most common knee injury encountered in practice. Mid portion is the most common site of disruption and there is forceful anterior translation of the tibia against the femur.

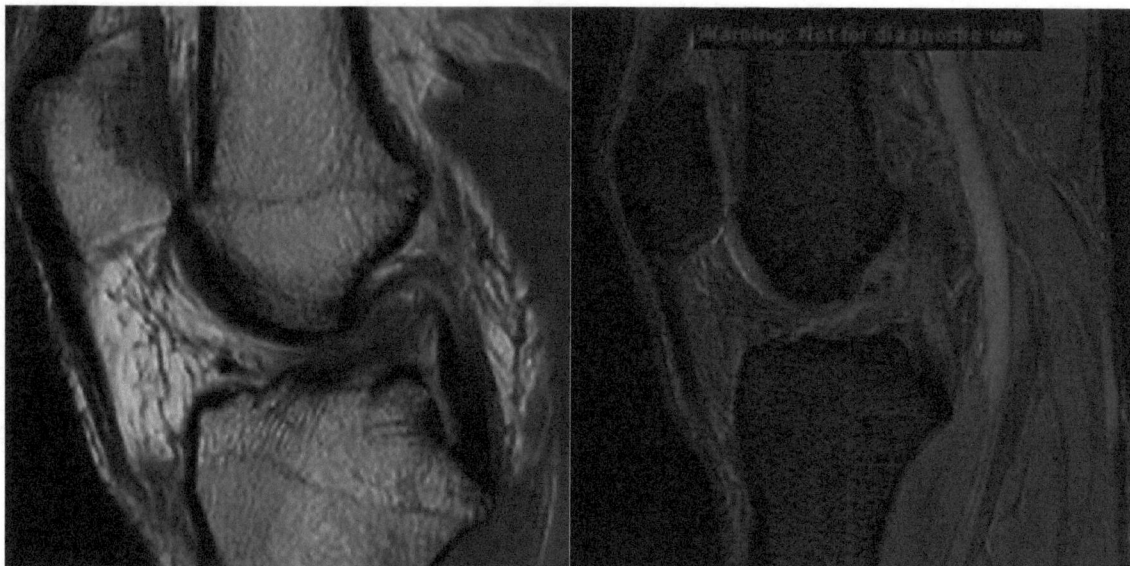

Midline sagittal images show lack of tendon fiber integrity with a frayed tendon on T1 – partial tear and complete absence of fibers on T2 – complete tear

Fun Fact: ACL should normally have some increased signal in it, especially near the attachment sites because it is a more fibrous tendon. The PCL should be a solid black band, it is like a steel cable, signal in the PCL is a sign of tear. Remember that the ACL and PCL are associated with Segond and reverse Segond injuries respectively.

Bucket Handle Tear: is a vertical long axis tear of the meniscus that causes a fragment of the meniscus to flip medially into the intercondylar notch creating a "double PCL" sign and a truncated appearance to the meniscus on coronal views.

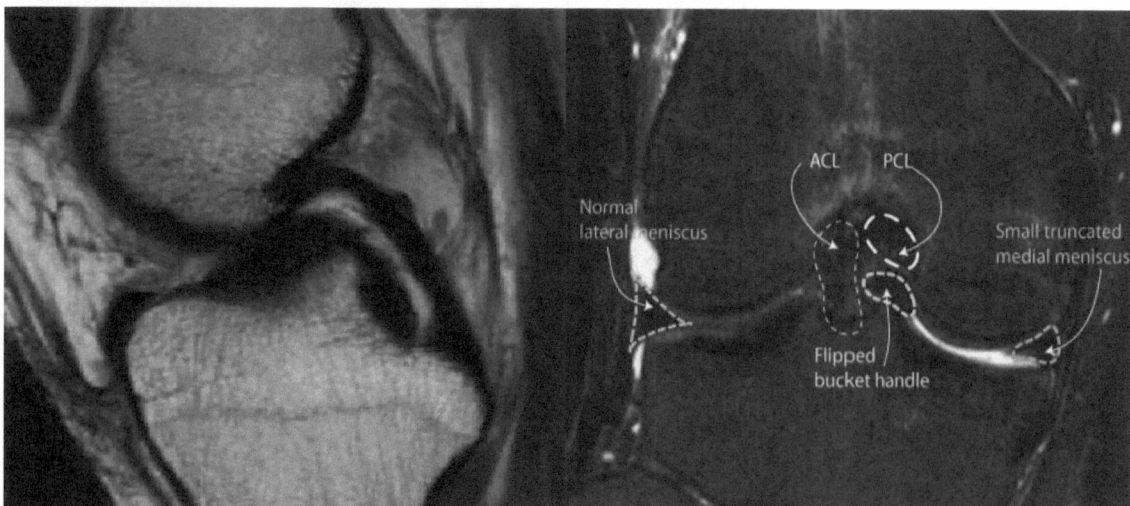

Patellar Tendon Rupture: occurs almost invariably at the proximal insertion of the tendon in trauma or in stressful athletic injuries (jumper's knee). If the midportion is torn, think about DM and chronic degenerative changes.

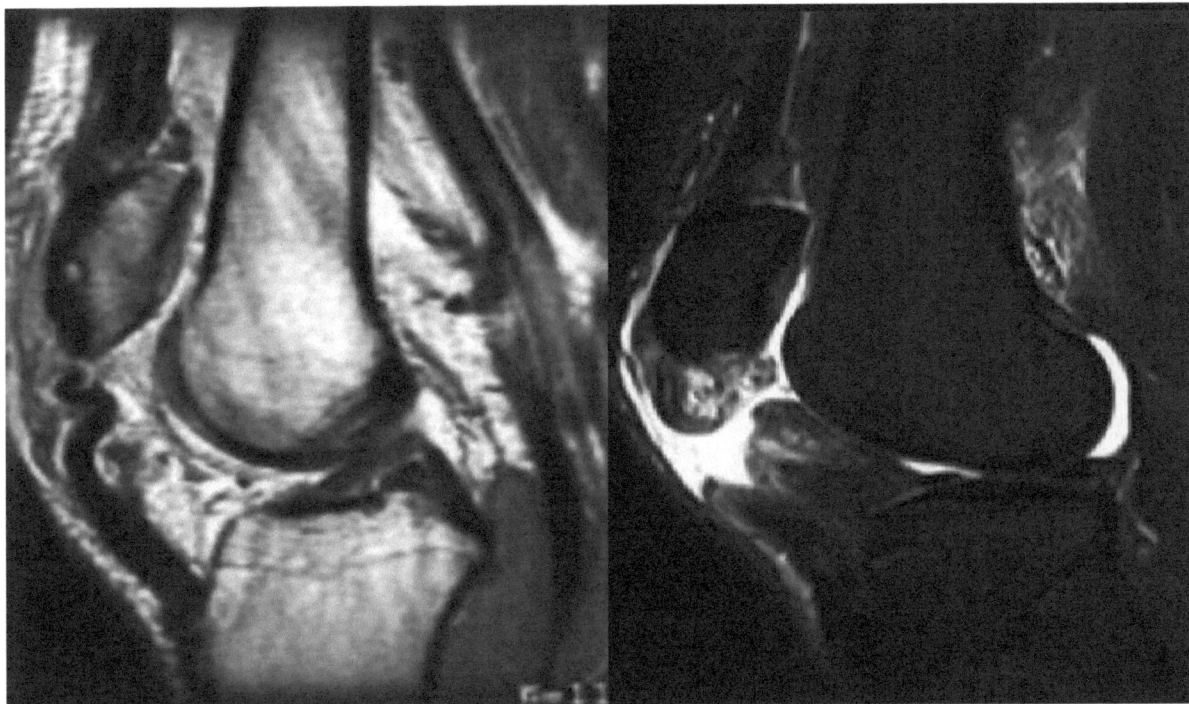

High Ankle Sprain: is an acute sprain of the distal tibiofibular syndesmotic ligament. This sidelines my running backs every year in fantasy football.

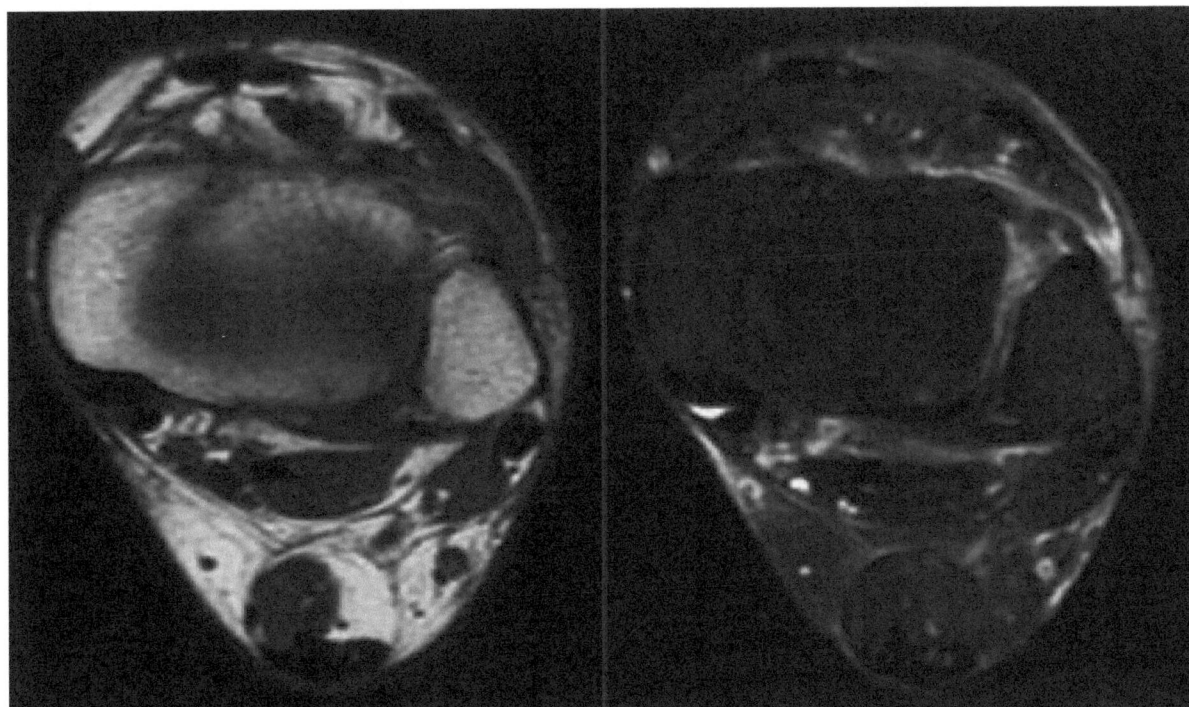

Plantar Fasciitis: inflammation of the plantar fascia of the foot and is considered the most common cause of foot pain. Look for plantar fascial thickening on the sagittal views that typically extends to the calcaneal insertion. There will be edema of the adjacent fat pad and underlying soft tissues.

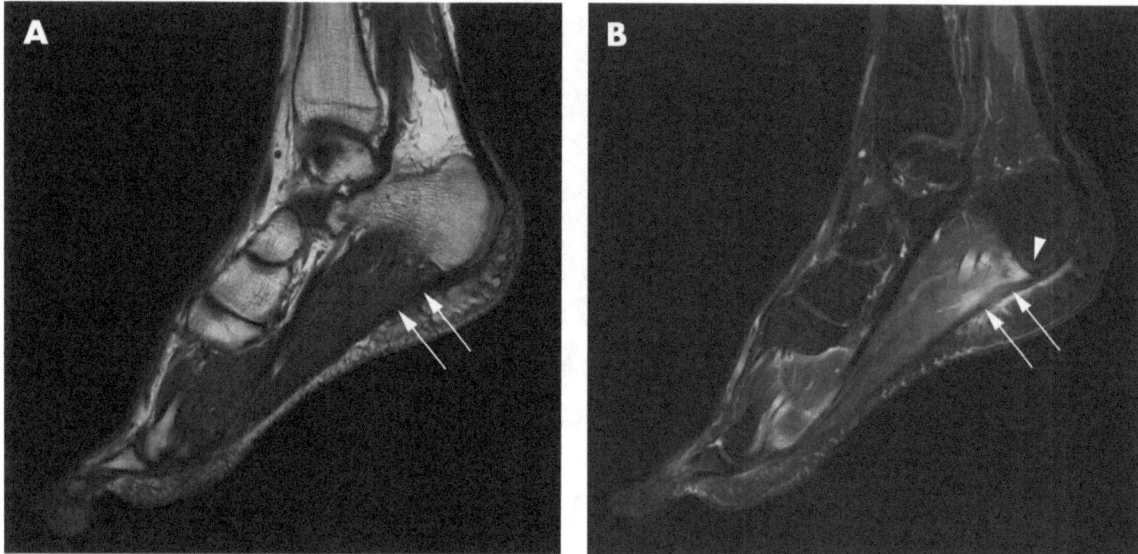

Something to keep in mind is that patients may complain of pain that is worse after a night of resting and then bearing weight, which eases up as the day goes on.

Posterior Tibial Tendon Tear: The PT tendon is the most commonly torn tendon in the medial aspect of the foot. Patients have pain and swelling. The PT tendon will have an oblong bulbous contour with a diameter 2–3 times that of the adjacent flexor digitorum longus tendon. The precursor to this is tendinosis and a complete rupture can lead to pes planus deformity.

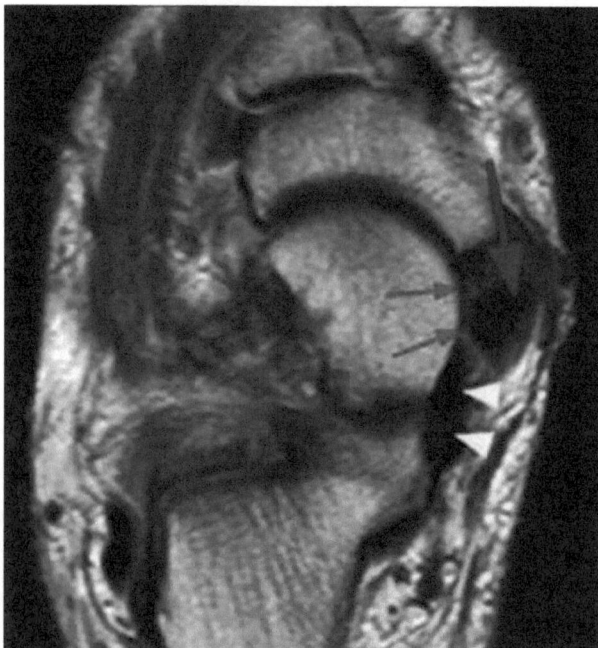

Morton's Neuroma: symptomatic peineural fibroma of a plantar digital nerve that most often occurs between the 3rd and 4th metatarsal heads or 2nd and 3rd metatarsal heads (2nd most common). Look for a T1 hypointense soft tissue mass between the metatarsal heads that enhances.

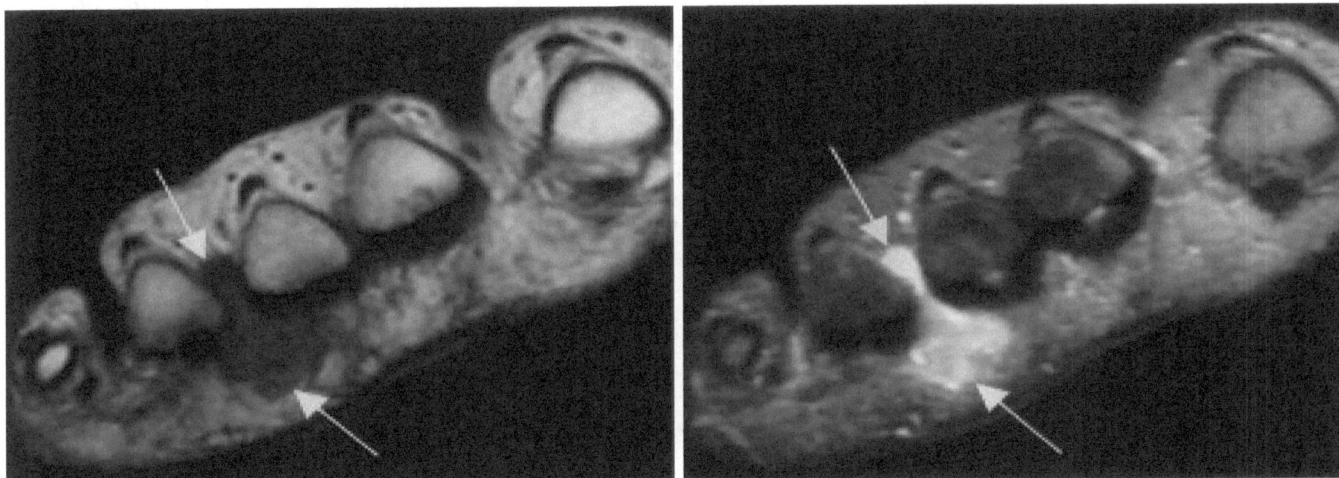

Osteomyelitis: bone infection with characteristic MRI findings. Low T1 intensity and T2 hyperintensity from marrow edema and reactive changes. Intense post contrast enhancement and may have an abscess. Surrounding soft tissues will enhance from cellulitis.

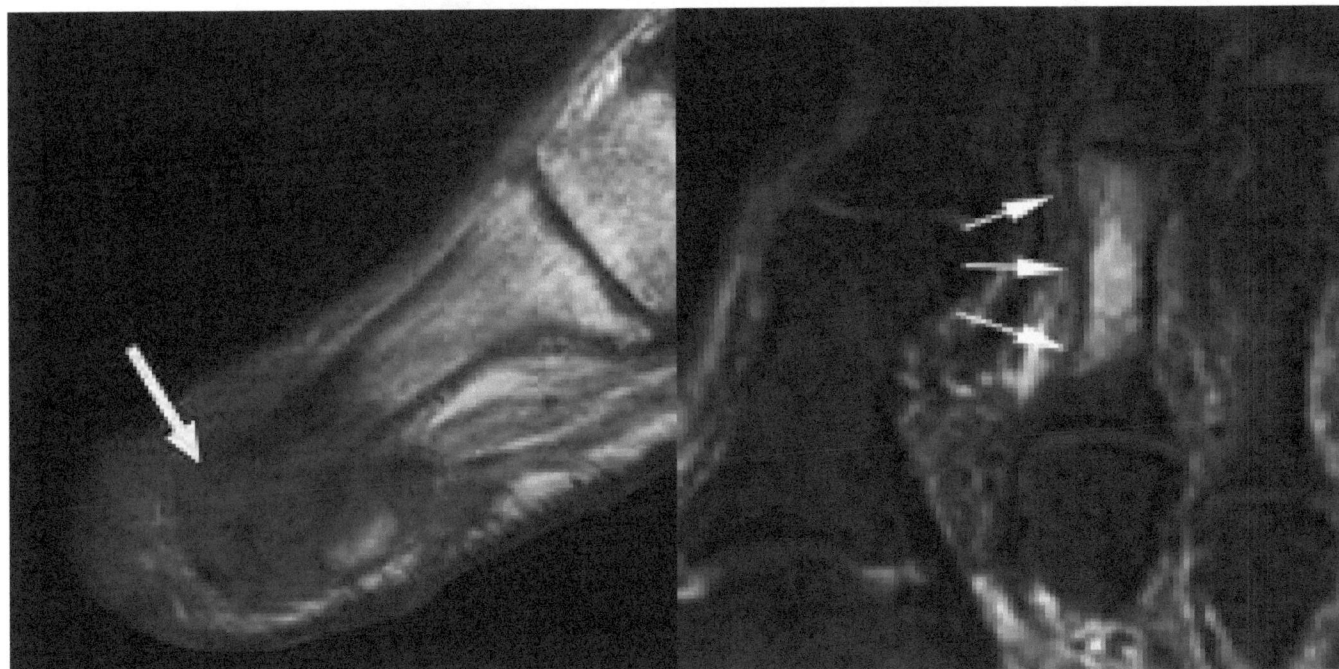

RANDOM DISEASES:

Hereditary Multiple Exostosis: autosomal dominant condition characterized by the presence of multiple exostoses (sessile and pedunculated). The exostoses grow with the patient until skeletal maturity then they should stop growing. They have a characteristic cartilage cap that should never be thicker than 2 cm. An abnormally thick cap, interval growth, or new onset pain without trauma are indications for malignant degeneration.

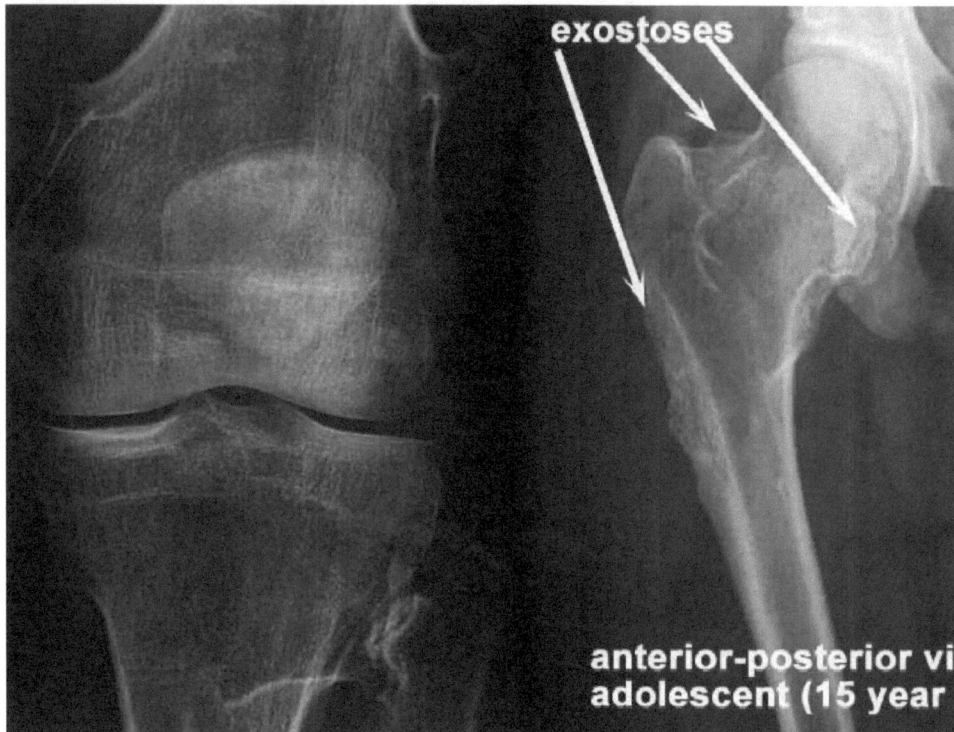

AVN Femoral Head: the hip is one of the most frequent sites and this can be due to trauma, ischemia, steroids, etc.

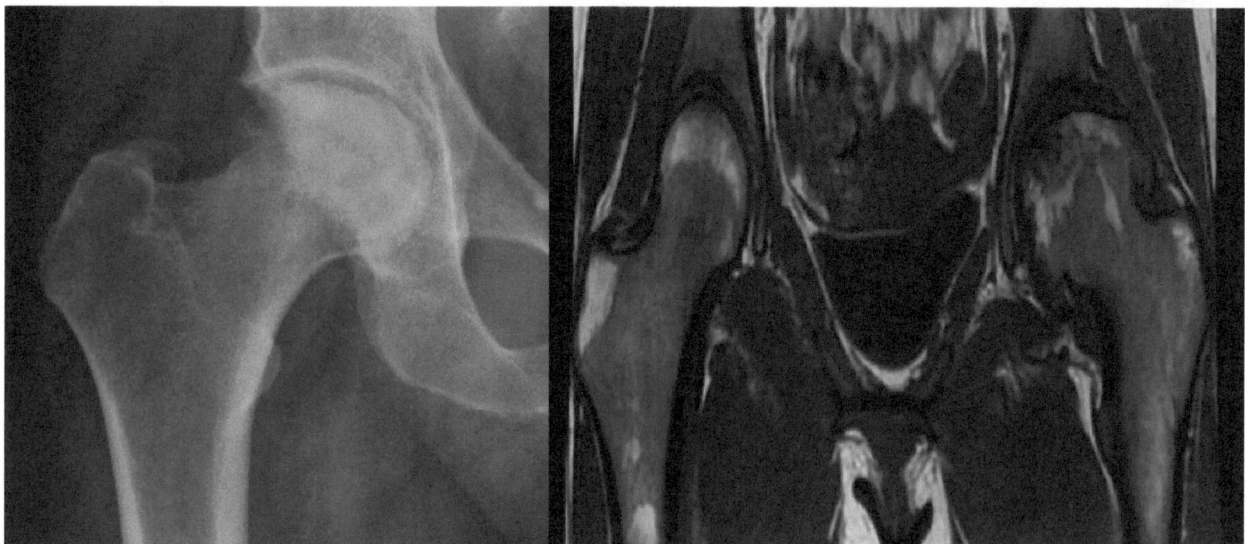

FICAT Staging:

1 – normal x–ray or slight sclerosis   2 – mixed sclerosis and osteopenia

3 – subchondral collapse (crescent sign)   4 – articular surface collapse

5 – djd

Tarsal Coalition: the **most common variant is the talocalcaneal** and the next most common is the calcaneonavicular coalition. A bony bar between the two bones characterizes an osseous coalition and a fibrous coalition is one where there is eburnation present but no bony bar.

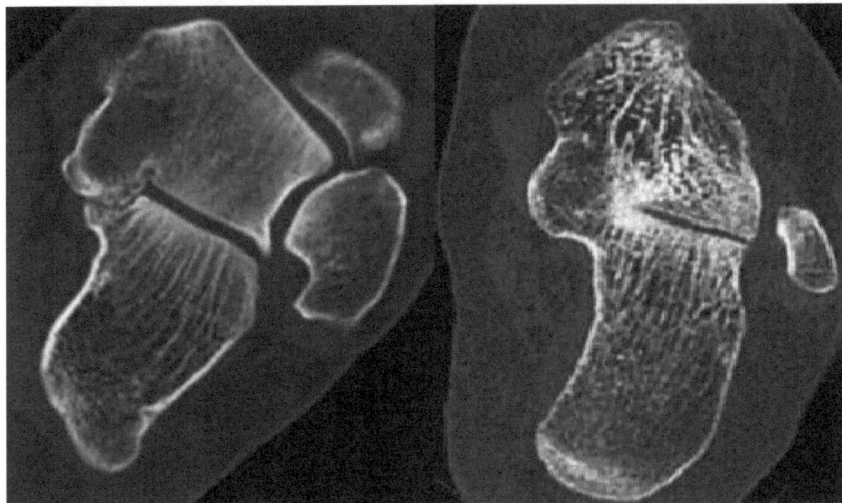

Osteopoikilosis: is an autosomal dominant condition with multiple bone islands that develop during childhood and do not regress – no malignant degeneration. Typical appearance, so do not mistake for malignany. Most lesions are going to be diffusely distributed around the pelvis. On MRI they are low signal on all pulse sequences. "Polka dot bones"

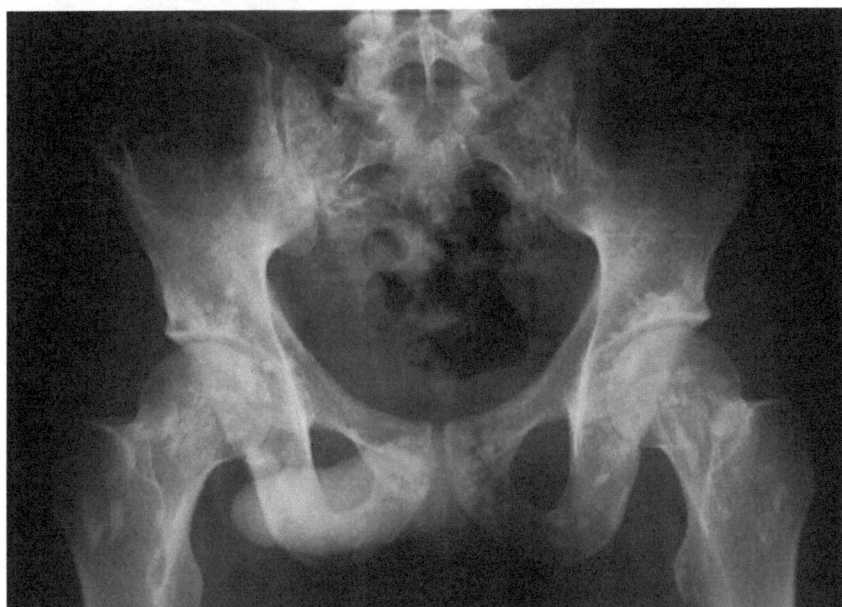

Calcific Tendinitis: due to the deposition of hydroxyapatite within tendons, usually the rotator cuff. Most symptoms occur when the calcium is fluffy rather than sharply defined. The fluff designates active inflammatory changes.

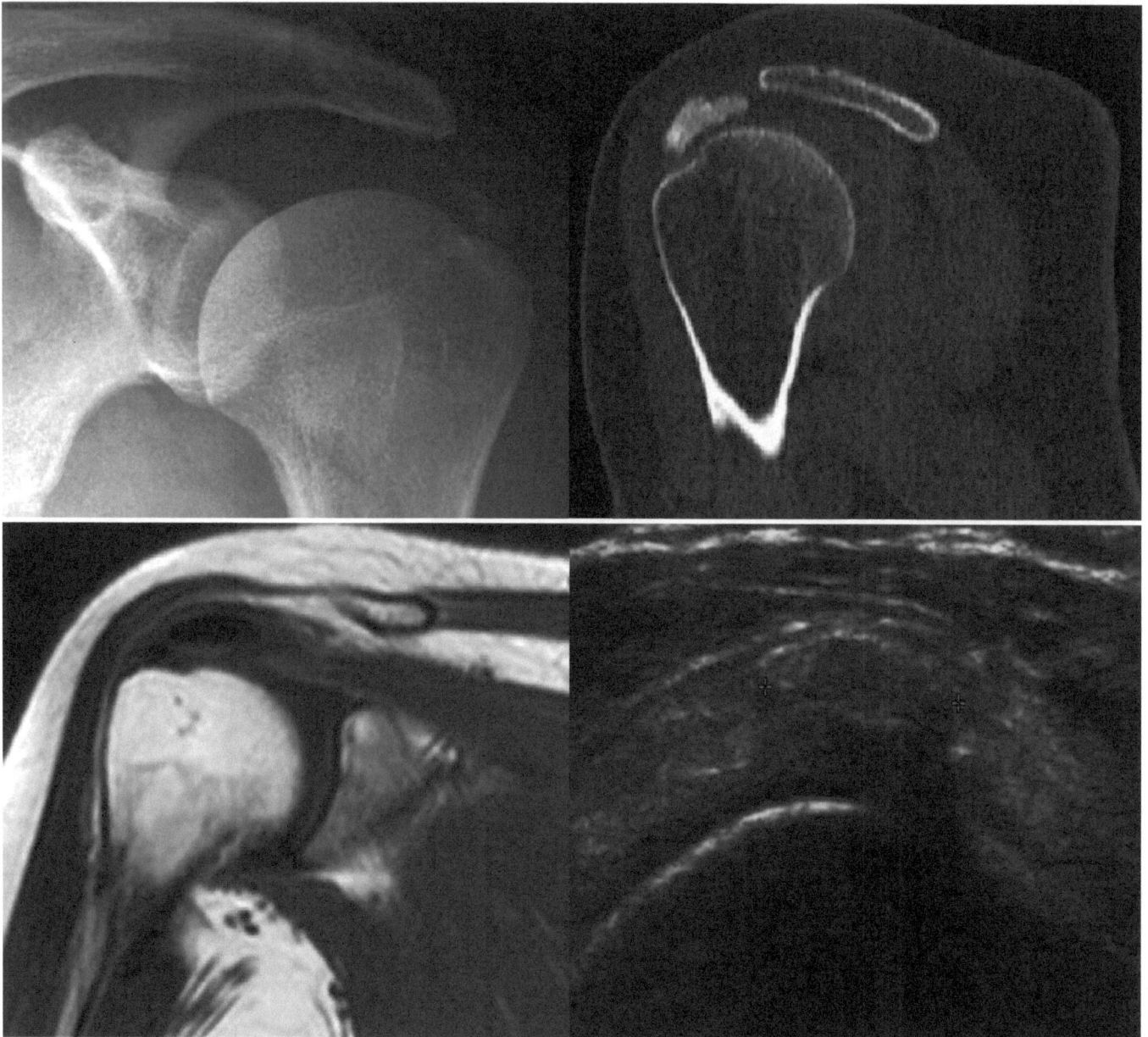

Melorheostosis: is a rare condition characterized by progressive hyperostosis of one bone or a series of bones in the same axis of the skeleton. It looks like dripping candle wax. It starts as linear hyperostosis and then demonstrates uniform cortical thickening on one side of a bone and progresses towards the center.

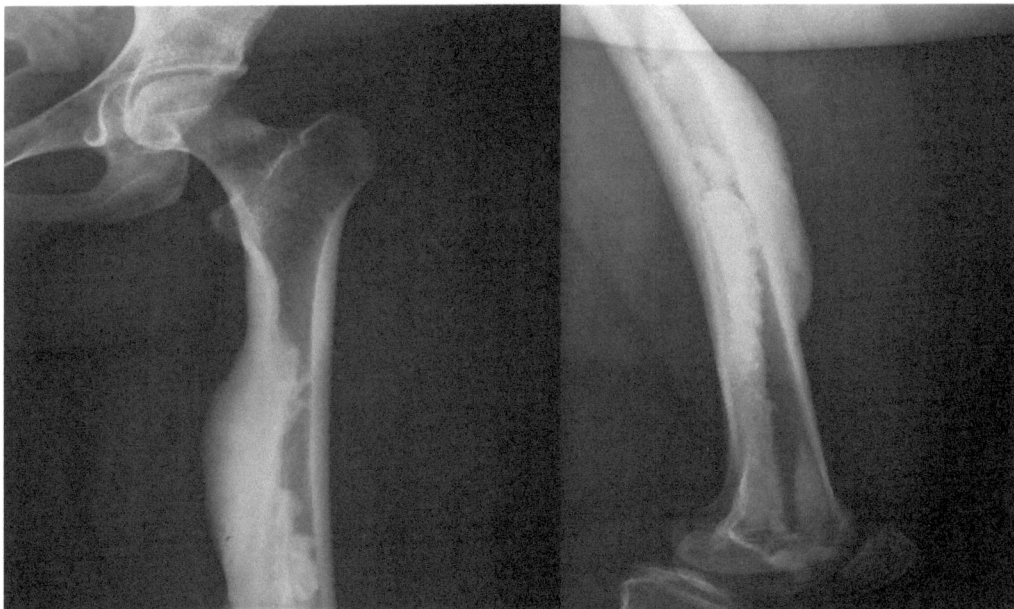

Vertebral Paget's Disease: causes enlargement of the vertebral body and posterior elements. The thickened cortex has a "picture frame" appearance and the trabecular pattern becomes coarse. If this involves the skull base it can lead to basilar invagination because the bone is soft and the skull settles.

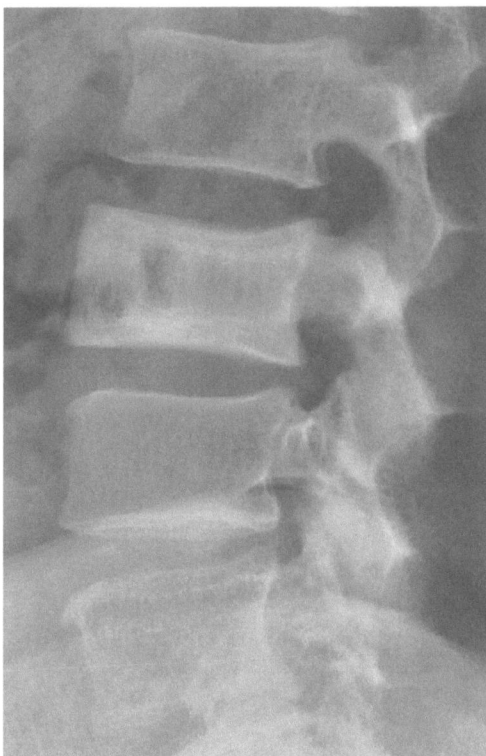

Engelmann's Disease: Typical age of onset is between 4–12 years old. Look for symmetric cortical thickening along the shaft of a tubular long bone involving both the periosteal and endosteal surfaces. This produces fusiform thickening of the cortical bone while narrowing the medullary cavity.

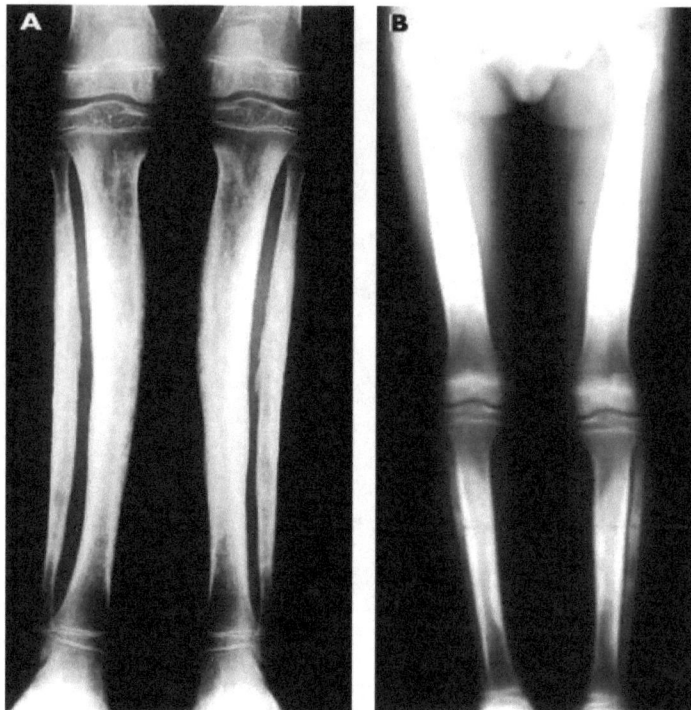

Sickle Cell: inherited disorder characterized by reversible sickling of RBCs. Oxygen tension is the most important factor in patients with this disease, when oxygen tension drops below 40 mm Hg they start to sickle. Increased blood viscosity causes thrombosis and infarction in end vessels, which may present as dactylitis in infants. Acute dactylitis is called hand–foot syndrome. **Vertebral bodies** will have a **biconcave** appearance and hip and shoulder AVN is common.

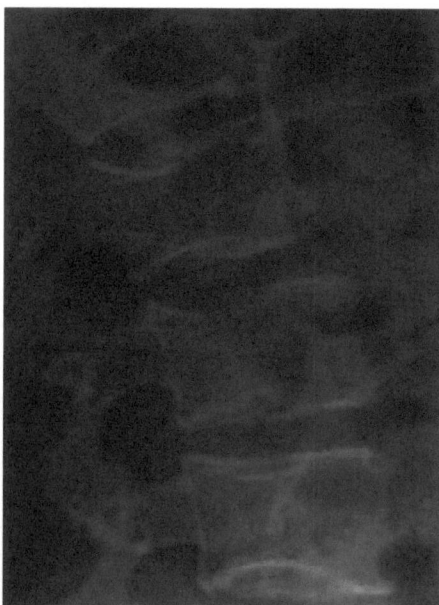

Parosteal Osteosarcoma: slow-growing malignant tumor arising from the periosseous tissues adjacent to the cortex and is most common around the knee. Characteristic appearance on x-ray is an osteoblastic, exophytic lesion encircling the bone. Treated with wide regional en-bloc resection and chemotherapy. If it recurs, it tends to be more aggressive.

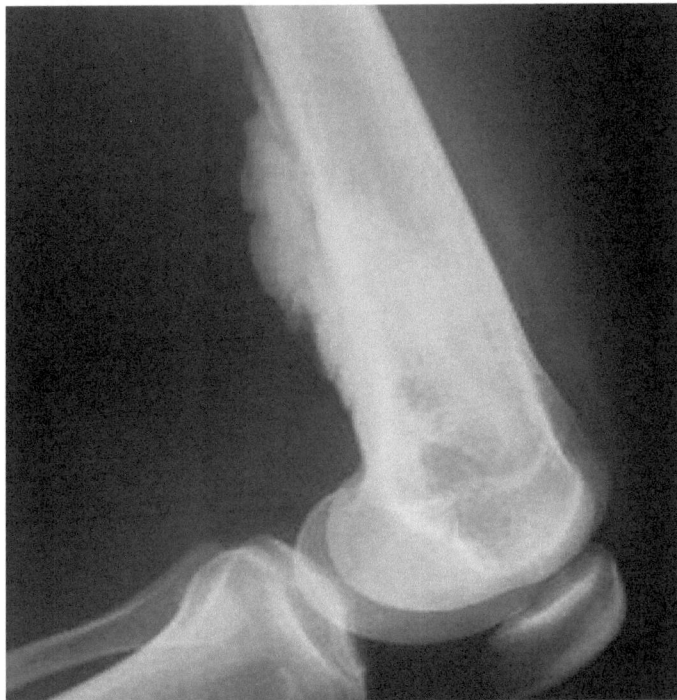

Paget's Disease: chronic disorder of excessive bony remodeling. Three phases: lytic (active), mixed (active), sclerotic (inactive). Polyostotic disease is more common than monostotic disease.

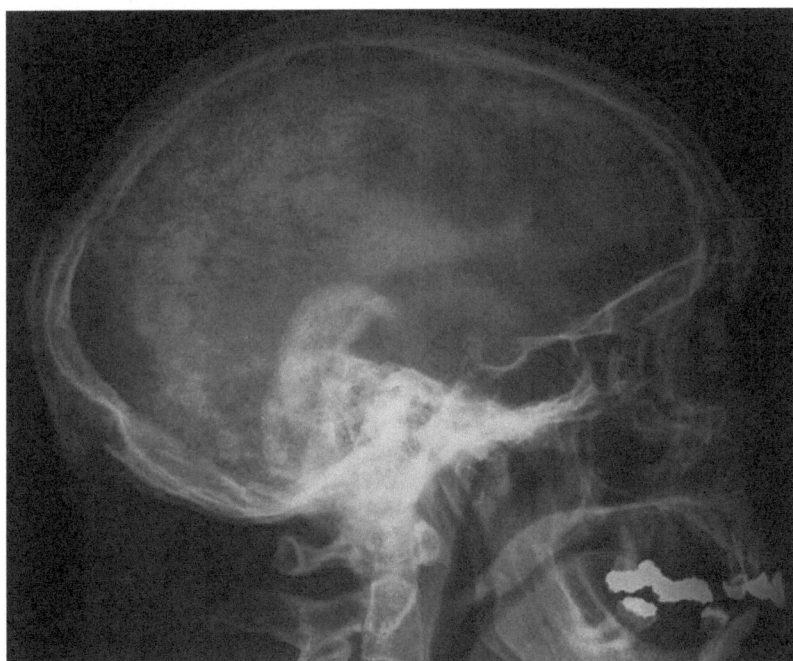

Skull – osteolysis is frequently seen as well-defined large areas of lucency usually in the frontal and occipital bones – osteoporosis circumscripta.

Spine – was discussed above, but cortical thickening and vertebral body enlargement is noted.

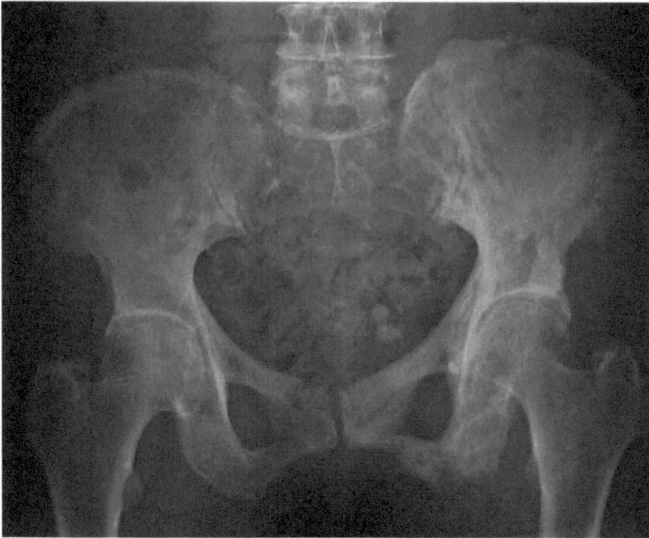

Pelvis – cortical thickening and sclerosis of the iliopectineal and ischiopubic lines in an asymmetric fashion with enlargement of the pubic rami as well.

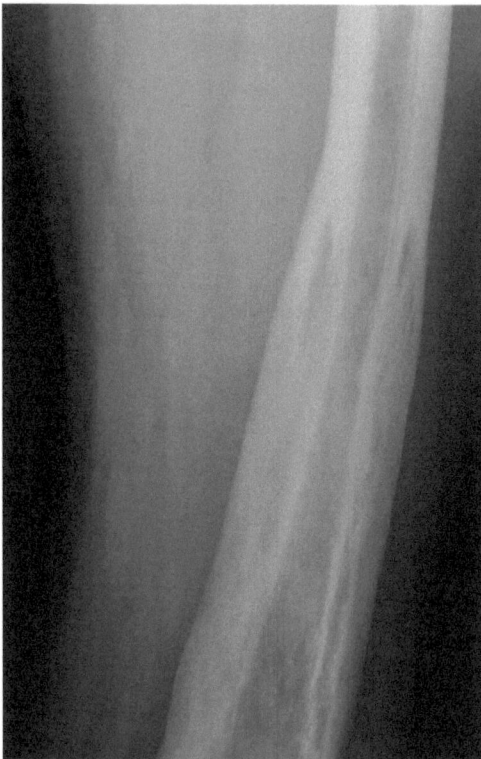

Long bones – osteolysis begins as a subchondral lucency with progression in a wedge shaped defect forming a "blade of grass" margin.

Paget's can have sarcomatous transformation, more common in patients older than 60 years old. The most characteristic finding in sarcomatous transformation is osteolysis causing focal destruction.

Bisphosphonate Bump: look for this in the characteristic location of the lateral subtrochanteric femoral cortex. Bisphosphonates are commonly given to patients with multiple myeloma and a bump in this region is at risk for pathologic fracture.

MSK ULTRASOUND: US displays the internal architecture of tendons better than any modality. A normal tendon when imaged appropriately should be a bright closely spaced bundle of linear reflections.

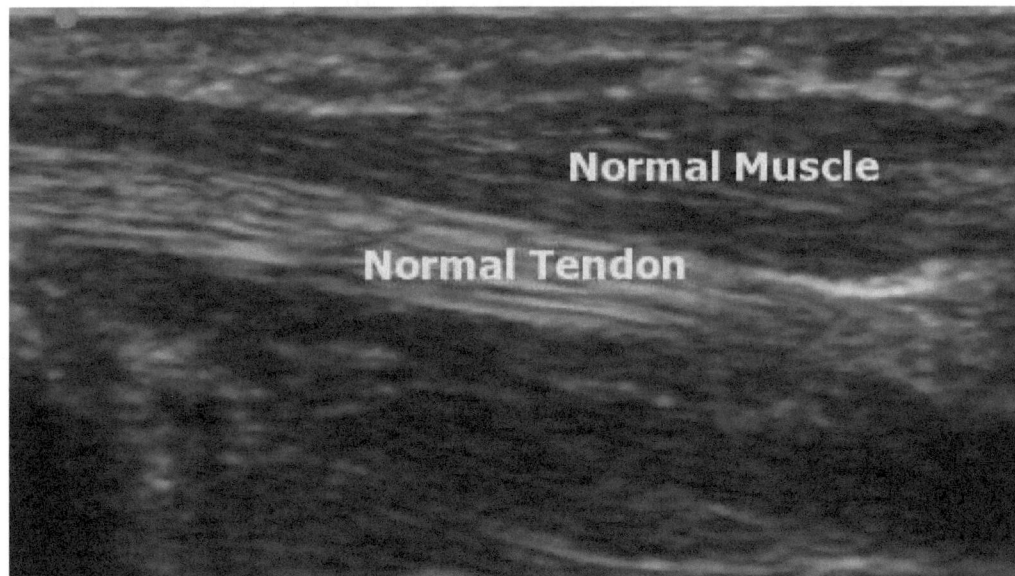

Shoulder: this basic image is going to be enough to answer many questions about the shoulder. Most questions I've encountered are geared towards supraspinatus injury, calcific tendinopathy, or bursitis.

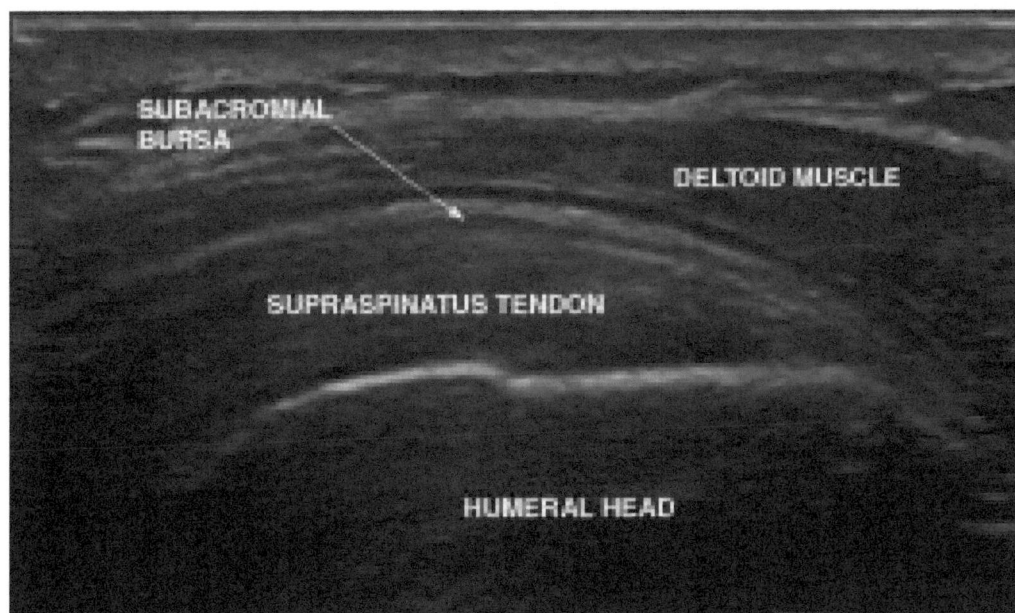

Calcific Tendinitis: patients can develop calcification within the substance of the rotator cuff, which can be painful. Ultrasound is the most accurate way to identify, quantify, and characterize rotator cuff calcifications. Like calcium anywhere in the body, this will be hyperechoic with posterior shadowing.

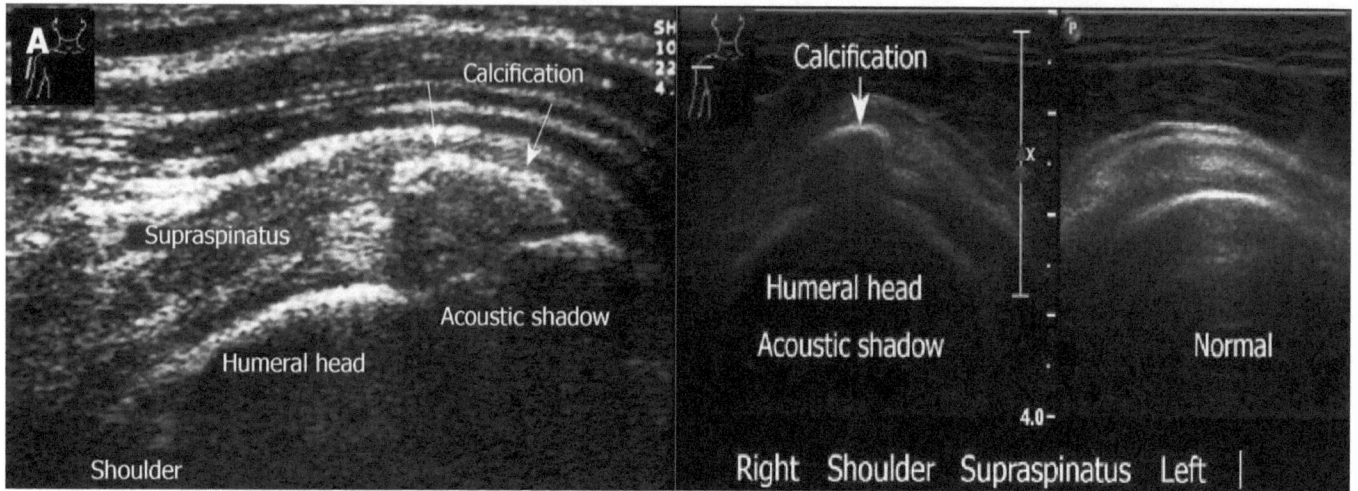

Supraspinatus Tear: can be partial thickness (left) or full thickness (right). The key is to look for fluid in the subacromial subdeltoid bursa, which would point to a full thickness tear. Also look for a retracted tendon – full thickness.

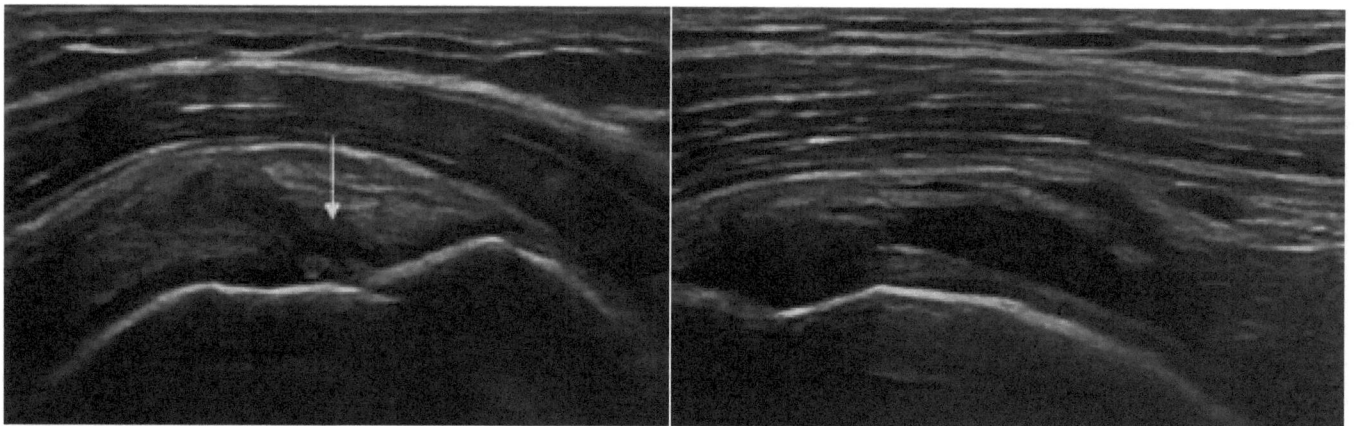

Subscapularis Tear: the significance of this tear is that the subscap holds the biceps tendon in place; if it is torn the biceps tends to sublux medially (arrows in both images).

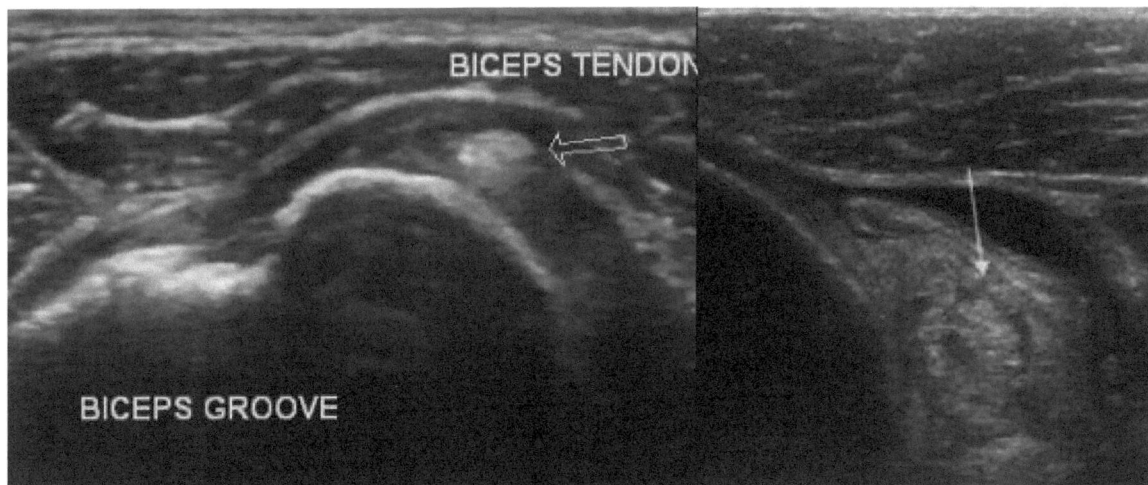

Ganglion Cyst: is the most common cause of cysts in the hands and wrists with the dorsal wrist being the most common location. Dorsal ganglia usually arise from the scapholunate joint and are comprised of thick gelatinous liquid. They will be anechoic with well–defined walls and through transmission.

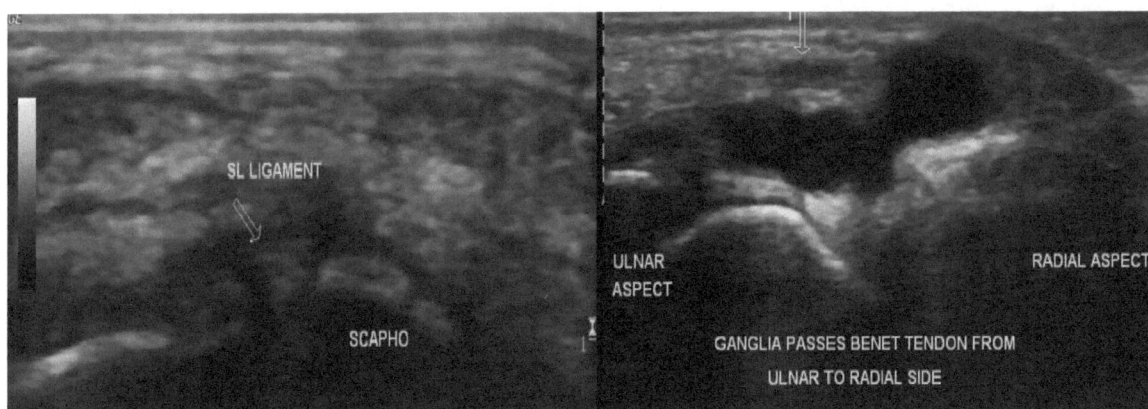

Trigger Finger: stenosing tenosynovitis that develops from repetitive microtrauma due to frequent flexion and extension movements of the fingers. This results in thickening of the A1 pulley leadding to stenosing tenosynovitis of the flexor tendons. Patients find it difficult to straighten or bend the affected finger, the finger locks in flexion and snaps with extension. Arrow points to the thickened A1 pulley.

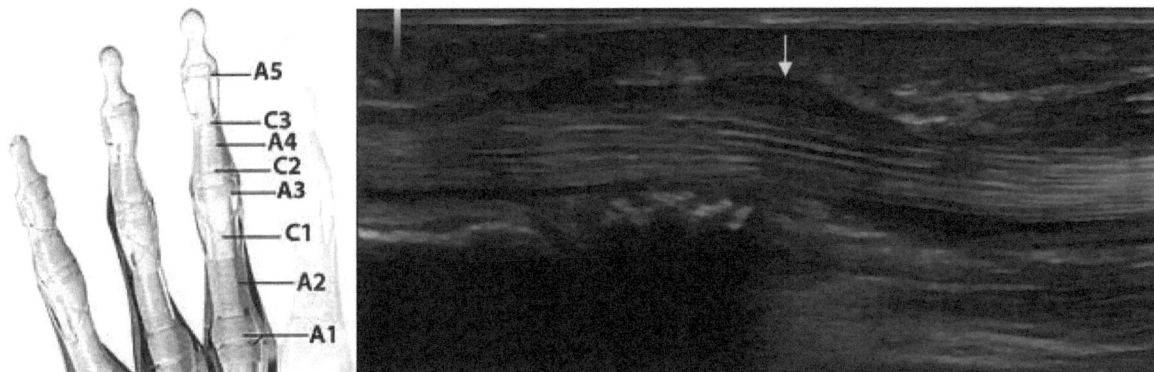

Rectus Sheath Hematoma: hemorrhage in the abdominal wall can be in the rectus sheath or in the muscle. It is limited to one side by the linea alba (seen in the image below) but when large it can extend below the umbilicus it can cross the midline. They are usually seen in patients on anticoagulation or those with trauma.

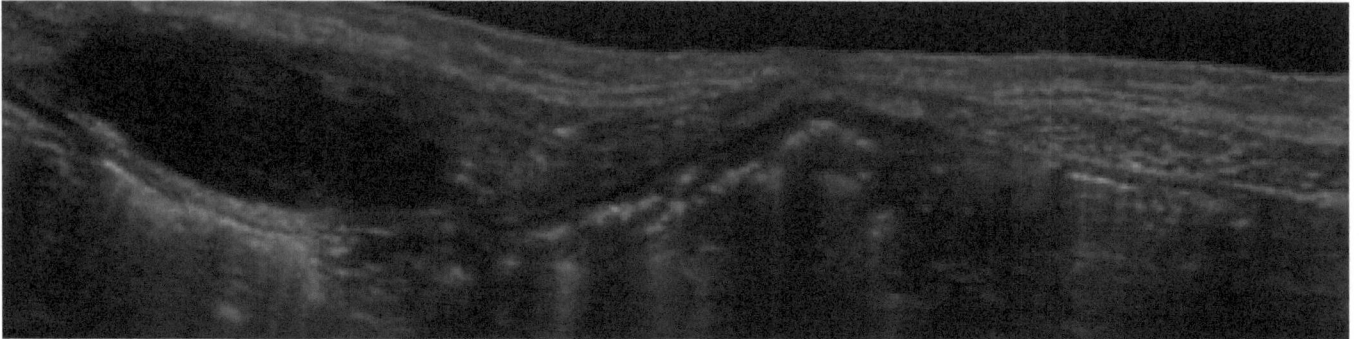

Soft Tissue Foreign Body: US is used to look for radiolucent foreign bodies: wood, glass, and plastic. Foreign bodies can be a source of pain and infection so it is important to find them and take them out. All foreign bodies appear as *linear bright reflectors*. Glass and metal can show ring–down artifact.

Surrounding hyperemia may be present.

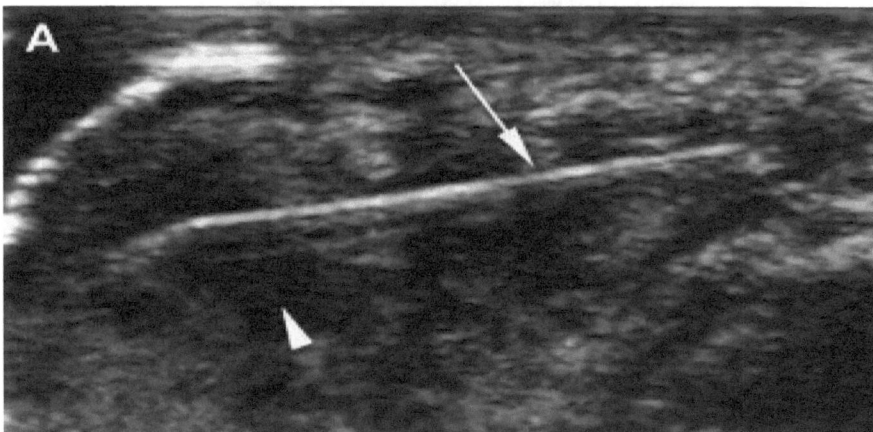

Baker's Cyst: is a cystic distention of a bursa located posterior and medial to the knee arising between the gastrocnemius and semimembranosus muscles communicating with the knee joint. The key diagnostic feature is the neck of the cyst, which courses between the two muscles.

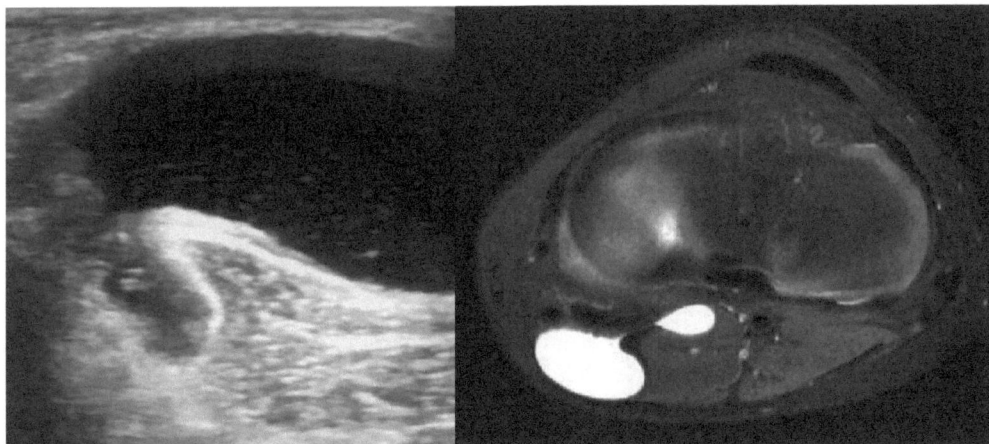

Tenosynovitis: refers to an inflammation of the tendon sheath and can be due to a variety of etiologies. This includes primary inflammatory disorders (RA), trauma, gout, or foreign bodies. Look for fluid distending the tendon sheath and thickening of the tendon sheath. A simple tenosynovitis should have clear anechoic fluid, infectious fluid would have echoes, the case below shows pannus due to RA.

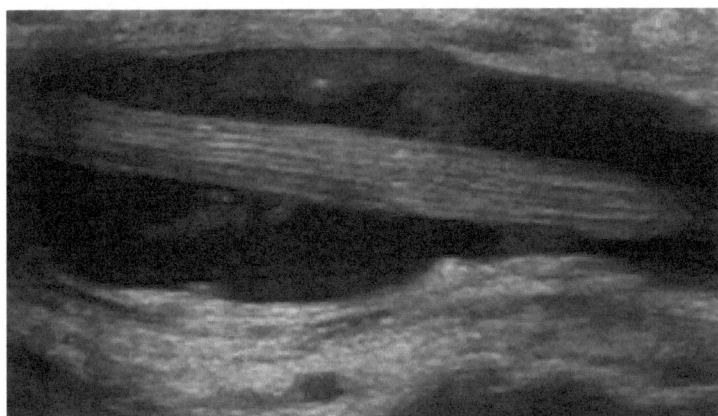

Achilles Tendinosis: this is a chronic condition due to mucoid degeneration causing tendon thickening and scarring. The Achilles is the most commonly injured tendon in the body. The first image shows a thickened tendon while the second shows a thick tendon with calcification.

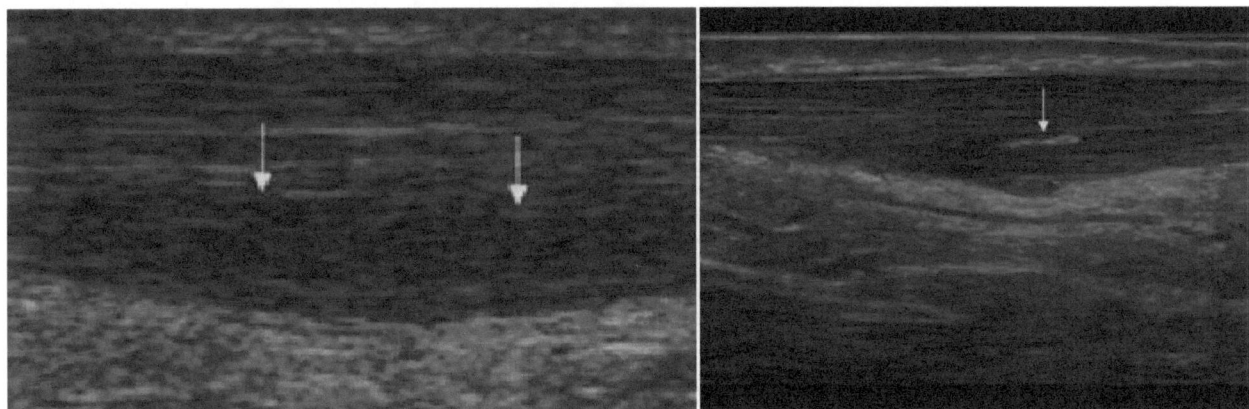

Plantar Fasciitis: is the most common cause of inferior heel pain and results from repetitive microtrauma in athletes. It is exacerbated by prolonged weight bearing and obesity. US findings are thickening and decreased echogenicity in the fascia (> 4–mm is too thick). The left image is a normal plantar fascia and the right is a thickened slightly less echogenic fascia consistent with fasciitis.

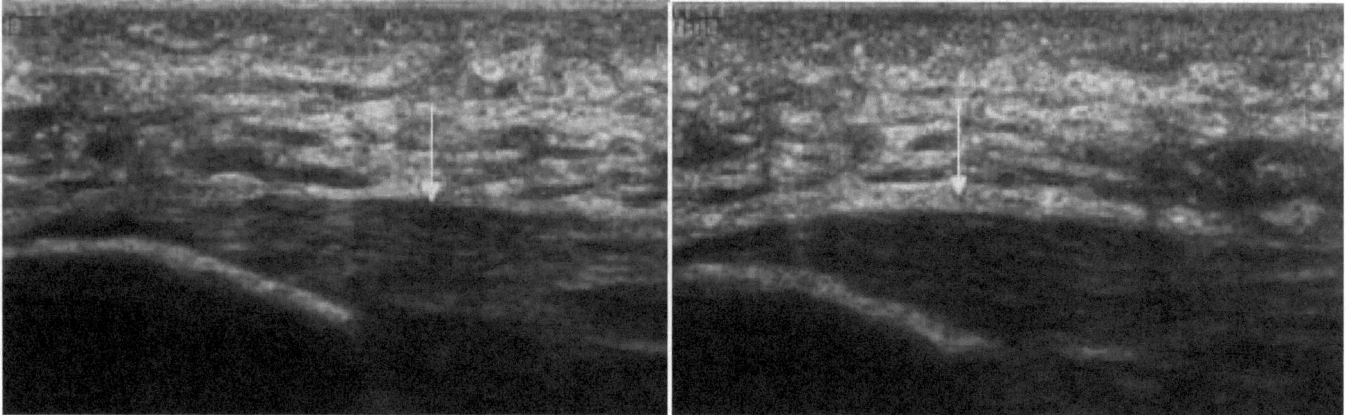

Plantar Fibromas: benign disease of fibroblast proliferation of the plantar fascia. Can be seen in kids and adults. The nodules are located in the middle of the plantar arch and may extend to involve the skin, they can be symptomatic because of mass effect and invasion of adjacent structures.

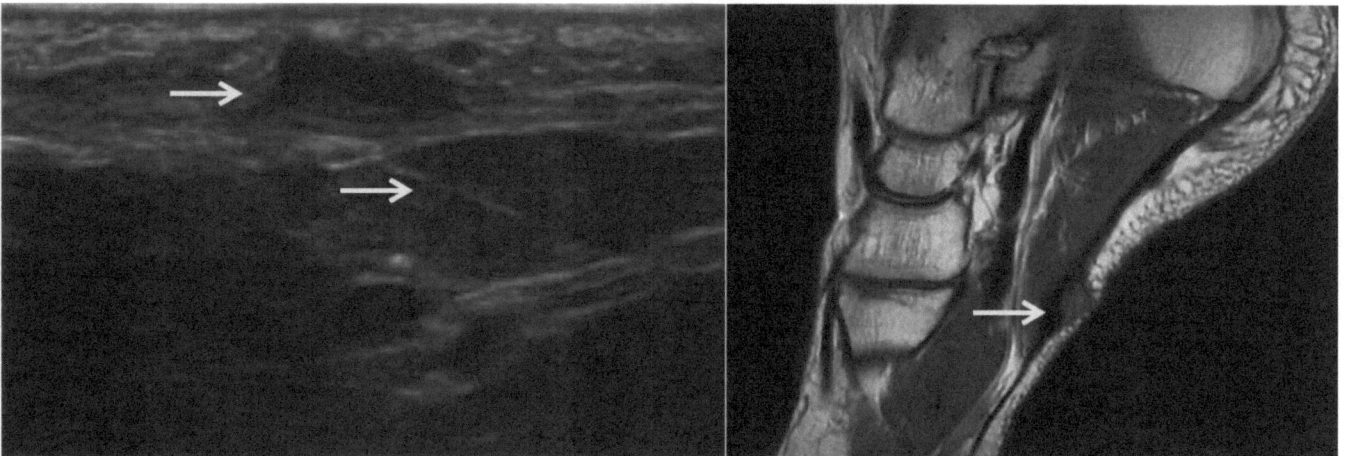

Neuro

BRAIN TUMORS: Always use location and patient age to help guide your differential. These two things above all others will help guide you in the right direction. Remember, brain tumors wont have restricted diffusion except in rare circumstances.

Adults:

Intra-axial - Supratentorial	Extra-axial
Glial Tumors (GBM is king)	Meningioma (dural tail, CE +)
Metastases (>1 lesion)	Metastases
Lymphoma (periventricular with solid CE in normal person or ring enhancing in HIV)	

Below are the adult supratentorial tumors. Starting with Gliomas of which there are 4 types.

1. Astrocytomas: most common and deadliest is GBM and most benign is Pilocytic Astrocytoma

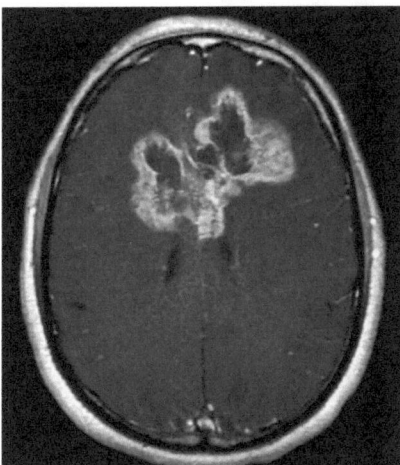

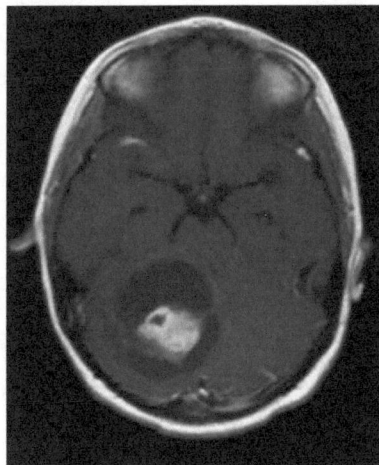

GBM   Pilocytic Astrocytoma

2. **Oligodendroglioma:** prefers the frontal lobes, calcifies, and demonstrates little edema as it is a slow growing tumor.

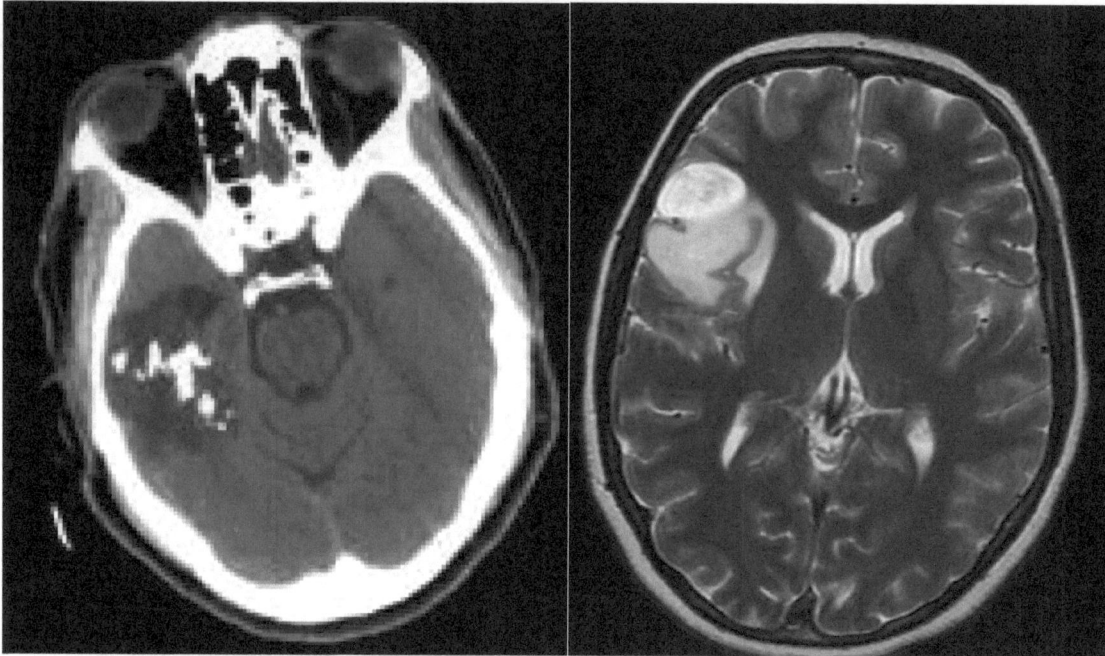

3. **Ependymoma:** Most often in the fourth ventricle, but when supratentorial, they are in the parenchyma. Will have variable appearance but, very heterogeneous with areas of cystic change, calcification, and contrast enhancement. In the 4th ventricle it tends to go out the foramen of Luschka and Magendie "plastic tumor".

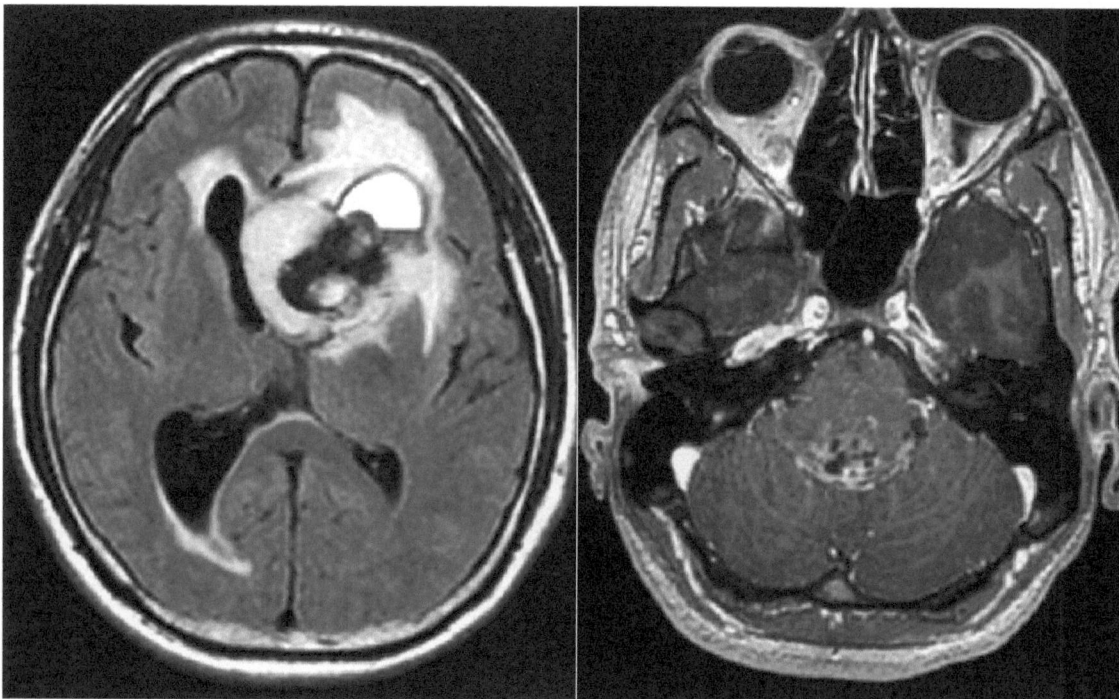

4. **Choroid Plexus Tumor:** key feature is *intraventricular location* (threw it in here because it is a glial tumor) and avid enhancement. Look for a frond like morphology. Causes significant hydrocephalus as it leads to CSF overproduction. Has an association with VHL.

Fun fact: In adults this tends to be in the 4th ventricle, but in kids it'll be in the lateral ventricle.

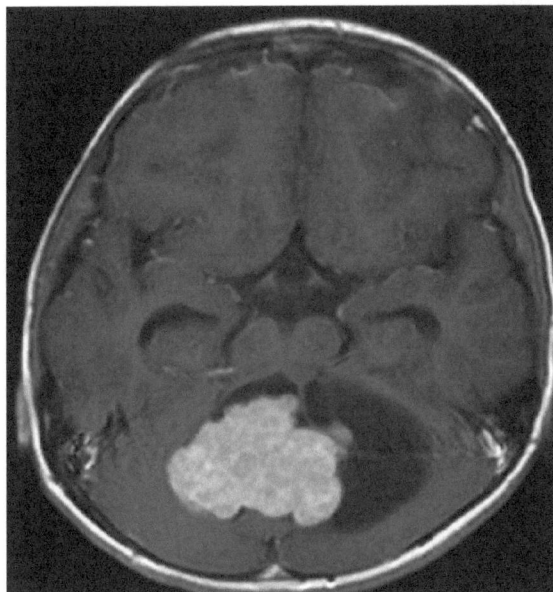

5. **Brain Metastases:** The number one intracranial neoplasm. 80% are from lung, breast, melanoma, renal cell, and GI tumors. Variable appearance, likes the grey-white interface and likes to bleed. Usually marked CE and surrounding edema. If you see multiple masses, think mets!

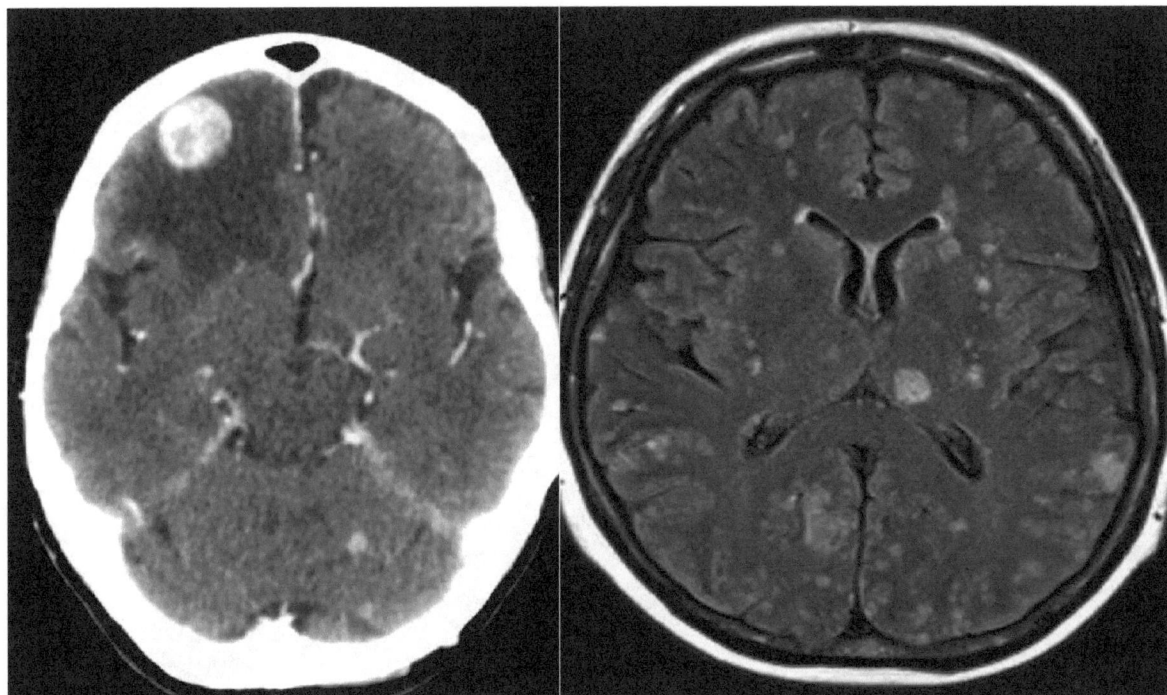

6. **Lymphoma:** involves the corpus callosum and periventricular regions. In fact when you see a corpus callosum lesion, think GBM or Lymphoma! *Homogeneous low signal on T2*, enhances variably in normal person, ring enhanced in HIV.

Important to remember that a ring-enhancing lesion in the brain of a HIV infected individual is either toxo or lymphoma. So get a Tl-201 scan – it'll be hot in lymphoma.

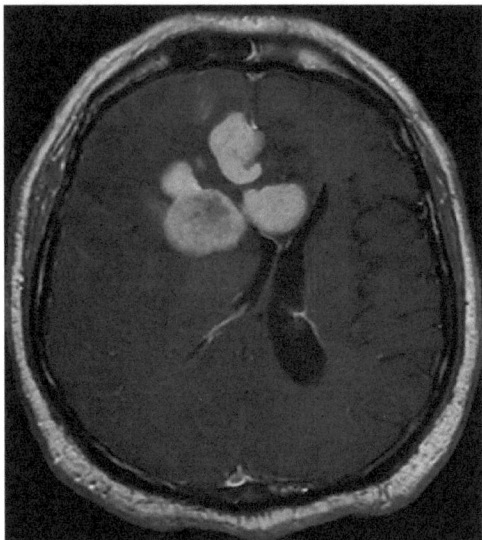

7. **Meningioma:** the most common extra-axial tumor of the brain. This is a non-glial tumor of the meninges occurring more often in women than men. Multiple meningiomas in a person under 40 should make you think of MISME and think NF-2. Intensely enhancing mass with a dural tail. RF: female, prior XRT, syndromic.

Intraventricular meningioma is almost always located in the **trigone of the ventricle.**

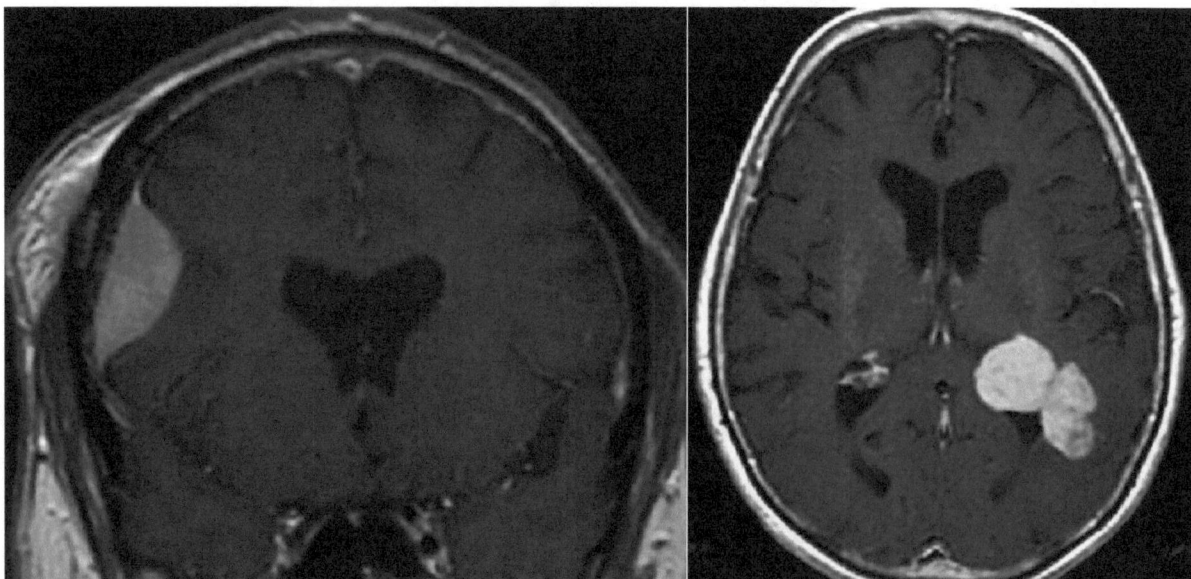

Infra-tentorial Intra-axial
Metastases – see above
Hemangioblastoma – cyst with mural nodule, seen in VHL
Astrocytoma – see above

Hemangioblastoma: Uncommon tumor overall (but most common adult primary infratentorial mass), associated with VHL (patient will have multiple). Majority are in the cerebellar hemisphere. Typically a sharply demarcated mass composed of a cyst with an enhancing nodule. Nodule enhances brightly, cyst wall doesn't enhance. Calcium is uncommon.

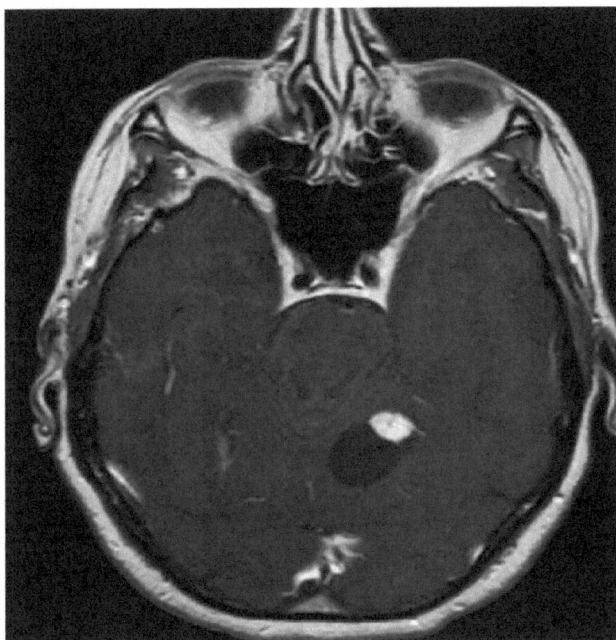

PEDIATRIC:

Supra-tentorial Intra-axial
Pilocytic Astrocytoma – by far the most common
Ependymoma – review discussion above – most common 4th ventricle mass in kids
Atypical Rhabdoid Tumor (ATRT) – bad apple, very aggressive

1. **Pilocytic Astrocytoma:** low grade WHO Grade I tumors with good prognosis. If you see optic nerve involvement, especially bilaterally (optic gliomas) – think NF-1. Tend to have a large cyst with enhancing mural nodule – textbook appearance.

Remember these are more common in the posterior fossa, but because they are the most common childhood brain CA, I put it here to start the discussion.

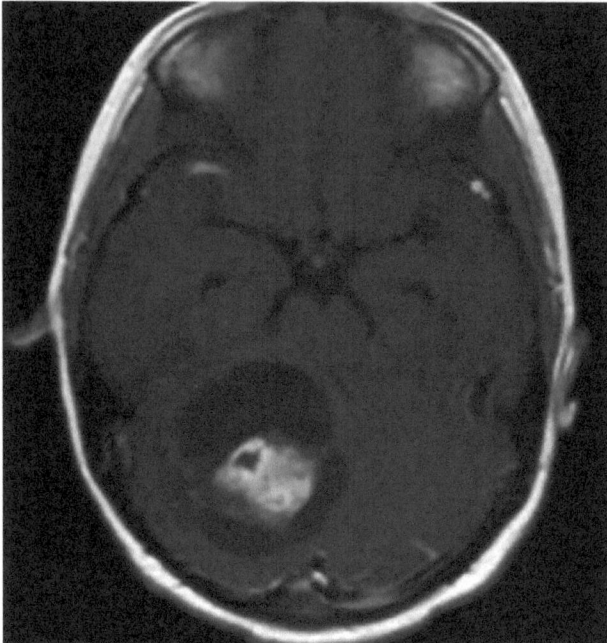

2. **ATRT:** WHO Grade IV tumor, very aggressive, looks like it is shredding the brain apart. Heterogeneous appearing mass with cystic necrosis, hemorrhage, enhancement, vasogenic edema, and calcifications.

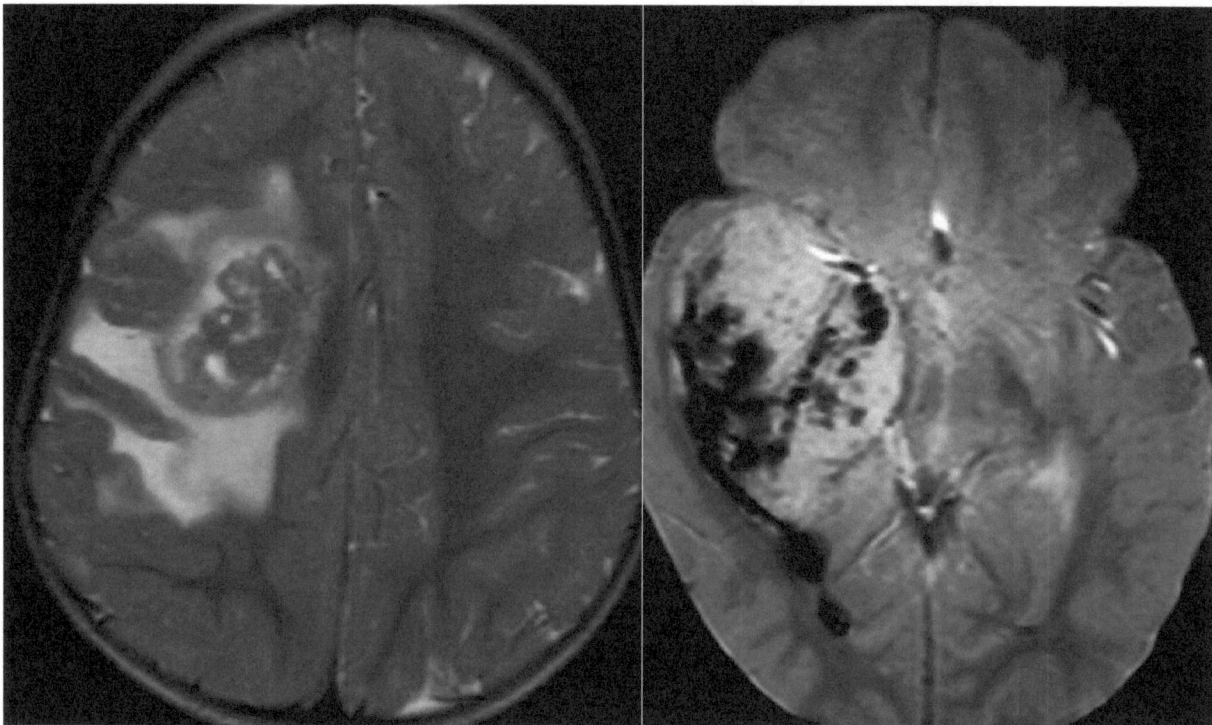

Infra-tentorial Intra-axial
Medulloblastoma – 4th ventricle invasion with leptomeningeal spread
Ependymoma – discussed above
Pilocytic Astrocytoma – tends to displace the 4th ventricle forward

Medulloblastoma: is the most common pediatric posterior fossa tumor. Rapidly growing tumor with symptoms of increased intracranial pressure from obstructive hydrocephalus.

Tends to arise from the vermis and pushes into the 4th ventricle from the roof (displaces the ventricle down and back). Hyperdense mass on NCCT. Enhances heterogeneously and has areas of calcification, necrosis, and hemorrhage.

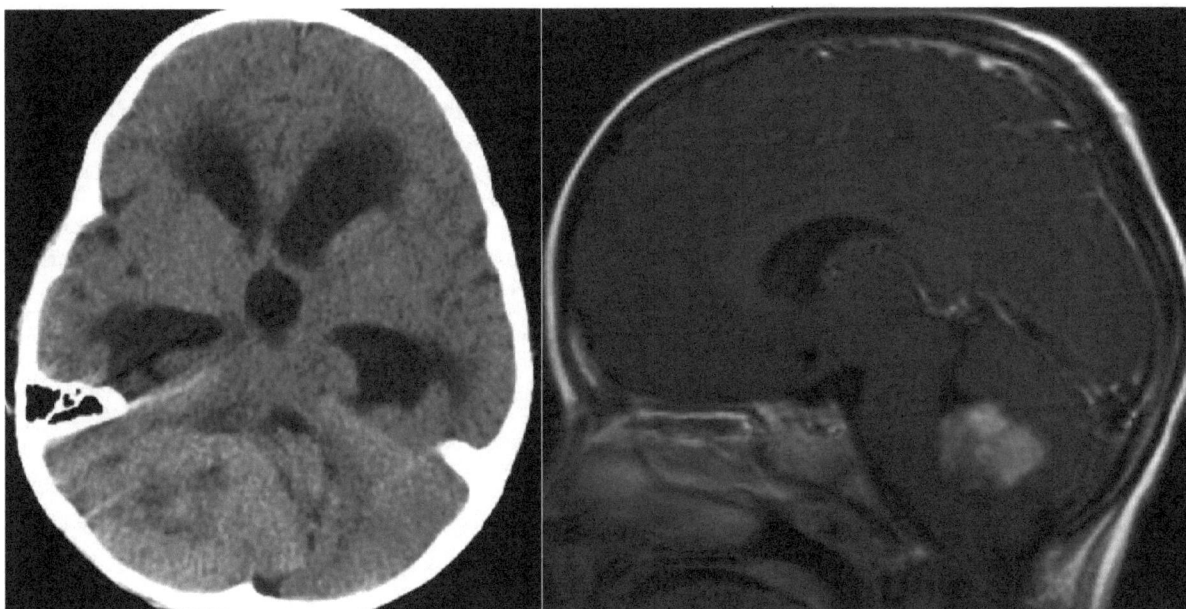

Sellar and Suprasellar
Pituitary Adenoma – benign tumor < 1 cm micro and > 1 cm macro. Symptoms based on size of lesion and hormonal activity (i.e. prolactinoma). Macroadenoma can encase carotid artery – usually only one side
Optic Glioma – strong association with NF-1
Meningioma – enhancing mass with dural tail
Germinoma – midline masses that either occur in the pineal gland or suprasellar region. Demonstrates calcium and homogeneous enhancement.
Cranipharyngioma – midline heterogeneous with suprasellar extension, enhancing mass with mass effect on adjacent structures causing headaches and visual symptoms. On CT appreciate the calcifications. Bimodal distribution: 5-10 yo adamantinomous type and > 60 yo squamous type.
Lymphoma – enlargement of pituitary gland and enhancement. Remember that lymphoma is low intensity on T2.
Rathke's Cleft Cyst – mucoid containing cyst most often in the pars intermedia (center of the gland). High T1 and T2. No contrast enhancement.

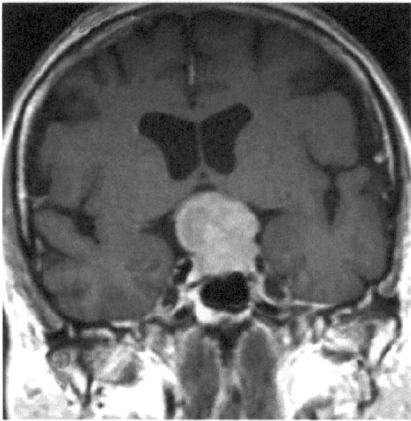

Macroadenoma

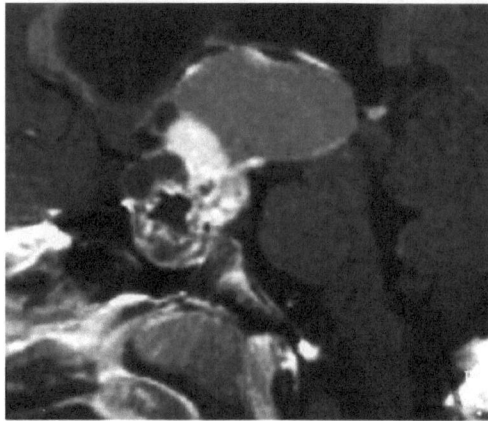

Craniopharyngioma

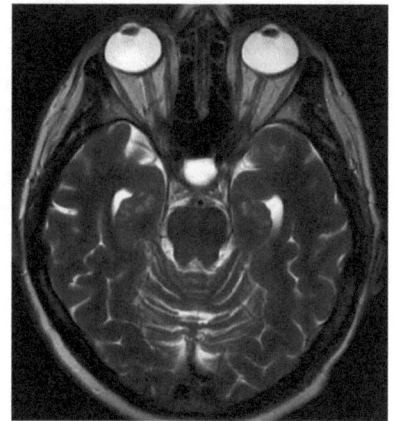

Rathke Cleft Cyst

Pineal Region – calcifications in this region in kids are a good indicator of mass because kids shouldn't have calcifications of the pineal before age 7 and only in 10% up to age 14
Pineocytoma – most often in the **second decade of life**, clinical presentation is from obstructive hydrocephalus and Parinaud syndrome. CT shows **peripherally dispersed calcifications** and soft tissue mass isodense to brain. Solid components will enhance!
Pineoblastoma – most aggressive and highest grade pineal tumor. Tends to disseminate in CSF. Can be associated with retinoblastoma (triretinal retinoblastoma). Similar symptoms to pineocytoma. Peripheral calcifications similar to pineocytoma. Present as much larger than pineocytoma > 4 cm. Heterogeneous enhancement. Kids.
Germinoma - midline masses that either occur in the pineal gland or suprasellar region. Demonstrates **central calcium** and homogeneous enhancement. Kids.

Patterns of calcification of pineal tumours

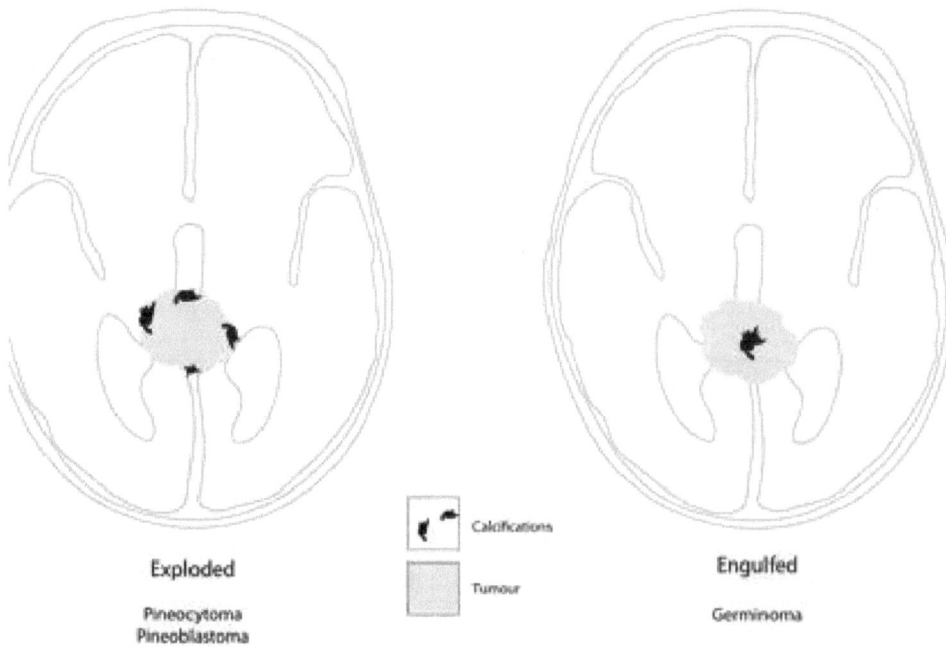

Exploded

Pineocytoma
Pineoblastoma

Calcifications

Tumour

Engulfed

Germinoma

Fun Facts:

I.   Tumors that disseminate:

  – ATRT
  – Medulloblastoma (tons of leptomeningeal nodules)
  – Pineoblastoma
  – Germinoma
  – Ependymoma
  – Choroid Plexus CA

II. Tumors that calcify:

  – Pineal tumors
  – Oligodendroglioma
  – Meningioma
  – Ependymoma

III. Tumors that demonstrate restricted diffusion:

  – Epidermoid
  – Mucinous adenoCA
  – Lymphoma

IV: Dermoid tumors are fatty tumors that are typically in the midline. They can rupture and cause a chemical meningitis. Look for high T1 signal droplets in the cisterns.

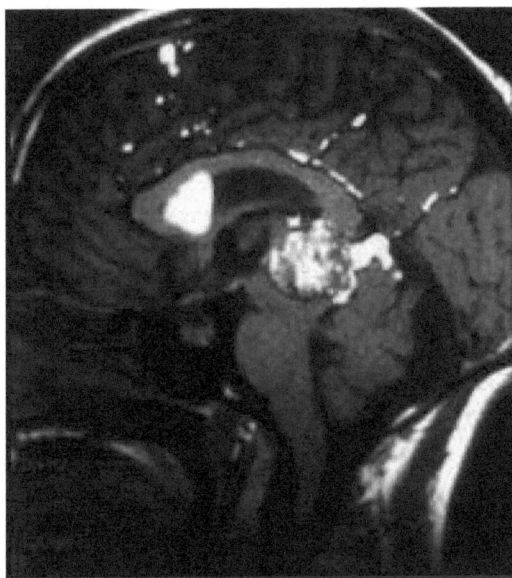

Lipomas are also midline masses with high T1 signal. Can sit on top of the CC and follow its contour. Ant – ass with CC dysgenesis and more tumefactive than posterior ones which tend to be more ribbon like.

HEAD and NECK: Breaking the spaces of the H&N into their anterior and posterior divisions as they surround the pharynx best approaches this difficult subject.

Pharynx: center of the neck around which all other spaces exist. The pharynx is lined by mucosa and lymphoid tissue (Waldeyer's Ring).

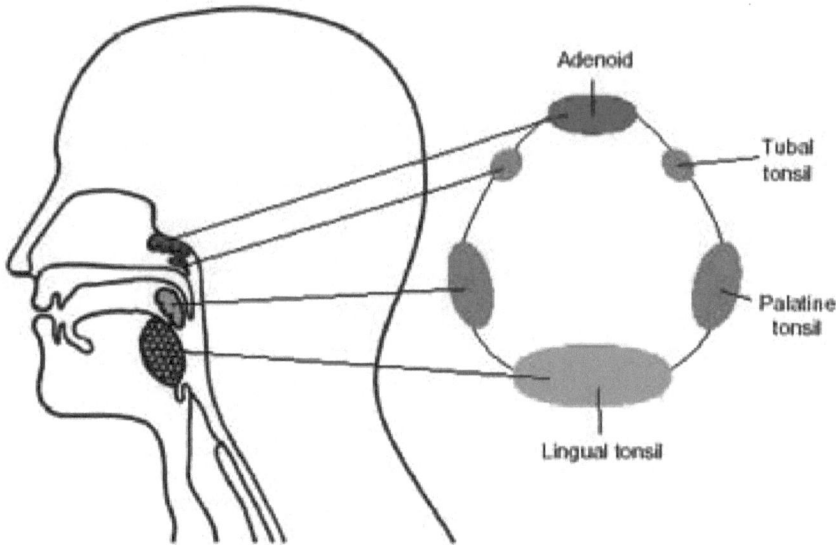

The components of the pharynx from top to bottom:

– Nasopharynx: nasal cavity to soft palate
– Oropharynx: soft palate to hyoid bone (base of tongue with lingual tonsils is part of the oropharynx)
– Hypopharynx: hyoid to cricoid

Lesions that arise in the pharynx are – SCC (99%) and LAD (mets or lymphoma)

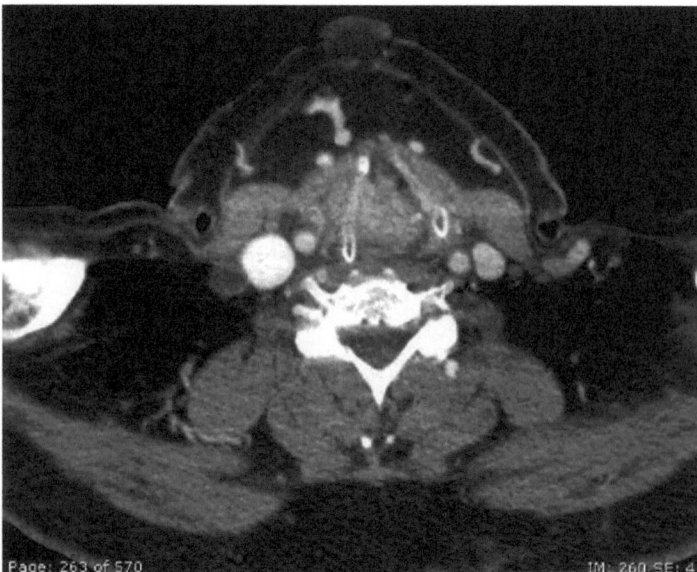

There are four anterior spaces and three posterior spaces in the neck all lined/formed by layers of the deep cervical fascia. Lesions arise from structures in the compartments.

ANTERIOR:

Masticator Space – most lateral space surrounding the muscles of mastication and extends up the temporalis muscle. Superficial layer of deep cervical fascia.

- Muscles of mastication (masseter, pterygoids, temporalis)
- Mandible (teeth and bone)
- CNV3 (mandibular division which comes through the foramen ovale)

Most of the time this will be a dental abscess, it could be a rhabdosarcoma in kids, or nerve sheath tumor.

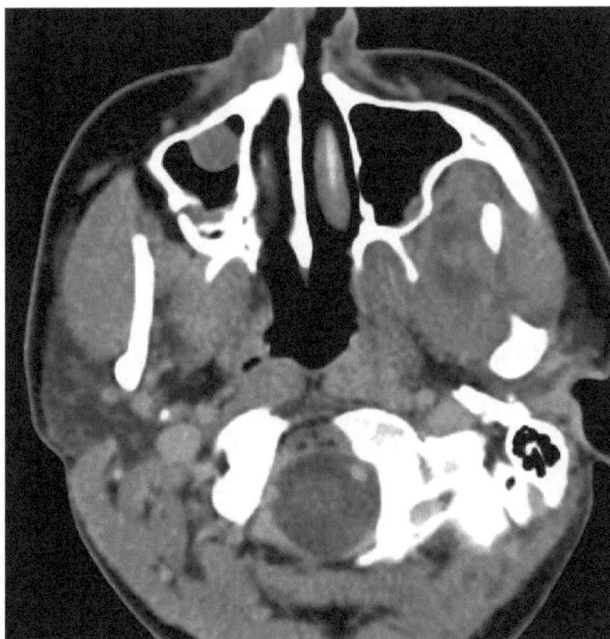

Parotid Space – Has a deep and superficial component which are relative to the location of the retromandibular vein. Superficial layer of DCF.

- salivary gland (parotid)
- lymph nodes (intra-parotid)
- CN VII (exits the stylomastoid foramen and courses lateral to the retromandibular vein – superficial lobe)

Pleomorphic Adenoma: is the most common parotid tumor and is benign. It has a small chance of malignant degeneration over time, so surgery is treatment. Warthin is also a common benign tumor. The most common tumor to have *perineural spread is a cystic adenomatoid tumor.*

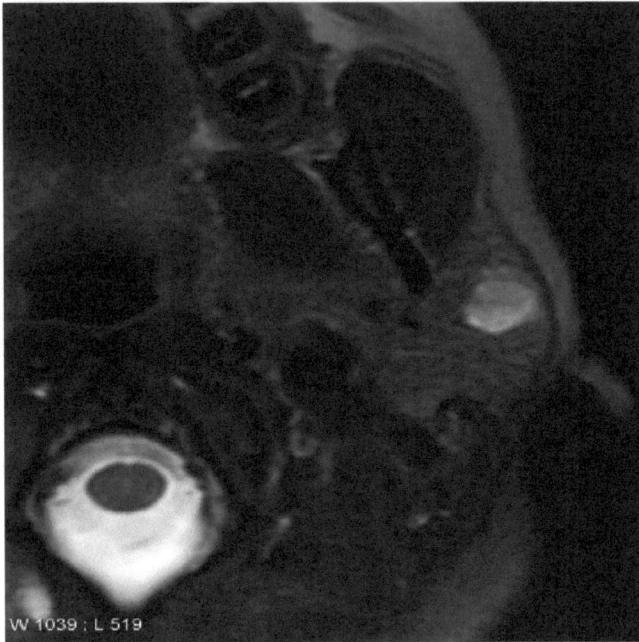

Pleomorphic adenoma is well defined and hyperintense on T2 imaging.

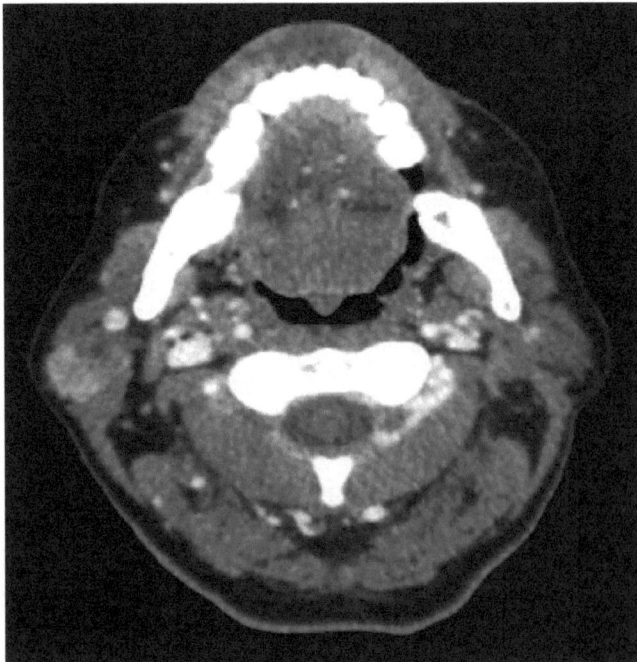

Warthin tumors are cystic masses with solid nodules and often occur bilaterally. They also tend to be in the parotid tail.

Carotid Space - Is composed of all three layers of the DCF.
- Carotid artery (carotid body tumor)
- Jugular vein (thrombosis)
- CN IX-XII (nerve sheath tumors)
- LN (LAD)

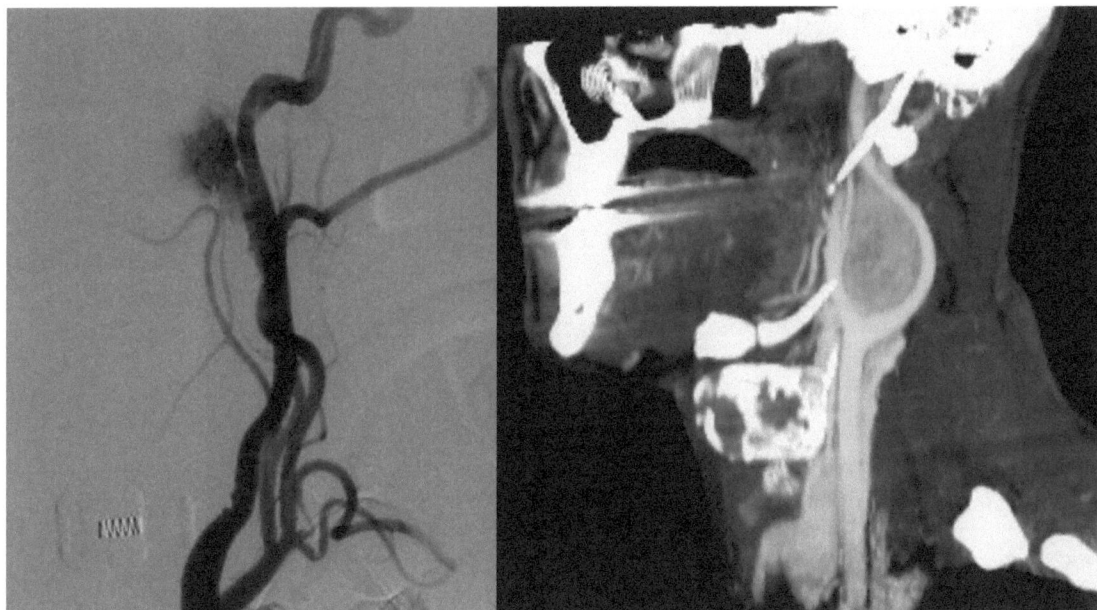

Carotid body tumors splay the ICA and ECA apart and enhance as brightly as the vessels. Fed mainly by ECA.

Parapharyngeal Space - predominantly fat composed and is located lateral to the pharyngeal mucosal space. Use the displacement of this space to localize the origin of the other masses. Most common tumor here is the pleormorphic adenoma.

POSTERIOR:

Perivertebral Space – contains the longus colli and longus capitus muscles. This is surrounded by the deep layer of the DCF.

- Vertebral bodies
- Discs
- Paraspinal muscles
- Nerves

The deep layer of the DCF is so tough that it contains masses and infections and pushes them back into the spinal canal. Look for discitis-osteomyelitis, neurofibromas and schwannomas of the nerves.

Retropharyngeal Space – this is an important area to look at because fluid and infection can track down this space and enter the mediastinum (danger space).

– LN
– Fat

Posterior Cervical Space – is located directly behind the parotid space "posterior triangle". This is where cystic hygromas happen.

– LN
– Fat

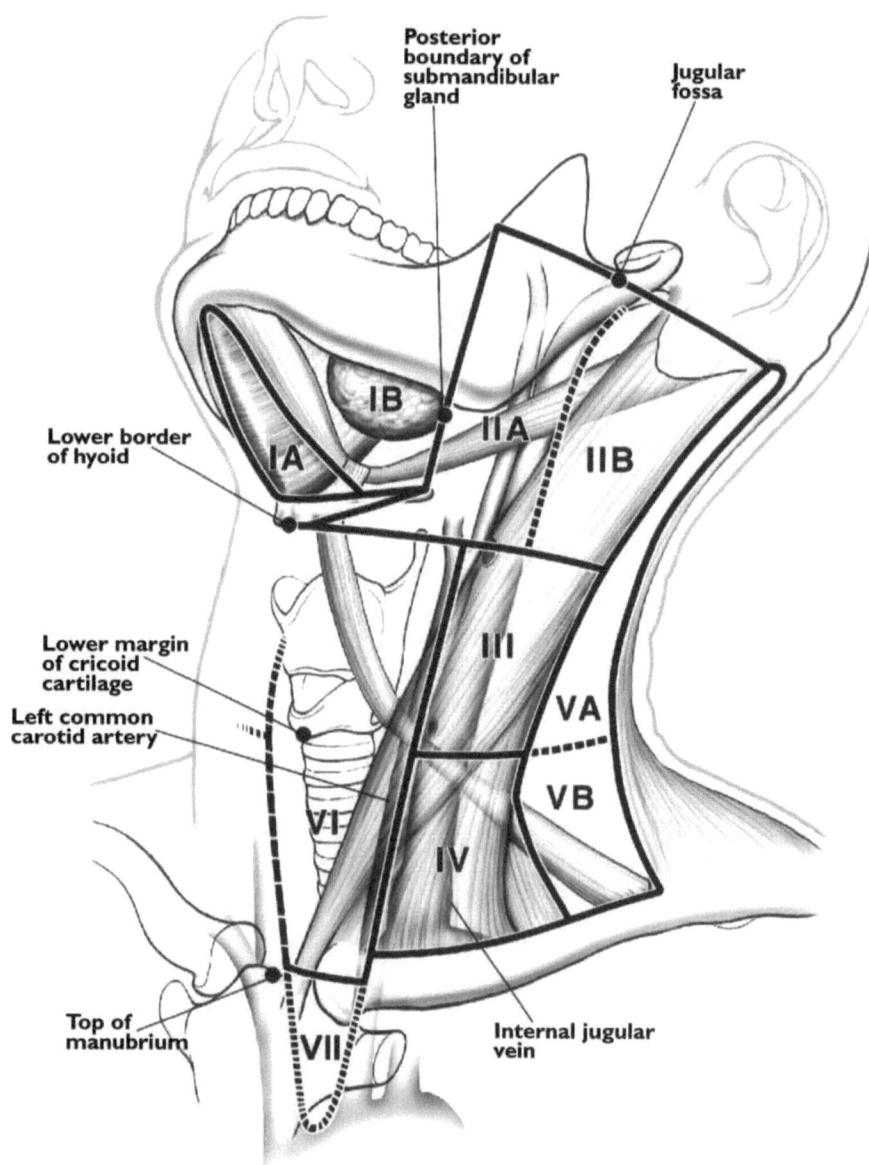

Be able to identify cervical lymph node levels on imagin

CNS INFECTION:

Basilar Meningitis: can be due to a variety of causes: TB, coccidiomycosis, cryptococcus, sarcoid and metastasis. Look for meningeal caking and enhancement. CSF needs sampling and a CXR should be checked to look for apical mass, cavity, or hilar nodes.

TB: the most common presentation of intracranial TB is meningitis. There will be diffuse basal enhancement with enhancing exudates.

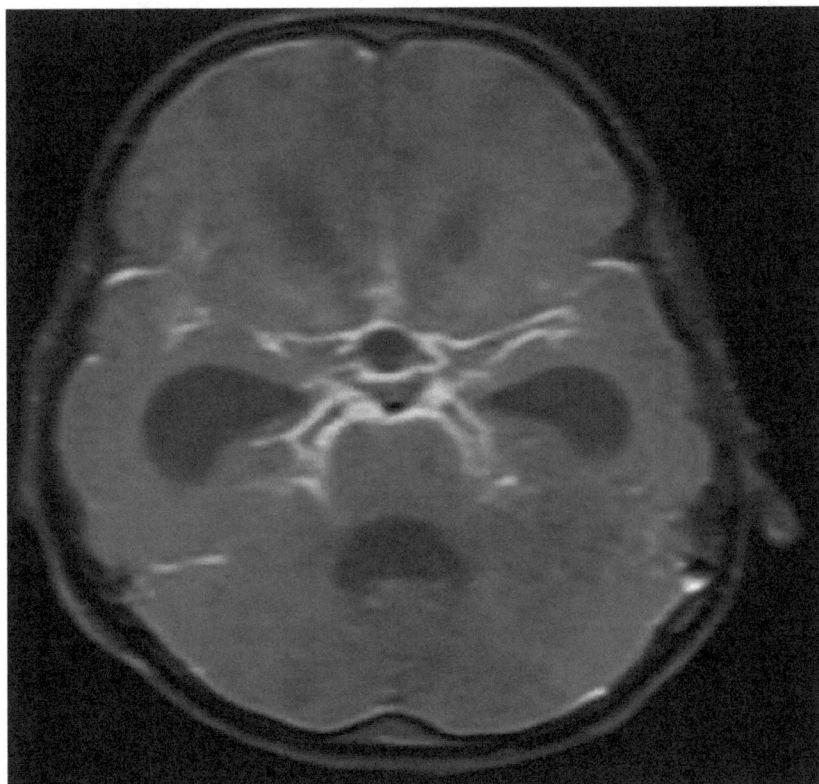

Ring Enhancing Lesions: MAGIC DR

- Metastases
- Abscess (pyogenic) – look for restricted diffusion
- Glioma
- Infarct/ Infection
- Contusion
- Demyelinating disease
- Radiation

Abscess: ring enhancing lesion with surrounding vasogenic edema and restricted diffusion.

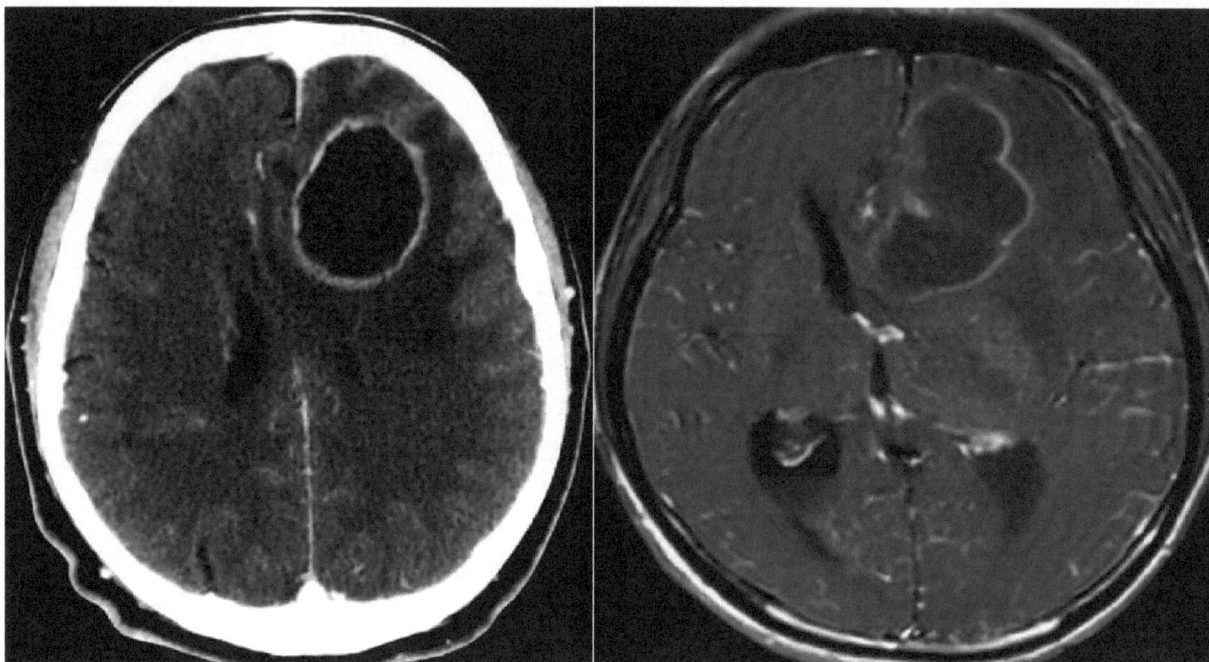

Neurocysticercosis: caused by the pork tapeworm *T. soleum*. Look for a cyst with a dot (scolex). There are usually calcifications all over the parenchyma. No restricted diffusion. Patients with hydrocephalus will commonly show a lesion in the fourth ventricle. This is the #1 parasitic infection of the CNS.

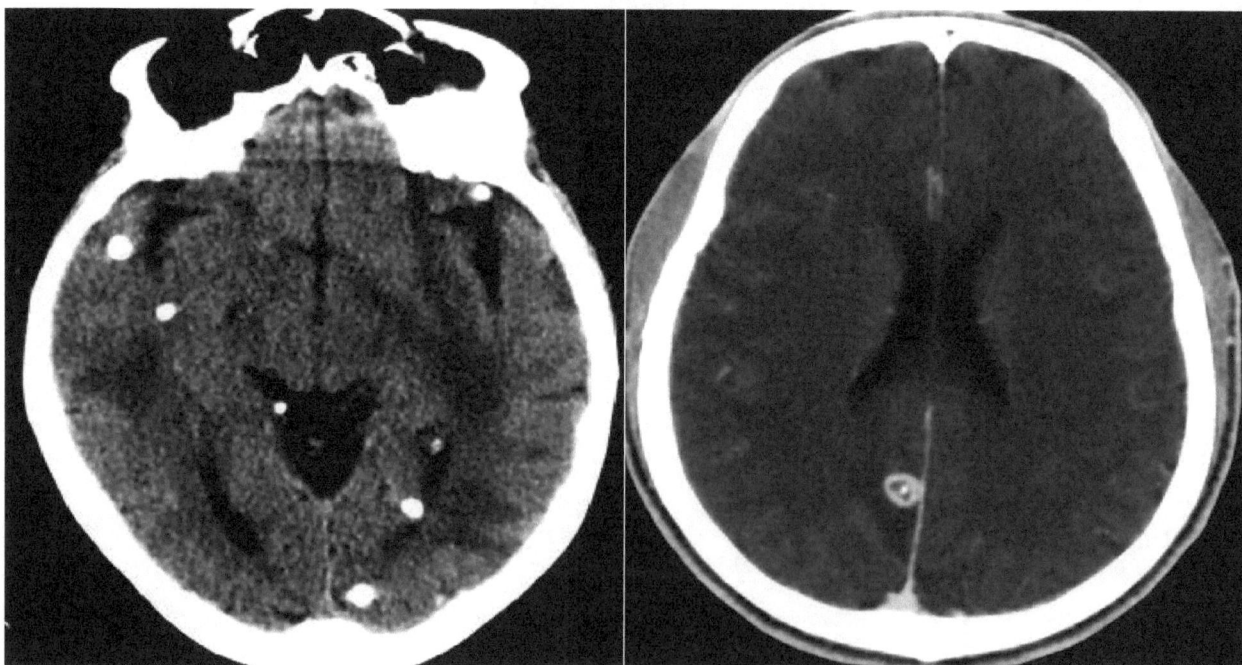

Epidural Abscess: lentiform appearance with peripheral enhancement and central fluid and restricted diffusion. Always look for adjacent brain abscess and call neurosurgery ASAP.

Herpes Encephalitis: is the most common cause of fatal sporadic viral encephalitis. HSV 1 in adults and HSV 2 in kids. The virus hides in Meckel's cave in the gasserian ganglion. Bilateral asymmetric temporal lobe involvement (limbic system).

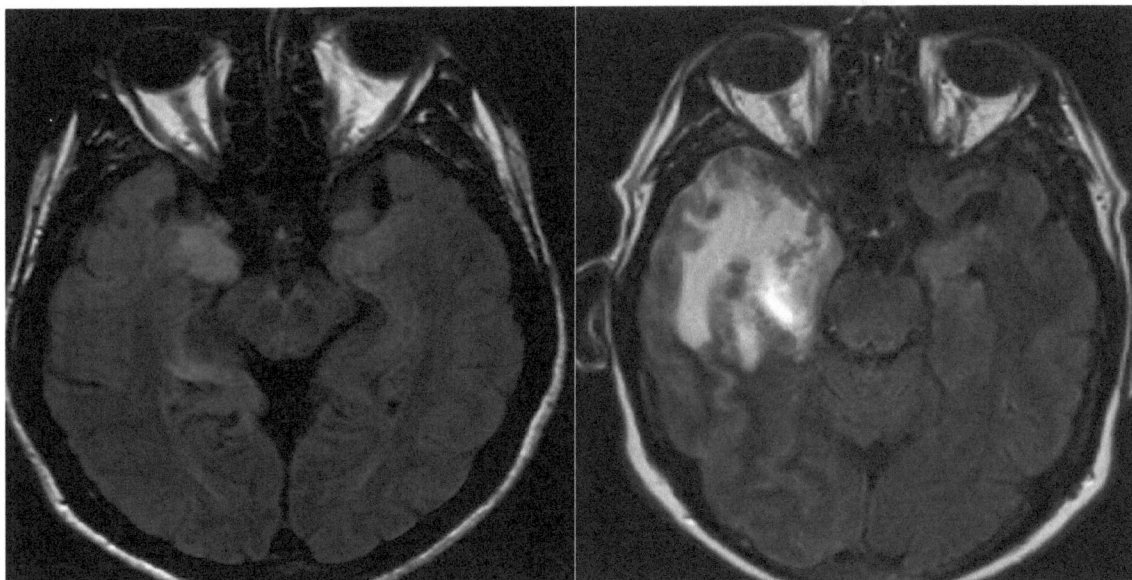

Basal Ganglia Lesions: Tricky, big differential

Infection	Toxic/Metabolic	Vascular	Neoplasm
Cryptococcus	CO Poisoning	Hypoxia	Lymphoma
Toxoplasmosis	Drugs	Infarct	
CJD	Mitochondrial		

Cryptococcus: seen in AIDS with CD4 < 100. Can cause basilar meningitis. Look for dilated perivascular spaces. Shouldn't enhance.

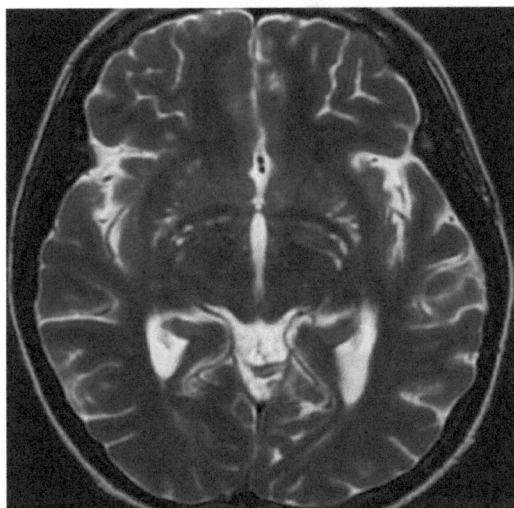

Toxoplasmosis: AIDS with CD4 < 100. Variable sized lesions with rim enhancement and eccentric target sign. No Tl-201 uptake (this is how you differentiate from lymphoma).

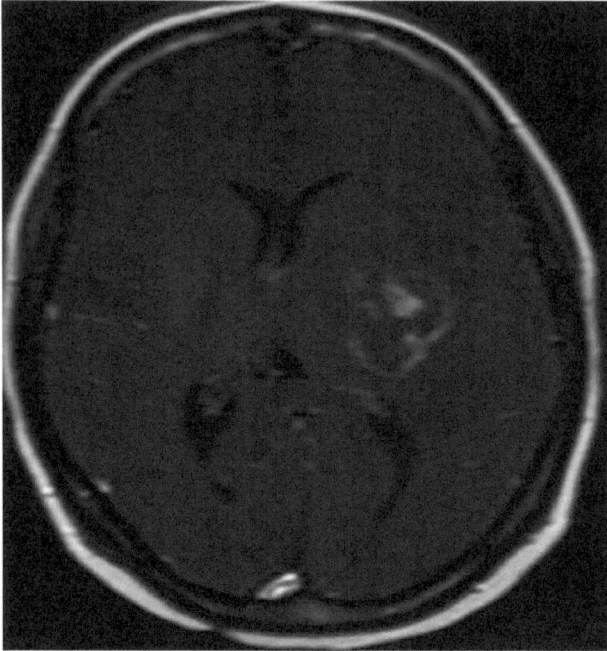

CJD: rapidly progressing dementia with basal ganglia and cerebral cortical involvement. Ribbon-like appearance with brightening of the cortex on FLAIR and DWI. Caused by prions.

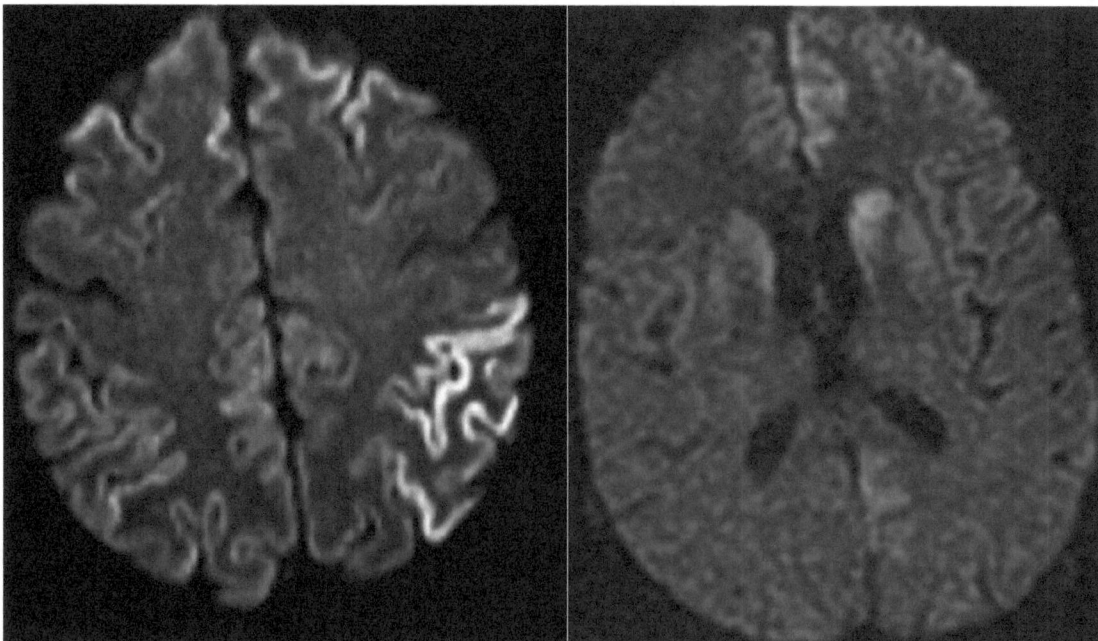

WHITE MATTER: Broad differential here as well

Infection	Vascular	Demyelination	Neoplasm
PML	Radiation	MS	Lymphoma
HIV	PRES	ADEM	
CMV			

PML: **asymmetric** white matter disease (U-fibers) caused by the JC virus. No mass effect, no enhancement. This is a fatal disease. Immunocompromised. **Patchy and peripheral!**

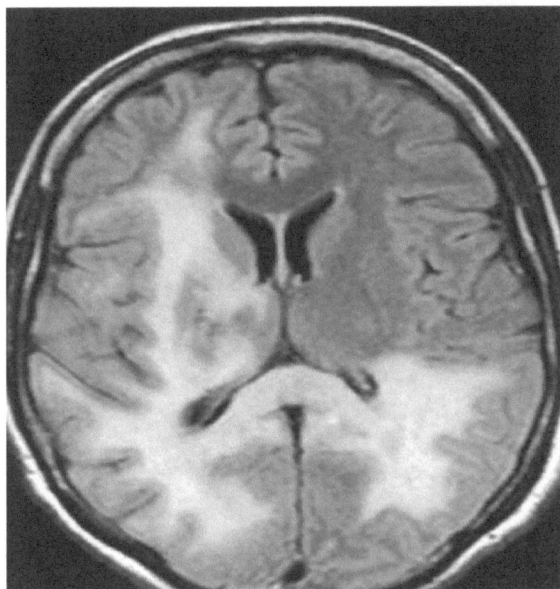

HIV Ecephalopathy: bilateral, **symmetric** white matter lesions with associated atrophy. Likes the **frontal lobes**.

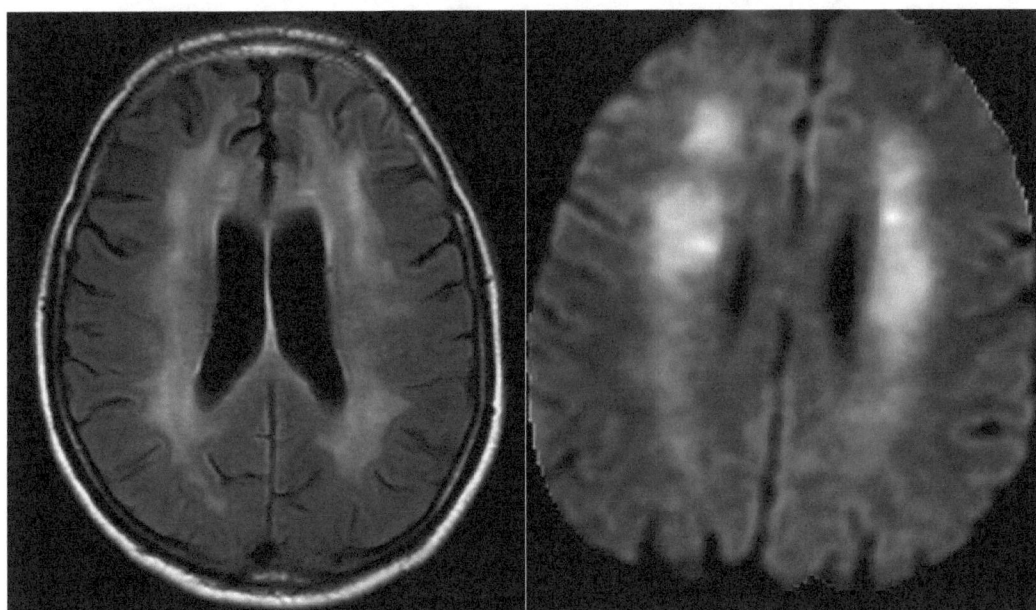

CMV: AIDS patients with CD4 < 50. It infects the entire neuroaxis (brain, cord, meninges, nerve roots, and eye). Can cause a ventriculitis that shows up as thin ependymal enhancement and hydrocephalus. Look for periventricular white matter lesions.

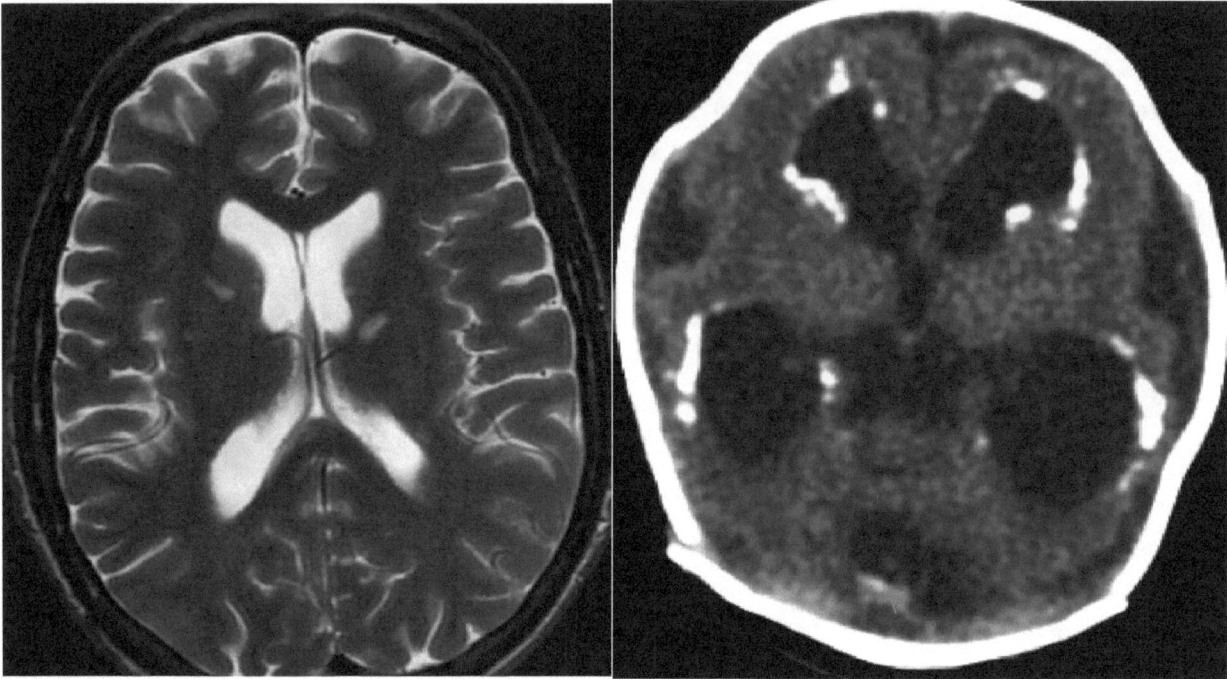

ADEM: post-vaccination or post-viral process with enhancing multiple bilateral WM lesions. Should improve with steroids. If you see it in the spine it will always be in the brain too. Increased myelin basic protein.

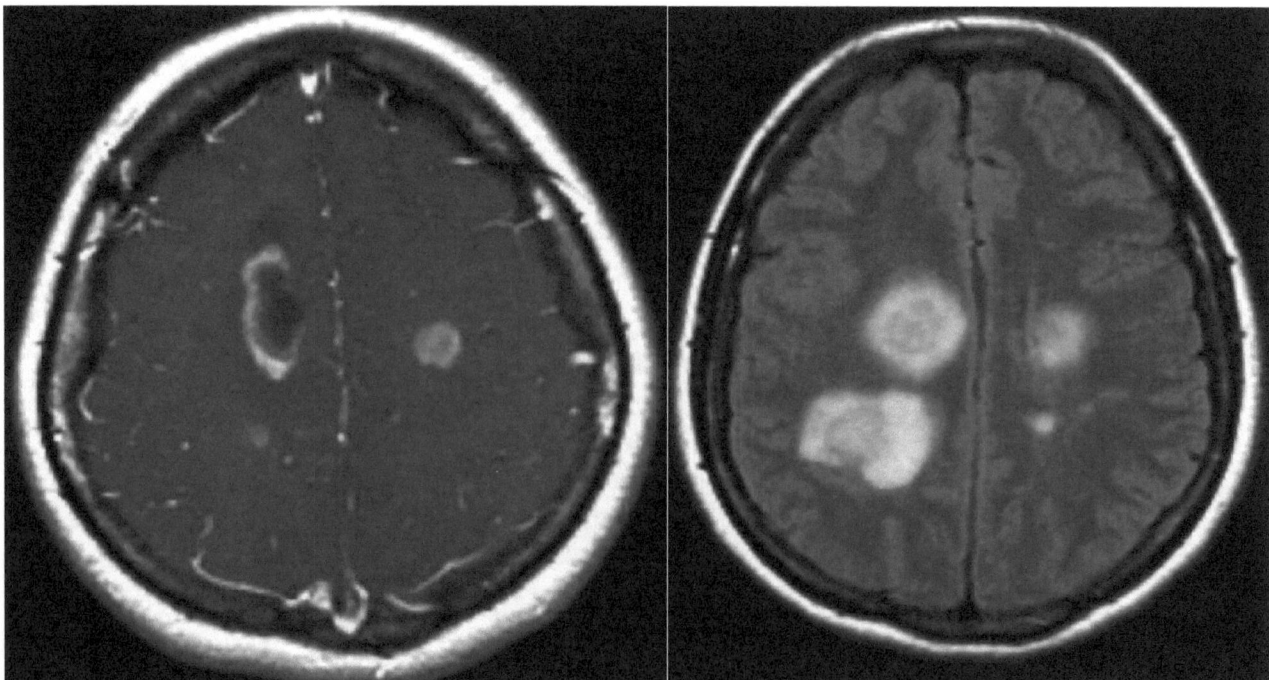

MRI Appearance of Blood:

- **Diamagnetic** materials create a magnetic field opposing B_0
- **Paramagnetic** – have an unpaired electron and these augment B_0 with slight positive susceptibility (deoxy- Hgb, metal chelates [Gadolinium], and Fe3+)
- **Ferromagnetic** – due to large groups of atoms with unpaired electrons and large local fields with positive susceptibility. These can have residual magnetization once removed from B_0 (Fe3+, Ni, Co). - **Superparamagnetic** – small particles of Fe3O4 that do not have magnetic memory like ferromagnetic materials.

Hemoglobin breakdown after hemorrhage: Oxy →→ deoxy →→ methemoglobin →→ hemosiderin →→ ferritin

Hyperacute (0-6 hours):

T1	T2	SWI
Iso- to hyperintense – protein	Hyperintense – edema	Hypointense – deoxyHgb

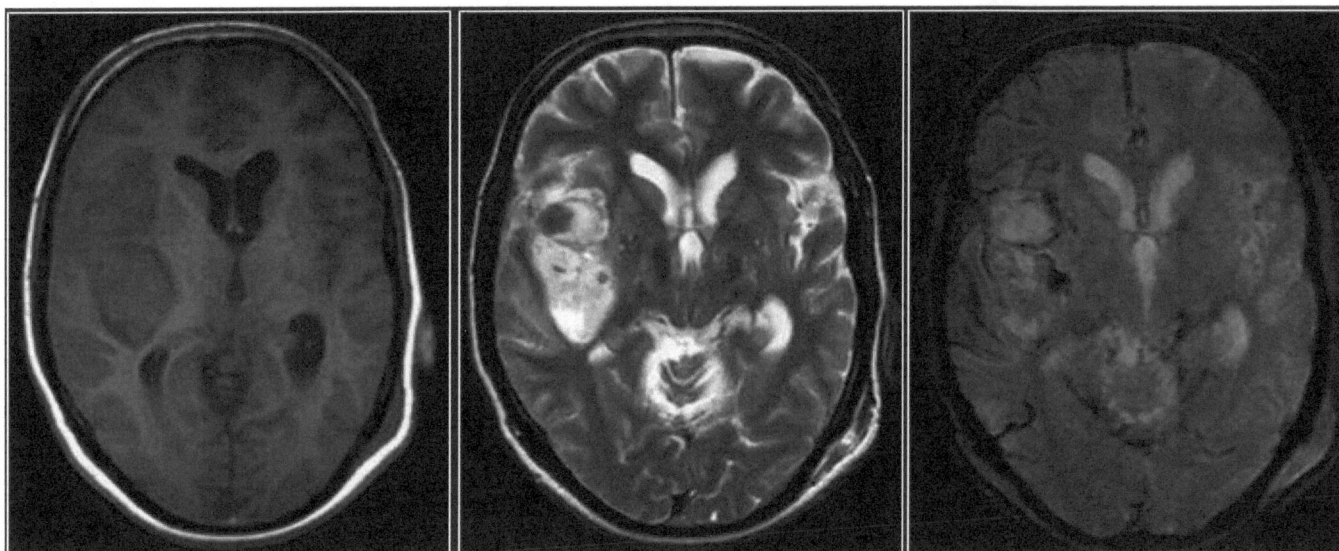

Acute (6-72 hours): progressive conversion of oxy →→ deoxy with decreased water

T1	T2
Hypointense	Hypointense

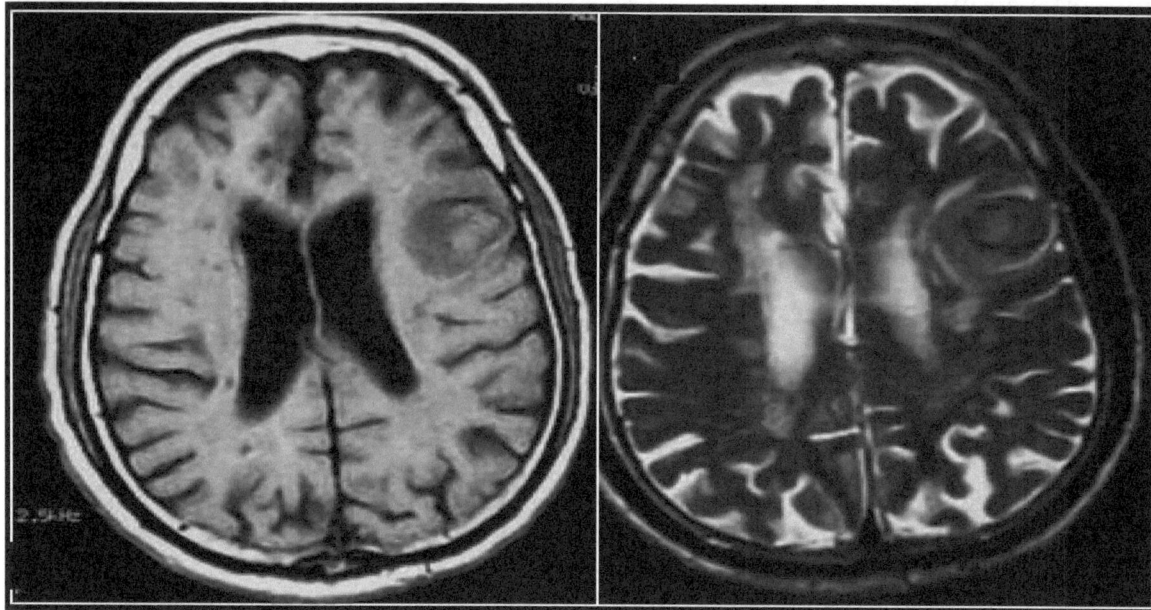

Early Subacute (3-7 days): methemoglobin with superparamagnetic effects

T1	T2
Hyperintense	Hypointense

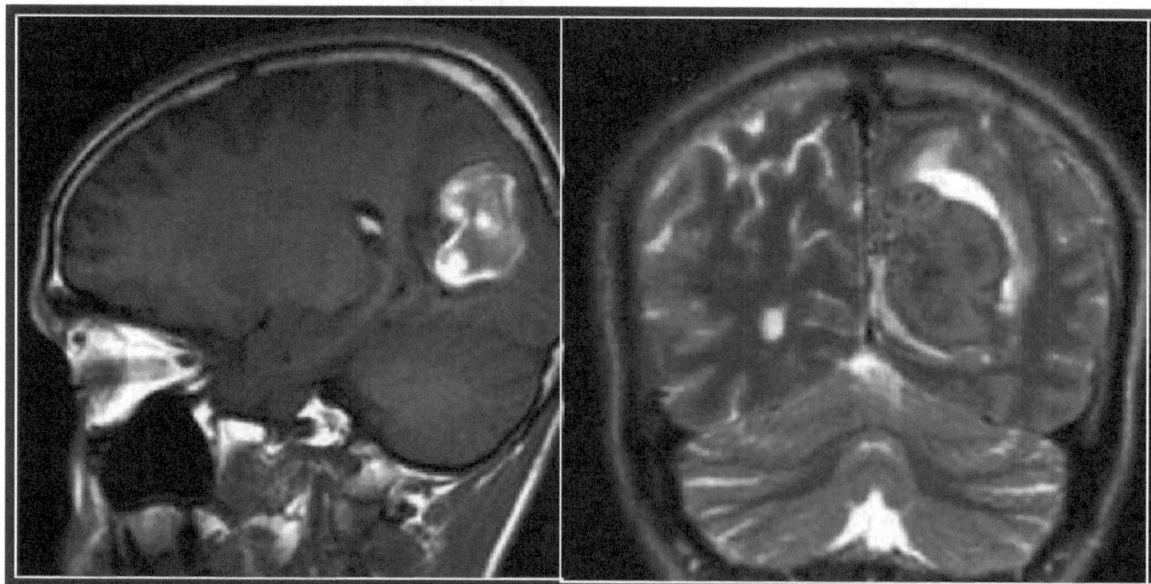

Late Subacute (7-14 days): accumulation of hemosiderin and ferritin

T1	T2
Hyperintense	Hyperintense with Hypointense periphery

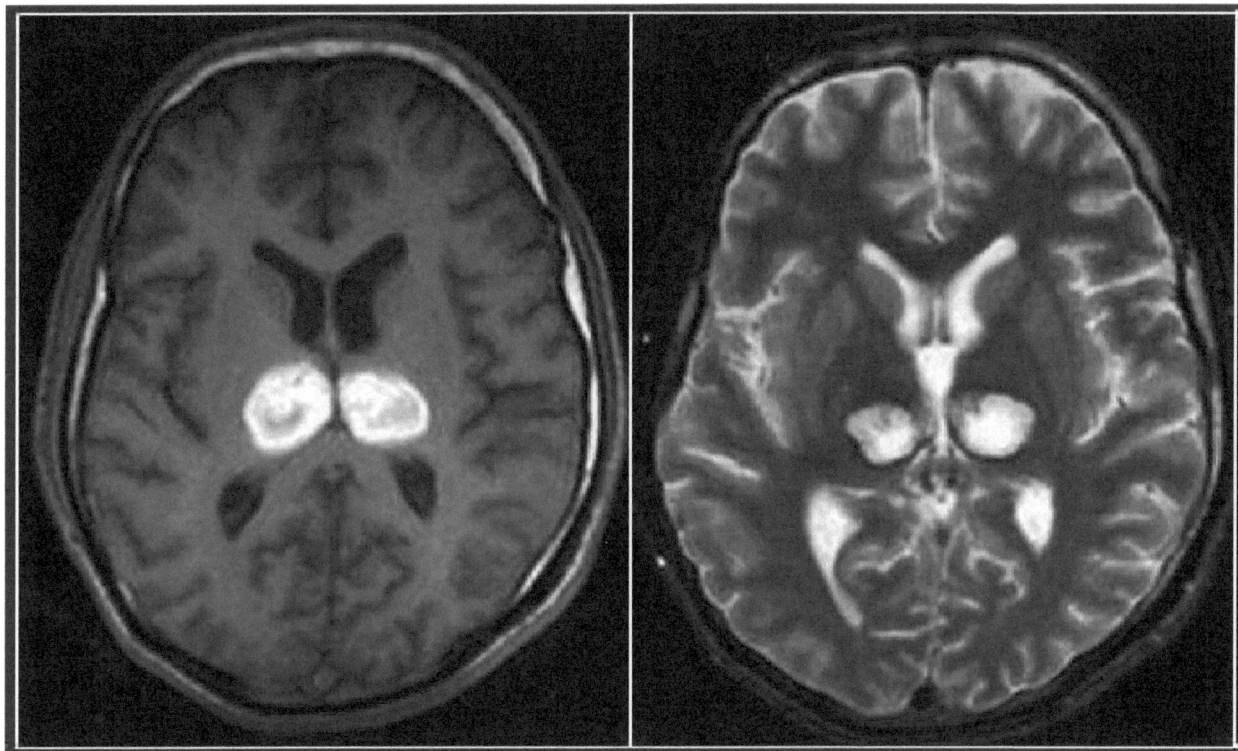

Chronic (> 2 weeks): hematoma shrinks

T1	T2	SWI
Central hyperintense, peripheral hypointense	Central hyperintense, peripheral hypointense	Trapped hemosiderin causes blooming

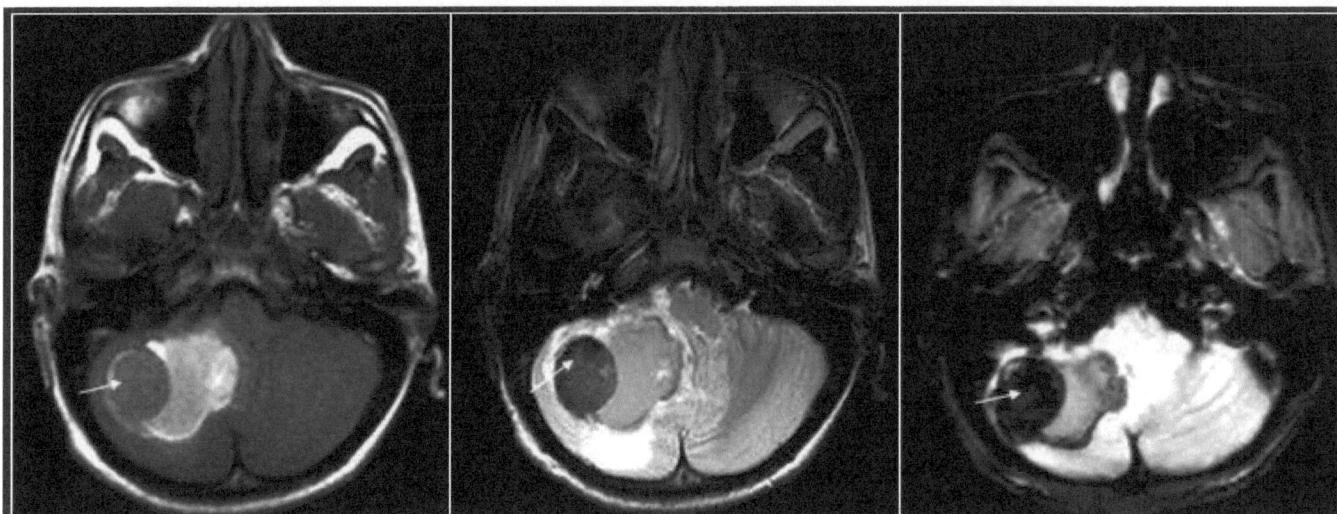

ORBITS:

Periorbital Cellulitis: is a preseptal process limited to the soft tissues anterior to the orbital septum. It most often arises from contiguous spread of infection from adjacent structures. This is typically treated with antibiotics on an outpatient basis.

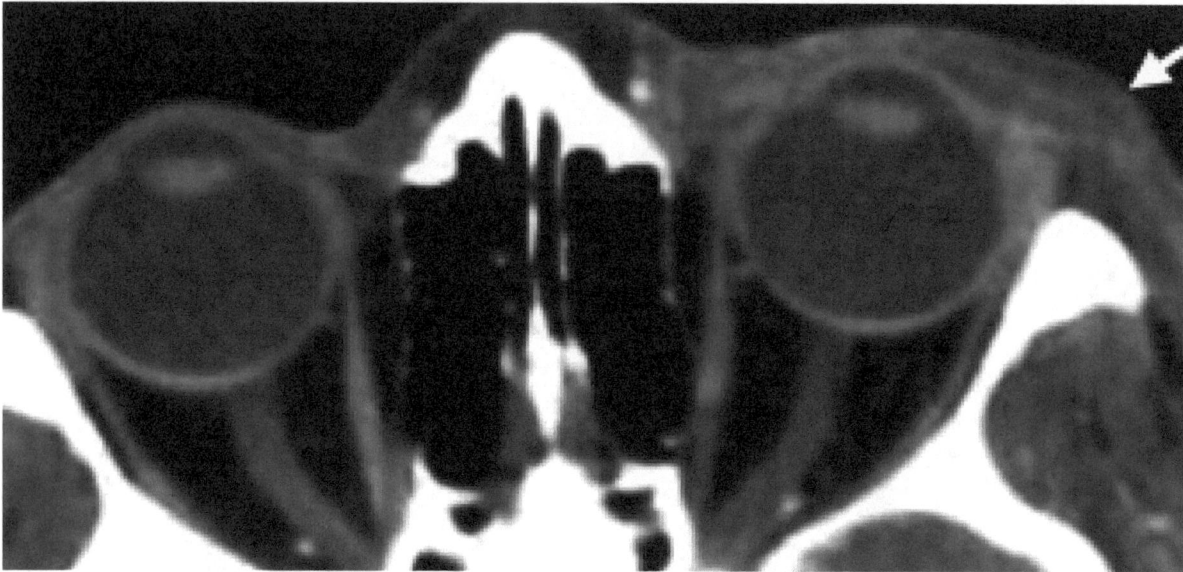

Orbital Cellulitis: is a postsetptal infectious process most common caused by paranasal sinus infection spreading to the orbit via a perivascular pathway, so bone destruction isn't present. This requires intravenous antibiotic treatment.

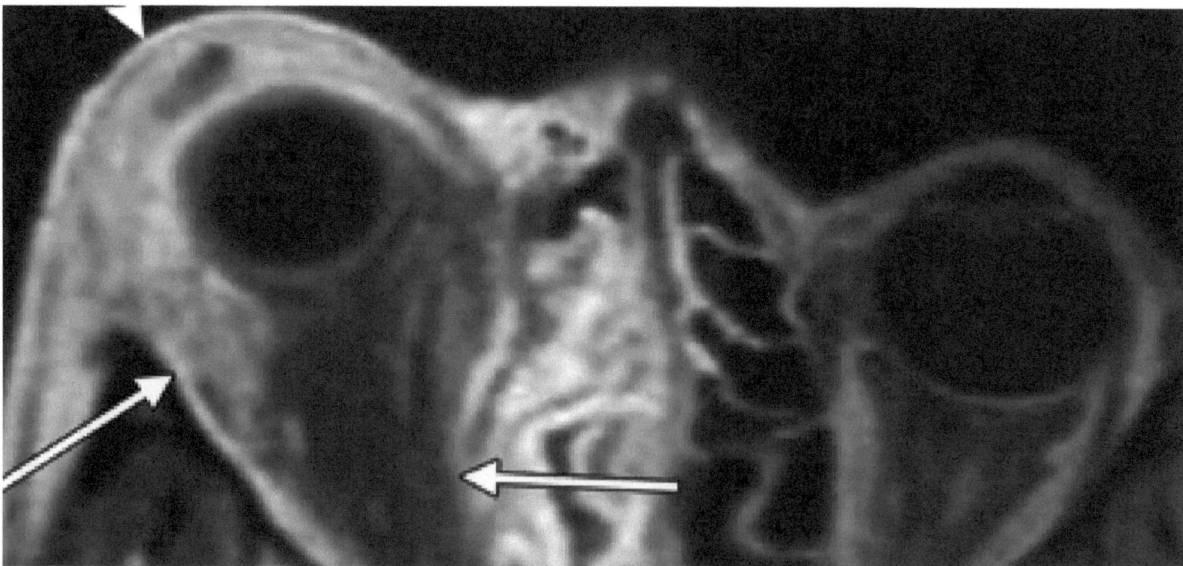

Subperiosteal Abscess: this is a complication of ethmoid sinusitis, the abscess can cause mass effect on the medial rectus muscle. There is proptosis, chemosis, and opthalmoplegia with decreased visual acuity. This is a surgical emergency.

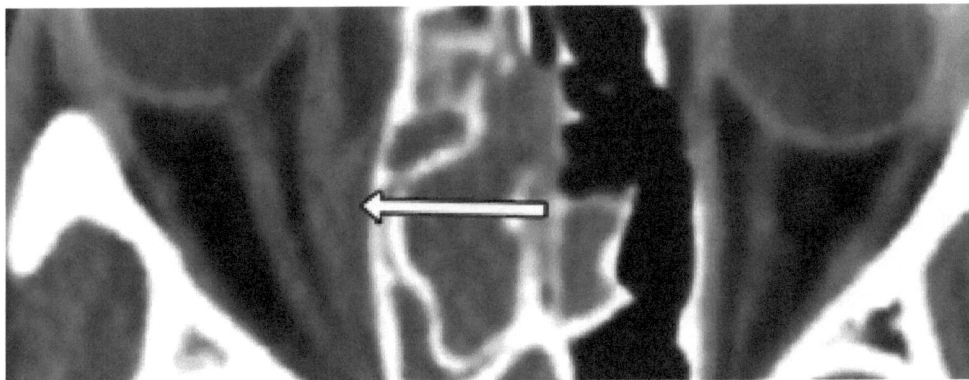

Retinal and Choroidal Detachments:

Retinal Detachment: is a separation of the sensory retina from the pigmented epithelium. These have a characteristic V-shape with the apex of the V at the optic disc.

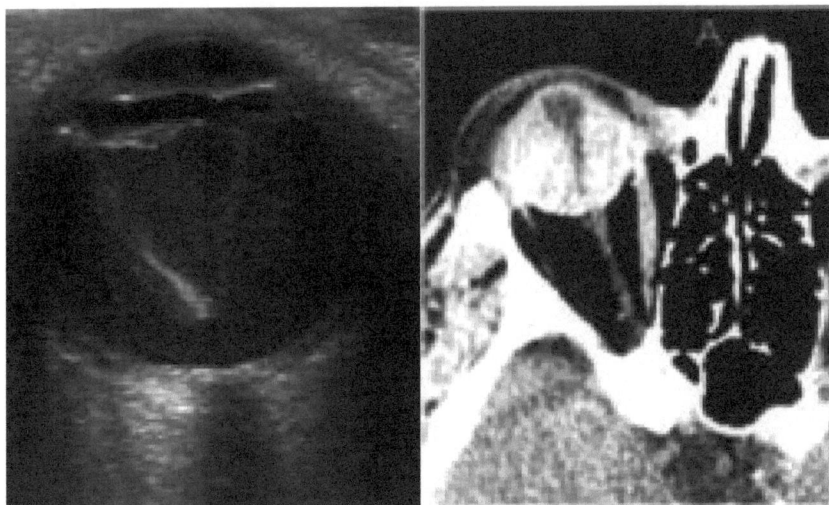

Choroidal Detachment: is the accumulation of fluid in the subchoroidal space, a condition that may occur after surgery, trauma, or uveitis. It spares the region of the optic disc and has a classic appearance "tennis ball".

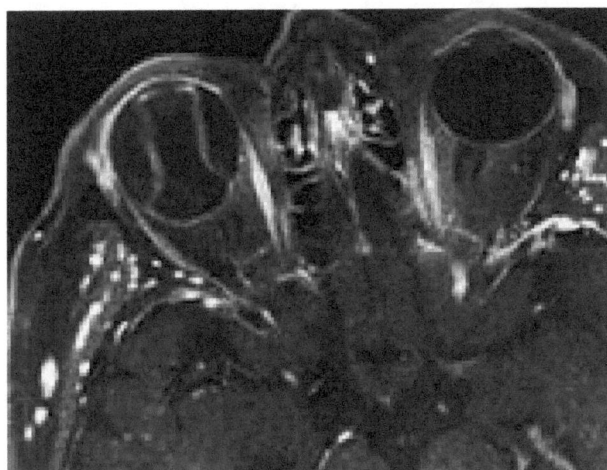

Calcifications:

Trochlear Calcifications: occur as a normal variant and are located in the superomedial location within the orbit.

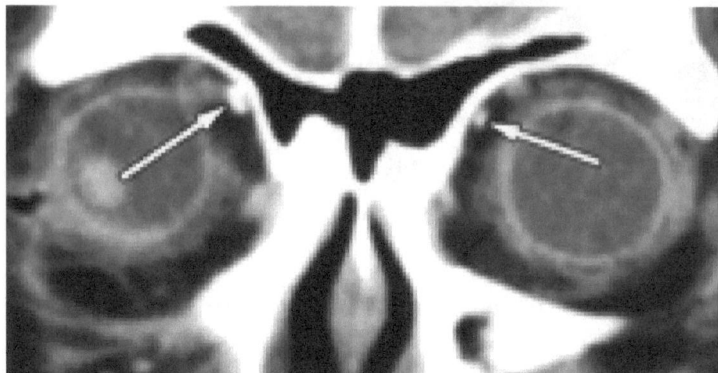

Optic Drusen: are punctate calcifications near the optic disc and are a benign cause of pseudopapilledema. They are typically seen in patients with age related macular degeneration.

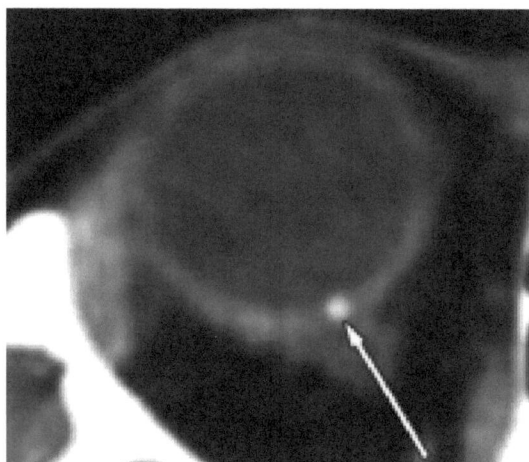

Phthisis Bulba: is a shrunken globe with ocular calcification or ossifications and is the sequela of processes such as: infection, inflammation, and trauma. Image below shows a scleral plaque in the right eye, and phthisis bulba on the left.

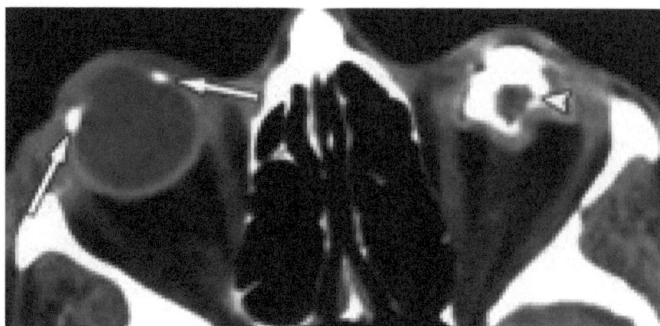

Orbital Masses and Tumors:

Rhabdomyosarcoma: is the most common extra-ocular orbital malignancy in childhood. These tumors mostly occur in the first decade of life but have been seen in all ages. It is an aggressive, rapidly growing tumor manifesting with proptosis. These are always unilateral and typically located in the superonasal quadrant.

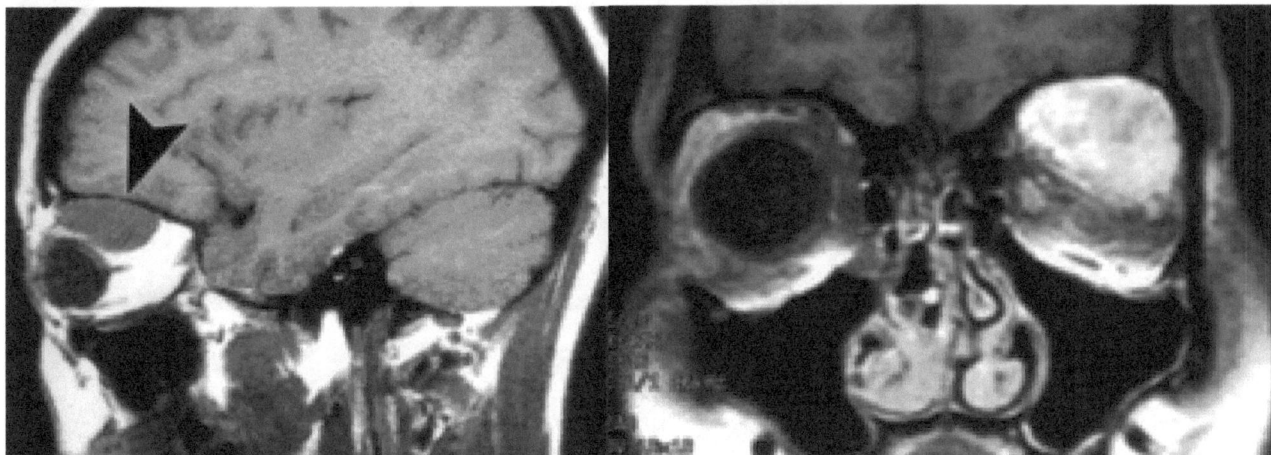

Small lesions can appear isointense to muscle on CT and well-circumscribed. As they enlarge, they can erode bone and have areas of hemorrhage giving them a more heterogenous appearance.

Retinoblastoma: is the most common intraocular neoplasm in kids. This presents as leukocoria on physical examination and can be unilateral or bilateral. When bilateral it is associated with an autosomal dominant inherited mutation. The mass tends to have calcification and enhancement.

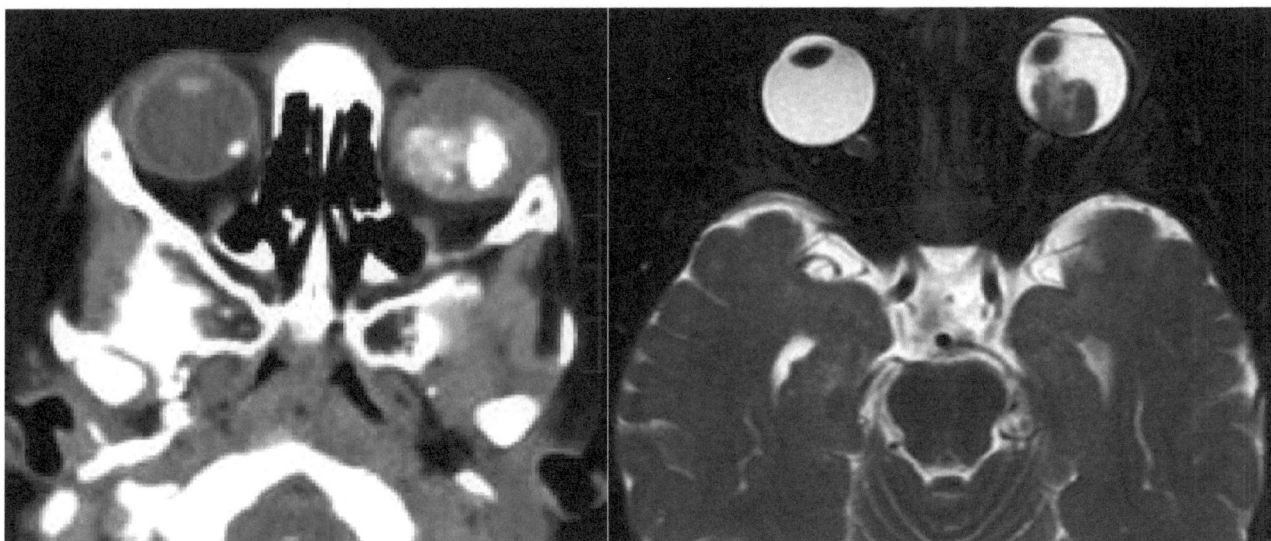

Trilateral Retinoblastoma: is bilateral retinoblastoma plus a pineoblastoma

Hemangioma: is the most common vascular mass in the orbit of an adult. Patient presents with a slowly growing orbital mass resulting in proptosis, diplopia, and sometimes visual field defects. These are well circumscribed masses bounded by a capsule and composed of dilated vascular spaces (*cavernous*). Since flow is slow, areas of thrombosis are common and it fills in with contrast gradually.

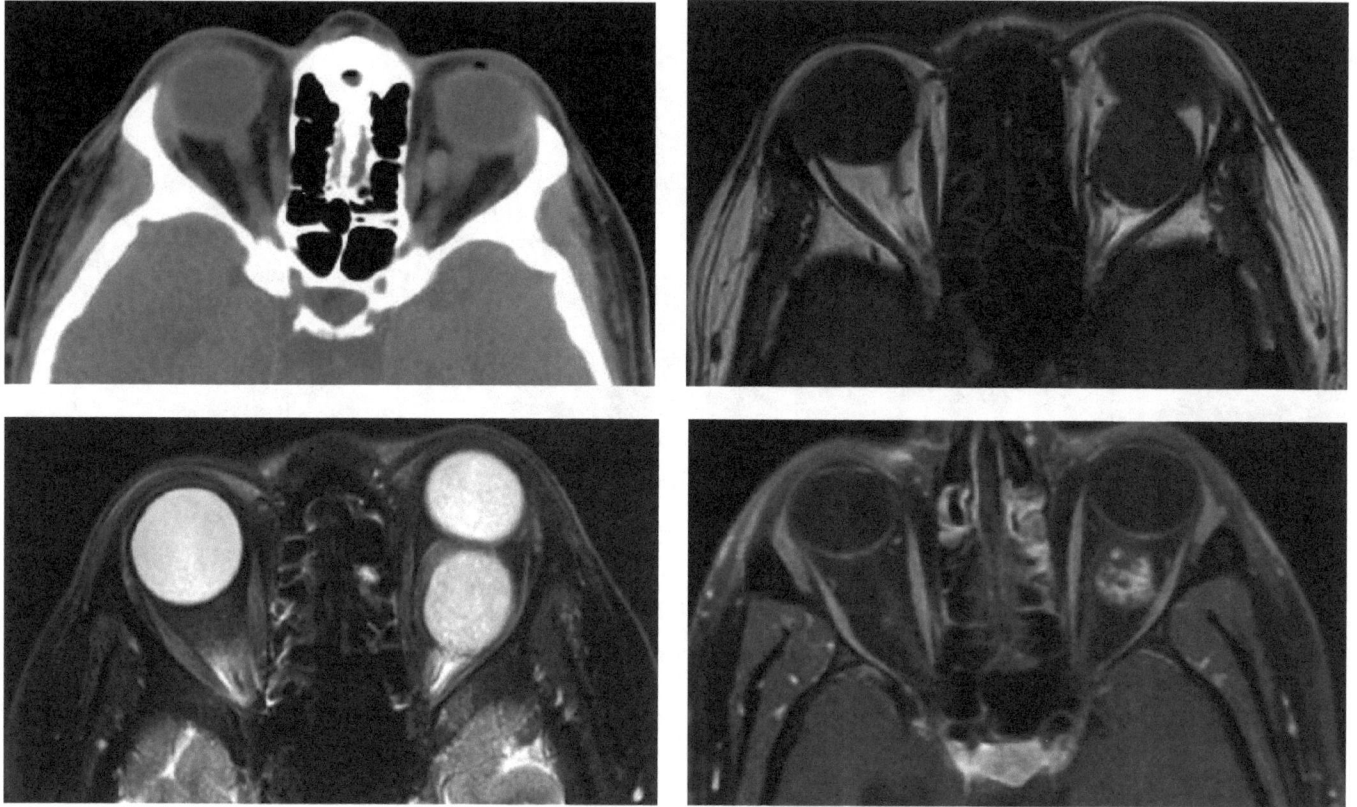

TEMPORAL BONE: by far and above the hardest thing to interpret is a CT IAMS, let's break it down.

EAC: this is mostly skin, cartilage and bone. It extends from the tympanic membrane (medially) to the external auditory meatus (laterally).

Microtia – refers to small pinna of the ear. Most often associated with ossicular dysplasia (branchial cleft 2) and EAC stenosis/atresia (cleft 1).

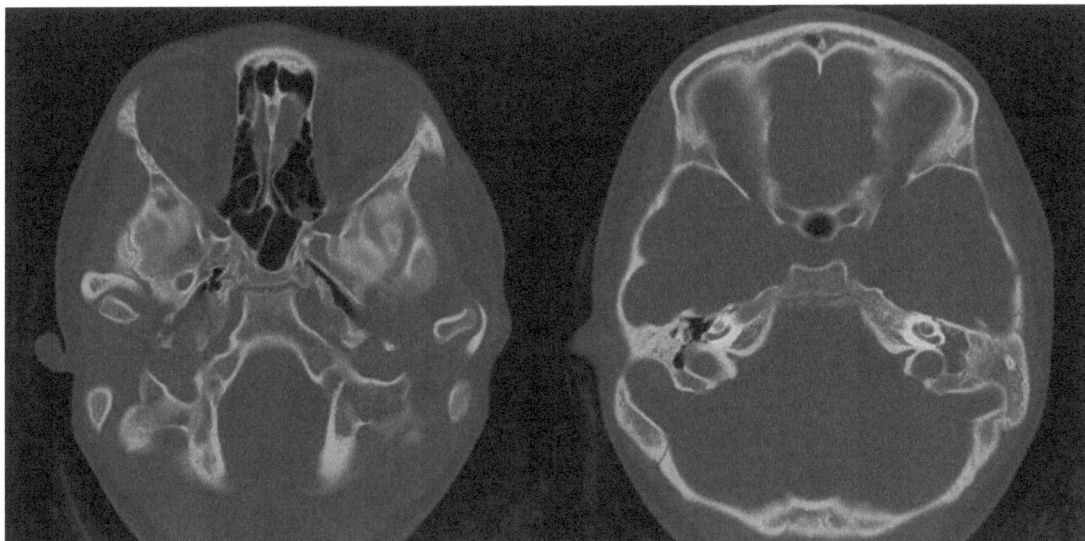

EAC Atresia: complete or partial bony atresia of the EAC.

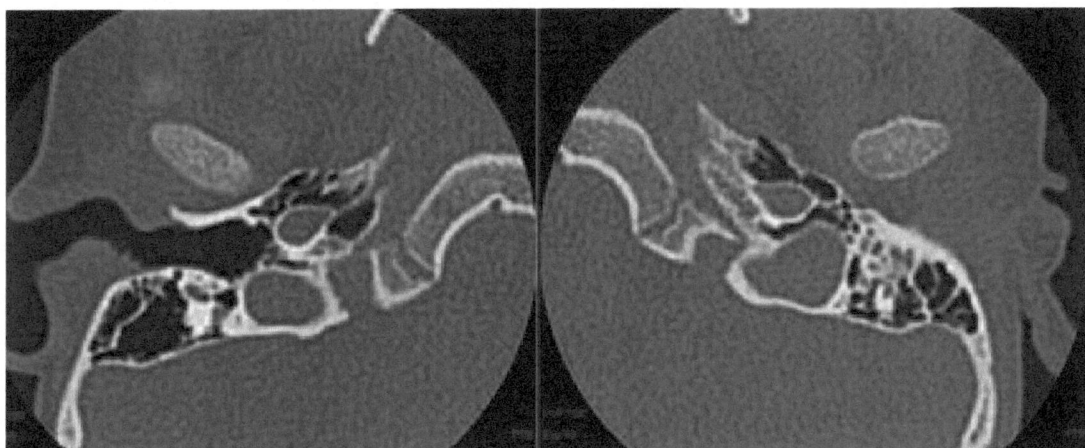

2nd branchial cleft cyst: cystic dilation of the remnant of the 2nd branchial apparatus. Characteristic location is posterior to SMG, lateral to carotid space, and anterior to the SCM.

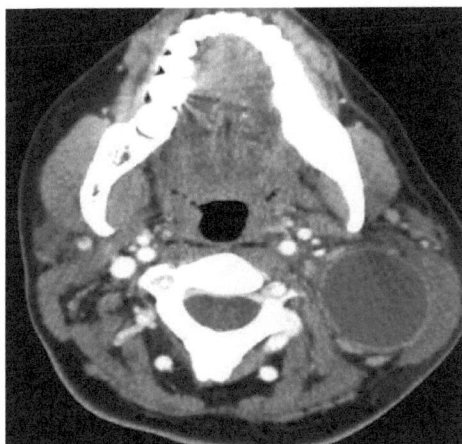

Other lesions:
- Malignant otitis externa: elderly diabetic patients with infection, inflammation, and bony erosions. Can cause CN palsies and venous sinus thrombosis.
- SCC: most common tumor in the EAC, usually see early involvement of the facial nerve and necrotic

LAD
- Adenoid cystic CA: perineural spread via CN VII

MIDDLE EAR: broken down by its relationship to the tympanic membrane. Epitympanum, Mesotympanum, and Hypotympanum.

Facial nerve normally enhances at: geniculate ganglion, anterior tympanic segment, and posterior genu.

Tegmen tympani – roof
Prussak's space – medial to the scutum
Aditus as antrum – connection to the mastoid air cells, serves as a route of spread for infection

Tensor tympani mm – CN V, attaches to manubrium of malleus
Stapedius mm – CN VII, attaches to the stapes to dampen loud noises

Tympanic membrane has two parts: pars flaccida (upper 1/3rd) and pars tensa (lower 2/3rd). The pars flaccida is attached to the scutum and the pars tensa is attached to the tympanic annulus.

Ossicles: Malleus, Incus, Stapes

In trauma, the incudostapedial joint is most often disrupted.

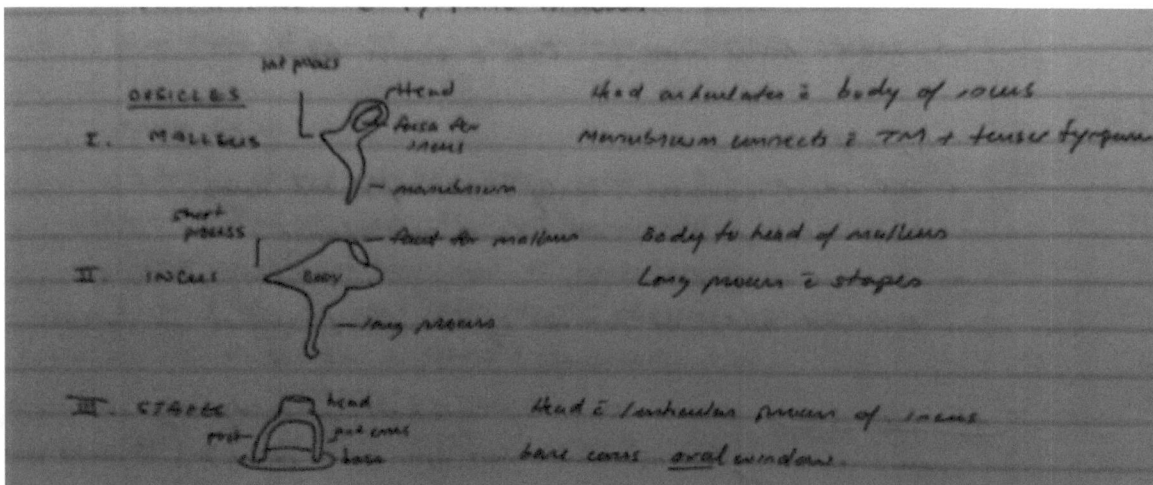

Lesions to be aware of:

Cholesteatoma: erosive collection of debris growing through the tympanic membrane. Look for erosive changes of the scutum and ossicles. This does **not enhance.** That's how you tell it apart from granulation tissue. Erodes the tegmen tympani and can have intracranial extension.

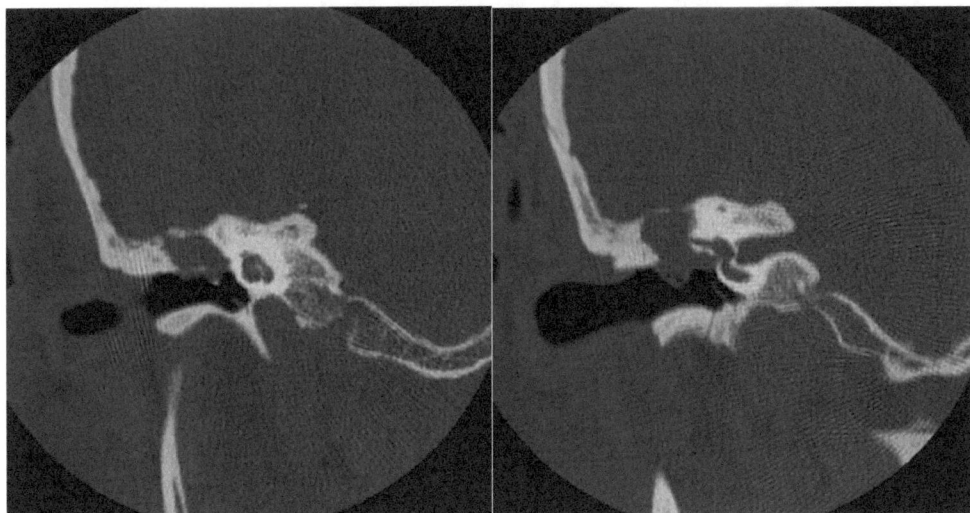

Glomus Tympanicum: arises from the cochlear promontory. It is a paraganglioma and is very vascular. It will **enhance** and is a pulsatile mass causing tinnitus. Physical exam will show a red retrotympanic mass.

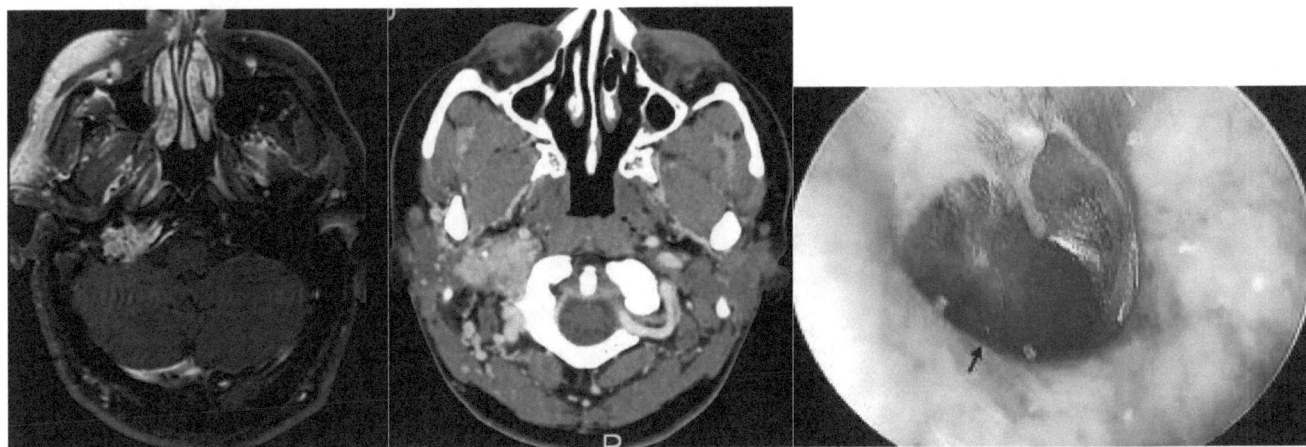

Avid contrast enhancement because of vascularity.

Congenital Cholesteatoma: is an epidermoid. Appears as a pearly white mass in the middle ear on physical exam +/- erosions. **Avascular** mass behind an intact tympanic membrane.

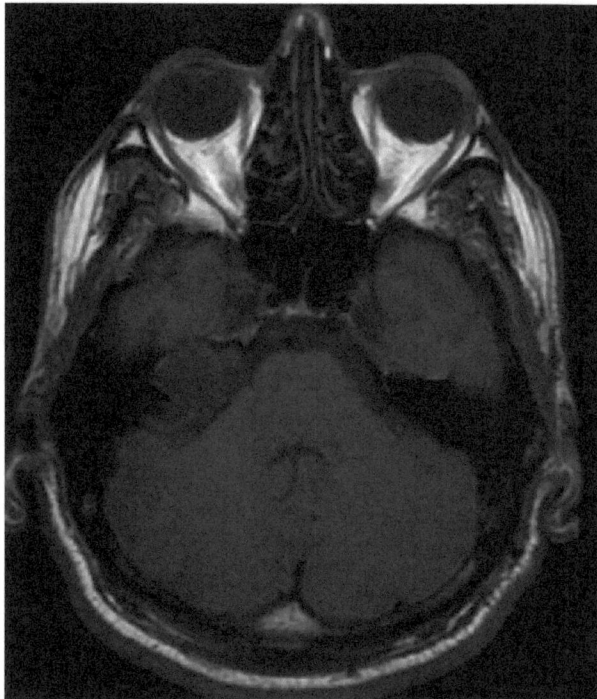

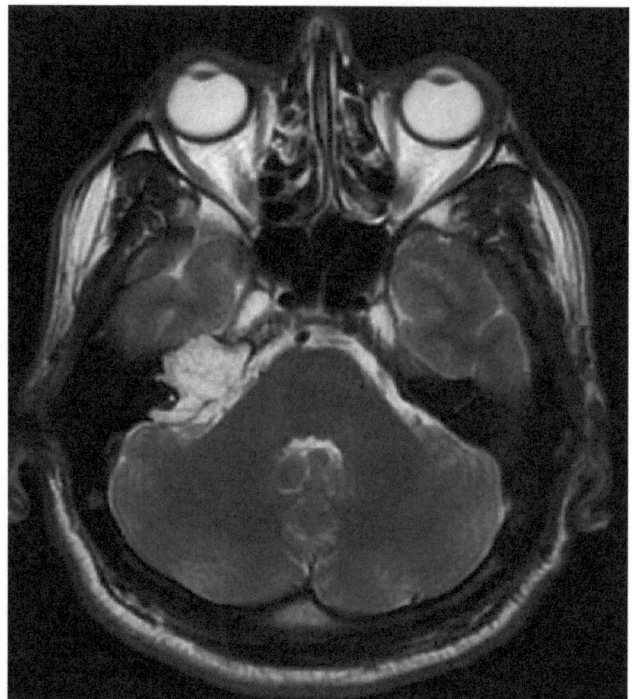

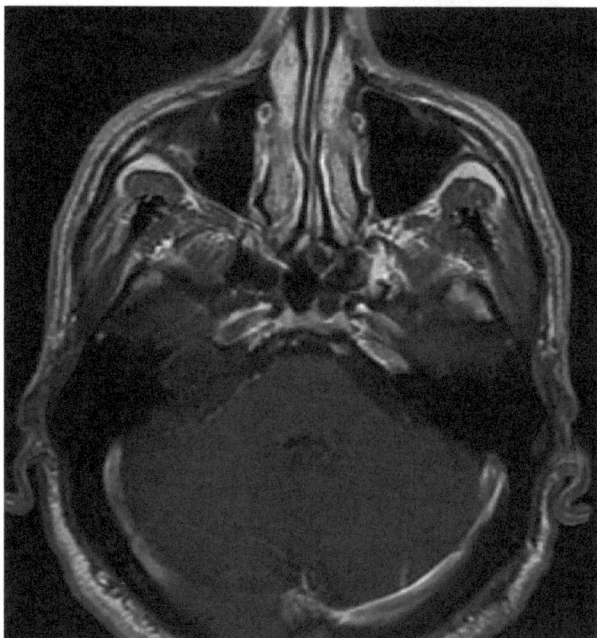

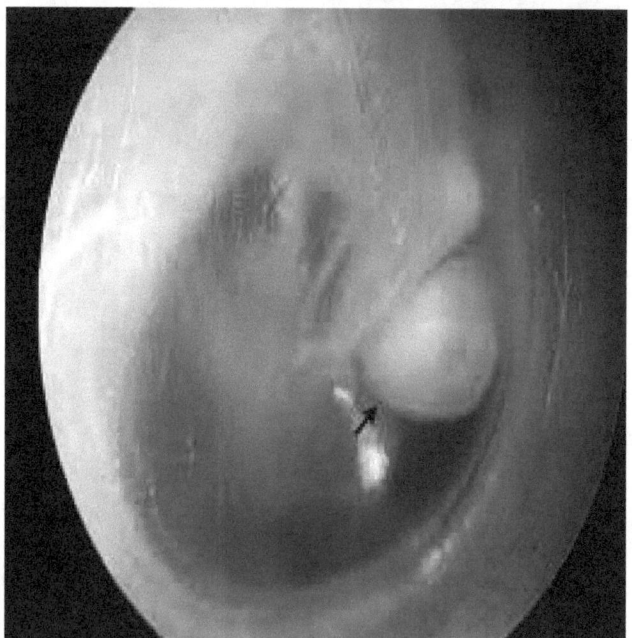

Low T1 High T2 no CE

Cholesterol Granuloma: caused by recurrent hemorrhage and formation of granulation tissue. Will appear as a non-pulsaile bluish mass. The mastoid air cells are the most common location and it is also seen at the petrous apex.

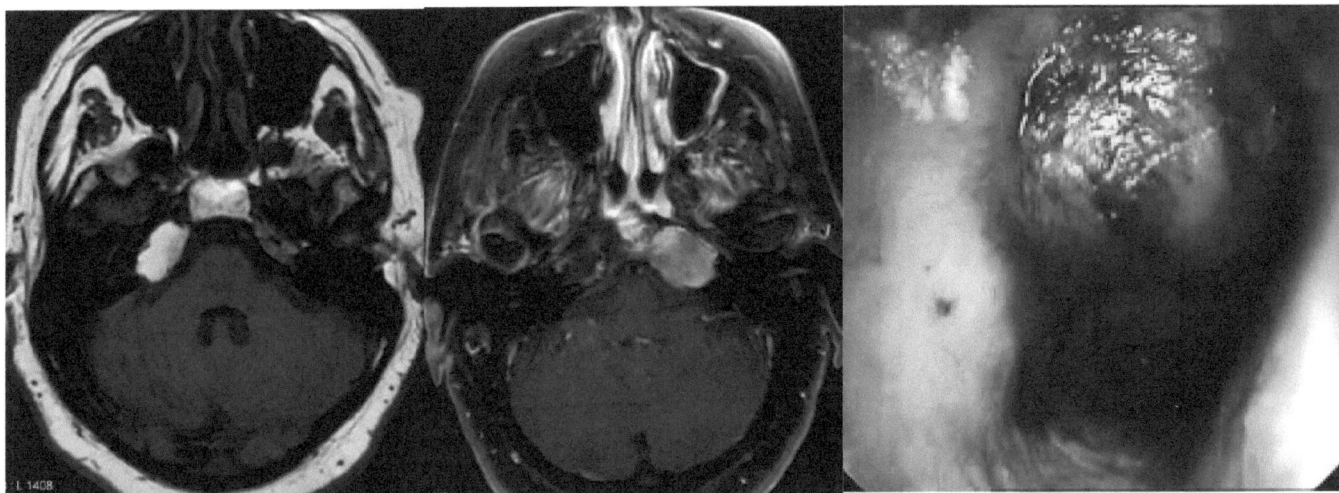

T1 – high signal with minimal enhancement, but it's hard to see because the intrinsic high signal of the lesion.

Aberrant Carotid: red pulsatile mass through the tympanic membrane. Often seen in the setting of absent foramen spinosum (so no middle meningeal artery). These people will have persistent stapedial artery 30% of the time.

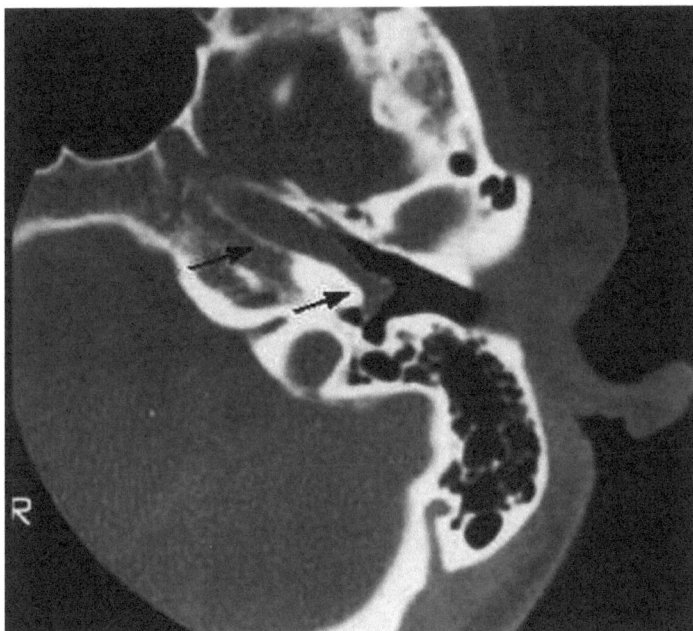

INNER EAR:

Osseous labyrinth – cochlea, semicircular canal, and vestibule
Membranous labyrinth – perilymph and endolymph
Cochlea – 2.5 turns connects to the round window – bony center is the modiolus Vestibule – articulates with the stapes at oval window

Vestibular Aqueduct Enlargement: normal is between 0.5 – 1.5 mm, and enlargement is the number 1 cause of congenital sensorineural hearing loss.

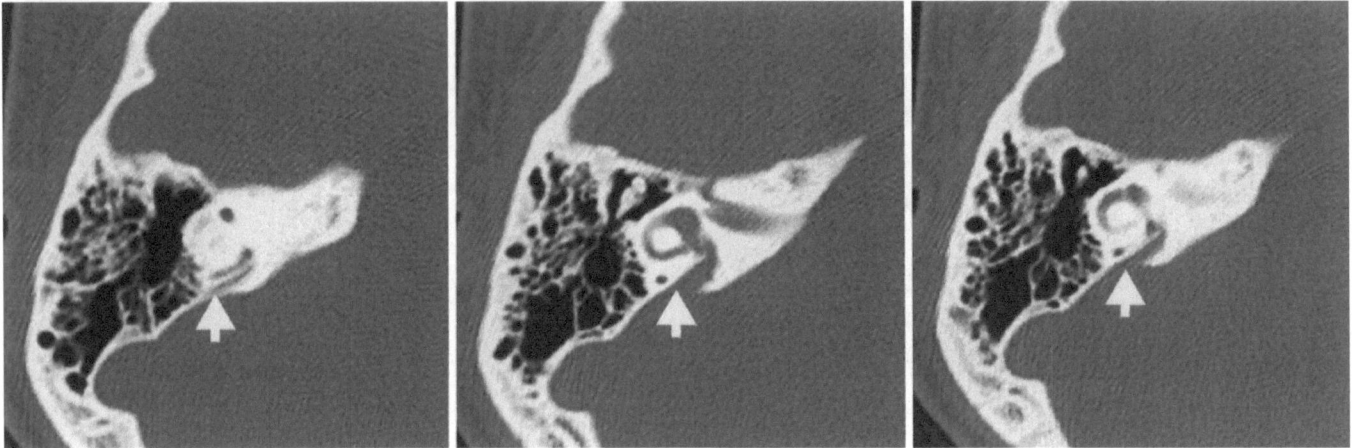

Mondini Malformation: is incomplete spiralization of the modiolus, less than 2.5 turns.

Ramsey Hunt Syndrome: is reactivation of varicella zoster in CN VII. Virus lies dormant in the geniculate ganglion. CN VII should never enhance except in the tympanic and mastoid portions. Painful ear and periauricular vesicles are present.

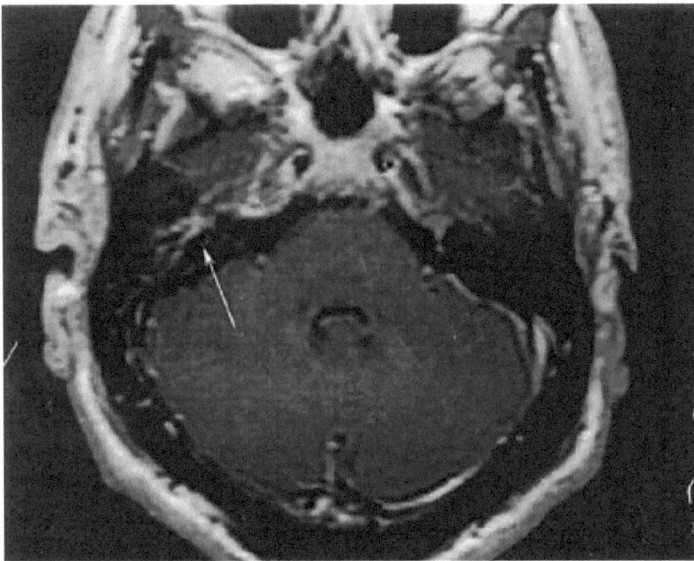

SPINE: The spinal cord is a reversed brain with the gray matter centrally and the white matter on the outside. So when you see a lesion in the cord, think about what your differential would be if that same lesion involved the brain. That will help guide your differential.

Extradural	Intradural Extramedullary	Intramedullary
Degenerative changes	Schwannoma	MS
Hemangiomas	Neurofibroma	Astrocytoma
Metastasis	Meningioma	Ependymoma
Paget's Disease	Metastases	Hemangioblastoma
Lymphoma	Arachnoid Cyst	Cavernous Malformation
Chordoma	Paraganglioma	AV fistula
ABC	Ependymoma	Syrinx
Giant Cell Tumor		Metastases
Osteoid Osteoma		Infarct
Osteoblastoma		

Metastases: They can be anywhere and enhance avidly. Look for a history of prior malignancy. Tumors that like the spine are lung, breast, renal cell and thyroid to name a few. Most mets are extradural and involve the vertebral body because of its vascular nature. Drop mets are intradural and commonly from: ependymoma, germinoma, pineoblastoma, choroid plexus CA, medulloblastoma and ATRT. To differentiate mets from fracture look for posterior element enhancement and marrow signal loss.

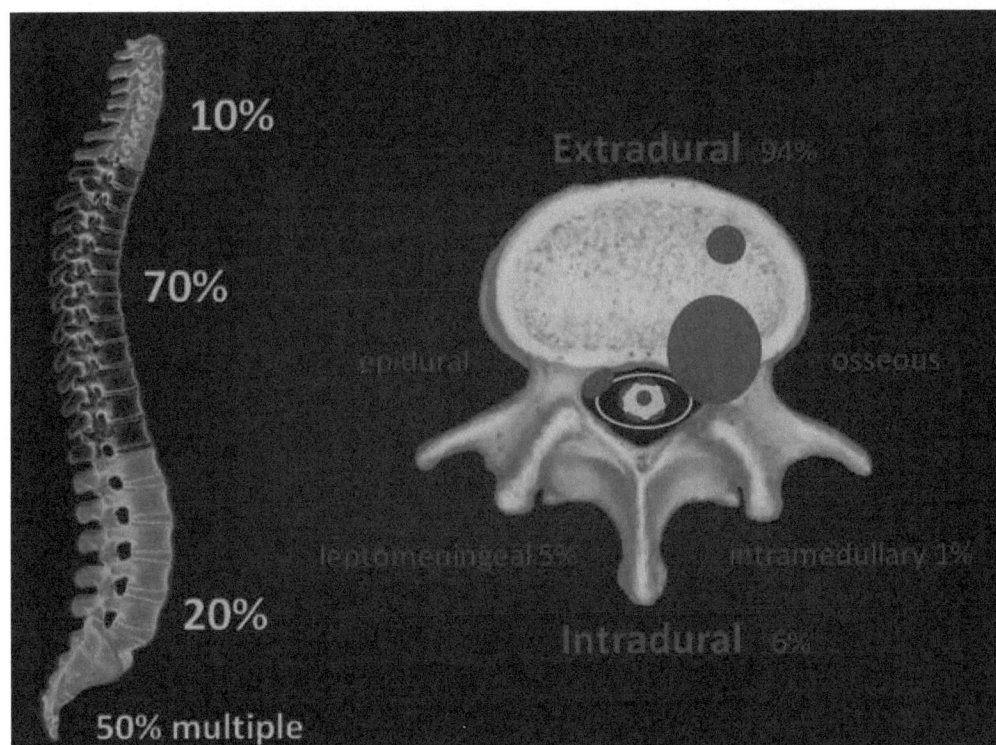

INTRAMEDULLARY: these are intra-cord lesions with expansion of cord from inside out.

Astrocytoma: expands the cord and extends greater than one segment with enhancement. Look for this in kids, not adults. There is an association with NF1.

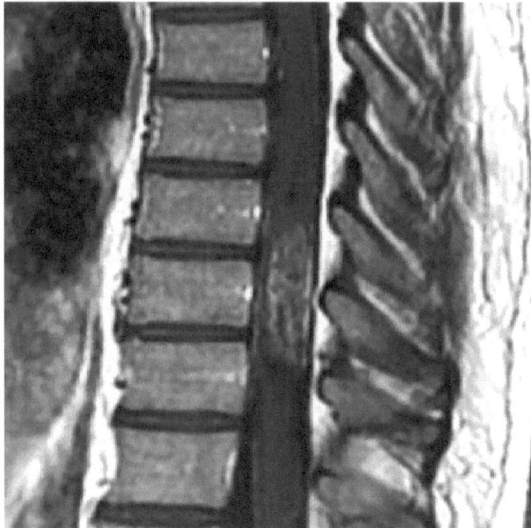

Ependymoma: most common spinal cord tumor overall; seen in both the adult and pediatric population. More common in distal cord. Expands the cord as it arises from the central ependymal cells. Myxopapillary ependymomas are found in the filum terminale.

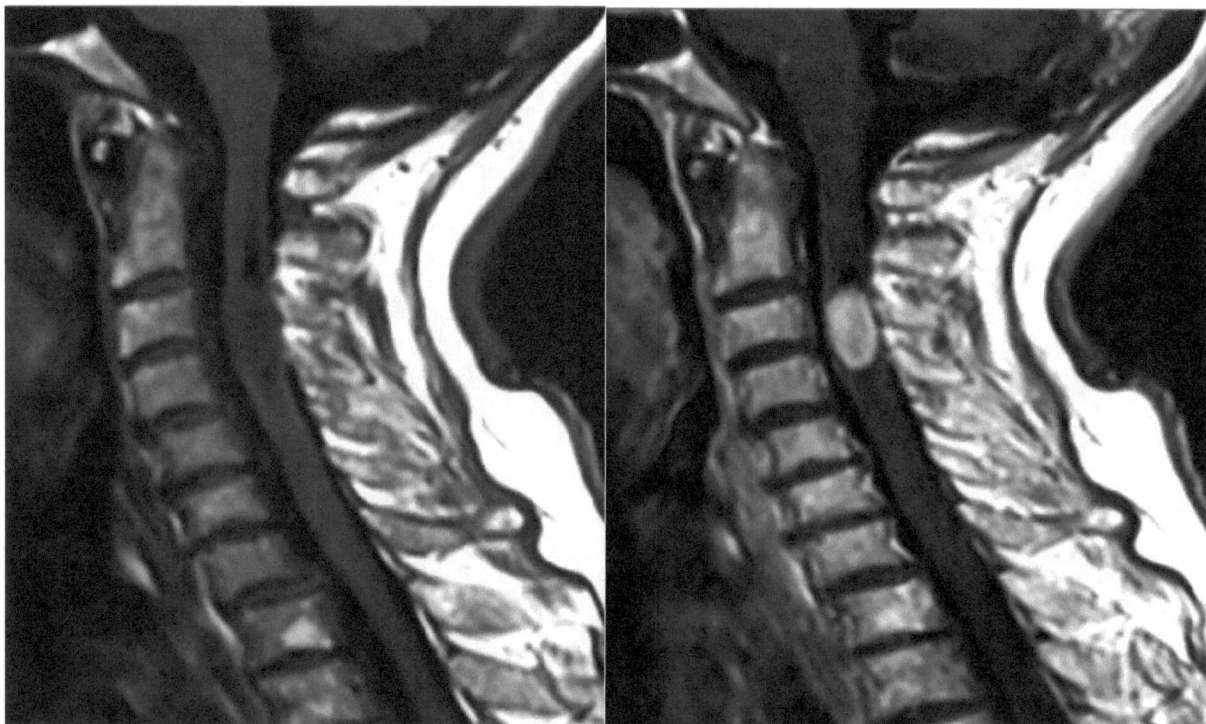

Hemangioblastoma: is the third most common primary intramedullary tumor after ependymoma and astrocytoma. It is more often seen in adults. It is very common to see a cyst with enhancing nodule (similar to presentation in brain). It is associated with VHL.

Remember that a cyst with nodule in a kid is probably an astrocytoma.

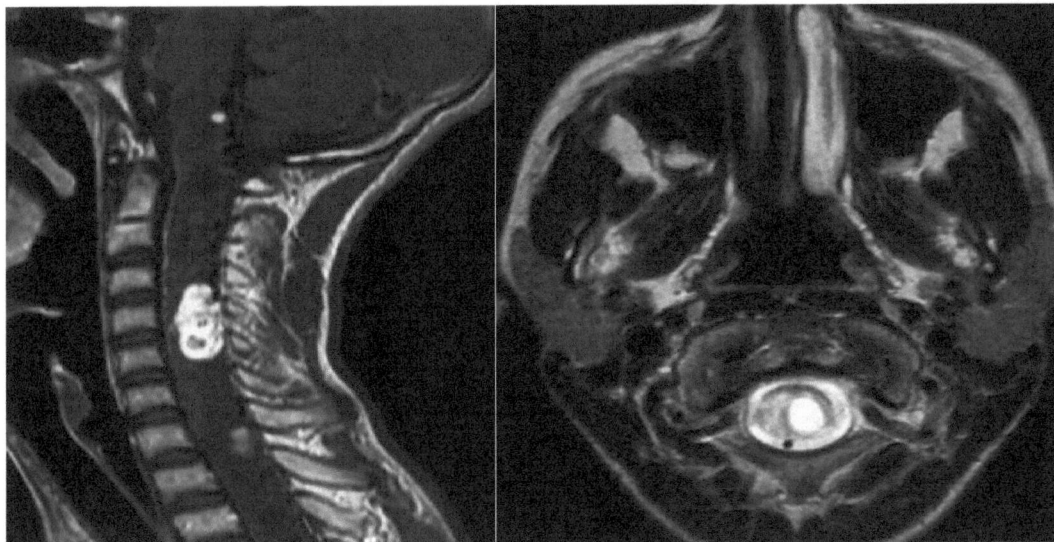

MS: relapsing remitting WM disease. Young females are the typical patient. Hyperintense on T2 and FLAIR with incomplete peripheral enhancement in active lesions. Typically multifocal.

Bad variant of MS is Devic's disease (neuromyelitis optica): transverse myelitis plus optic neuritis with a paucity of intracranial lesions. Tends to span several segments and it will not have any intracranial lesions except the optic nerves.

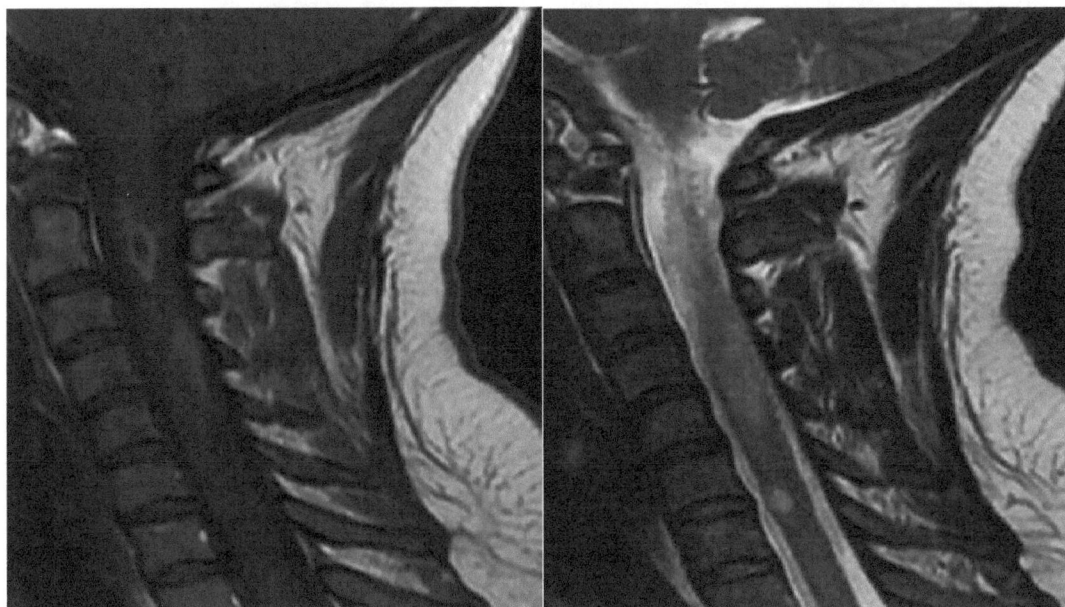

Spinal Cord Infarct: usually due to anterior spinal artery insult that knocks out the gray matter giving a characteristic "owls eye" sign (this is BS it looks more like a Tai Fighter.

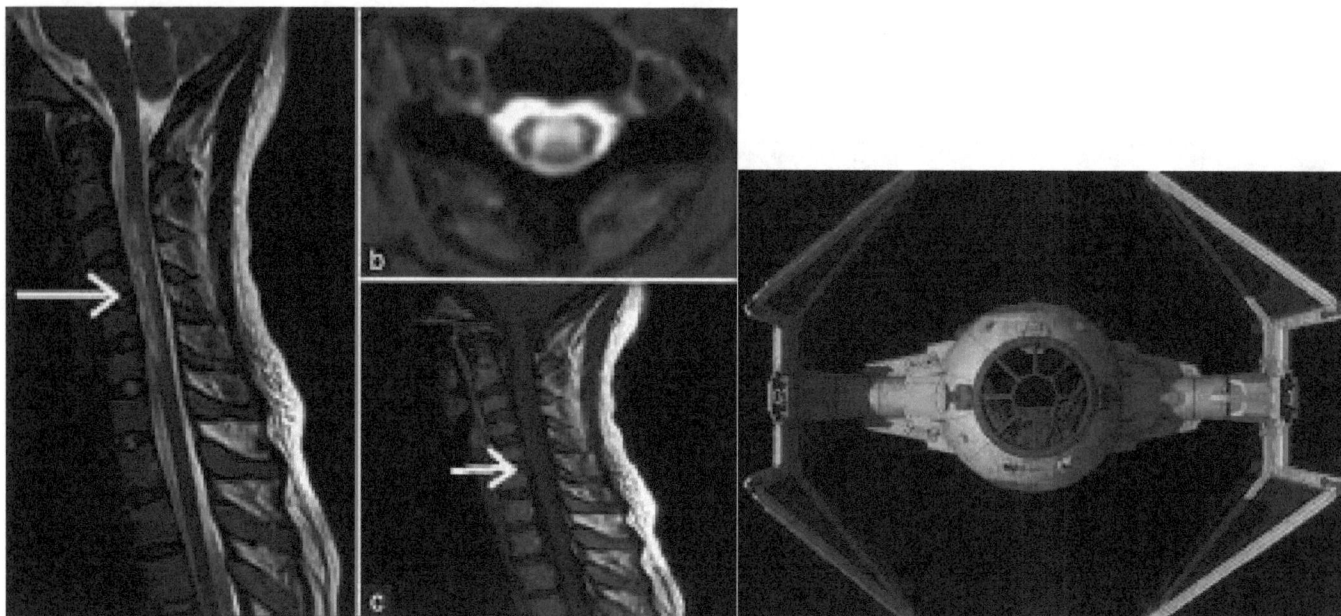

INTRADURAL-EXTRAMEDULLARY:

Schwannoma: represents 30% of intradural-extramedullary lesions and as such is the most common tumor of this type. It is most often found in the cervical and lumbar regions. Tends to be a slow growing process that causes foraminal expansion and radiculopathy. Enhances more than a neurofibroma. Can be heterogeneous because it can get big. Most are solitary and sporadic, but if multiple, think NF2. Shaped like a dumbbell.

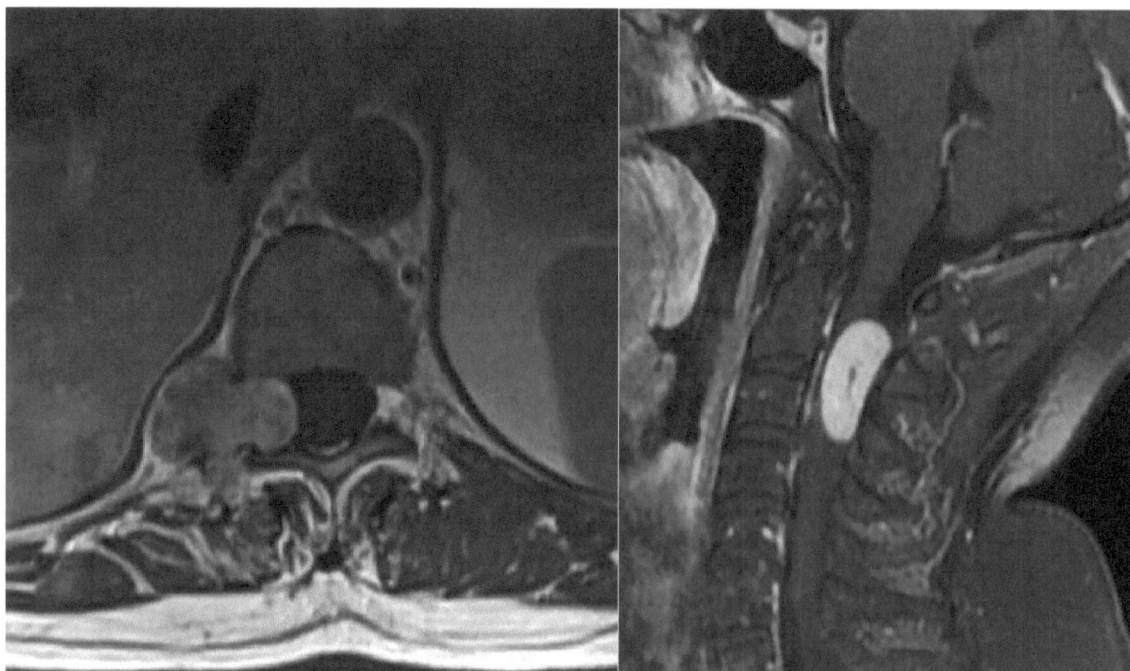

Meningioma: account for 25% of intradural-extramedullary tumors and are the second most common tumor of this type. The have avid enhancement with a dural tail. If you see multiples, think MISME and NF2.

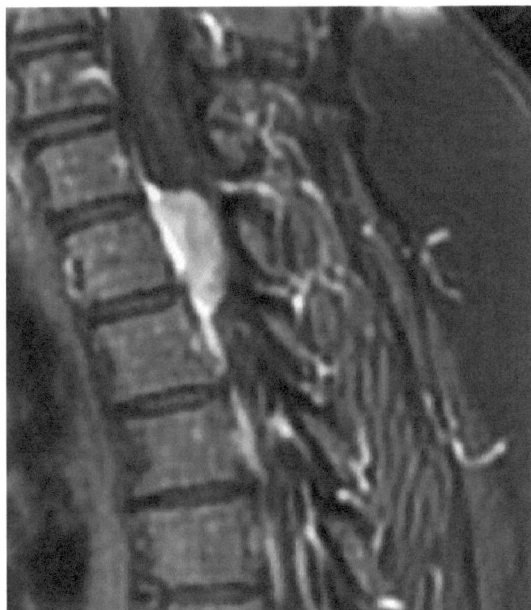

Neurofibroma: benign peripheral nerve sheath tumors. Hard to differentiate from schwannoma, but these enhance less. If you see multiple foraminal masses think NF1.

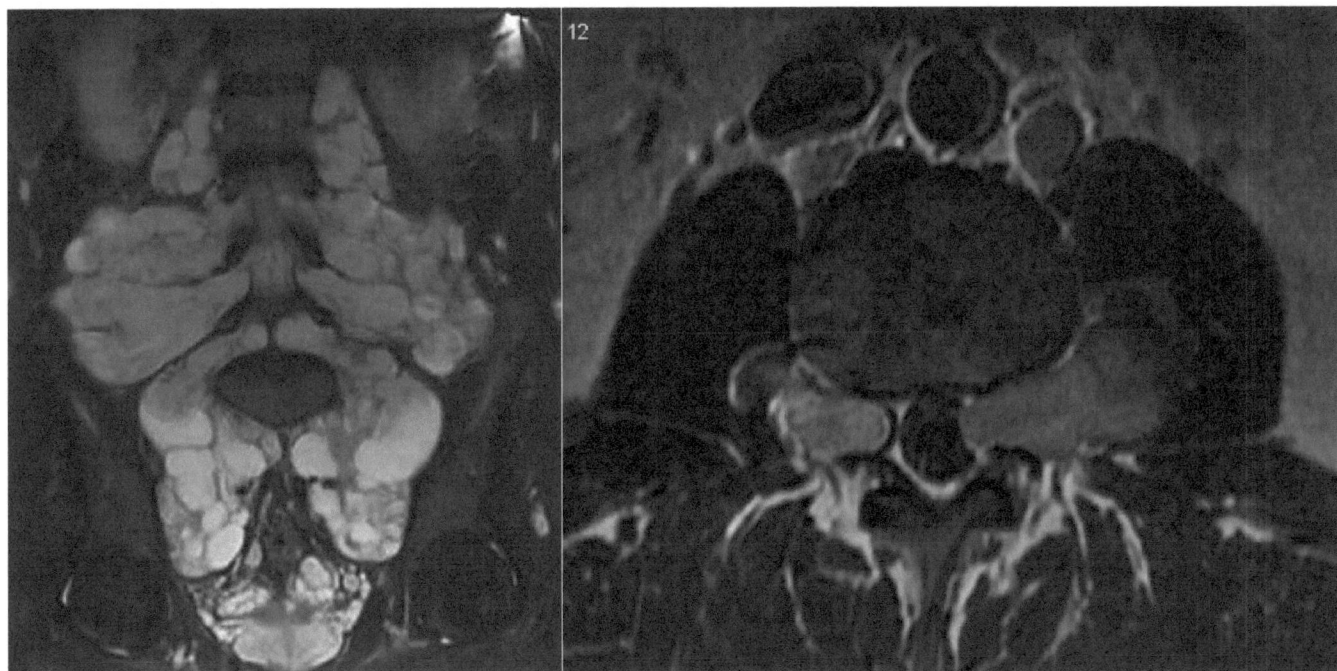

EXTRADURAL:

Metastases: if it involves the vertebral bodies, it is unlikely to be a primary brain malignancy, look elsewhere for tumor. Low signal on T1 replacing fatty marrow with enhancement and soft tissue masses that can break through the cortex.

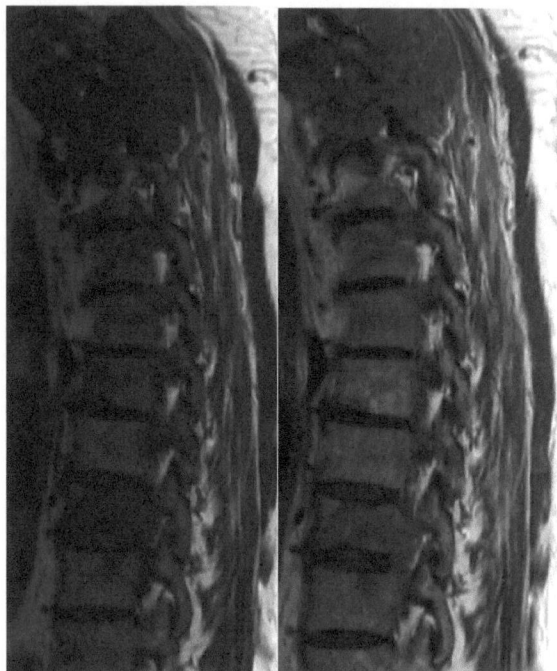

INFECTIONS:

Discitis/Osteomyelitis: hematogeneous infection with destruction of adjacent vertebral endplates. Soft tissue inflammation, enhancement and abscesses are associated findings. In kids it starts in the disc and in adults it starts in the endplate.

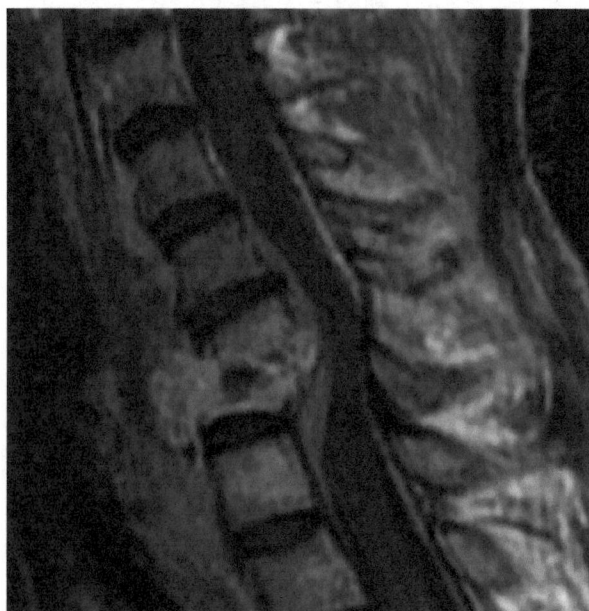

Tuberculous Spondylitis (Pott's Disease): is a disc sparing multi-level infection by mycobacterium tuberculosis. Intravertebral abscesses and enhancement of the vertebra and soft tissues are common findings. Look for a gibbus deformity.

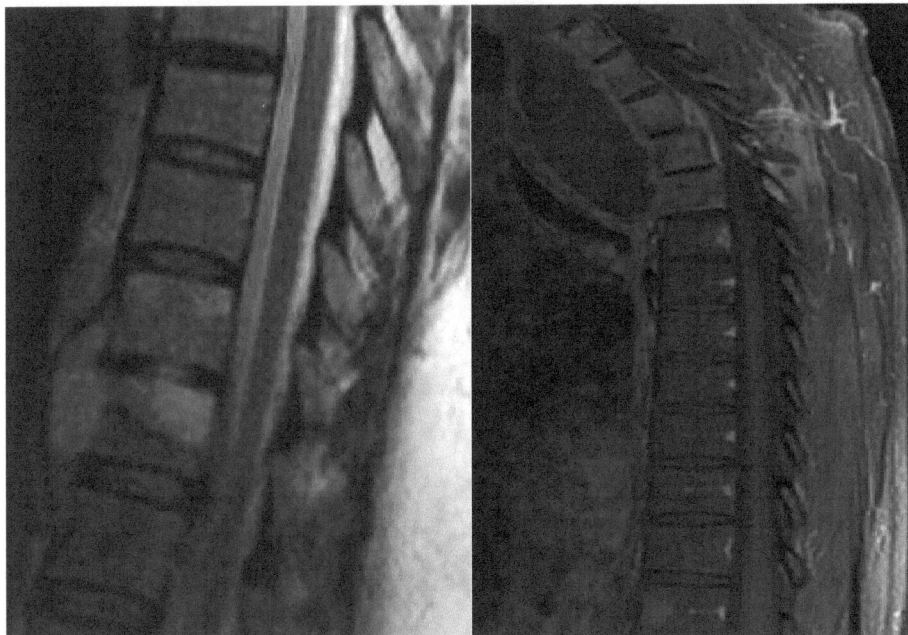

OTHER STUFF:

Epidural lipomatosis: can be due to endogeneous (Cushing's), exogeneous (steroids) or idiopathic causes. Excess fat accumulation in the epidural space with compression of the cord is the classic finding. On axial view the thecal sac will have a "stellate appearance".

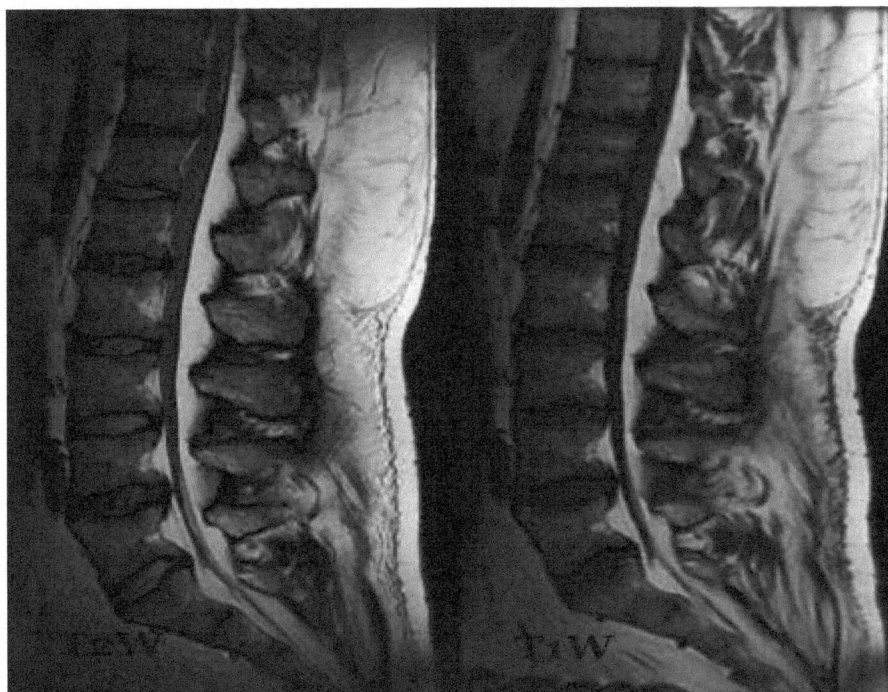

Diastometamylia: "split cord syndrome", usually seen below T8. Can have fibrous or osseous septum.

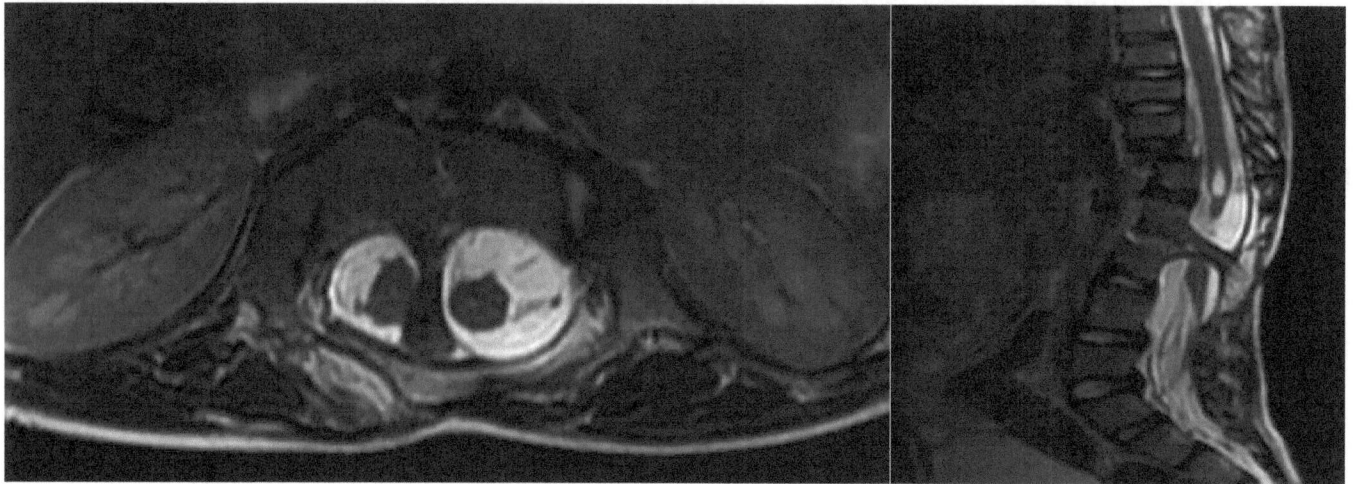

Arachnoiditis: is a broad term that is used for inflammation of the meninges and subarachnoid space. Caused by SAH, infection (post-op or otherwise), trauma, and sarcoidosis to name a few.

Three types:

1. Central clumping
2. Empty sac sign with the nerves around the periphery
3. Soft tissue mass in central cord

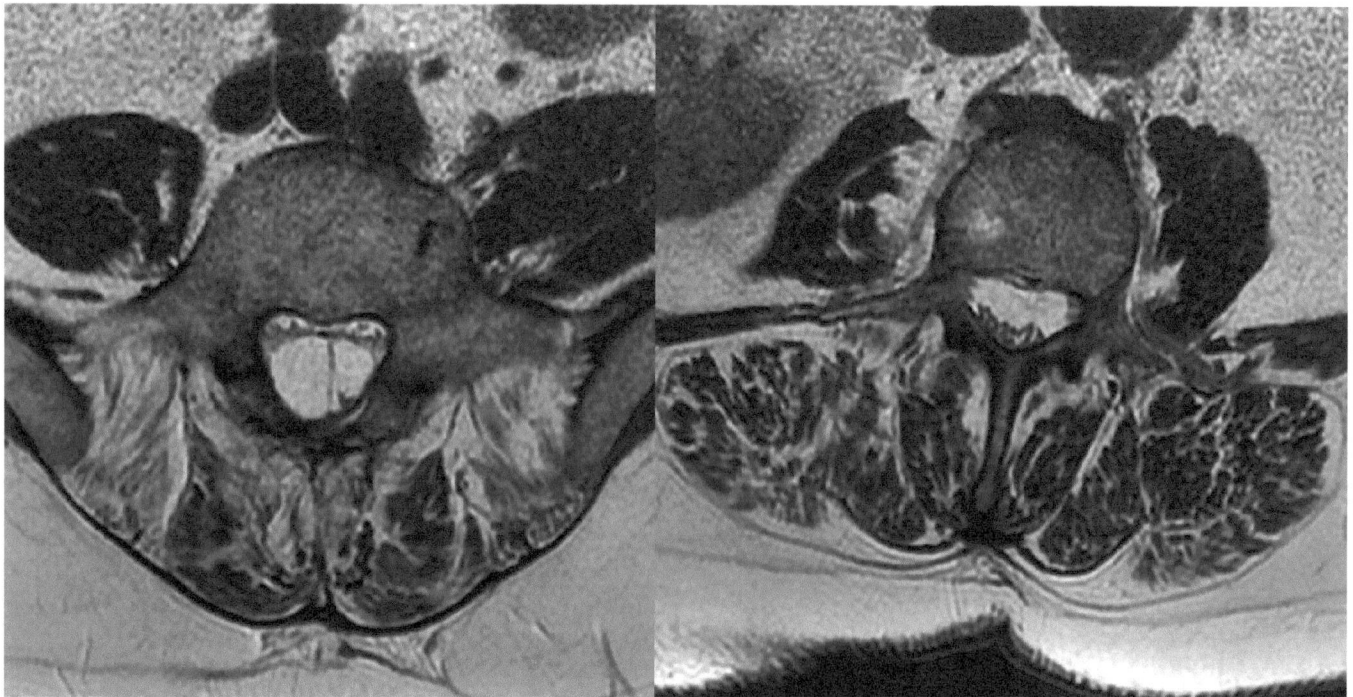

FUN FACTS:

1. Conditions associated with dural ectasia – NF1, Marfan's and Ehler-Danlos
2. Currarino's Triad – presacral mass, sacral bony defect, and anorectal anomaly
3. Plexiform neurofibroma is more likely to have malignant degeneration than a schwannoma.
4. Cystic conus lesion: epidermoid, terminal ventricle, syringohydromyelia
5. Lumbar plexus is formed from the ventral rami, with injury, think psoas muscle atrophy
6. Leptomeningeal sarcoid prefers the cervical spine.
7. Callosal dysgenesis is the most common midline defect seen with other CNS malformations.
8. Brainstem glioma is a death sentence. It is an expansile tumor in kids that typically affects the pons. Should not enhance, if it does, poor prognostic sign.
9. Esthesioneuroblastoma – cyst formation at tumor margin where there is intracranial extension is a helpful identifying feature.

Important Anatomy:

Supraorbital Foramen	Supraorbital artery and vein	Supraorbital nerve
Cribiform Plate		Olfactory nerve bundles (CN I)
Optic Canal	Ophthalmic artery	Optic nerve (CN II)
Superior Orbital Fissure	Superior ophthalmic vein	CN III, IV, V_1, VI
Foramen Rotundum		CN V_2
Inferior Orbital Fissure	Inferior ophthalmic artery	Infraorbital branch of CN V_2
Foramen Ovale		CN V_3
Foramen Spinosum	Middle meningeal artery	
Foramen Lacerum	Internal carotid artery	
Internal Acoustic Meatus	Labyrinthine artery	CN VII and VIII
Juduglar Foramen	Inferior petrosal and sigmoid sinus	CN IX, X, XI
Hypoglossal Canal		CN XII
Stylomastoid Foramen		CN VII

Cavernous Sinus: receives blood from the inferior ophthalmic vein, superior ophthalmic vein, superficial middle cerebral vein, inferior cerebral veins, and sphenoparietal sinus. It drains via:

- superior petrosal sinus to the transverse sinus
- inferior petrosal sinus to the jugular bulb
- to the pterygoid plexus

Contains CN III, IV, V1, V2, and VI as well as the ICA. From superior to inferior I use the pneumonic **OTOM** and then remember that the abducens is medial to these and posterolateral to the ICA.

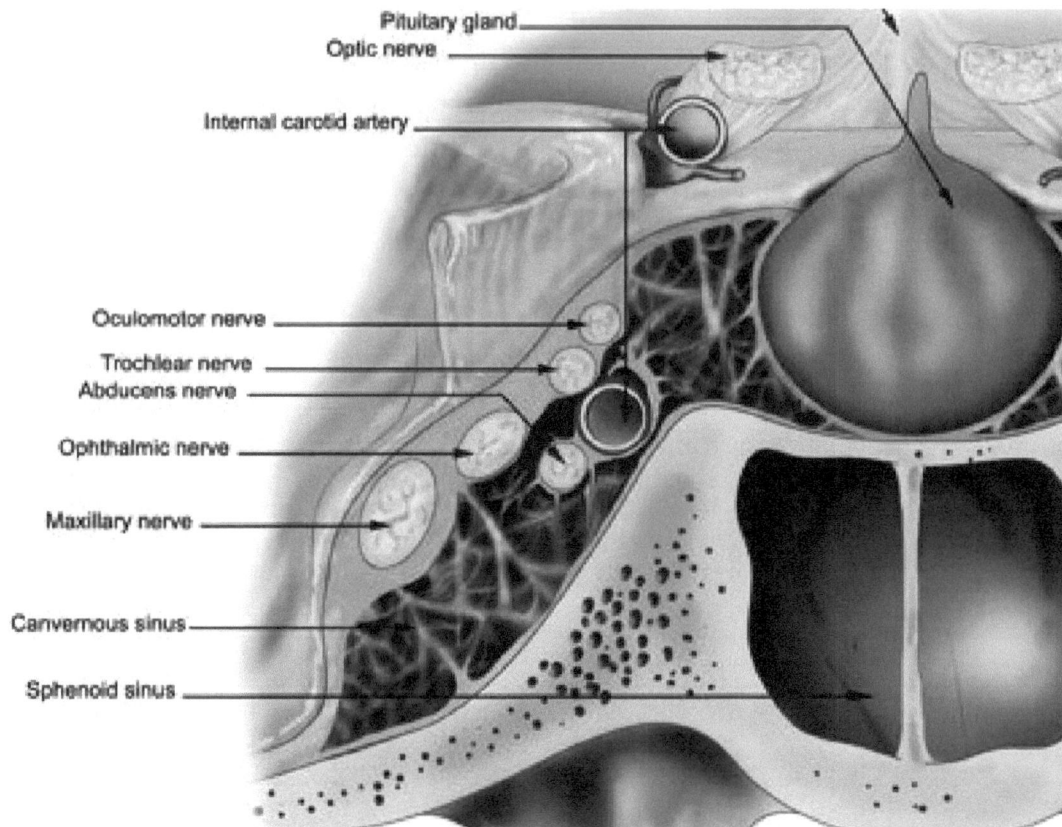

Labeled diagram (top):
- Pituitary gland
- Optic nerve
- Internal carotid artery
- Oculomotor nerve
- Trochlear nerve
- Abducens nerve
- Ophthalmic nerve
- Maxillary nerve
- Cavernous sinus
- Sphenoid sinus

Cranial Nerves on MRI:

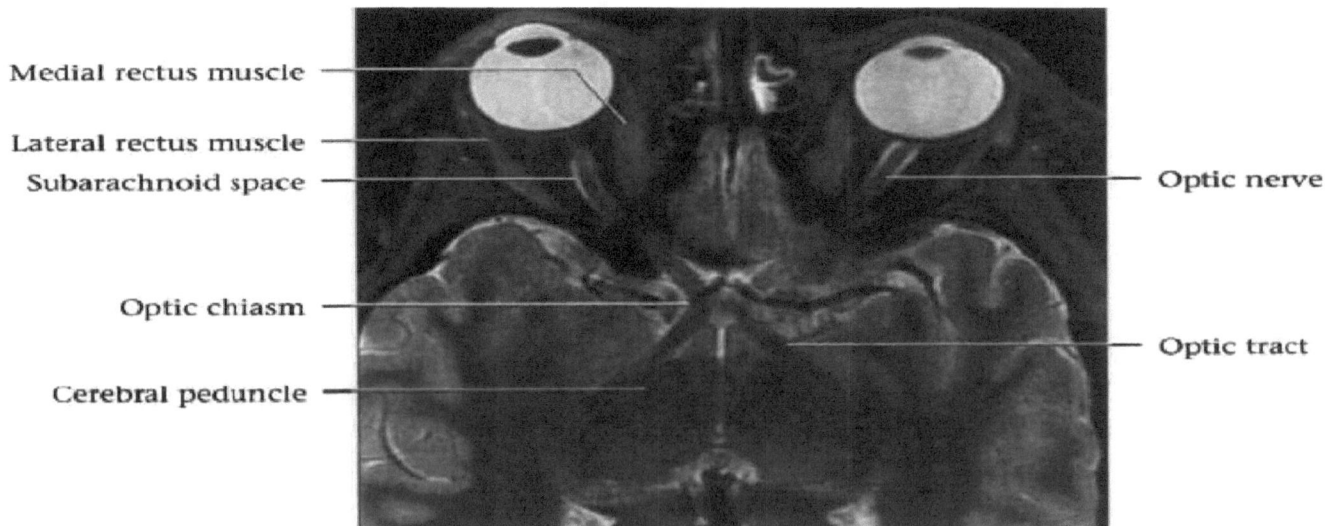

Labeled MRI (bottom):
- Medial rectus muscle
- Lateral rectus muscle
- Subarachnoid space
- Optic chiasm
- Cerebral peduncle
- Optic nerve
- Optic tract

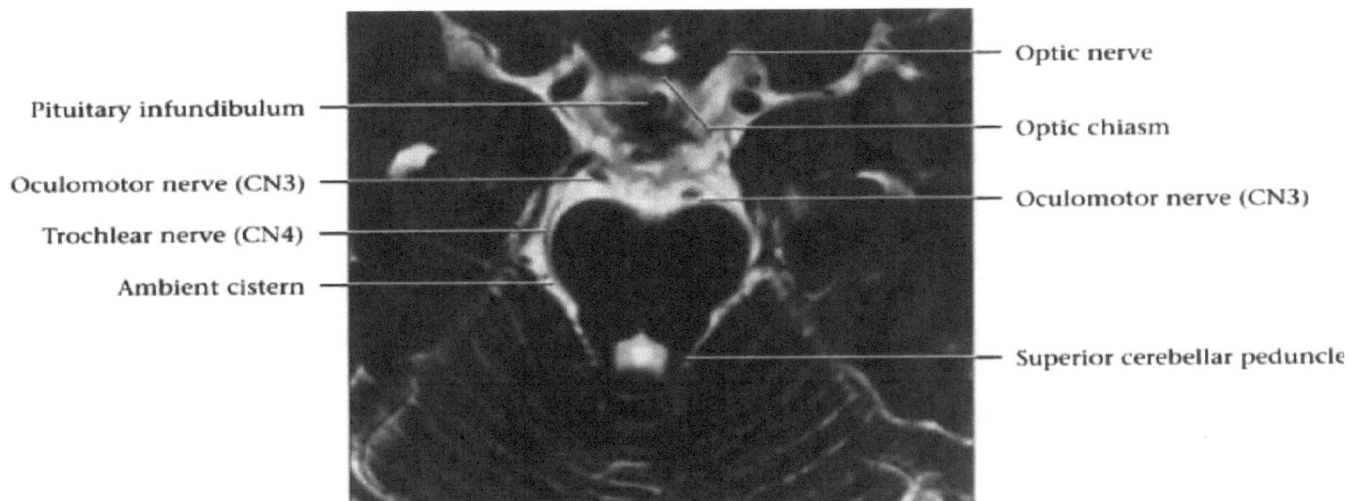

Pituitary infundibulum — Optic nerve

Optic chiasm

Oculomotor nerve (CN3) — Oculomotor nerve (CN3)

Trochlear nerve (CN4)

Ambient cistern

Superior cerebellar peduncle

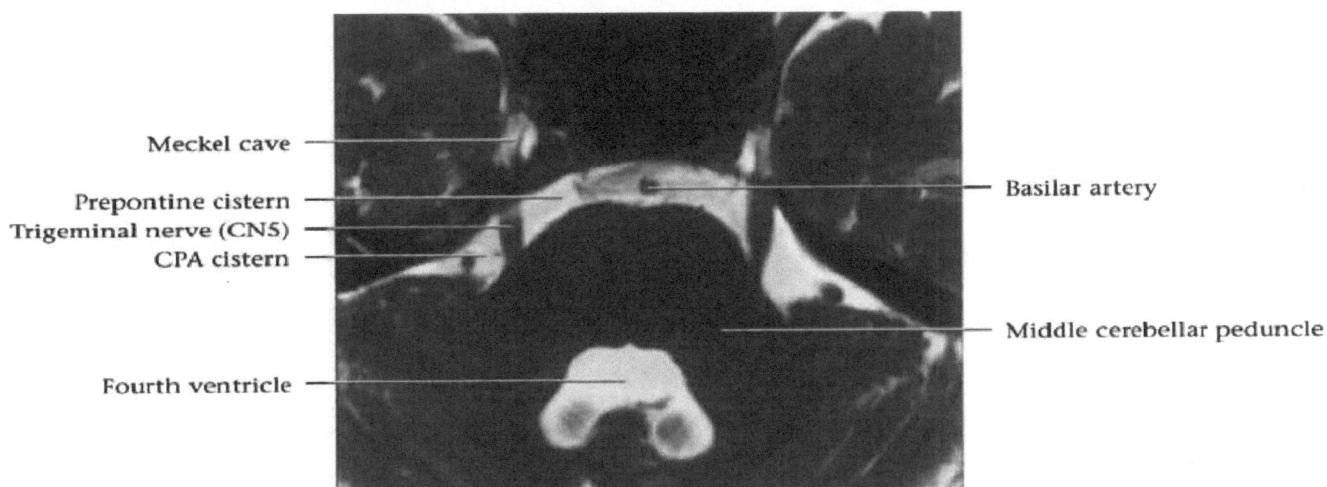

Meckel cave — Basilar artery

Prepontine cistern

Trigeminal nerve (CN5)

CPA cistern — Middle cerebellar peduncle

Fourth ventricle

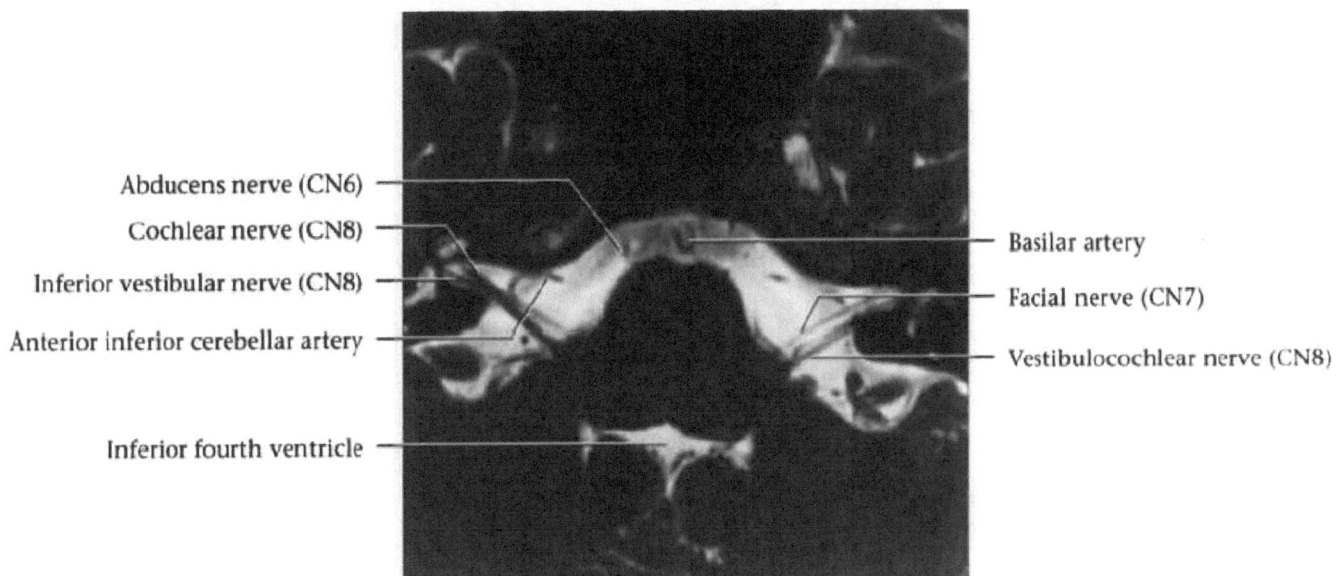

Abducens nerve (CN6) — Basilar artery

Cochlear nerve (CN8)

Inferior vestibular nerve (CN8) — Facial nerve (CN7)

Anterior inferior cerebellar artery — Vestibulocochlear nerve (CN8)

Inferior fourth ventricle

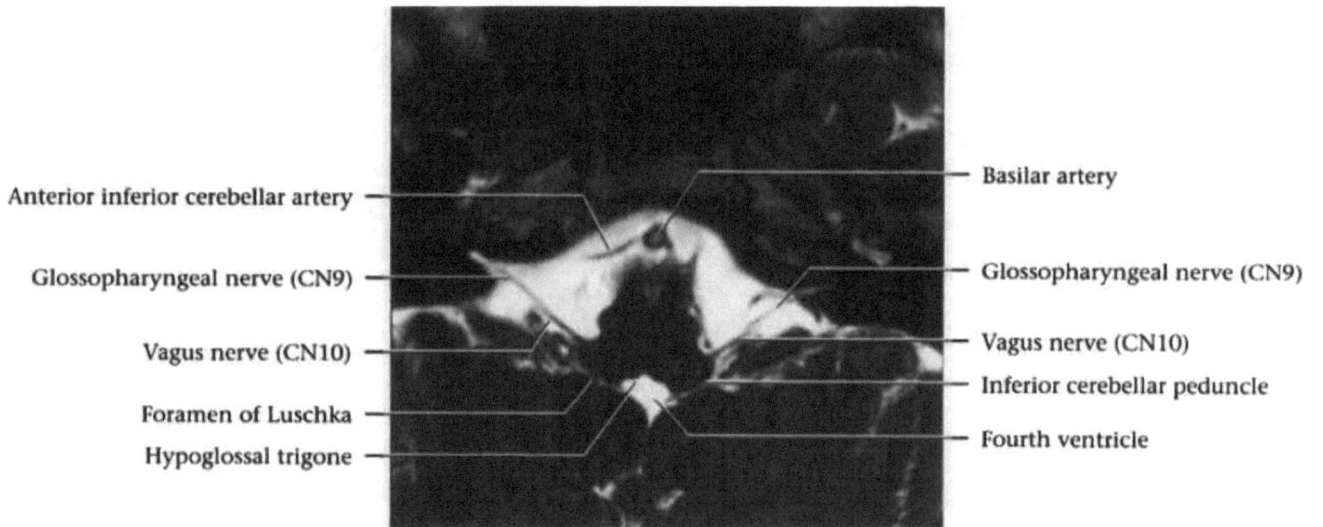

Anterior inferior cerebellar artery

Glossopharyngeal nerve (CN9)

Vagus nerve (CN10)

Foramen of Luschka

Hypoglossal trigone

Basilar artery

Glossopharyngeal nerve (CN9)

Vagus nerve (CN10)

Inferior cerebellar peduncle

Fourth ventricle

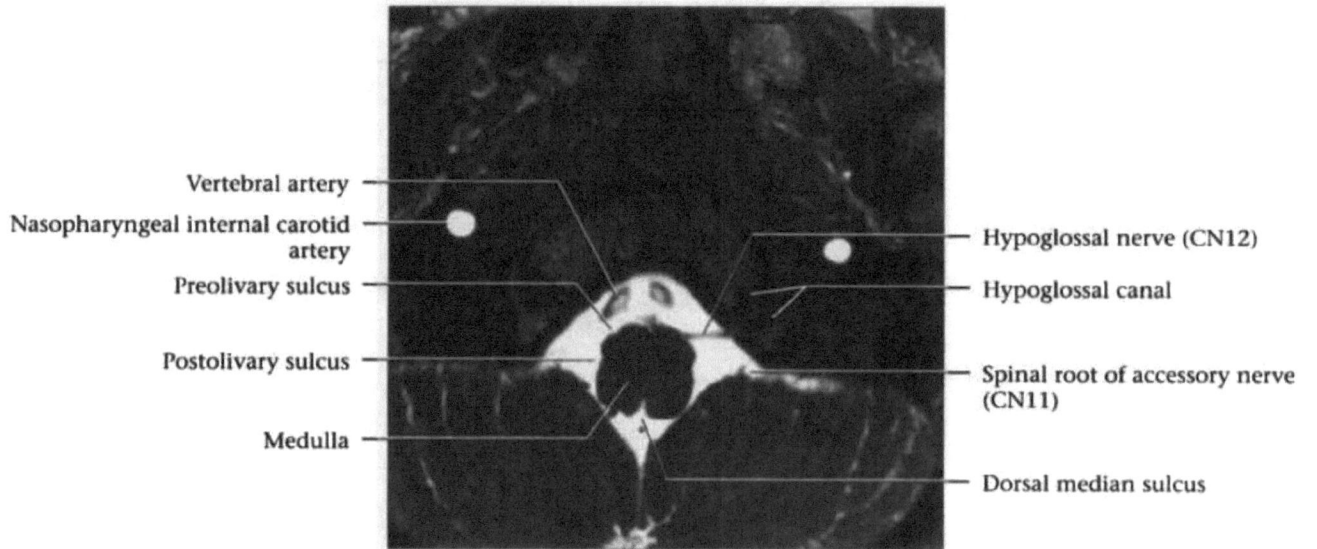

Vertebral artery

Nasopharyngeal internal carotid artery

Preolivary sulcus

Postolivary sulcus

Medulla

Hypoglossal nerve (CN12)

Hypoglossal canal

Spinal root of accessory nerve (CN11)

Dorsal median sulcus

Nuclear Medicine

Brain Imaging: the main tracers used in brain imaging are FDG (hexokinase mediated facilitated diffusion), HMPAO (Ceretec) and ECD (Neurolite) – both of these have active transport across the BBB and bind irreversibly to cerebral cortex. Remember that tumors wont take up HMPAO and ECD.

Brain Death: is a **clinical** diagnosis, we can infer this based on the findings of the study. The clinical criteria are coma, lack of brainstem activity, reflexes or spontaneous respiration with the exclusion of reversible causes. The brain death study shows the physiology of brain death – no intracerebral blood flow. This is the only brain study where SPECT is not mandatory.

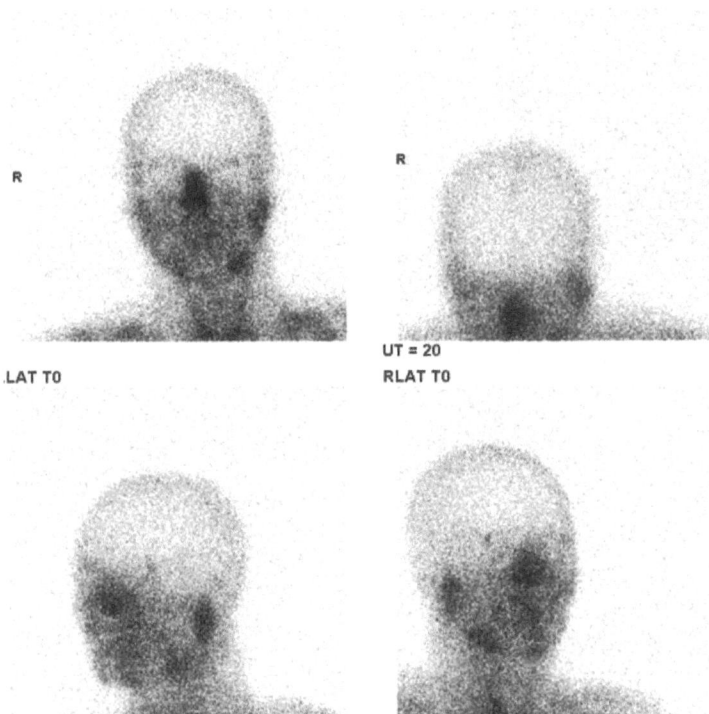

R

.LAT T0

R

UT = 20
RLAT T0

The 'hot nose' sign shows ECA flow, we wrap a tourniquet around the scalp to prevent scalp activity from throwing us off.

Tumor Imaging: done with FDG but remember that MRI is more sensitive for picking up brain tumors than PET. The more important use of this study is to check a tumor bed post–op. On MRI both granulation tissue and post–radiation changes as well as tumor can enhance, but only tumor will take up FDG.

– Vasogenic edema surrounding a tumor actually makes it more conspicuous on PET because the edema suppresses normal parenchyma
– Pituitary adenoma is FDG avid, so always glance at the sella before you close the study

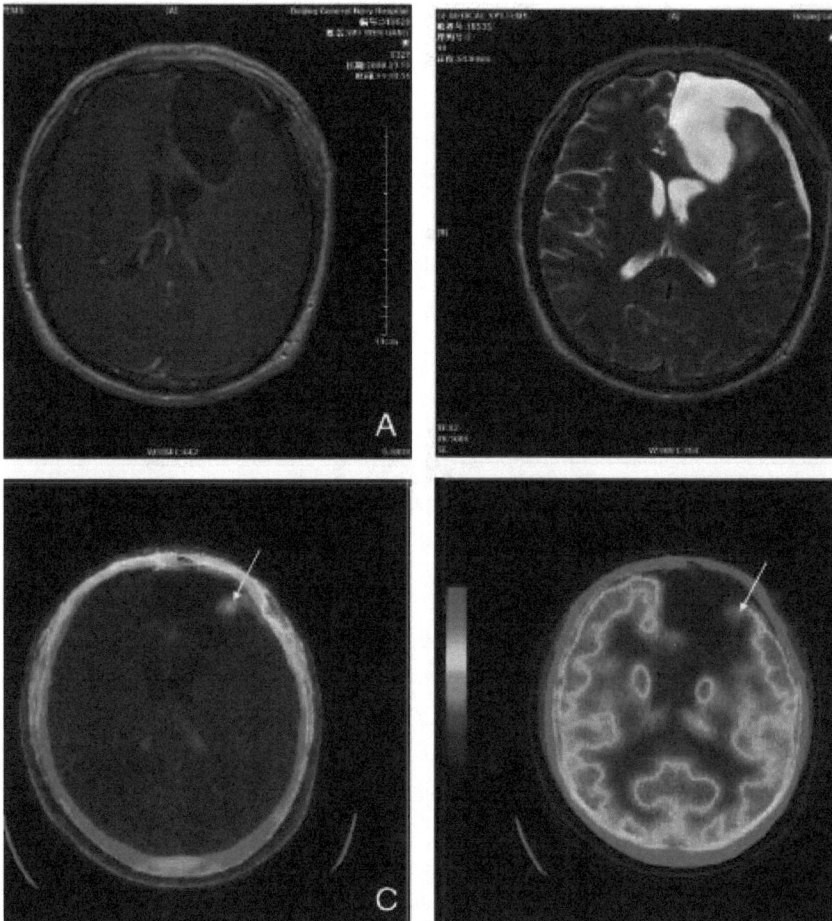

A – T1–Gad MRI shows peripheral enhacement in the post–op left frontal lobe

B – T2 image shows fluid signal and surgical defect with edema in the brain parenchyma

C, D – PET imaging shows increased focal activity in the left frontal lobe at an area of enhancement consistent with tumor

Seizure: patients with partial complex seizures that are poorly controlled with medication may benefit from surgical lobectomy. When related to mesial temporal sclerosis, excision of the focus typically eliminates the seizure activity. The patient undergoes continuous video EEG monitoring to catch seizure activity. Once it happens the radiotracer is injected within 2 minutes of onset (FDG has better image quality than HMPAO, but because of its two hour half life, it is hard to use in this scenario, so we use the Tc–99 agents with the 6 hour half life).

– During the ictal state there will be increased uptake at the seizure focus
– In the post–ictal state there is decreased activity in the seizure focus

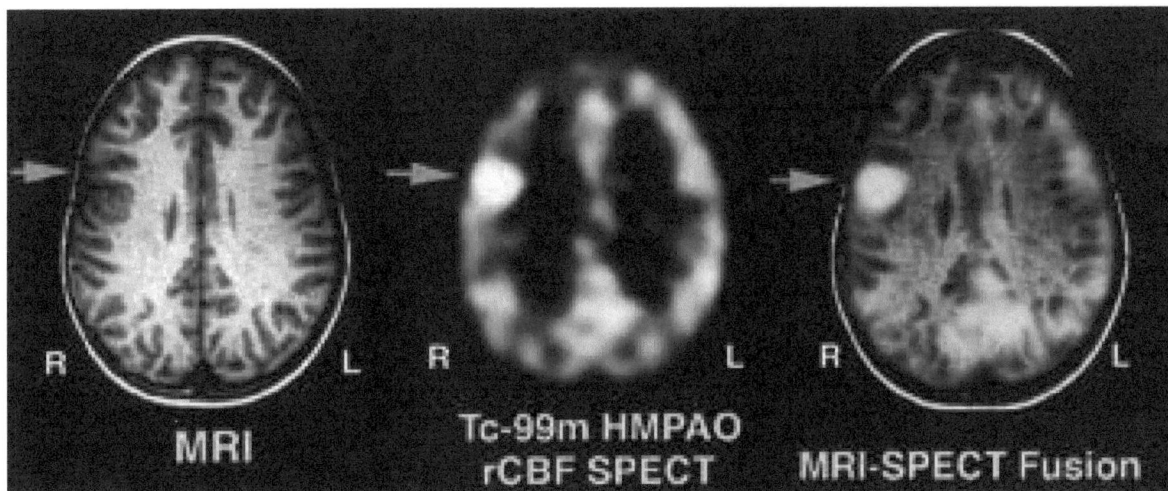

Dementia: the pattern of hypoperfusion and hypometabolism demonstrated corresponds to the clinical disease

Alzheimer's Disease	Bilateral posterior parietal and temporal lobes
Picks' Disease	Bilateral frontal and temporal lobe
Multi-infarct Dementia	Random distribution
Lewy Body	Occipital lobe – this is the key defining feature of this disease

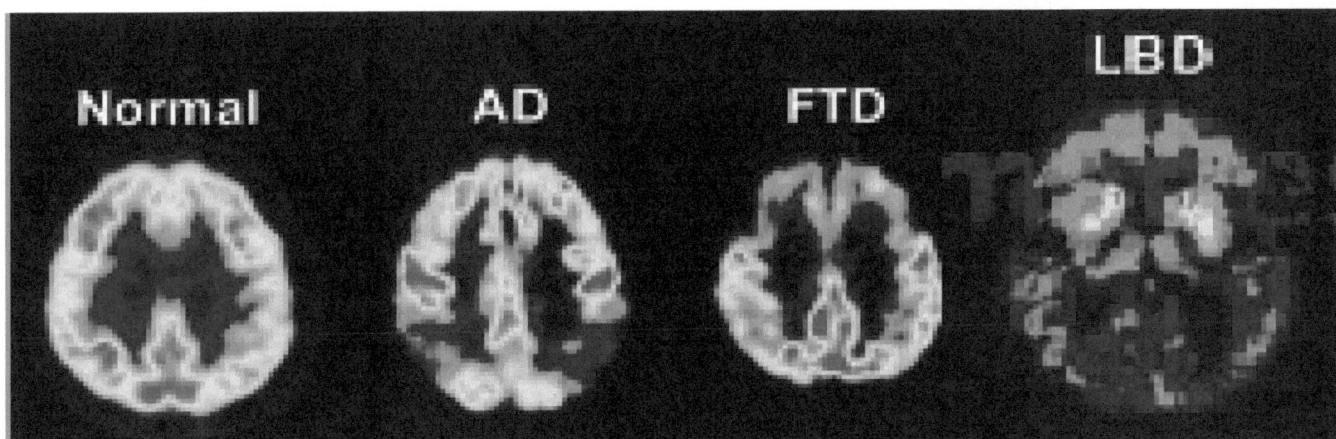

Parkinson's Disease: is caused by a loss of pigmented neurons in the substantia nigra and is characterized by bradykinesia, tremor, and rigidity. We now use DaTSCAN (ioflupane–I–123 injection). Ioflupane is a cocaine analog that has an affinity for the presynaptic dopamine transporters, which are abundant in the striatal region. Since it is an I–compound, use KI 2 hours before and 24 hours after the scan to block thyroid uptake.

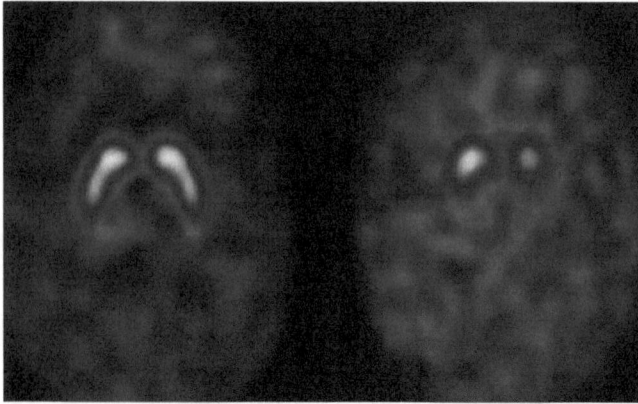

Easy to interpret – image on the left is normal, the caudate looks like a "comma" while the image on the right is abnormal, the caudate looks like a "period" or truncated comma. It can be unilateral or bilateral.

Nuclear Medicine Cisternographys: done to check for CSF leaks in patients post–surgery or post–trauma. Use 500 microCi In–111 DTPA and inject it intrathecally. 4 hours post LP the patient comes to NM and four planar images are acquired (Ant, Post, RL, LL) and the following day four more planar images are acquired.

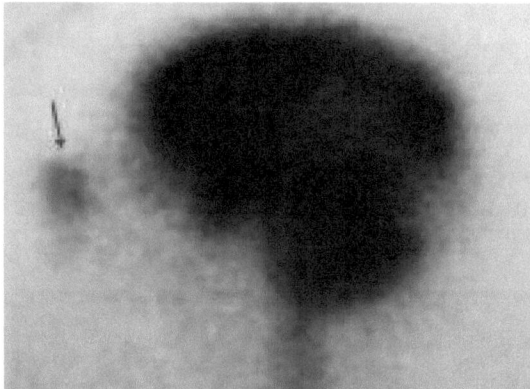

Cisternography can also be used to evaluate for NPH. Injected tracer fails to leave the subarachnoid spaces at 24 hours, pools in the ventricles consistent with obstruction to CSF outflow.

<u>Thyroid:</u> this is going to be a lengthy discussion not only of nuclear medicine imaging techniques but also of thyroid malignancy since it isn't covered anywhere else in this study guide.

Tracers we use are Iodine based

- I–123 [159 keV, 13.5 hour T½, diagnostic only]
- I–131 [360 keV, 8 day T½, diagnostic or therapeutic]

These agents are affected in their efficacy by certain drugs: PTU, exogeneous iodine, synthroid, lugols solution, amiodarone, and iodinated contrast

Normal Scan: should show homogeneous uptake throughout the gland with a butterfly shape. The right lobe is often larger than the left. Normal Iodine biodistribution is esophagus, stomach, salivary glands, and blood pool. The 24–hour RAIU should be 10–30%. Use a pinhole collimator to image (also this reduces star artifact – caused by septal penetration of the parallel collimator).

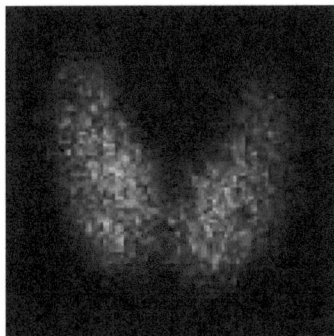

Thyrotoxicosis: thyroiditis and graves disease are the most common causes of thyrotoxicosis and can sometimes be difficult to clinically distinguish. A suppressed TSH (<0.1) is diagnostic of thyrotoxicosis. We can use a RAIU to differentiate conditions with increased uptake vs. those with decreased uptake.

Grave's Disease: is an autoimmune disease of the thyroid most often responsible for thyrotoxicosis (85%) and is more common in females. Results from antibody mediated stimulation of the TSH receptor with increased production and release of T3 and T4 (TSH is decreased). This is a hyperthyroid state.

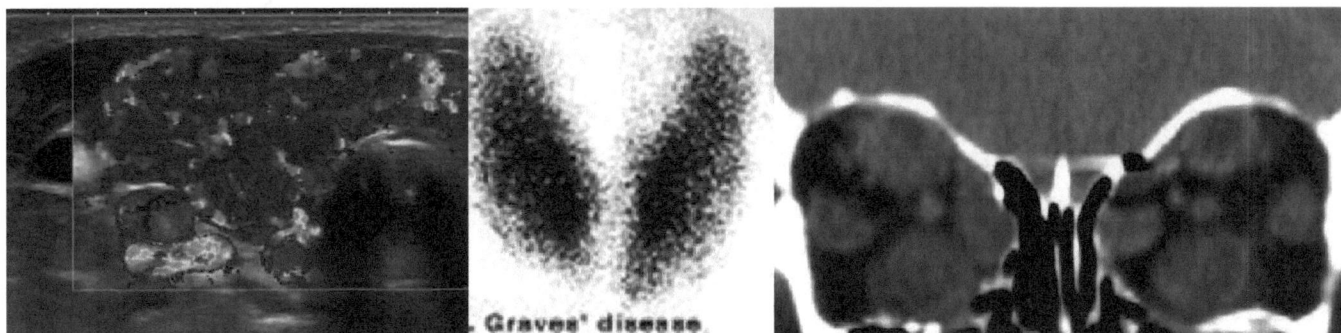

Left – US image shows hyperemic enlarged left lobe during thyrotoxicosis, this is the "thyroid inferno" pattern
Middle – NM 1–123 scan shows diffusely enlarged gland with increased RAIU
Right – Grave's opthalmopathy with enlarged extraocular muscles. These enlarge in a predictable manner: inferior, medial, superior, lateral, and obliques (IM SLO).

Hashimoto's Thyroiditis: is an autoimmune thryroiditis that affects middle aged females. Patients present with hypothryroidism and a goiter, however, a small subset of patients will present with "Hashithyrotoxicosis" – an acute hyperthyroid phase sometime during the disease which can be confused with Grave's. Look for anti–thyroglobulin and thyroid peroxidase antibodies.

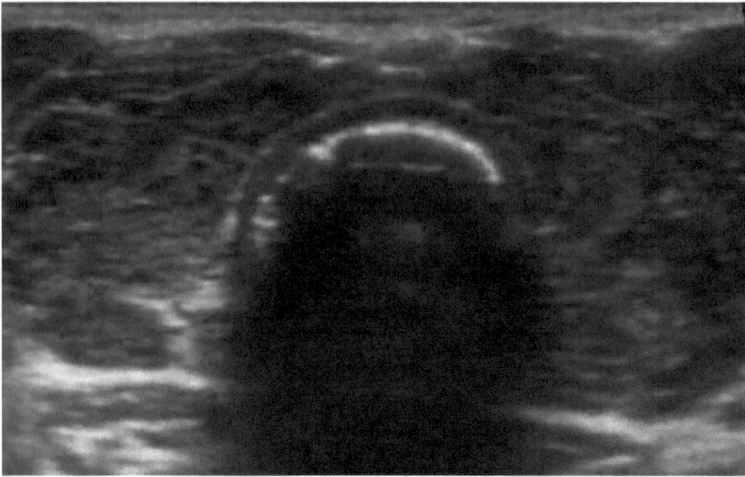

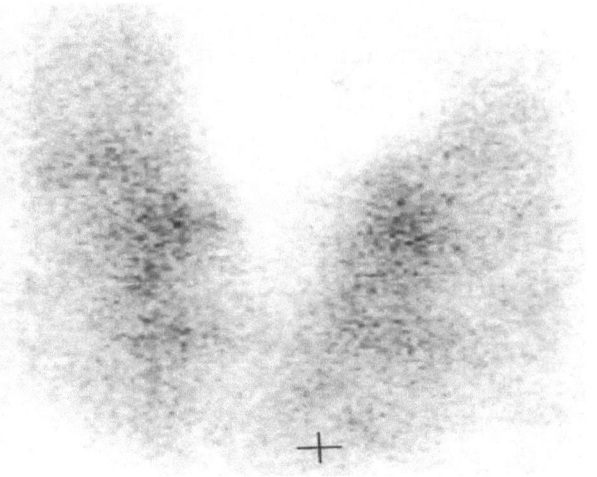

Left –US shows coarsened echogenicity and enlargement of the thyroid gland

Right – Scintigraphy demonstrates heterogeneous uptake with multiple areas of decreased activity relative to background

Subacute Thyroiditis: seen in young females as clinical hyperthyroidism. In the acute phase of this disease, there is very low RAI uptake (< 1% at 24–hours). The lack of uptake is how we separate this from Grave's disease because both conditions are hyperthryroid but Grave's has high uptake. After the acute phase the patient is hypothyroid and then they recover. As the patient recovers the thyroid uptake also improves. RAI therapy is contraindicated as this is a self–limiting process.

The physiology is based on: an inflammatory insult to the thyroid causes release of Iodine (T3/T4) which in turn cause the HP axis to stop secreting TSH.

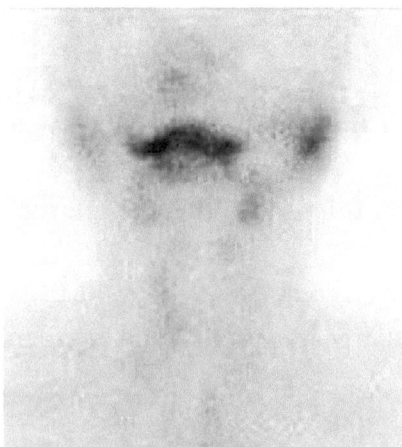

Nodules: usually an incidental finding, but we biopsy nodules > 1.5–cm. A cold nodule is more worrisome than a hot nodule. Most cold nodules are colloid or simple cysts, but up to 20% can be malignant. Hot nodules are less worrisome, they are typically adenomas and some can suppress the rest of the gland.

Plummer Disease: solitary toxic nodule that suppresses the rest of the gland can also be seen in the setting of multinodular goiter. The autonomous nodule can cause thyrotoxicosis by releasing thyroid hormones. To treat we give PTU to get patient euthyroid then either ablate with 25–30mCi of I–131 or a lobectomy.

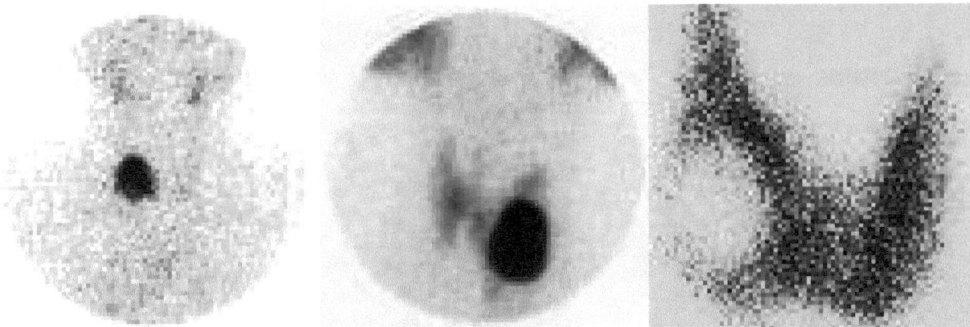

Multinodular Goiter: seen in euthyroid patients as an enlarged lumpy thyroid gland due to adenomatous hyperplasia. The incidence of thyroid cancer in these patients is less than 5%, but this increases if there is a dominant nodule. A history of radiation therapy to the head and neck increases the risk of CA to 30%. If goiter suddenly enlarges and the patient is hyperthyroid think toxic multinodular goiter.

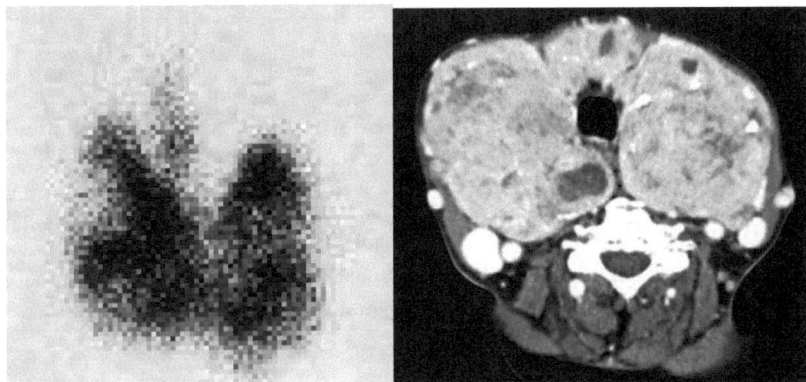

RAI Therapy (I–131):

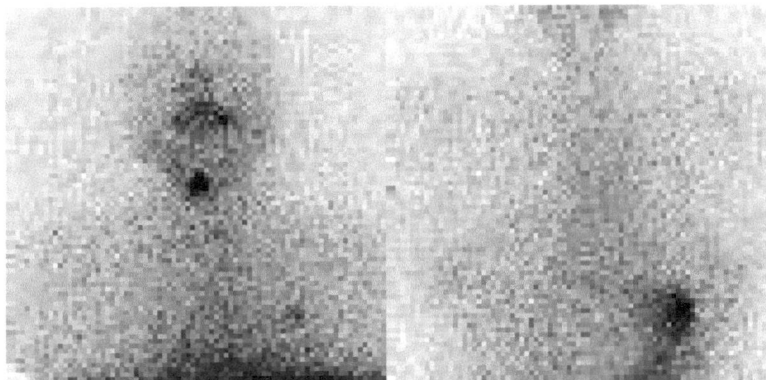

Case:

Image on left shows increased activity in the thyroid bed and in a left mediastinal node. Patient was treated with 200 mCi of I–131 and the image on the right shows resolution of disease.

I–131 is a po beta and gamma emitter. Prior to therapy the patient has to avoid iodine for 4–6 weeks and be off their thyroid medications for 1 week. The patient should be NPO 24–hours prior to and 2–hours post therapy. If female, make sure they have a negative pregnancy test. Women cannot get pregnant for 6 months after therapy.

Treat papillary and follicular cancers, medullary and anaplastic will not respond to this. RAI recommended for:

- Patients post thyroidectomy
- Carcinoma > 1.5–cm
- Extra–thyroid extension
- Metastatic LAD

The goal is to eliminate all diseased and normal remaining thyroid tissue. Follow patient with serial thyroglobulin levels (TG) because TG should not be present in a patient without thyroid tissue.

Thyroid scan administered dose is 50 microCi Thyroid cancer scan dose is 1.5 mCi
100 mCi I–131 for initial disease
125–200 mCi for recurrence/residual disease 200–300 mCi for metastasis
Limit to < 1000 mCi to decrease risk of pulmonary fibrosis

Treated patients are admitted in to a radiation safety room prepped by the radiation safety officer.

Thyroid Ultrasound: risk factors for a thyroid nodule being malignant are counter–intuitive: young, male patient with a solitary nodule that is cold on thyroid scan. Also, prior radiation therapy to the head and neck is an important risk factor. It is very common to see elderly women with benign thyroid nodules.

Most nodules are going to be benign colloid nodules, cysts, or hyperplasia. Cancer nodules will be papillary (70%), follicular (20%), medullary, anaplastic, or thyroid lymphomas.

Papillary: spreads to local lymph nodes Follicular: spreads hematogeneously

US Features:

Hyperechoic solid nodule	This is the "white knight" a good guy, < 5% chance of malignancy
Isoechoic solid nodule	25% of these will be papillary or follicular CA
Hypoechoic solid nodule	These have a good chance of being malignant, anaplastic CA or lymphoma
Large cystic components	Cysts favor benign process, but some papillary CA can have cystic areas
Comet tail artifact	Colloid cyst – benign
Intranodular flow	Soft tissue nodule flow favors malignancy
Halo around an isoechoic nodule	Typical of follicular CA

Benign Features	Malignant Features
Large cystic component	Hypoechoic solid
Hyperechoic solid	Intranodular blood flow
Comet tail	1–cm with micro–Ca2+ 1.5–cm with coarse Ca2+
Halo	Microcalcification – need biopsy

Papillary Cancer: is the most common cancer of the thyroid and frequently has nodal metastases. It appears as a solid mass with punctate regions of calcification. This will be hot on Iodine scan but does not concentrate pertechnetate. Good prognosis with surgical excision and RAI ablation.

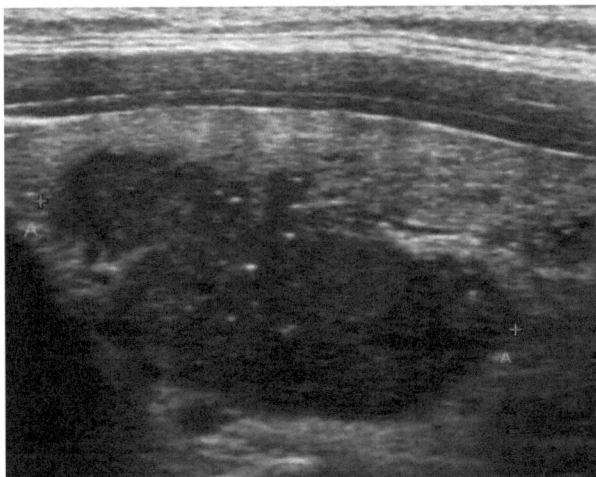

Follicular Cancer: the second most frequent thyroid cancer occurring in a slightly older age group than papillary cancer. This tends to have hematogeneous metastases instead of nodal metastases. Lesions are typically hypoechoic and lack cystic changes. Interestingly this concentrates pertechnetate but not Iodine.

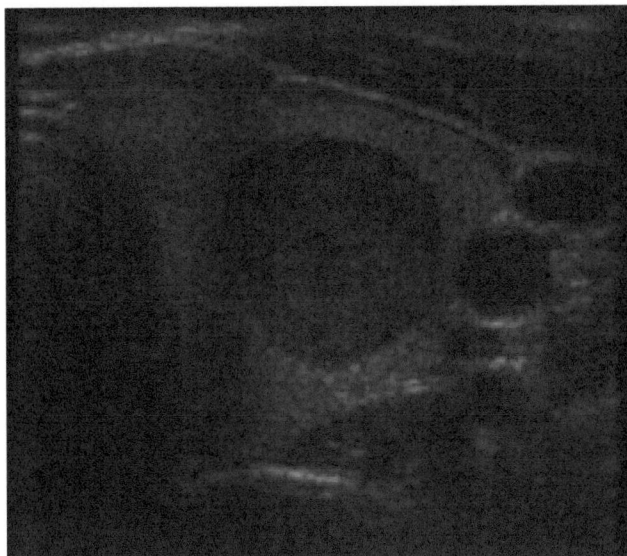

Medullary Thyroid Cancer: is characterized by the production of calcitonin and calcification of both the primary cancer and metastatic sites. It is associated with MEN II, VHL, and NF–1.

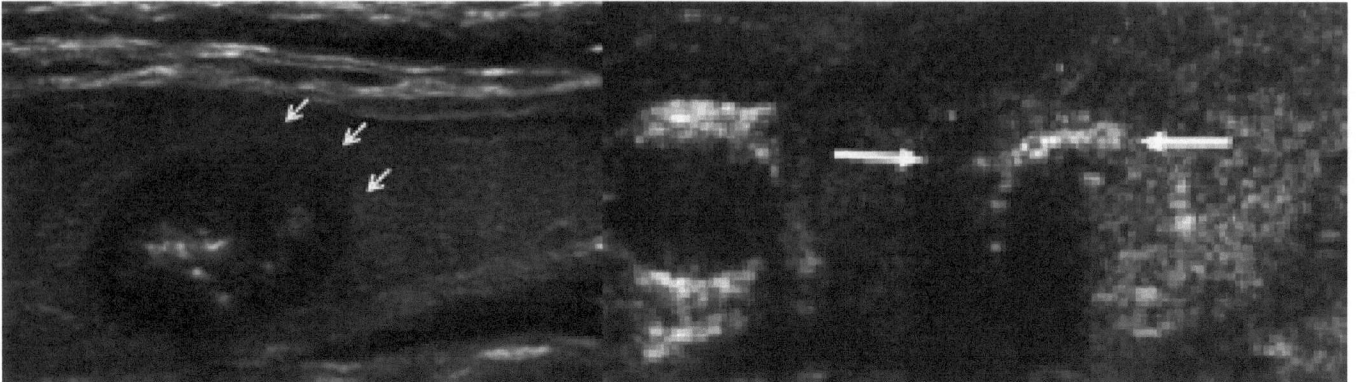

Anaplastic Thyroid Cancer: highly aggressive and carries the worst prognosis. Typically occurs in the elderly, has an association with MNG, and more often in females. Becomes large and compresses other structures, very heterogeneous.

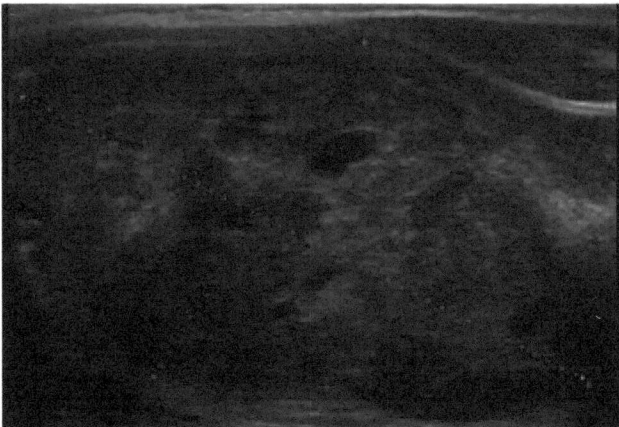

Benign Lesions of the Thyroid: look for cystic lesions, those with comet tail artifact, and solitary hyperechoid nodules "white knights" (pictured below – left to right, respectively).

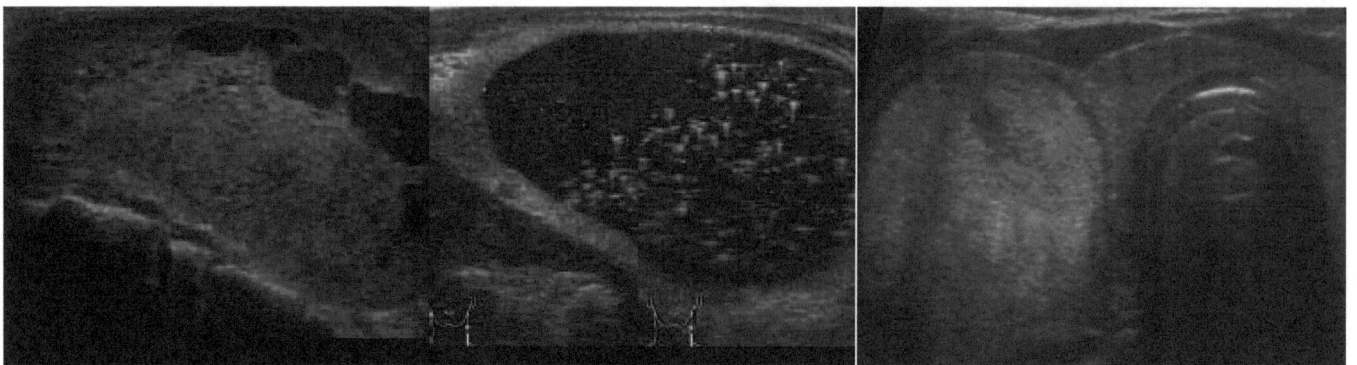

Parathyroid Adenoma: is a benign tumor of the parathyroid glands and is the most common cause of primary hyperparathyroidism. Patients have elevated Ca2+, decreased PO4, and elevated PTH. This tends to be a solitary process but can be multiple or ectopic.

Study is performed with Tc–99 Pertechnetate (20–25 mCi) and imaging is done at 20 minutes and 2 hours. Early concentration occurs in both the thyroid gland and parathyroid glands. The thyroid will washout and delayed retention is seen in adenomas.

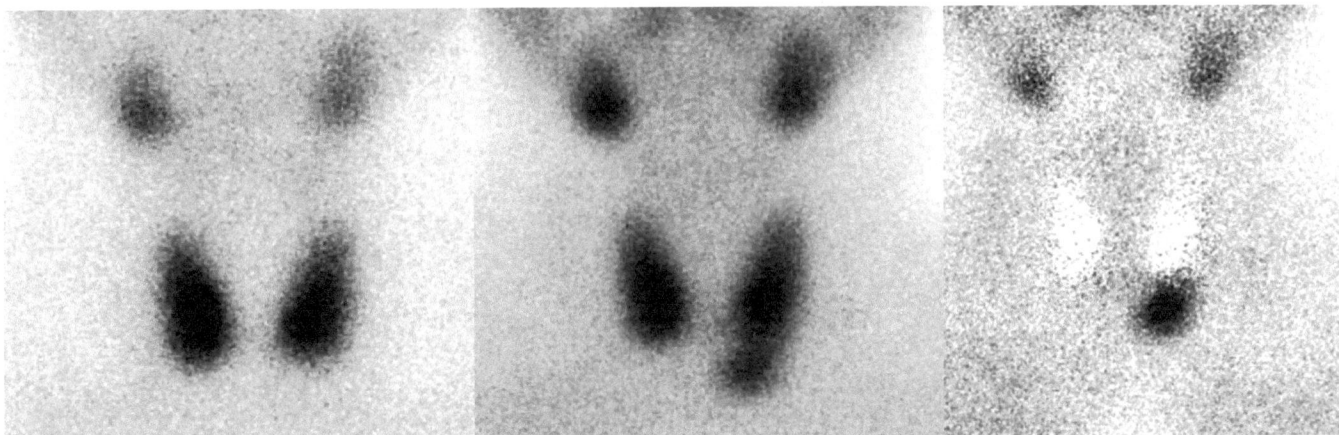

Cardiac & Chest:

Myocardial imaging is performed with tracers that get taken up by the heart during first pass via active transport (Na–K ATPase pump). These tracers accumulate in proportion to the amount of perfusion.

Overall thought, perfusion imaging shows us the worst defects and underestimates the amount of disease. The ideal exam is done using exercise testing with the patient achieving 85% max heart rate.

Pharmacologic Agents:

– Adenosine – vasodilator and causes bronchospasm, effects are short–lived but can be reversed with theophylline. Do not use in patients with heart block.
– Dipyramidole – vasodilator
– Regadenosen – vasodilator
– Dobutamine – vasopressor, increases cardiac work (ideal for those who cant exercise and have bronchospasm)

Tracer	Dose	Half–Life	Properties
Thallium–201	3–4 mCi	73–hours	Active transport
Tc–99 Sestamibi	20, 40 mCi (rest, stress)	6–hours	Passive diffusion
Rubidium–82		1.3–minutes	Active transport (K+ analog), made in a Sr–82 generator

Three axes are used to image the LV: short axis, vertical long axis, and horizontal long axis To SPECT the LV we only image 45–degrees RAO to 45–degrees LPO = 180–degrees

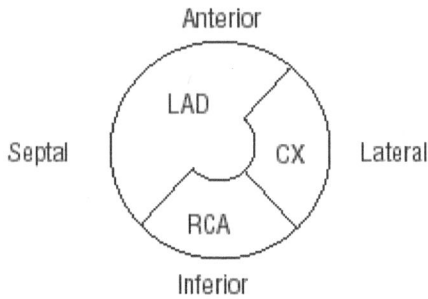

The trick is to detect perfusion defects and decide if they are ischemia (reversible) or infarct (fixed). Some confounders are artifacts.

Breast Attenuation: greatest along the antero–septal wall
Sub–diaphragmatic: greatest along the inferior wall (image below)

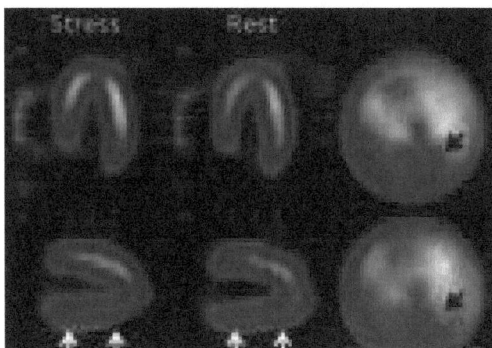

Indications to Discontinue a Stress Test:

1. Severe angina pain
2. Decrease in blood pressure
3. Frequent PVCs
4. ST–wave elevation
5. Patient cannot go on Normal myocardial perfusion scan:

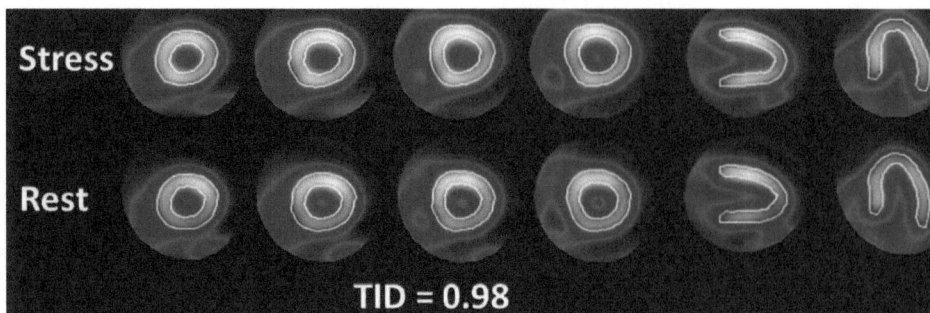

Stress–induced Ischemia: lateral wall w Infarcted Myocardium: apex of LV

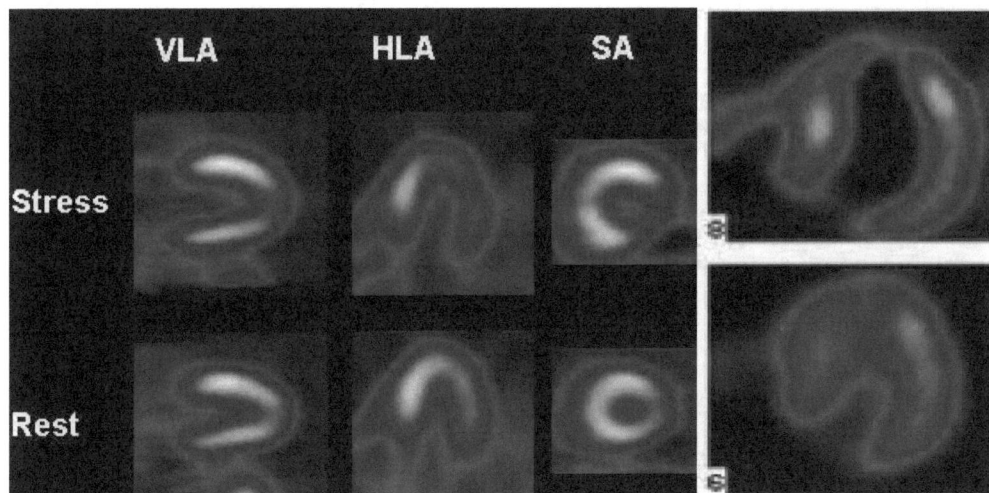

Hibernating Myocardium: this is chronically ischemic but not yet infarcted myocardium. It is important to recognize this because treatment varies. Revascularization can actually improve cardiac function.

Normally done with F–18 FDG PET imaging. On regular sestamibi imaging it looks like an area of scar.

Under normal circumstances the heart uses free fatty acids for metabolism, but when it is stressed (ischemia) it uses glucose, so with FDG imaging we will see increased FDG activity in areas of ischemia (hibernating myocardium), areas that show no activity are infarcted.

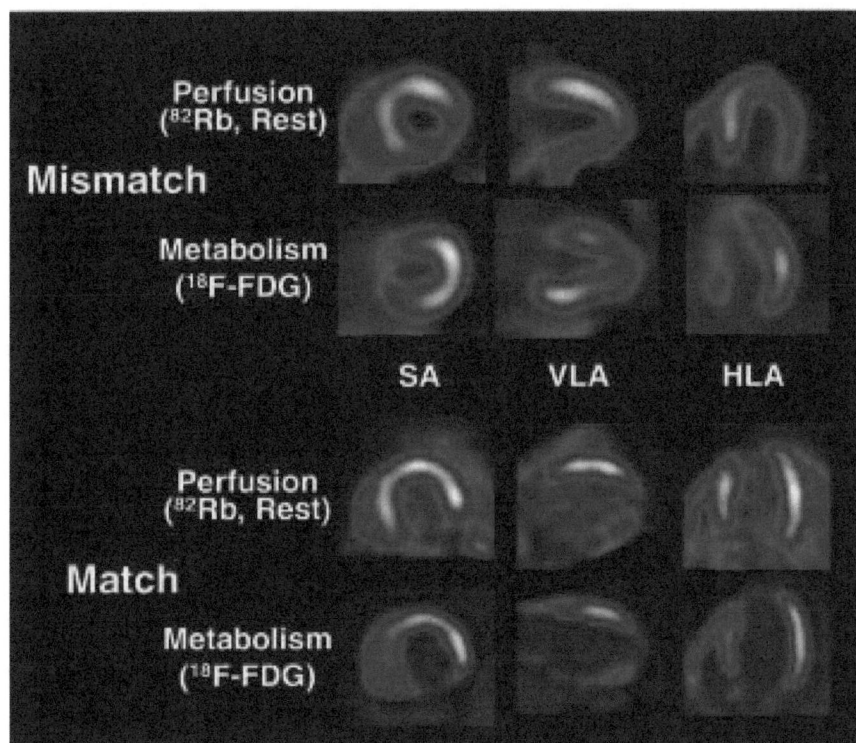

LBBB: exercise induced ischemia in the septum mimicking ischemia are seen in the septum in 30–90% of patients with a LBBB. Since the septum is perfused by the LAD, when it is ischemic the anterior wall and apex should be ischemic too. This is not the case in patients with LBBB and that is your clue to the diagnosis. Do not use exercise stress or dobutamine (increases cardiac work), instead use the other pharm agents – dipyramidole, regadenoson, and adenosine.

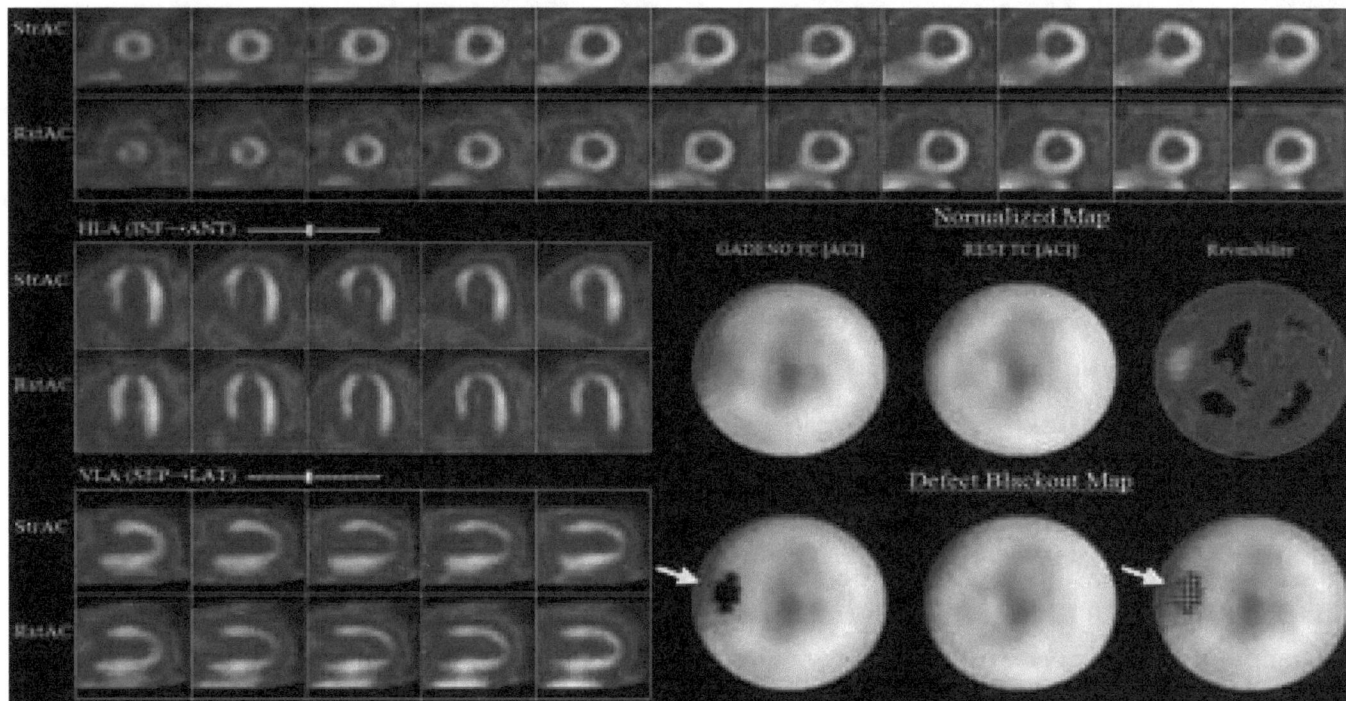

MUGA: accurate way to calculate LVEF and is used in patients undergoing chemotherapy with cardiotoxic drugs. The patient's heart rhythm is gated and each cardiac cycle is divided into 16 frames to maximize temporal resolution. Normal LVEF is 50–75%. Patient positioning and selection of ROIs is important because: EF = (ED–ES)/ED.

Example:
If the ROI is drawn to cover the LA or the spleen (overestimation of background) – falsely high LVEF If the ROI is underestimated then the LVEF is falsely low

Lungs: we are mainly going to discuss VQ scans and what accounts for defects in ventilation, perfusion, or both. Abnormal perfusion is not a specific finding because ventilation issues can lead to perfusion defects. So to diagnose a PE there has to be a mismatch.

Ventilation agents: this is performed first because the perfusion imaging has much higher counts

- Xe–133 is an gas that only allows for anterior and posterior imaging – needs negative P room
- Tc–99 DTPA allows for multiplanar imaging but tends to clump in the central airways b/c it's an aerosol

Perfusion agent:

– Tc–99 MAA is injected in the supine position (200–400k particles administered). We have to reduce the dose in patients with pulmonary HTN, right to left shunt, pediatric and pregnant patients.

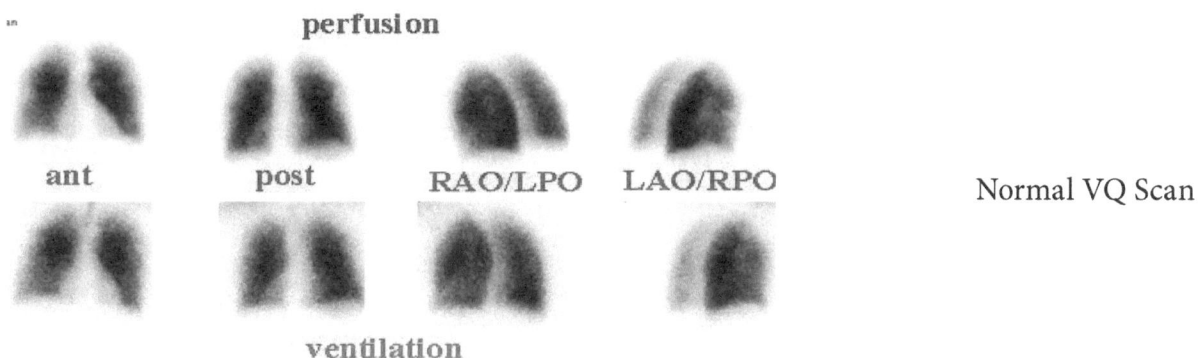

Normal VQ Scan

Below are two examples of positive VQ scans:

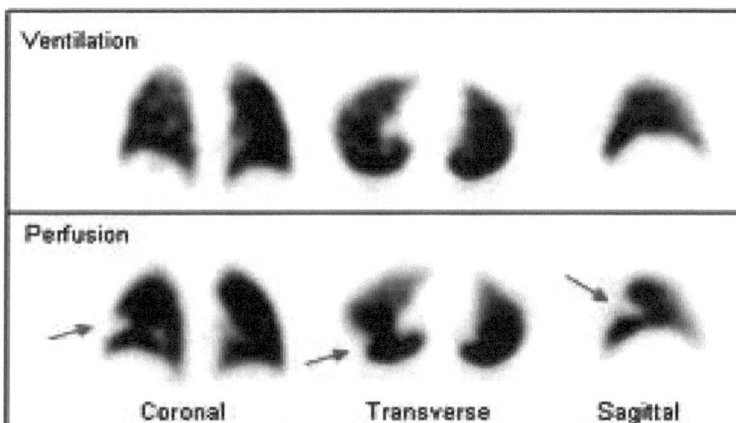

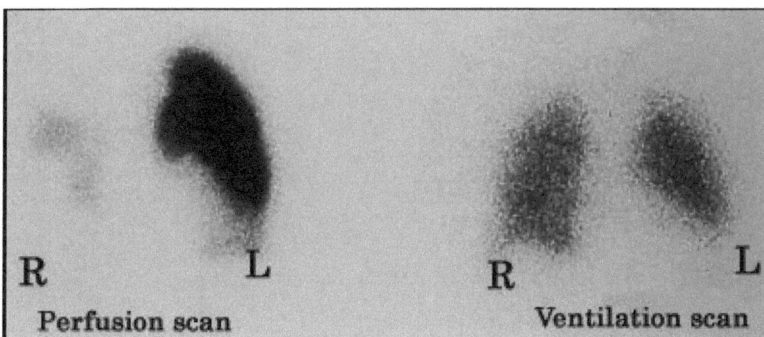

1. Matched Defect – underlying obstructive process (COPD, emphysema) with normal CXR – Low Probability
2. Mismatch – segmental perfusion defect with normal ventilation with a clear CXR – suspicious for PE
   a. High – two or more segmental perfusion defects
3. Triple Match – matched VQ defect as well as associated CXR finding – < 25% chance of being PE

<u>Hot Spots:</u> keep an eye out for this, it is basically multiple focal hot spots on the perfusion portion of the exam due to radioactive emboli. MAA accelerates blood clotting and the clots adhere to the MAA. The radioactive emboli are the result of the tech drawing blood back into the syringe containing Tc–99 MAA and then injecting.

GASTROINTESTINAL:

HIDA: is used to image biliary physiology, the tracer used is Tc–99 mebrofenin which gets cleared from blood pool by the liver and excreted by the biliary system. Most commonly we use it to assess for acute cholecystitis. Patient preparation is important. Ideally the patient should have fasted for 4 hours and should not be on opiates.

False Positive:

- GB overly distended by bile if patient has been fasting for > 24 hours
- Patient just ate and the GB is contracted

If the patient has been fasting for a long time, we can administer **Sincalide 0.02 mg/kg** to cause contraction.

We start imaging immediately after giving the Tc–99 membrofenin for one hour. At this time the GB should fill, if it doesn't we can either wait up to three hours or give **morphine 0.04 mg/kg** to cause sphincter of Oddi contraction and backfilling of GB and continue to image for 45 more minutes. Do not give morphine is there is any sign of CBD obstruction.

Acute Cholecystitis: non–visualization of GB confirms the diagnosis in the appropriate clinical setting.

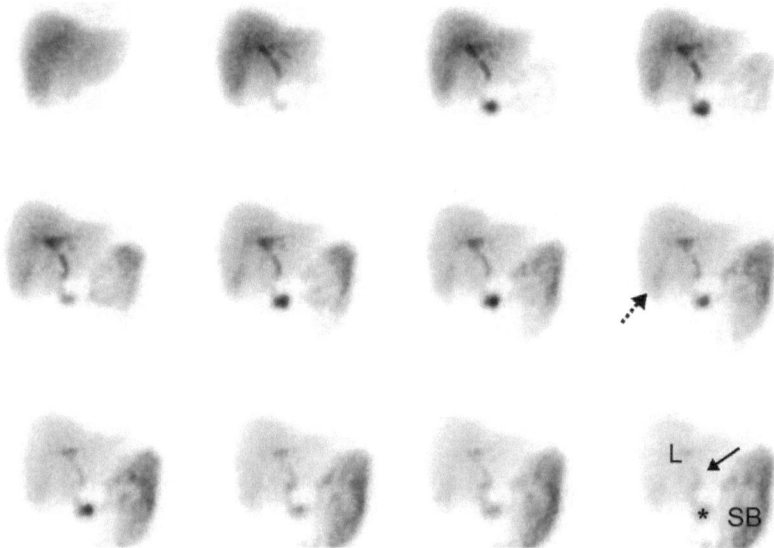

The most common causes of recurrent biliary pain after a cholecystectomy are retained or formation of new stones.

Chronic Cholecystitis: is prolonged inflammation of the GB almost always seen in the setting of cholelithiasis causing intermittent obstruction of the cystic duct. The GB will fill but EF will be low (<35%).

Acalculous Cholecystitis: GB dilated > 5–cm transverse in a sick ICU patient or those on TPN.

Bile Leak: easy diagnosis, surgeons will ask for this study after cholecystectomy in a patient with persistent abdominal pain and fluid in the abdomen that is new or increasing. Look for tracer accumulation in the GB fossa that then pours down the right paracolic gutter.

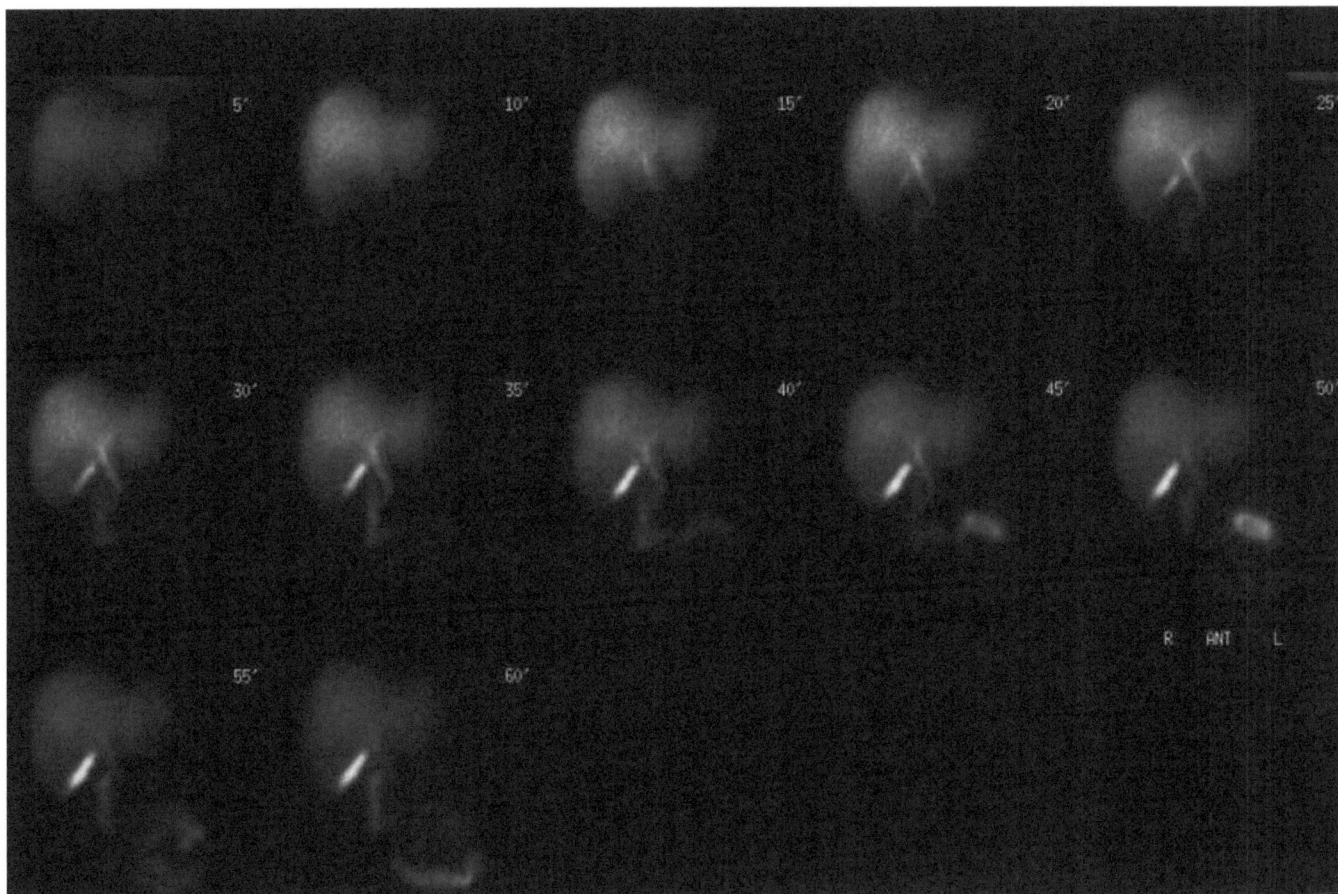

GI Bleed: performed with 20 mCi of Tc–99 RBC with continuous abdominal imaging. This can detect 0.1 ml/sec of bleeding. The diagnostic criteria are: sudden appearance of focal tracer activity, this will increase in intensity over time, and migrate with peristalsis. Sometimes the scan is negative initially, but because the tracer is good for up to 24 hours, you can bring the patient back and image again. It may show accumulated blood/tracer in the GI tract, but wont be able to localize since didn't see it happen from the get go.

The easiest way to label RBCs is in vivo but this has the lowest labeling efficiency. In vitro is the highest labeling efficiency.

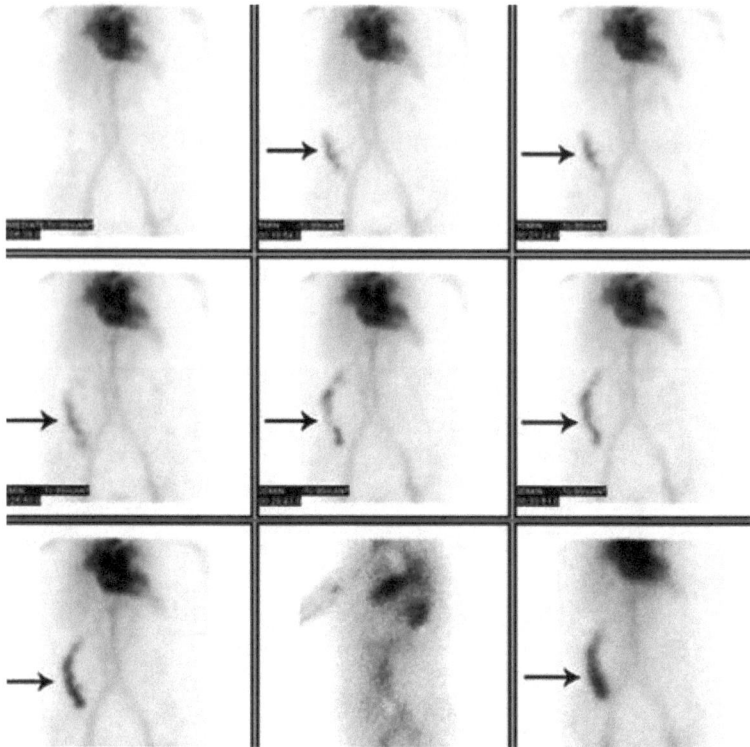

Meckel's Scan: done with 10 mCI of Tc–99 Pertechnetate with imaging for 30–45 minutes. Tracer gets taken up by gastric mucosa anywhere in the body and will be excreted into the stomach and will travel through the small bowel. It also has renal clearance. We can give H2 blockers prior to scan to increase efficacy. To make the diagnosis watch for a focus of tracer to show up in the abdomen at the same time as stomach activity. This ectopic focus, like the stomach will get more intense with time.

Fun Fact: Free pertechnetate has gastric, thyroid, and salivary gland activity.

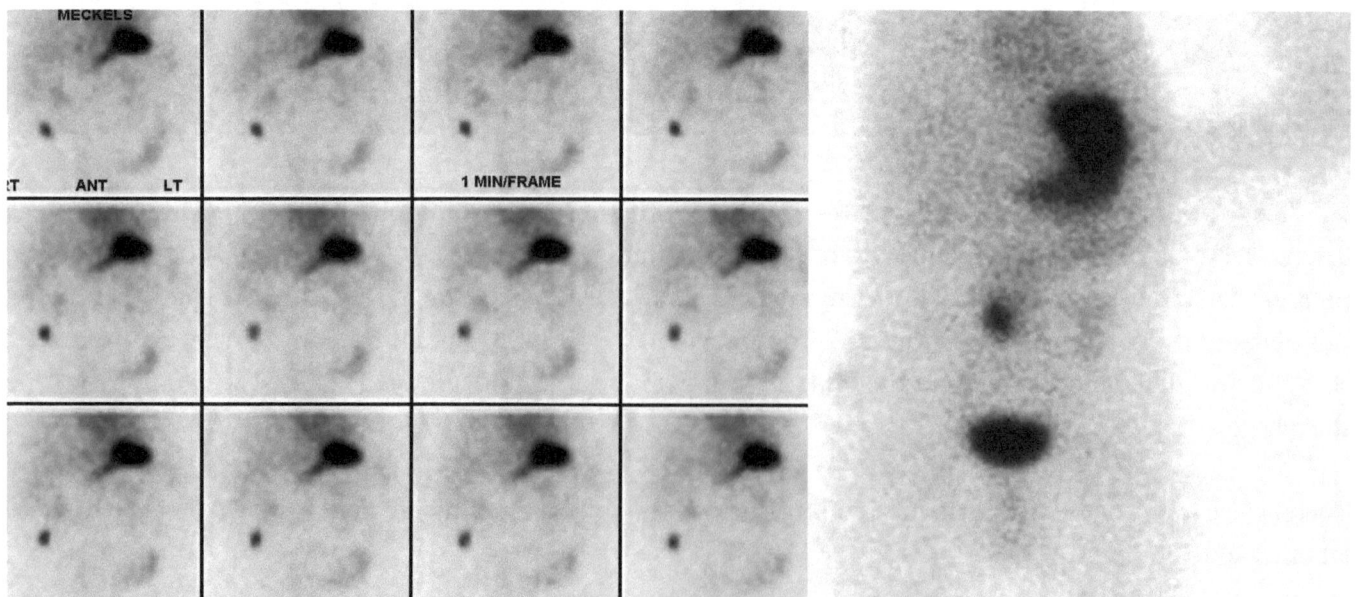

Meckel's Diverticulum – congenital intestinal diverticulum occurring most often near the distal ileum, considered the most common congenital anomaly of the GI tract. Approximately 2% of people may have it, presenting in the first 2 years of life, located 2 feet from the ileocecal valve. It is a remnant of the omphalomesenteric duct, contains ectopic gastric mucosa and can cause bleeding, intussusception, and small bowel perforation.

Gastric Emptying: performed with a solid meal consisting of scrambled eggs and Tc–99 Sulfur Colloid. Have patient eat the eggs and start imaging immediately in the anterior and posterior position. At 4 hours, > 90% emptying is normal. The normal time for half of a solid meal to empty is between 60–90 minutes.

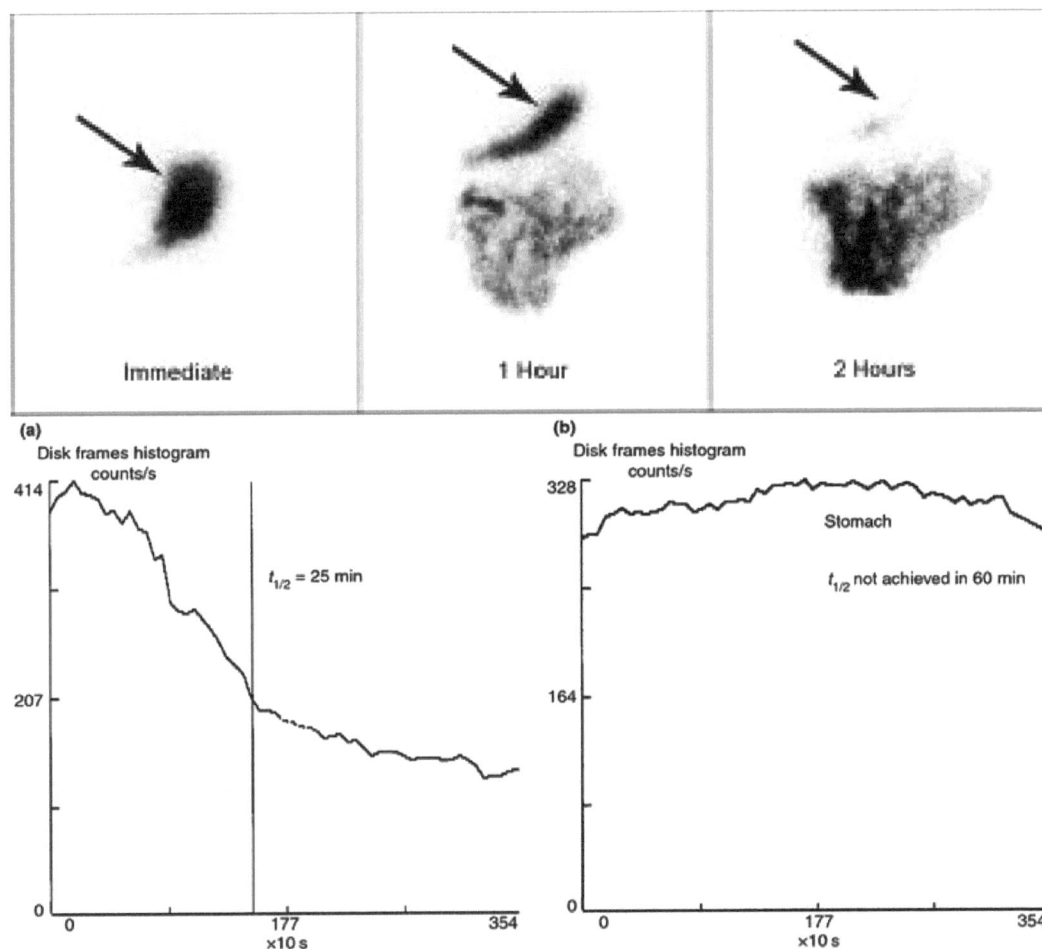

Top: shows normal imaging from a gastric emptying scan.

Bottom: two time activity curves, the left curve is normal emptying and the right curve is delayed emptying

GENITOURINARY: is used to view renal physiology and the two tracers we use are:

1. Tc–99 MAG3 – renal plasma flow agent that is taken up by active transport via tubular excretion
2. DMSA – binds the cortical tubules

Renal Scan: done by injecting 5–15 mCi of Tc–99 MAG3 and doing immediate dynamic imaging every 2–5 seconds for one minute (flow phase). Then continuous imaging every 30–60 seconds for 30 minutes for renal uptake and clearance (function).

– decreased perfusion to a kidney is almost always due to decreased function, except for in ATN
– ATN shows good renal perfusion but no excretion of tracer – oliguria

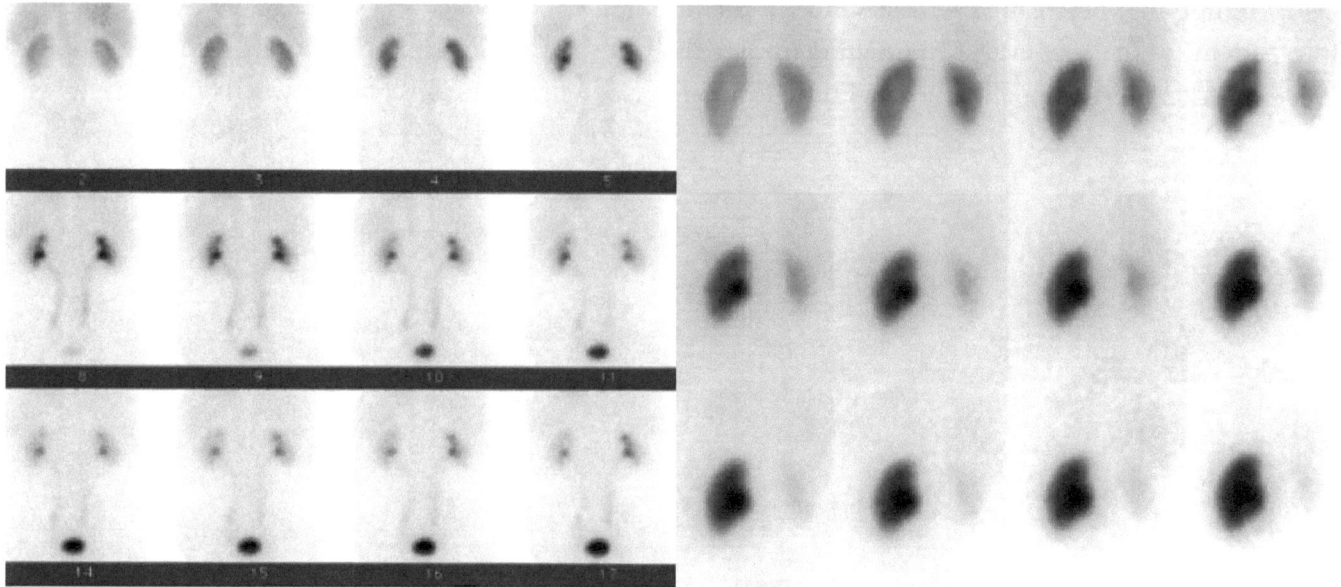

Left – normal renal scan showing renal uptake and symmetric rapid clearance

Right – abnormal scan showing persistent accumulation of tracer in the left kidney with distention of the collecting system – UPJ obstruction.

Renal Artery Stenosis: renal scan plus ACEI to block the constriction of the efferent arteriole inducing renal failure. A positive scan will show a drop in GFR in the abnormal kidney(s) and this is seen as a delayed nephrogram with MAG3 imaging. Since MAG3 is taken up by the tubules the initial uptake is normal, but **after we give the ACEI, there is a persistent nephrogram.**

DMSA: this binds the renal tubules in the cortex with very little excretion, it is used to look for pyelonephritis and renal cortical scarring. Procedure is simple, inject tracer, wait a few hours, then image the kidneys. There should be no collecting system activity. Areas of photopenia correlate with scar or acute pyelonephritis – clinical setting.

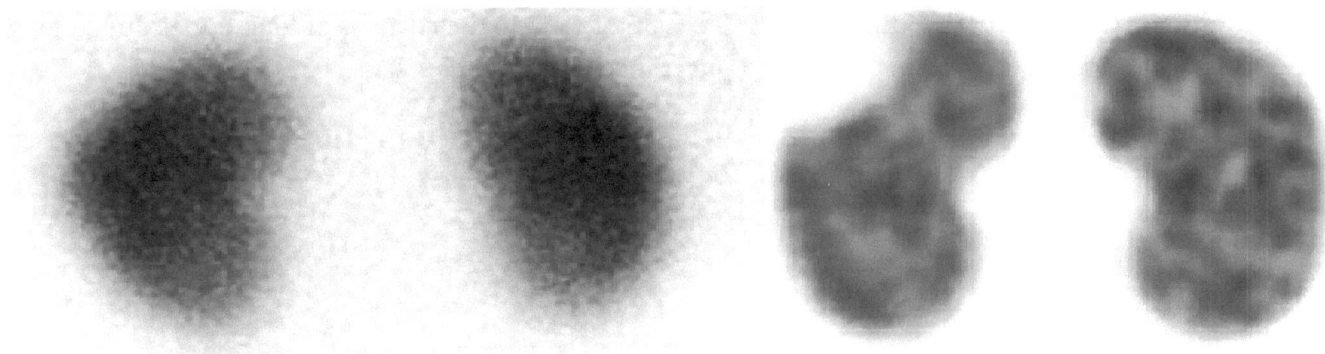

Left – normal DMSA scan with homogeneous cortical uptake. Right – focal defect in the superior pole of left kidney.

MSK:

Technique for Bone Scan is as follows:

The tracer used is Tc–99 HDP/MDP (20mCi), the tracer is taken up by "chemisorption" – binds to hydroxyapatite. After injection wait 3–4 hours to scan so the soft tissue activity is gone. Need a low energy, high–resolution collimator.

For three–phase:

1. Bolus injection with 3–5 second imaging for 1 minute (flow)
2. Blood pool images
3. Delayed images

Paget's Disease: intense uptake of tracer, can see the blade of grass appearance, likes the pelvis, hips, and femurs. Even osteoporosis circumscripta is hot – this is the active osteolytic phase of the disease

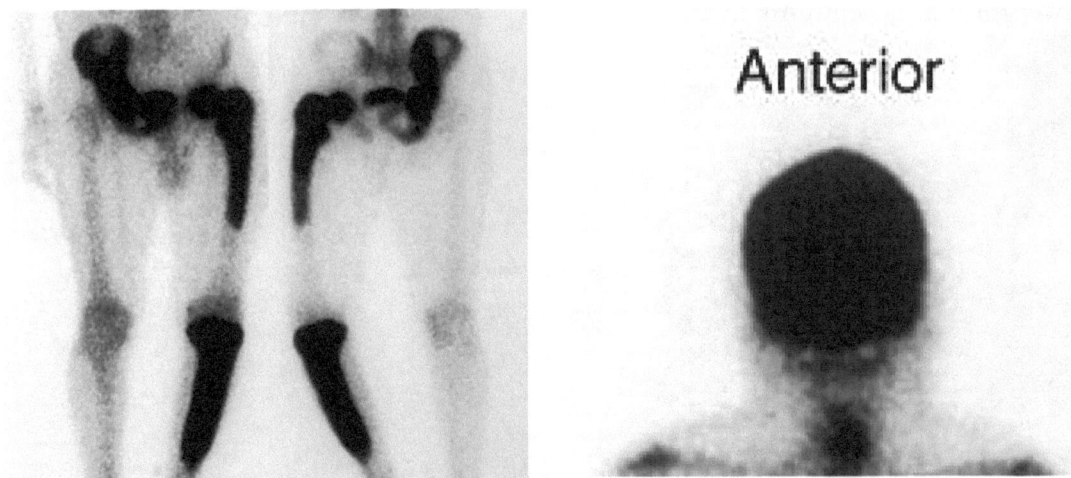

Hypertrophic Osteoarthropathy: diffuse tram–track uptake along the cortices of long bones due to lung cancer (most of the time), but can get a similar appearance with venous stasis.

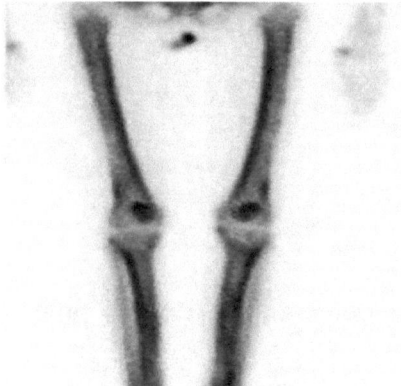

Fractures: get hot in 24–hours and stay abnormal for six months to three years. Stress fracture will be a focal cortical area of uptake and shin splint will be linear cortical activity. The patient shown below has right tibial stress fracture and left sided shin splints.

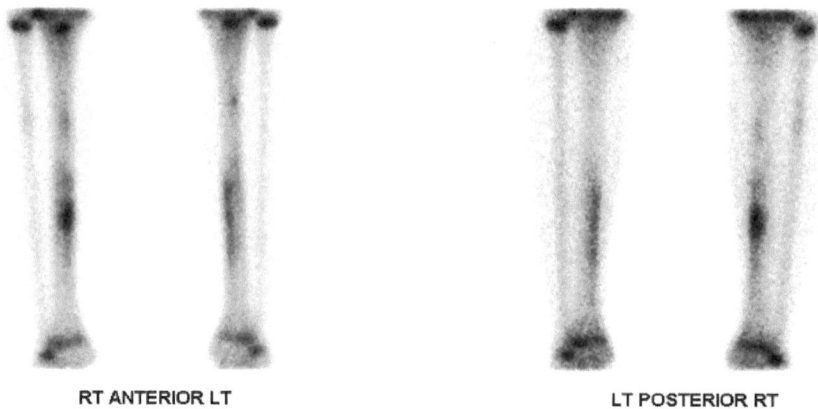

RT ANTERIOR LT   LT POSTERIOR RT

Rib fractures will be focal and contiguous over multiple segments; do not confuse this for metastases. Metastases will be all over the place, randomly distributed.

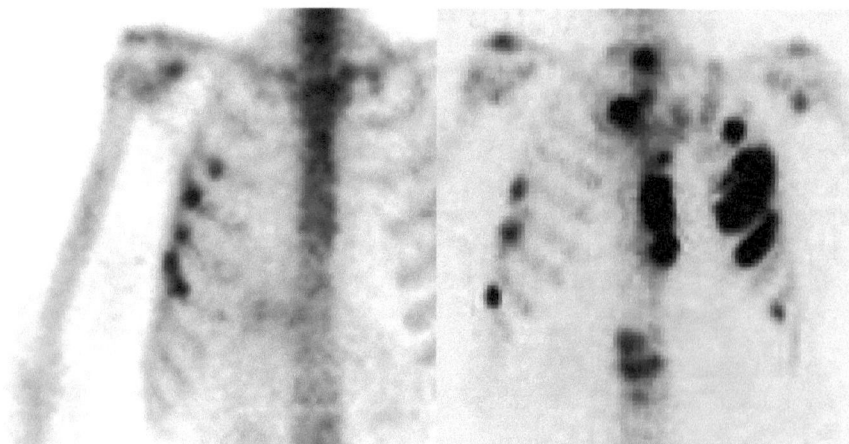

Flare Phenomenon: is increased sclerosis and activity in sites of prior bony metastasis after therapy. This will not persist for more than three months, so any increased activity after that point is a met, not flare phenomenon.

Special Cases:

1. Patient with abnormal bone due to prior fracture will be triple phase positive (if concerned for infection) so in these guys we have to do I–111 WBC scans
2. Ga–67 is used for spine infection imaging but needs to be correlated with a bone scan. If there is increased gallium uptake relative to HDP then it is positive for infection.
3. In–111 WBC is not sensitive for vertebral osteomyelitis.
4. If the bone shows increased I–111 WBC activity but you're still not sure if it's real, then get a Tc–99 SC scan, normal bone marrow will take up SC but infected abnormal bone will not.

Superscan: increased bony uptake in patients with extensive metastatic disease. There is a lack of normal kidney activity.

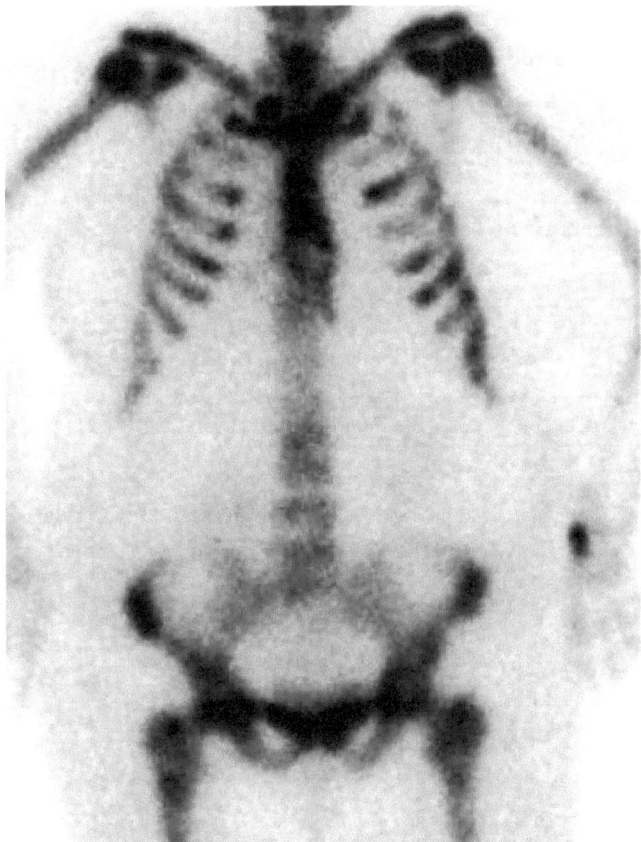

Prosthetics: normal uptake in a total hip replacement for up to one year and a total knee can be hot forever, but if there is hyperemia during the blood flow phase, that can be a problem. A loose femoral component will show activity at the distal tip.

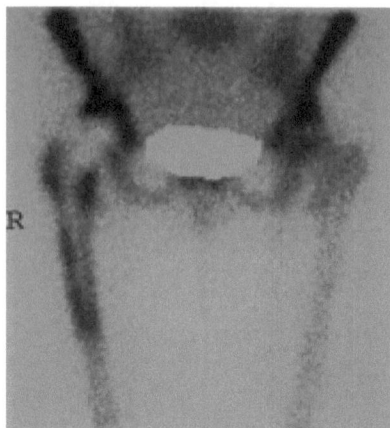

NaF PET: great for detecting bone mets, two times as much uptake as HDP, quicker clearance from soft tissues so we can image at one hour rather than waiting three hours. Increased patient dose – 20 mCi MDP = 5 mCi NaF.

Soft Tissue Uptake
Metastasis to the liver – focal
Excess Aluminum – diffuse, due to impurity during elution from generator
Infarctions – focal
Rhabdomyolysis – diffuse
Myositis Ossificans – focal
Metastatic Calcification – diffuse stomach, lung, kidney

Pars Defect: is a fracture of the neural arch of the vertebra involving the pars interarticularis and is believed to represent a stress fracture. Occurs most frequently in the lumbar spine at L5. Can be unilateral or bilateral. Can use bone scan + SPECT to localize injury and offer patient appropriate therapy.

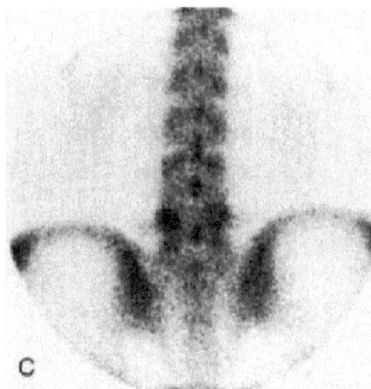

Sacral Insufficiency Fracture: seen in osteoporotic patients, those with hyperparathyroidism, and patients on steroids. Common sites include pelvis and vertebral bodies as well as the femoral neck and intertroch regions. Look for the "Honda sign".

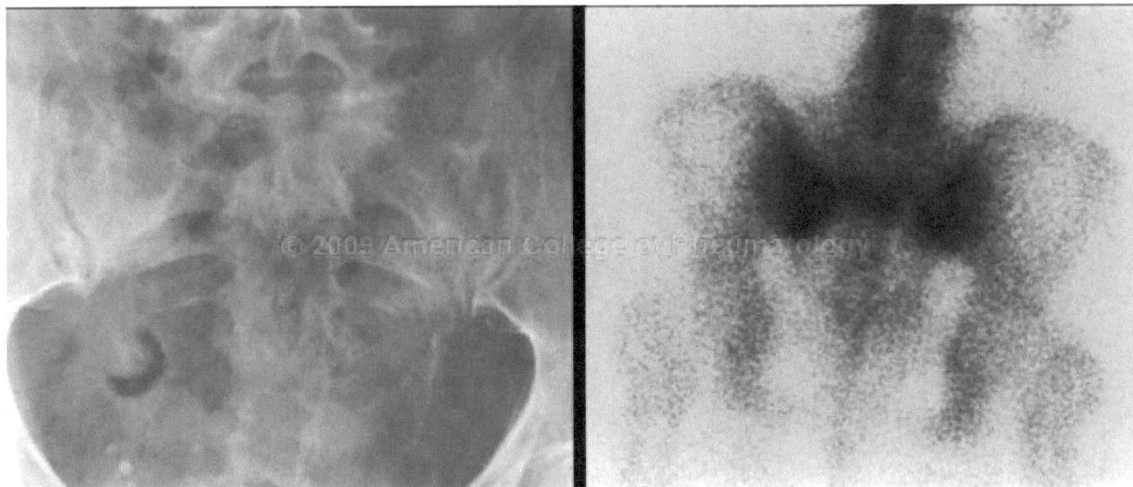

Tertiary Hyperparathyroidism: the mechanism of bone uptake of tracer is related to increase in bone resorption and subsequent turnover. Brown tumors will be focal hot spots. In long standing HPT, the patient gets calcifications in characteristic soft tissue locations: lungs, stomach, and kidneys. Look for prominent skull uptake, and the periarticular areas of large joints, sternum ("tie sign") and the AC joints.

Complex Regional Pain Syndrome: a paint producing entity with soft tissue swelling, periarticular osteoporosis, and late atrophy of the limb. Thought to be related to neurogenic, traumatic, or post– surgical issues. Typically the bone scan shows increased perfusion, blood pool, and uptake on delayed images (triple phase positive). Diffuse periarticular uptake is present. Look for it in the carpals and tarsals.

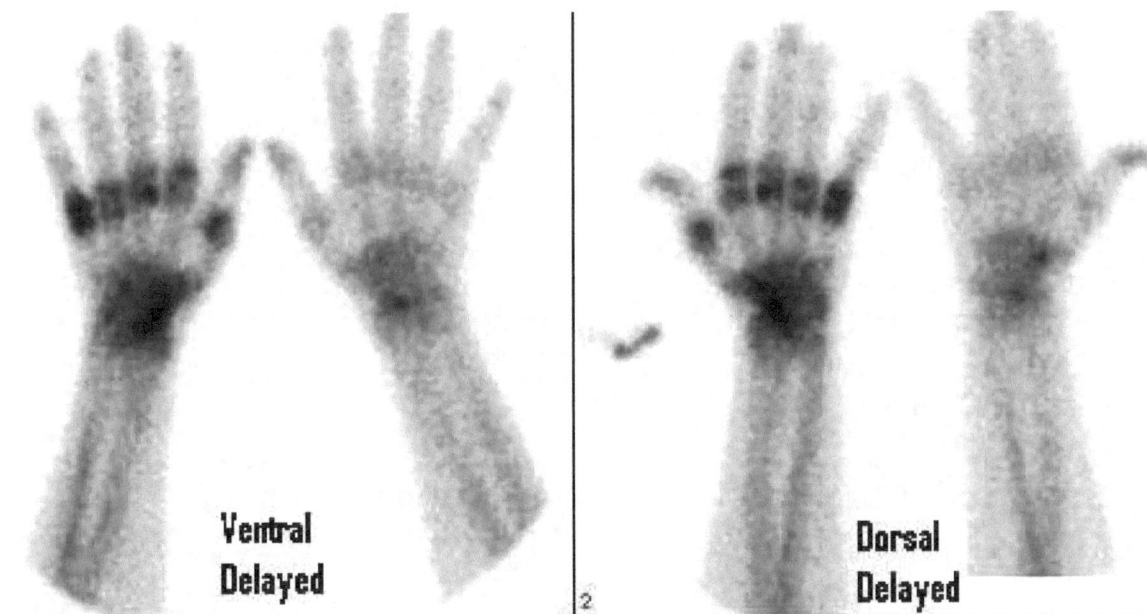

Idiopathic Osteonecrosis Knee: spontaneous disorder that occurs in the elderly, involves the medial femoral condyle preferentially. Bone scan abnormalities may precede the development of radiographic findings.

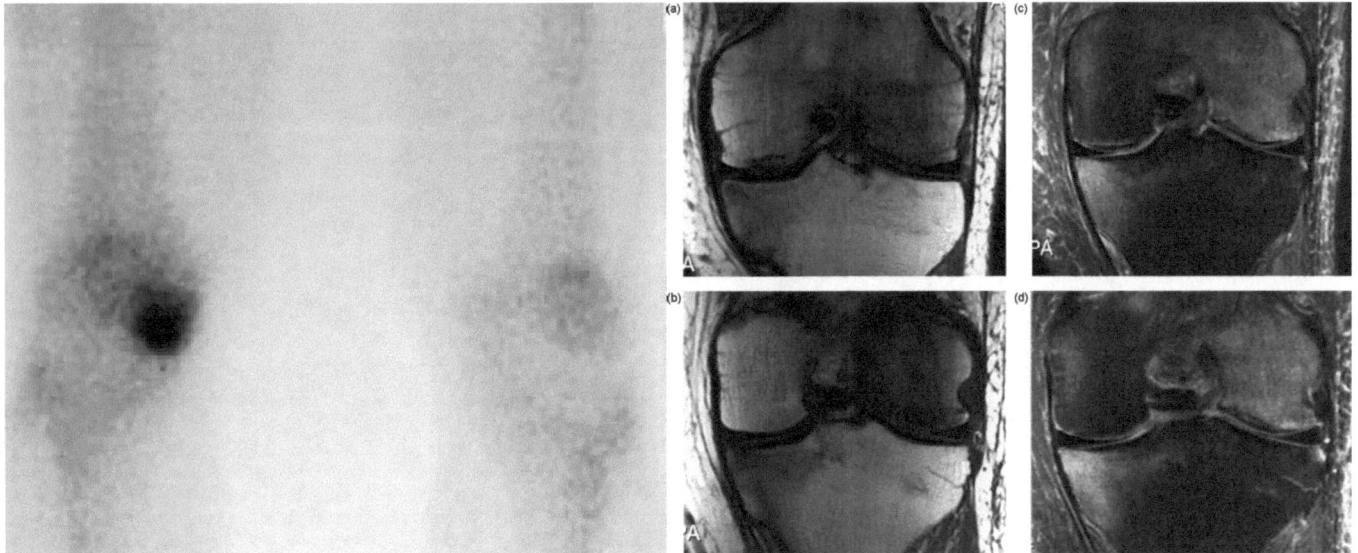

PET Scanning:

- Best for lesions > 10–mm
- Patient has to be fasting for 6–8 hours
- Do not perform if the glucose is > 200
- Do not perform immediately after GCSF therapy because bone marrow is very active
- FDG not good for prostate, renal cell, bladder cancers
- Be aware of brown fat

Standard Uptake Value (SUV) is a semi–quantitative value expressing intensity of uptake in an object relative to whole body distribution. It is a marker of activity but is not specific for one disease process.

Brown Fat: most common in females and kids, has a typical distribution of neck, chest, shoulders, and axilla. It is activated in people who are cold and shivering, obese people have less brown fat than thin people.

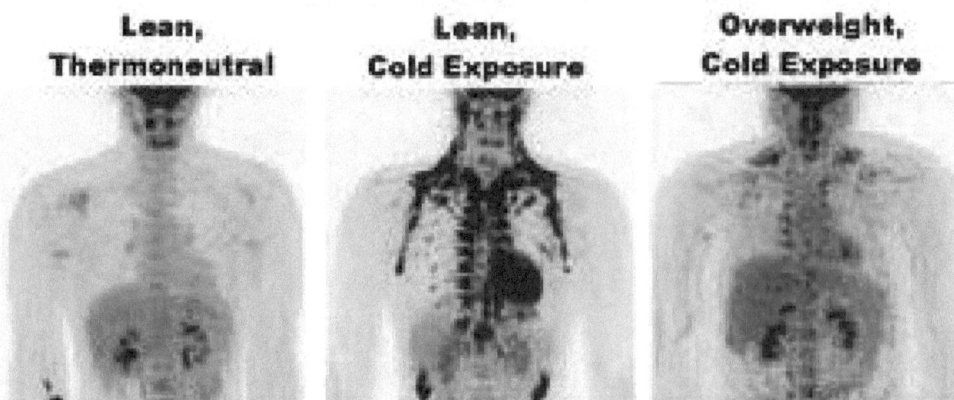

Key Points:

1. PET is used to stage and monitor therapy response in breast cancer
2. Lymphoma is PET avid and resolution of activity (not just declining) after therapy is a good prognostic sign
3. Metformin causes diffuse increased activity in the colon, start to worry if you see focal activity, get a scope
4. Tumors with low FDG uptake: renal cell, prostate, bronchoalveolar carcinoma, low grade gliomas, and neuroendocrine tumors
5. Do not perform FDG brain imaging within three months of surgery or XRT as it'll be a false +
6. Heavier patients have overestimation of SUV and lighter patients have underestimation

I–123 MIBG: is a nor–epinephrine analog that localizes in areas of sympathetic innervation and adrenergic tumors. Pretreat the patient with SSKI to block thyroid uptake and make sure patient is off their beta–blocker and amphetamines. We use this to look for neuroblastoma or pheochromocytoma.

A normal scan will have activity in: salivary glands, faint myocardial uptake, liver, spleen, and bladder excretion.

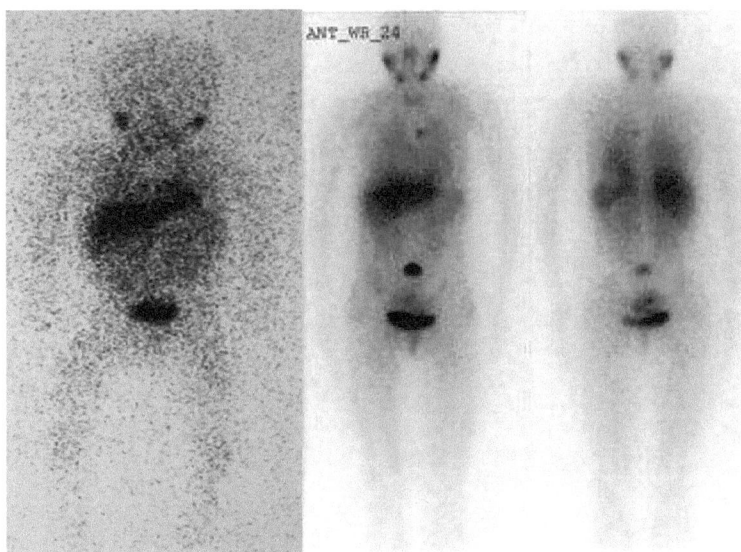

Left –normal MIBG scan distribution in a pediatric patient

Right – abnormal tracer activity seen in the low abdomen near the aortic bifurcation – likely a pheochromocytoma at the organ of Zukerkandahl.

In–111 Pentotreotide: is a somatostatin analong and is better for paragangliomas in the neck than MIBG. Patient has to be off of somatostatin prior to study. Use this to look for carcinoids and islet cell tumors.

A normal scan will have activity in: spleen and kidneys, liver, bladder excretion. No heart, salivary glands, or bone activity.

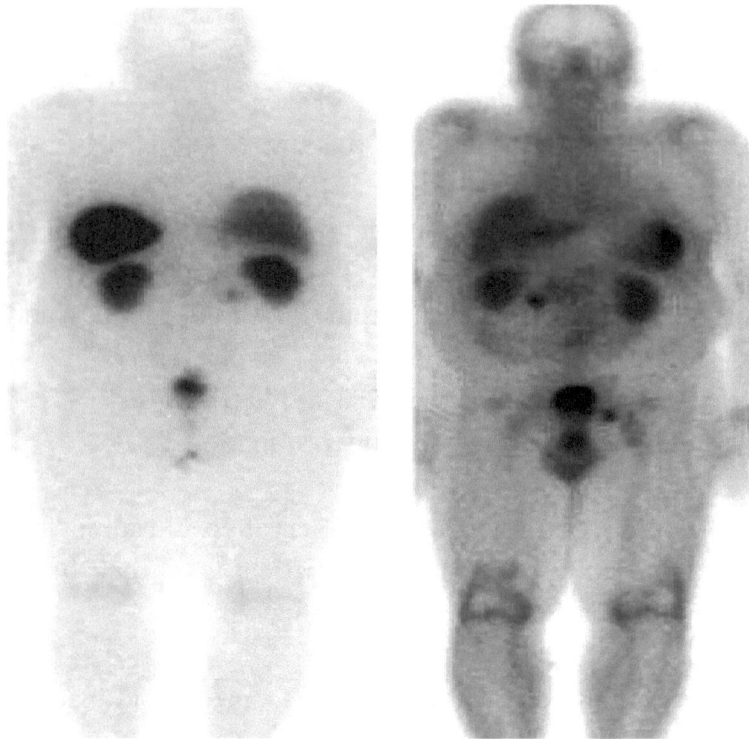

Ga–67 Scan: is used for tumor and infection imaging. It is used for spinal osteomyelitis and to detect lymphoma.

A normal scan will have activity in: bone, soft tissue, lacrimal glands, liver > spleen. No kidneys, ureter, or bladder, it's actually excreted in the colon. It looks smudgy, just kinda blurry.

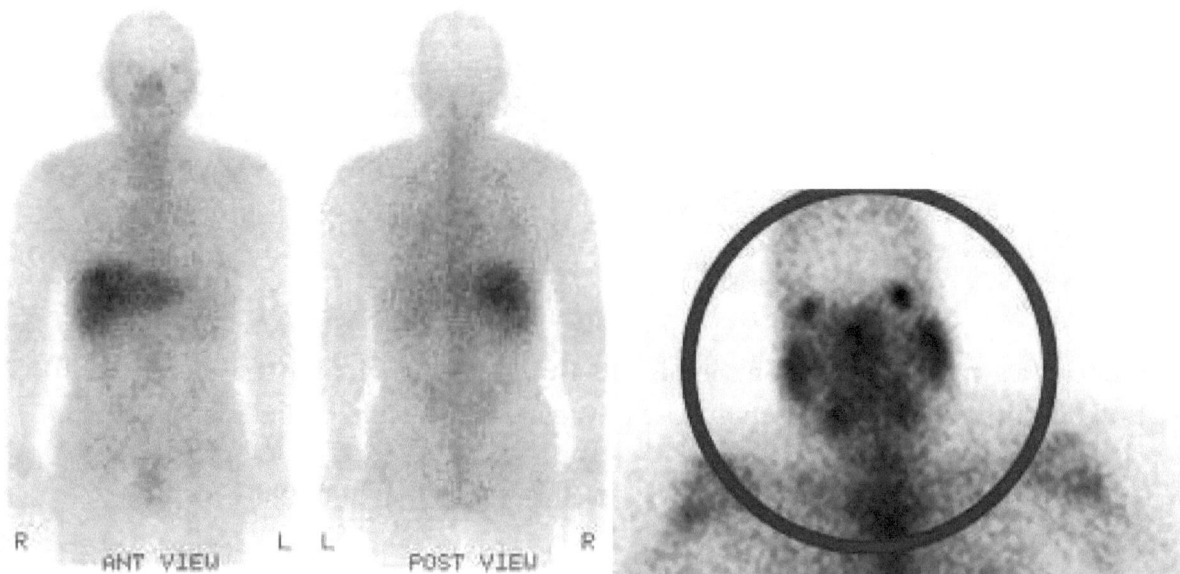

Panda Sign – Sarcoidosis

In–111 WBC or Tc–99 HMPAO WBC can be used: HMPAO needs to be imaged within 4–8 hours and only requires 10 mCi of tracer (lower radiation dose, preferred in kids). The In–111 has a 3–day T½, requires 500 mCi of tracer and is imaged at 24 hours. These are used to check for fever of unknown origin. The advantage over HMPAPO is that it has not GI uptake normally, so it is good for finding GI infections.

Normal scan In–111 spleen >> liver, bone marrow
Normal scan Tc–99 spleen >> liver, bone marrow and bladder

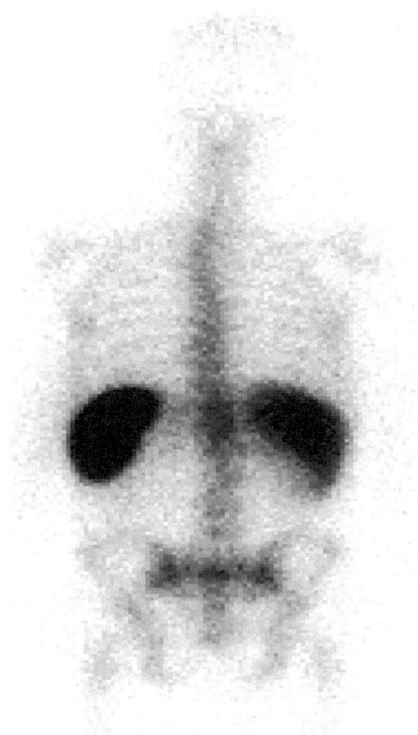

In–111 WBC

Fun Fact: common causes of cold defects on bone scan are AVN, radiation therapy, osteoclastic tumors, surgical changes, and sometimes osteomyelitis (especially in kids).

Lymphoscintigraphy: done to detect which lymph nodes are draining an area and in the OR that sentinel node is biopsied. For example, in breast cancer, metastasis to axillary LNs is the best predictor of post– treatment recurrence and death. If the sentinel node biopsy is negative no further LN dissection is needed.

The injection should be performed 1–cm from the primary lesion and a visible wheal should be produced. We inject between 100–250 microCi of Tc–99 SC and a small gamma probe is used to help localize the node in the OR.

This can also be done for melanoma imaging. The tracer is injected around the lesion we use a gamma camera to see the drainage path. Melanoma can have variable drainage, especially in the mid back.

Melanoma prognosis is dependent on skin depth, < 1–mm is good prognosis, > 4–mm is bad prognosis.

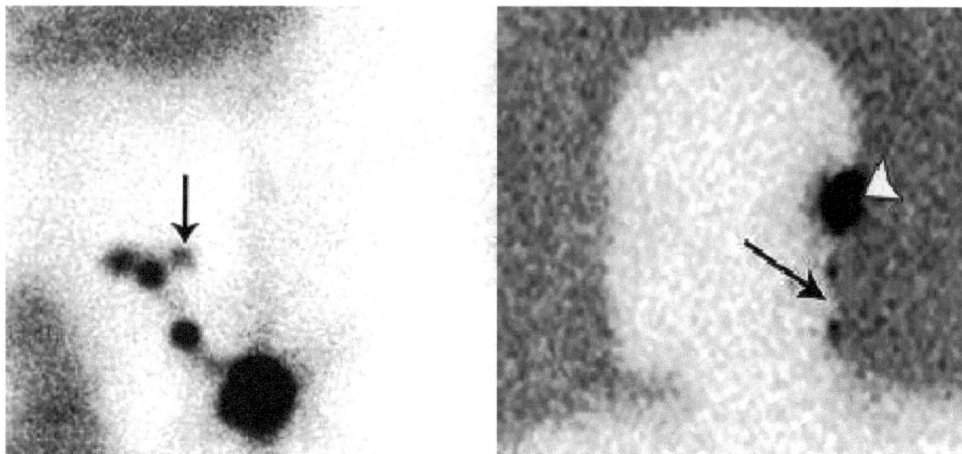

Left image shows typical breast lymphoscintigraphy with identification of axillary nodes. The image on the right depicts a cutaneous scalp melanoma with drainage to neck lymph nodes.

Quality Control:

Alpha particles – can be stopped by a sheet of paper
Beta particles – can be stopped by a layer of clothing or a few mm of Al
Gamma particles – need several feet of concrete to stop this bad boy or a few inches of lead
100 rad = 1 Gy – absorbed dose 100 rem = 1 sV – effective dose

Nuclide	Photon (keV)	Production Mode	Decay Mode	Half Life
Tc–99	140	Mo–Generator		6–hour
Ga–67	*91, 93, 185*, 296, 388	Cyclotron	Electron capture	78–hours
I–123	159	Cyclotron	Electron capture	13–hours
I–131	364	Fission	Beta–decay	8–days
In–111	173, 247	Cyclotron	Electron capture	68–hours
Xe–133	80	Fission	Beta–decay	5.3–days
Tl–201	70, 167	Cyclotron	Electron capture	73–hours
Rb–82		Sr–Generator	Beta–decay	3–minutes
F18–FDG	511 x 2	Cyclotron	Beta–decay	110–minutes

Mo–99 generator produces Tc–99 and we collect the Tc every 24 hours. Mo–99 is bound to Aluminum and Tc–99 is free floating in the saline solution.

1. Mo–99 impurity – 0.15 microCi of Mo per 1 mCi of Tc–99
2. Al impurity – 20 mcg per mL of eluate

Warning Signs:

1. Unrestricted area < 2 mrem/hour or < 100 mrem/7 days
2. Radiation area > 5 mrem/hour
3. High radiation area > 100 mrem/hour

Shipped package of radioactive materials needs to have wipe test performed and a survey for external exposure.

Dose Limits:

1. Public dose 100 mrem effective dose = 0.01 Sv (100 rem = 1 Sv)
2. Annual Occupational
   a. 5 rem to body – 50 mSv
   b. 15 rem to eye
   c. 50 rem to any one organ or tissue
   d. Minor dose is 10% of adult dose
3. Fetal dose 0.5 rem during entire pregnancy = 5 mSv

Breast Feeding:
1. F18 – no need to stop
2. Tc–99 – stop for 24 hours
3. Ga–67 – stop for 1–4 weeks
4. I–131 – stop for good

Major Spills: do not clean this up, call the RSO, cover spill, decontaminate, put up a sign

Greater than 100 mCi of Tc–99, Tl–201 Greater than 10 mCi of Ga–67, I–123 Greater than 1 mCi of I–131, Sr–89

After a Spill: immediately inform personnel in the area of the spill and the radiation safety officer. Contain the spill with absorbent paper towels and decontaminate personnel first then the area. Clean spills with soap and water while wearing gloves, disposable lab coats, and booties.

Medical Event: needs to be reported *within 24–hours of discovery* – tell the NRC, referring physician, and the patient (unless the referring physician says no). To qualify the dose difference has to exceed annual occupational exposure and one of the following:

- Dose given to wrong patient
- Wrong dose given to patient (differs by 20% of prescribed dose)
- Wrong nuclide given to patient
- Wrong exam performed

Cyclotron: accelerates particles to a high KE and they collide with a target. Uses H, 2H, and 4H. The product is rich in protons and decays by positron emission or electron capture.

Produces: Co–57, Ga–67, In–111, I–123, Tl–201, F18, Ga–68

Reactors: uses fission or neutron activation. U–235 atoms are bombarded with neutrons.

a. Fission – big atom splits into two smaller atoms and neutrons are emitted i. Produces: Xe–133, I–131, Mo–99
b. Neutron Activation – a target absorbs a neutron to form a new isotope and gamma rays are emitted

Generators: most common used is practice is Mo–99 →→ Tc–99. This is based on the parent–daughter equilibrium.

Dose Calibrator QC:

- constancy check daily
- accuracy and linearity checks quarterly
- geometry check at installation and after service G–M Detector QC:
- battery check daily
- background counting and constancy check daily
- calibration at install and after service (done with Cs–137)

<u>Gamma Camera QC:</u> below are two common artifacts, left is a cracked crystal and right is a photopenic defect from a malfunctioning photomultiplier tube

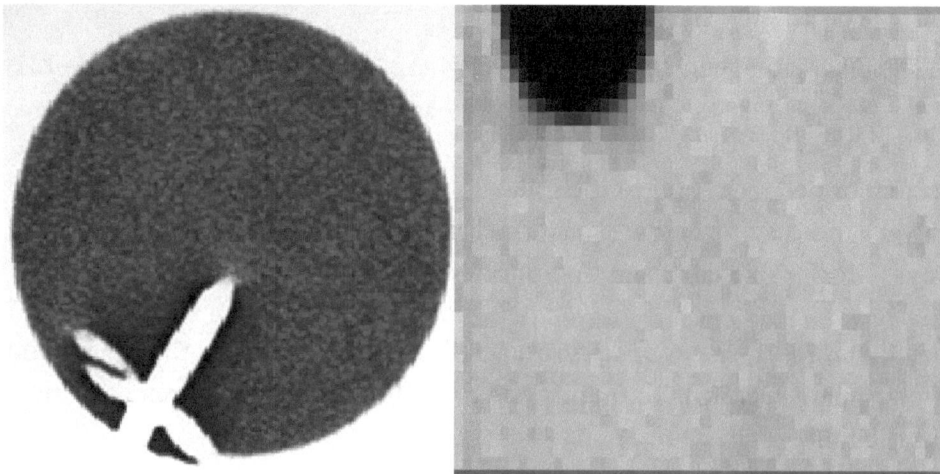

Pediatrics

PEDIATRIC NEURO:
Basic approach to the child's brain is easy and systematic. Look at the Sag T1 midline view to evaluate the CC, skull, brainstem, clivus, sella, and cerebellum. Next check your axial T1/T2 and look at WM tracts, check the cortex, and deep gray nuclei.

The brain develops to give us primitive functions first (breathing, heart rate, swallowing), so the brainstem develops first and then the more anterior cranial structures (caudal → → cephalad and dorsal → → ventral).

CORPUS CALLOSUM: actually pretty important. It develops in a predictable order – genu, body, splenium, then the rostrum. It may not form if something gets in its way i.e. lipoma. Also look at the parts that are formed to help you decide if it is a developmental problem or something that happened afterwards. If the genu and body are developed but the splenium and rostrum are not, then it is partial agenesis. However, if the splenium is gone, but the rostrum is present, then we know it was a post-developmental insult.

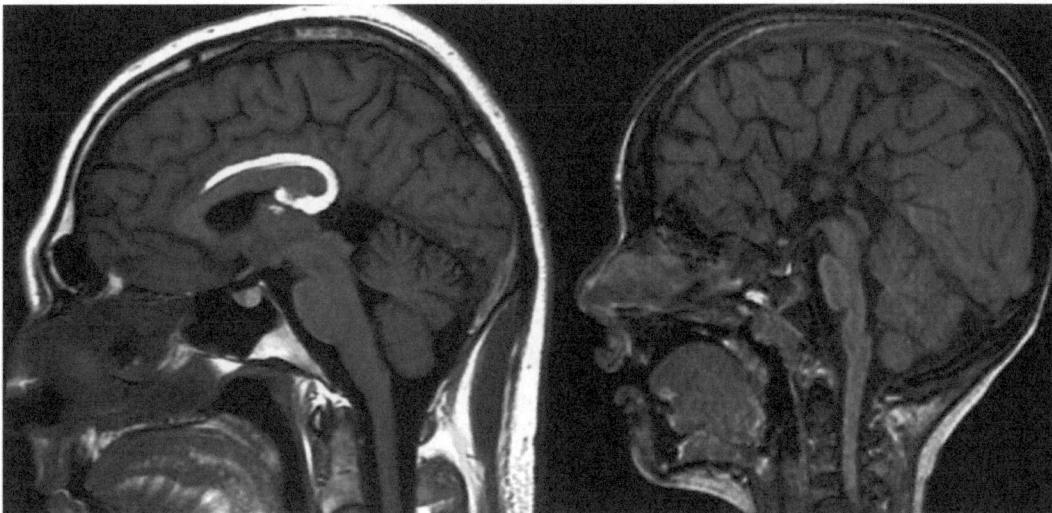

Lipoma   Agenesis of CC

Other things we can see on midline Sag T1: will not discuss sella masses or tumors here since that is covered in the peds brain tumor section in Neuro.

CHIARI I: Peg-like tonsils herniating 5-mm below foramen magnum. Often associated with cervical syrinx.

Have to r/o intracranial hypotension or increased ICP.

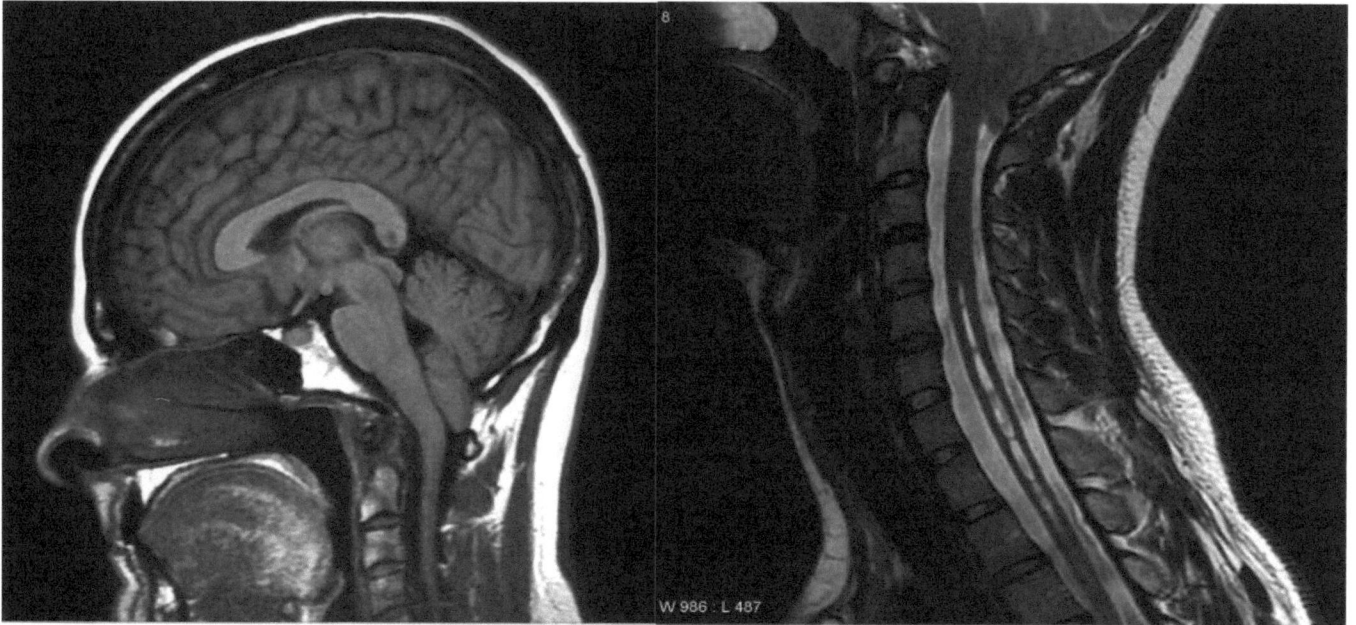

CHIARI II: Small posterior fossa due to a CSF leak at lumbar myelomeningocele (> 90%). Herniated tonsils, beaked tectum, agenesis of CC, towering cerebellum.

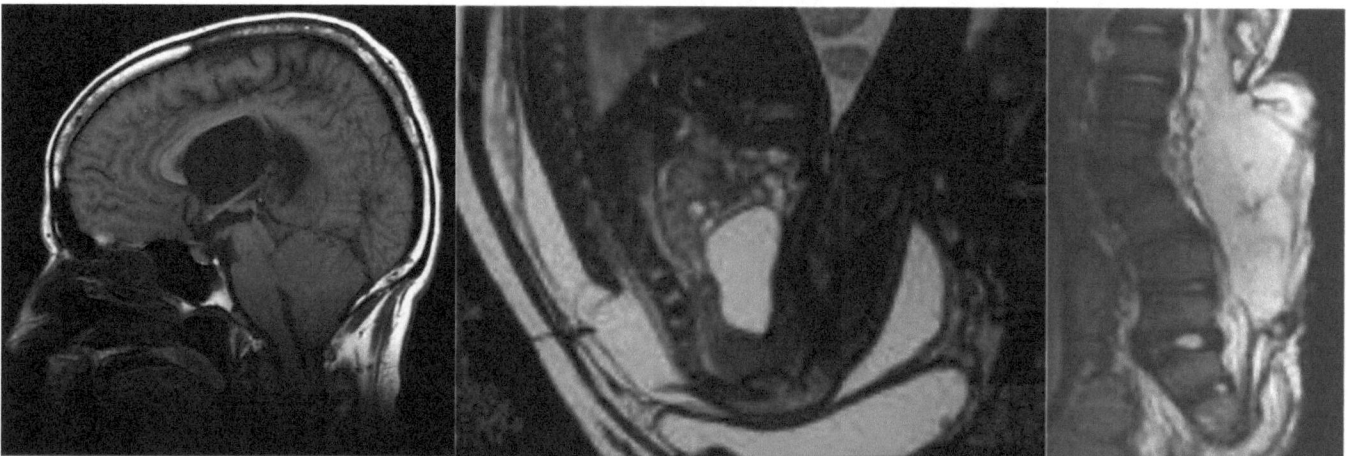

CHIARI III: is the most extreme end of the spectrum and has changes of Chiari II plus a high cervical or occipital cephalocele. Does not have a myelomeningocele.

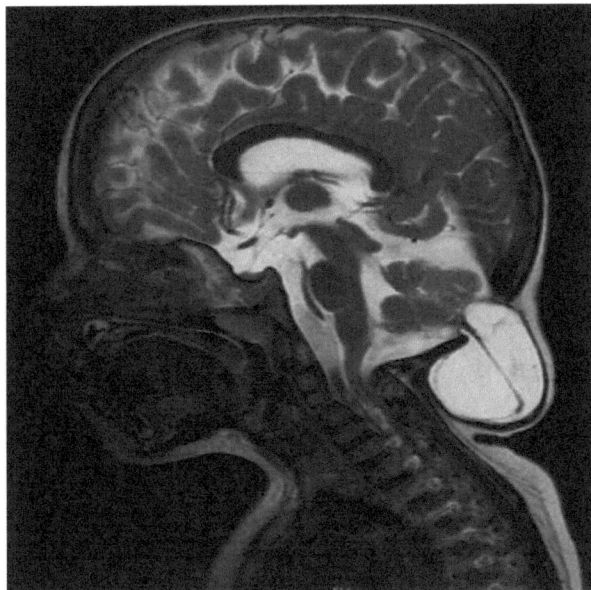

DW CONTINUUM: in contrast to Chiari where the posterior fossa is too small, in this **the posterior fossa is super big**. There is vermian hypoplasia or agenesis with a communication of the 4th ventricle with the enlarged cisterna magna.

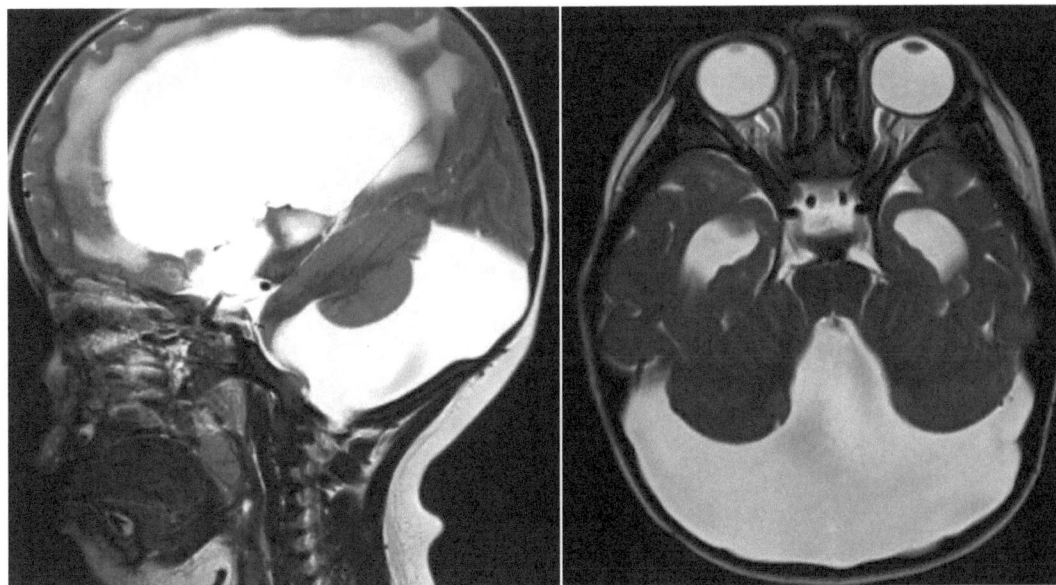

AQUEDUCTAL STENOSIS: congenital version is x-linked recessive and demonstrates dilated lateral and 3 rd ventricles with a normal 4th ventricle - due to webs or septa (intrinsic). Can be an extrinsic phenomenon due to mass effect from an adjacent mass.

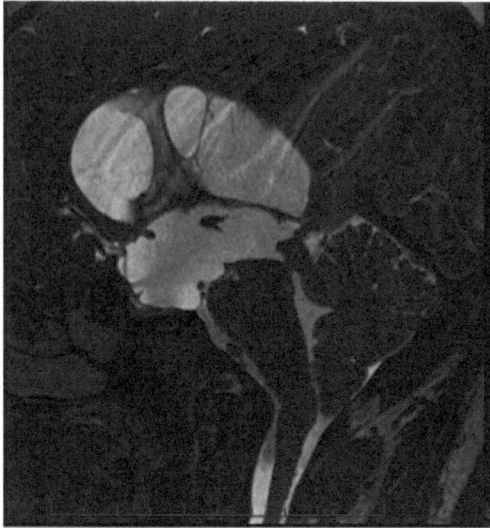

CEREBRAL MALFORMATIONS: switching gears here to talk about congenital anomalies of the cerebral hemispheres.

LISSENCEPHALY: paucity of sulci caused by arrested migration of the neurons from the germinal matrix. Can have a variable presentation i.e. pachygyria – few broad gyri

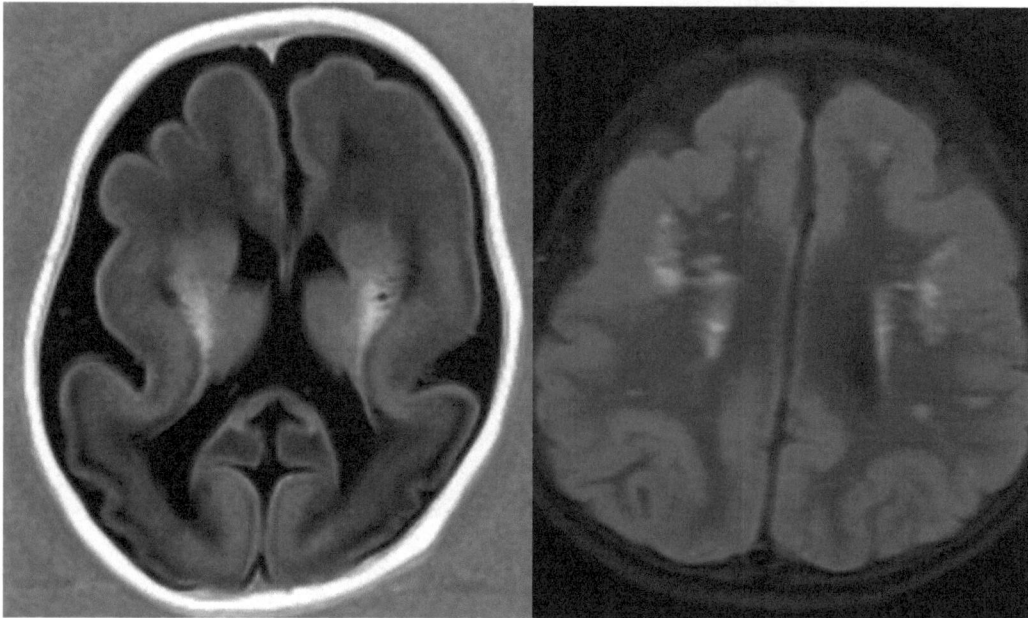

Notice how fat the gyri are and how few there are – Pachygyria

POLYMICROGYRIA: due to abnormal neuronal migration and organization. Thickened appearance to the cortex with multiple small gyri.

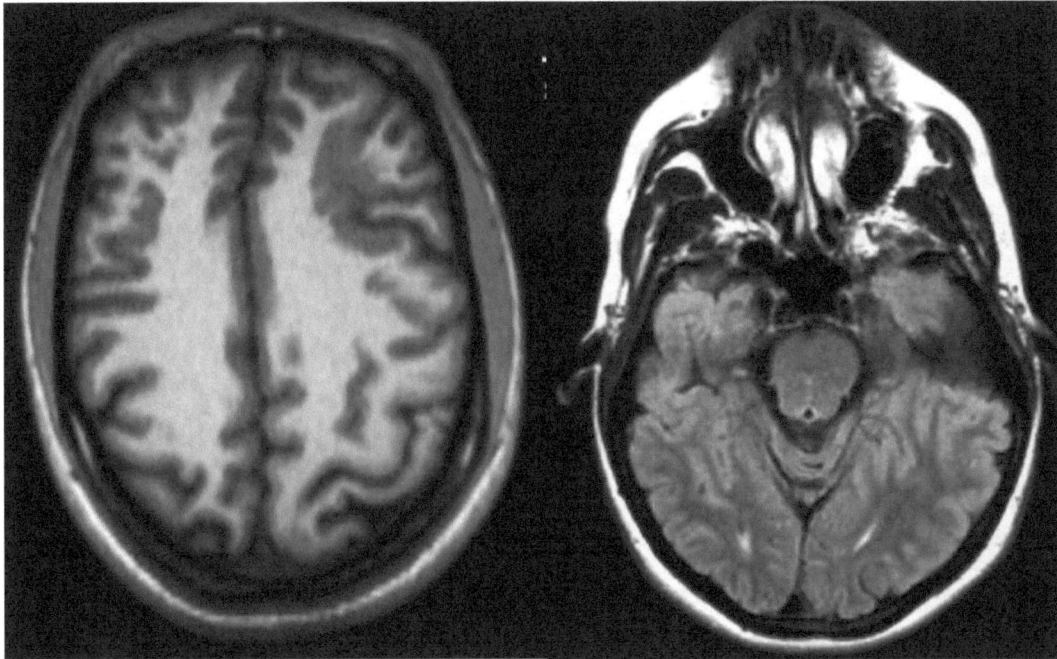

SCHIZENCEPHALY: can be a unilateral or bilateral finding of gray matter lining a cleft extending from the ependyma to the pia. Open vs closed lip defects. If bilateral, can be associated with septo-optic dysplasia – need to consult optho because they have to evaluate for optic nerve hypoplasia.

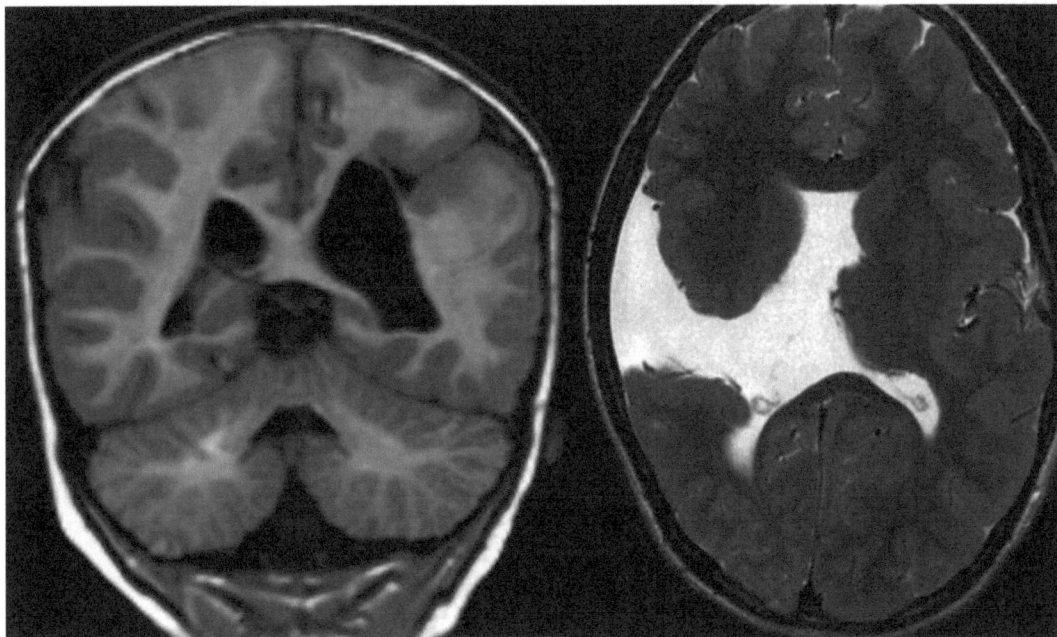

Closed Lip   Open Lip

HOLOPROSENCEPHALY: a condition where the anterior brain does not separate. **This is the only condition where the posterior CC forms but the anterior does not.** Look for monoventricle. Three varieties: alobar, semilobar, and lobar. There is **no falx**.

Alobar – the thalami are fused and there is a single large posteriorly located ventricle. Incompatible with extra-uterine life.

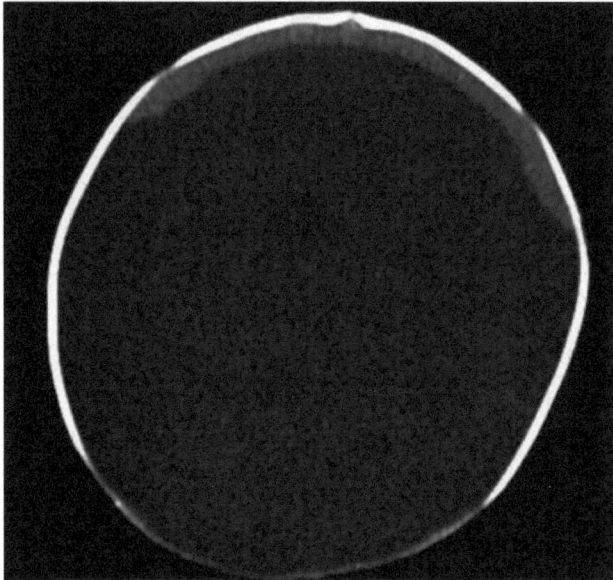

Alobar, as in lacking brain.

Semi-lobar – the basic structure of the cerebral lobes is present but they are fused anteriorly and at the thalami.
Associated with agenesis or hypoplasia of the CC. Incompatible with life.

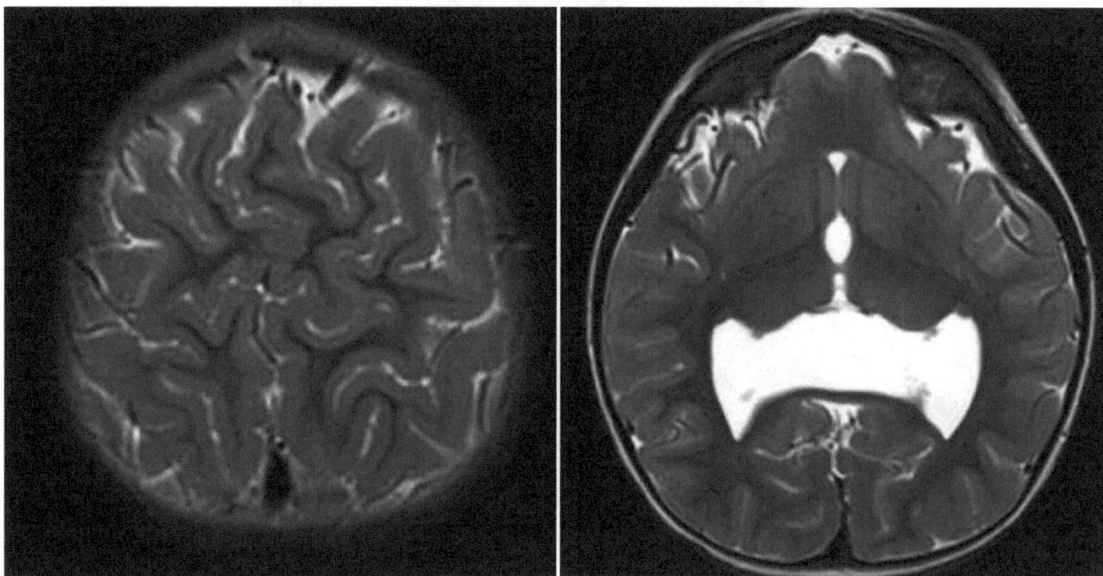

Lobar – least severe, subtle areas of fusion like the cingulate gyrus and thalami. +/- CC agenesis.

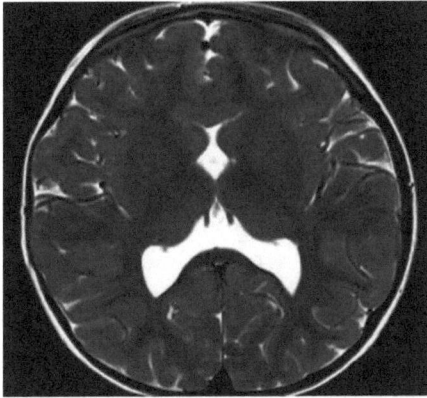

HYDRANANCEPHALY: ischemic insult to the anterior circulation in utero. Absent cerebral tissue, looks a lot like alobar holoprosencephaly except **there is a falx.**

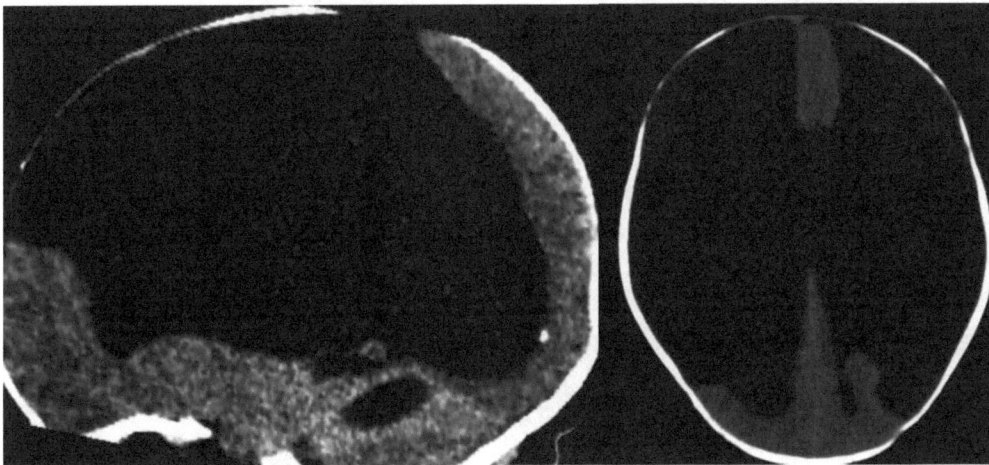

STURGE-WEBER: this is an aunt Minnie. Hypoplasia of cerebral cortex with intense meningeal enhancement. Ipsilateral port-wine stain and calvaria hyperplasia.

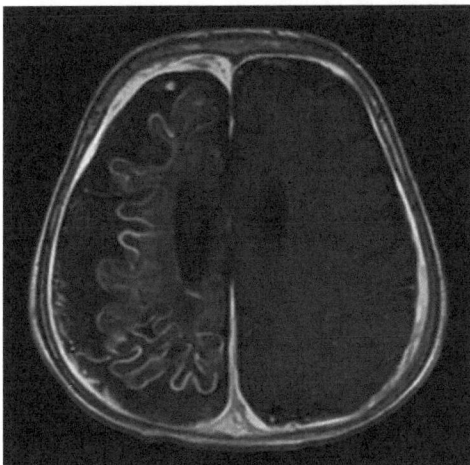

Germinal Matrix Hemorrhage: is primarily a disease of prematurity and most common in babies born before 32 weeks gestation. The germinal matrix is the site of fetal brain cell genesis and is located in the subependymal layers anterior to the caudothalamic groove. The bleed can extend into the ventricles and eventually into the parenchyma. More serious bleeds develop periventricular leukomalacia – necrosis and cyst formation.

Grading:

I – subependymal only

II. – intraventricular extension without hydrocephalus

III – intraventricular blood with hydrocephalus

IV – intraparenchymal hemorrhage and usually in the frontal or parietal lobes

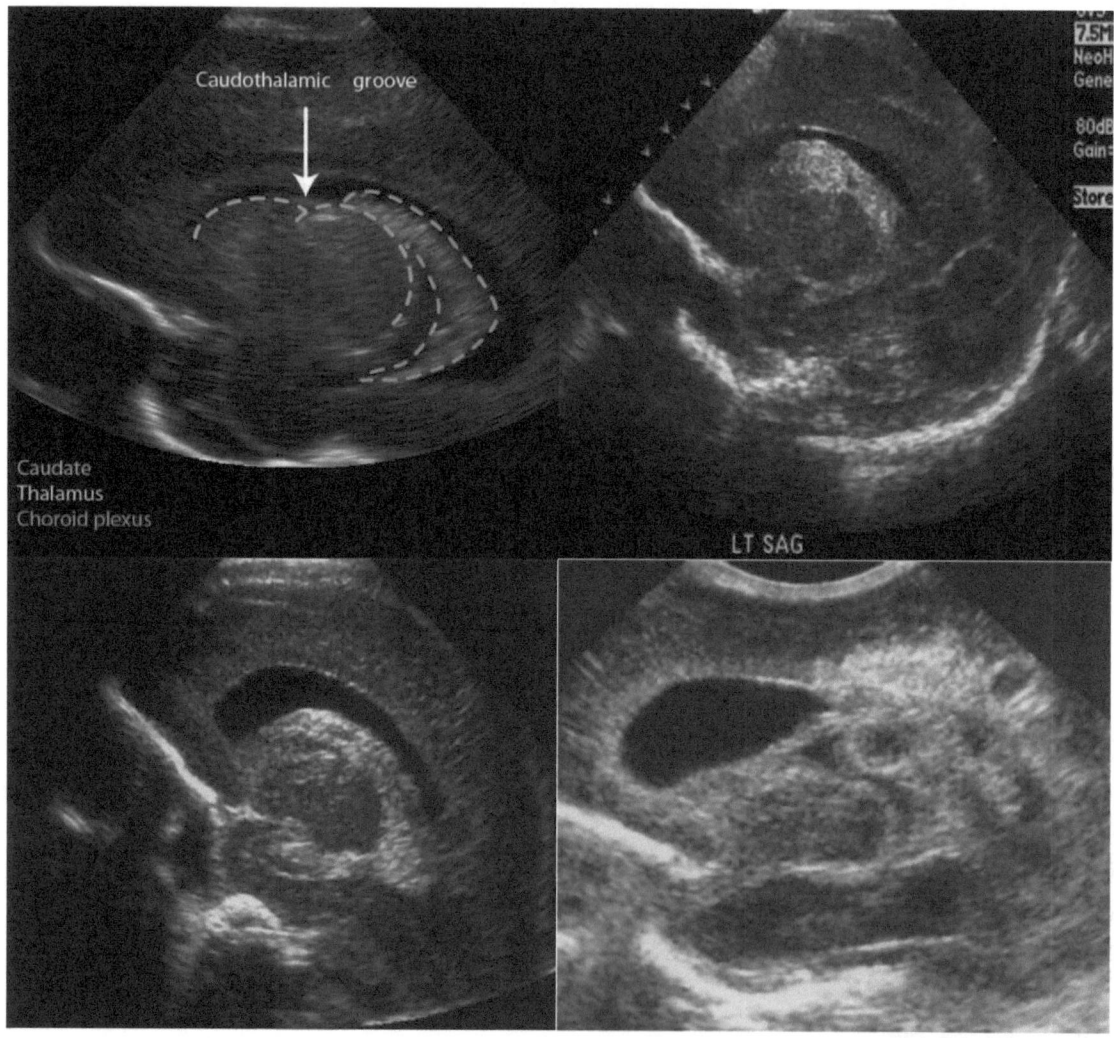

Top left – normal

Top right – grade II

Bottom left – grade III

Bottom right – grade IV

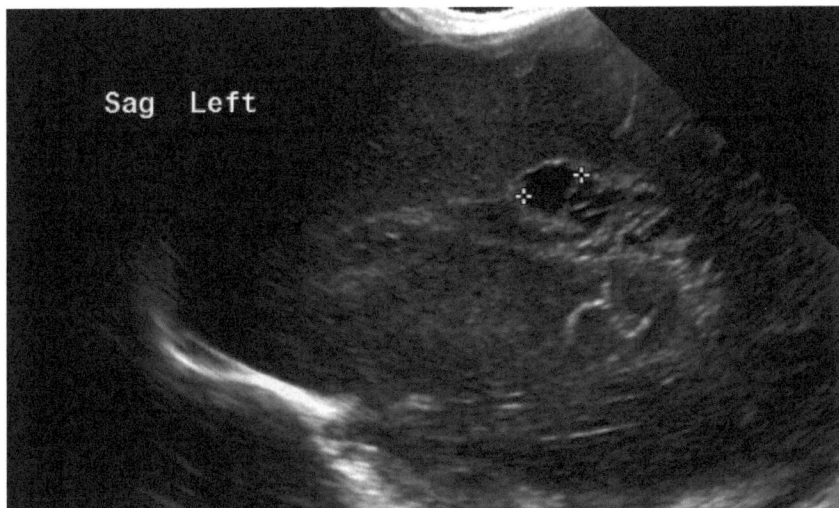

PVL

Juvenile NP Angiofibroma: benign but locally aggressive vascular tumor almost exclusively in males in their teens. Presentation is typically with obstructive symptoms, epistaxis, and chronic otomastoiditis due to an obstructed Eustachian tube.

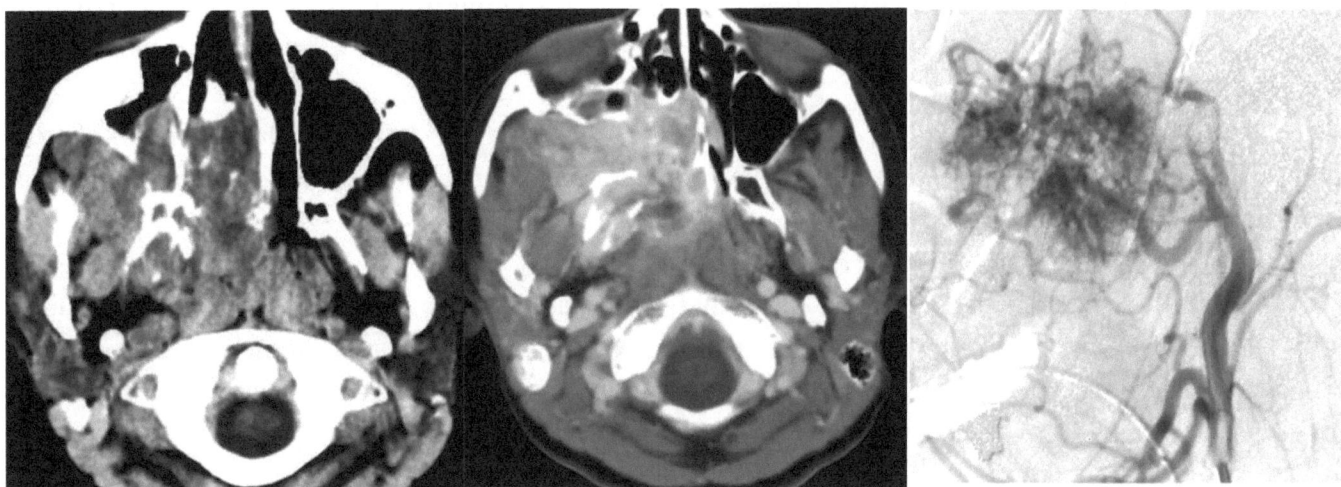

Wormian Bones: are small intrasutural bones seen between the cranial sutures in babies. These are most often found in the lambdoid suture. These can be a normal variant or associated with several diseases:

PORK CHOPS – pneumonic

Pyknodysostosis	Cleidocranial dysostosis	Down Syndrome
Osteogenesis imperfecta	Hypoparathyroidism	
Rickets	Otopalatodigital syndrome	
Kinky hair syndrome	Primary acroosteolysis	

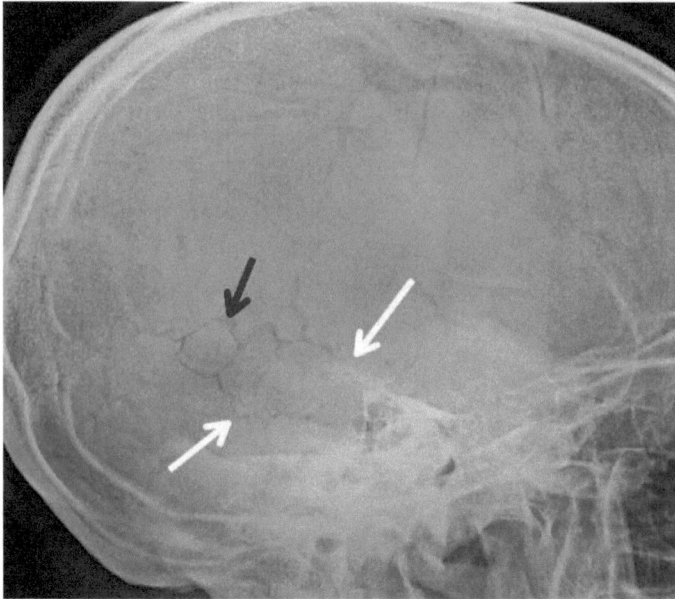

CHEST

Thymus: in relation to body size, it is biggest at birth and continues to grow as the child ages, it reaches maximum size in adolescence and starts to disappear after that. Thymus produces T-cells and a big thymus is a sign of health.

When looking at the neonatal chest x-ray first decide if the lungs are hypo- or hyperinflated. If hypoinflated, then surfactant deficiency disease and if hyperinflated – TTN, neonatal pneumonia, or meconium aspiration.

TTN: is seen in premature babies, babies of mothers who had sedation, and born by c-section. Babies will be tachypniec, with mild cyanosis, and grunting. Chest x-ray shows cardiomegaly and vascular congestion. There will be bilateral small effusions, but findings clear progressively peripheral to central and upper to lower within 48 hours.

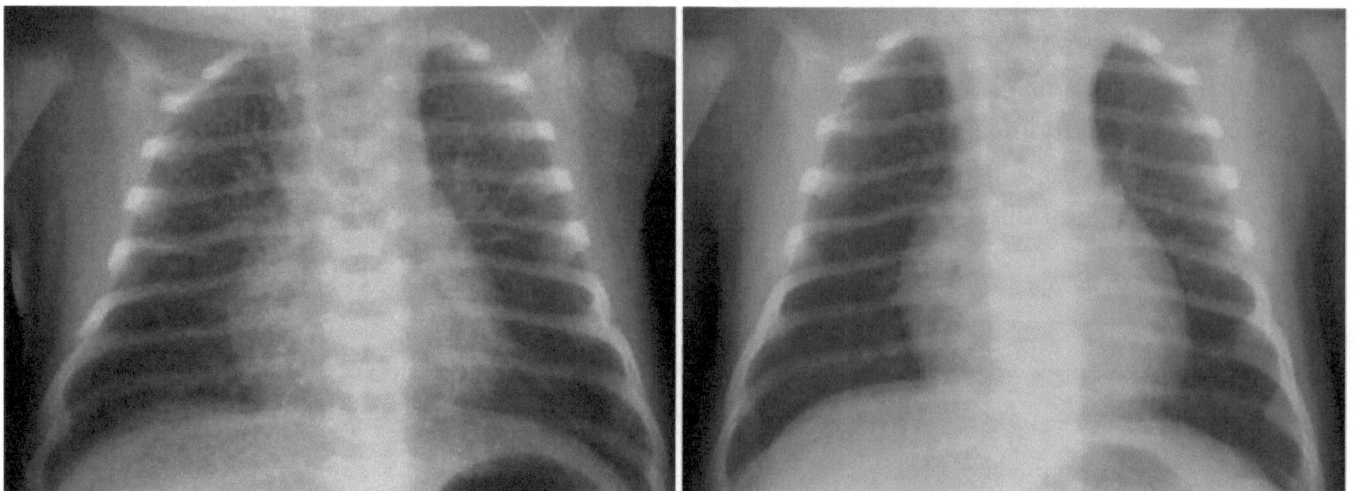

RDS (surfactant deficiency disease): commonly seen in premature babies due to a lack of surfactant causing acinar atelectasis. Membranes slough and hyaline membranes fill the alveoli. X-rays show low lung volumes, air bronchograms, but **no effusions**. Look for ground glass lungs and a bell–shaped thorax. Low lung volumes are because there is resistance to expansion. This is the number one cause of death in liveborn infants.

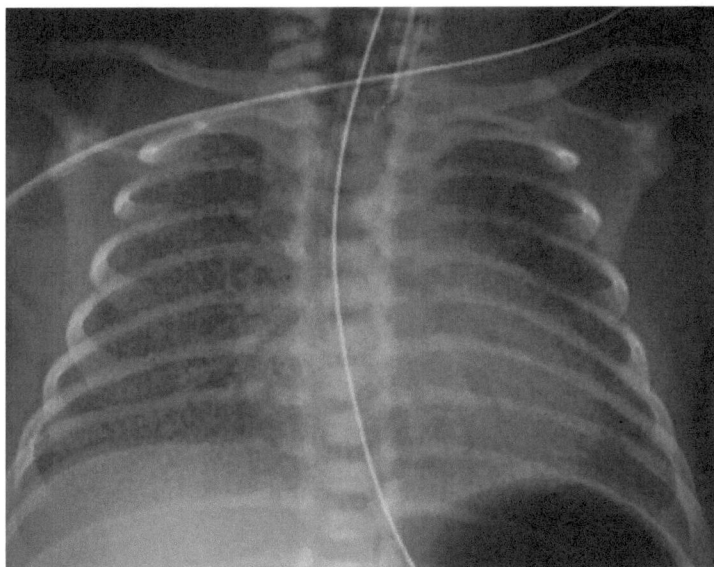

Pulmonary Interstitial Emphysema: refers to the pathologic lung changes that follow the rupture of overdistended alveoli. It typically follows barotrauma in infants with RDS. Following rupture of the alveoli, air tracks through the interstitium and may cause pneumothorax and pneumomediastinum. This is a restrictive lung disease. On x-ray look for bubbly lucencies radiating from the hilum– **asymmetric**.

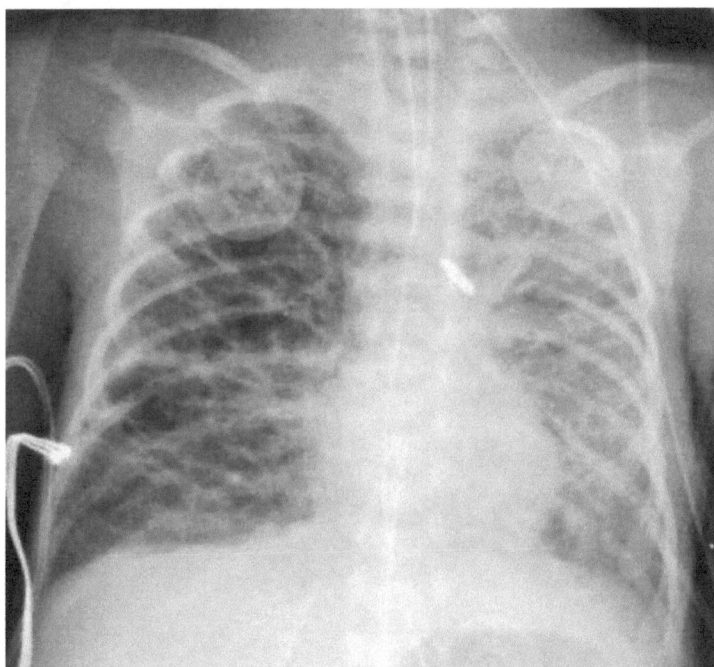

Bronchopulmonary Dysplasia: this is the late pathological change seen in infants on prolonged intubation. Results from barotrauma and oxygen toxicity while treating RDS. This is a combination of emphysema and scarring. Can improve over time. Hyperinflated lungs with ill–defined reticular markings with interspersed rounded lucencies **diffusely involving the lungs**.

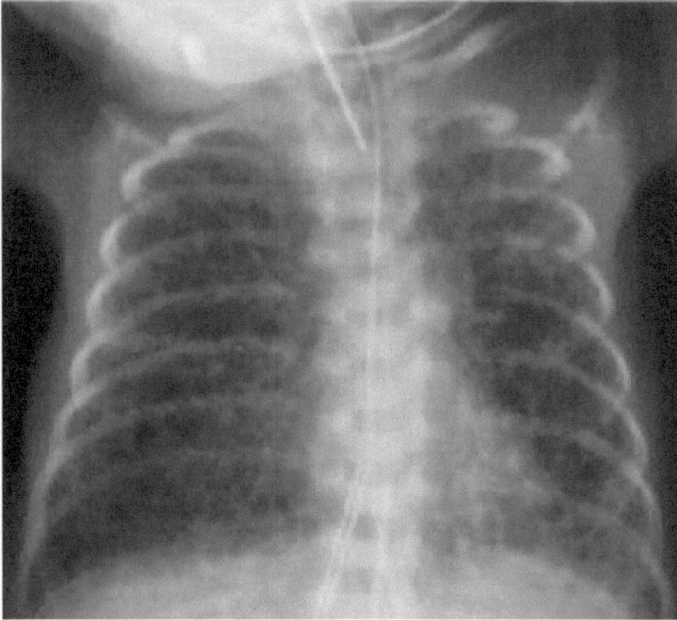

Meconium Aspiration: is due to in utero hypoxemia causing a simultaneous reflex where the child defecates and gasps causing aspiration. The meconium causes bronchial obstruction and chemical pneumonitis. X–ray shows patchy atelectasis, hyperinflation, and pneumonia.

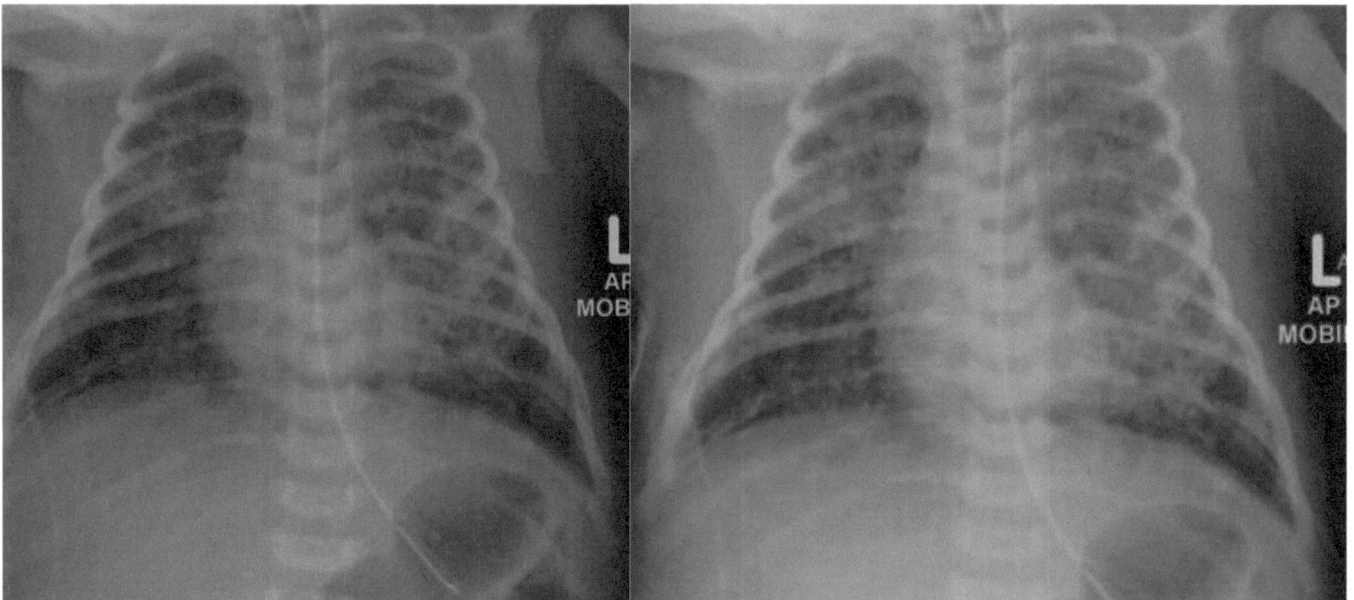

Neonatal Pneumonia: can occur in utero from a variety of causes (PROM – ascending infection, transplacental – TORCH, during delivery – vaginal flora: beta strep). This is **not a lobar process**, it is **diffuse**. Look for a growing pleural effusion (usually means beta strep) and patchy asymmetric opacities and hyperinflation.

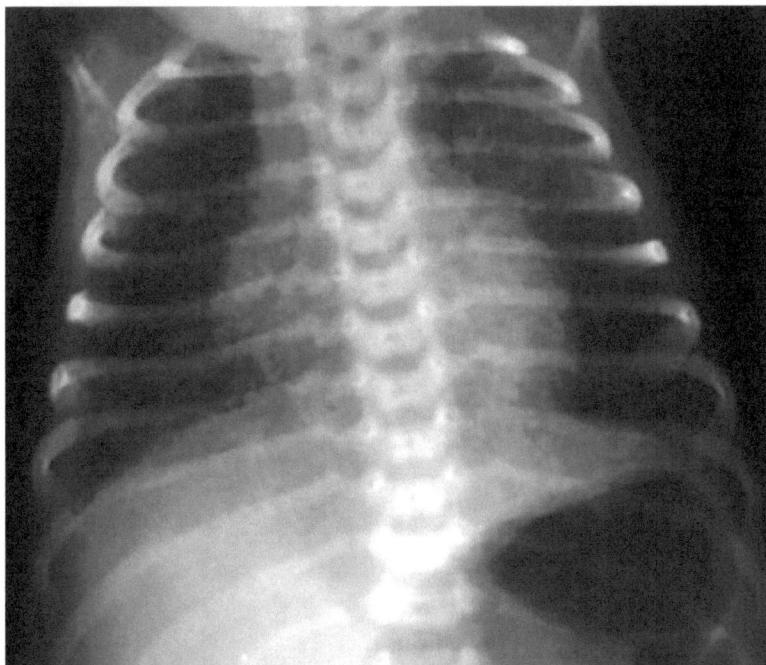

PNA: *Staph* pneumonia is more common in infancy, *H. flu* pneumonia is more common in 6–12 months of life, and *Strep pneumonia* is more common at 1–2 years of age. *Staph* is associated with consolidations and pneumatoceles,

Bonchopulmonary Foregut Malformations
Sequestration
Bronchogenic Cyst
Congenital Diaphragmatic Hernia (CDH)
Congenital Lobar Emphysema (CLE)
Congenital Pulmonary Airway Malformation (CPAM)

Sequestration: aberrant formation of segmental lung tissue with no connection to the bronchial tree occurring **preferentially in the LLL**. Can be divided into two distinct classes:

BA Intra–lobar: accounts for the majority of these and presents later in childhood with recurrent infection.

BB Extra–lobar: less common and presents in the neonatal period with cyanosis, respiratory distress, and infections. Can be infra–diaphragmatic in 10% of cases.

Both types derive an aortic blood supply, but differ in venous drainage. Inta–lobar drains commonly via the pulmonary veins but extra–lobar drains through the systemic veins into the right atrium. Extra–lobar sequestration has its own pleura. By definition neither connect to the bronchial tree.

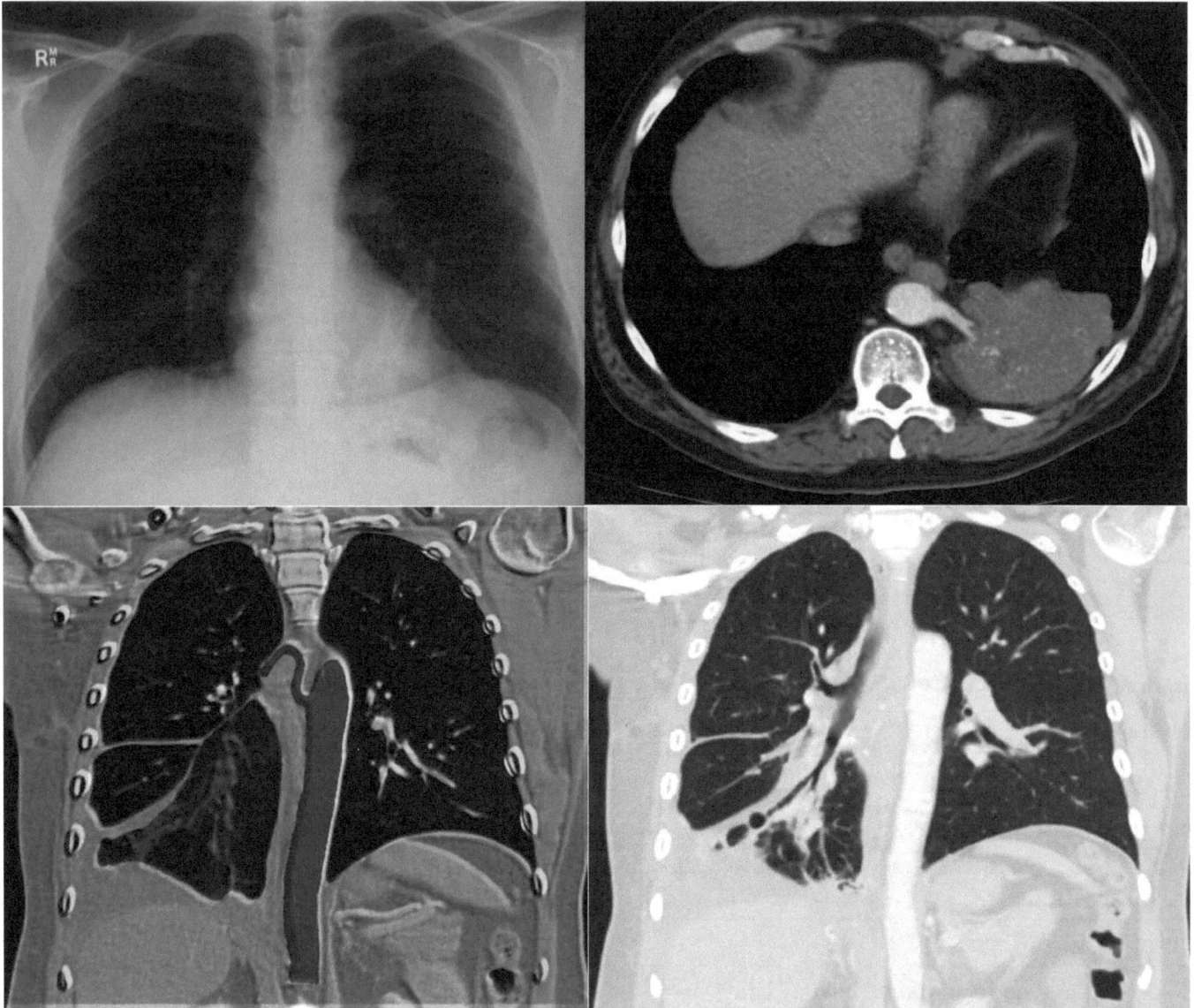

Bronchogenic Cysts: most often mediastinal and subcarinal in location, causes splaying of the bronchi. These are lined by bronchial epithelium and symptoms depend on the size, if you see an air–fluid level think of infection.

Congenital Diaphragmatic Hernia: usually due to a Bochdaleck hernia and occurs on the left far more often than on the right. Prognosis is dependent on the degree of pulmonary hypoplasia. This causes mediastinal shift. After the defect is filled, the thorax is filled with air and a small lung. Either discovered shortly after birth or on prenatal US as an echogenic chest mass. A good clue is when the NGT follows a normal course then turns up and goes into the left hemithorax.

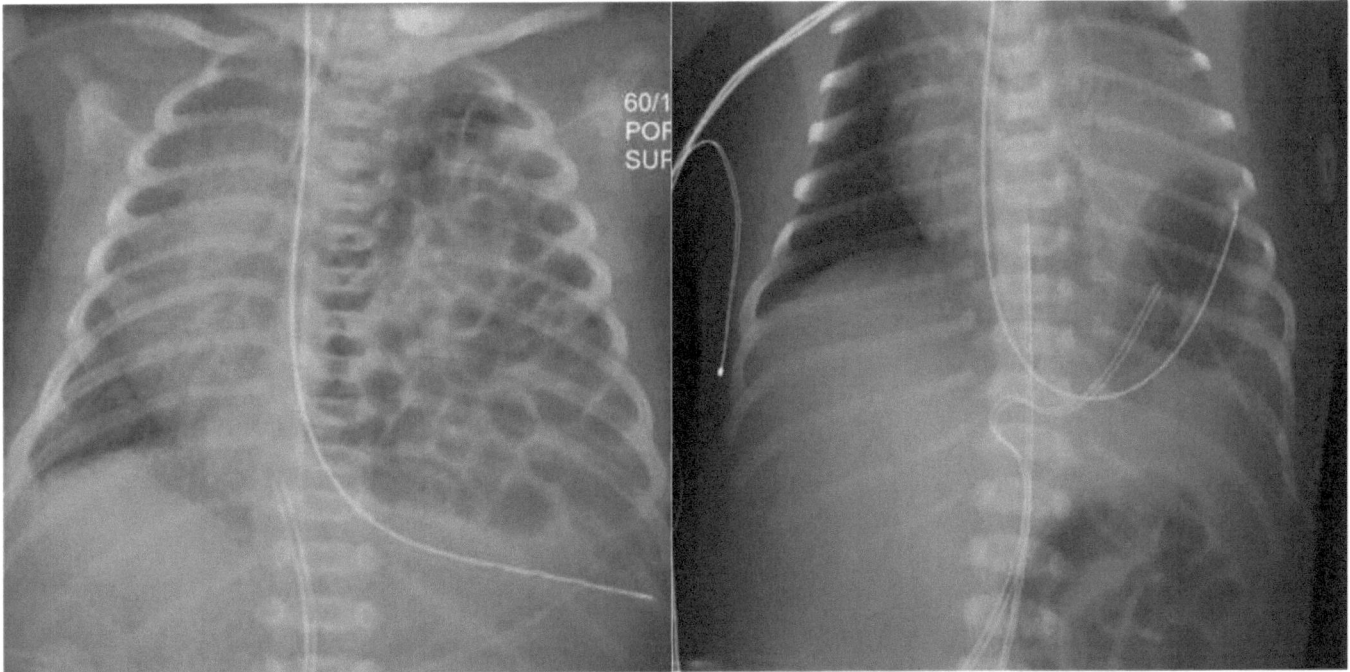

Congenital Lobar Emphysema: this is not truly emphysema, it is due to bronchial atresia. It is seen most often in the left upper lobe. This is initially fluid filled, then it becomes air filled. There is air trapping and hyperexpansion of the lobe with mass effect on the other structures. Surgical resection is curative.

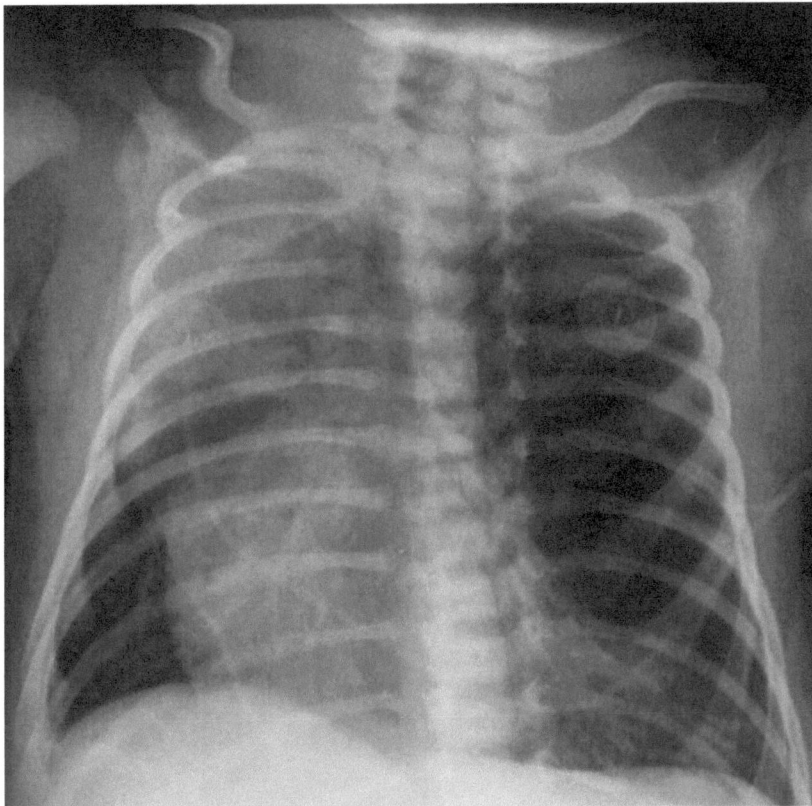

CPAM: this is a hamartomatous proliferation of terminal bronchioles composed of cystic and solid structures. The upper lobes are more often involved. There are three types categorized by cyst size:

Type I – most common and consists of one or more dominant cysts measuring 2–10 cm in size.
Type II – cysts are smaller than 2–cm in size
Type III – microcysts < 5–mm, looks more solid, and has a poor prognosis

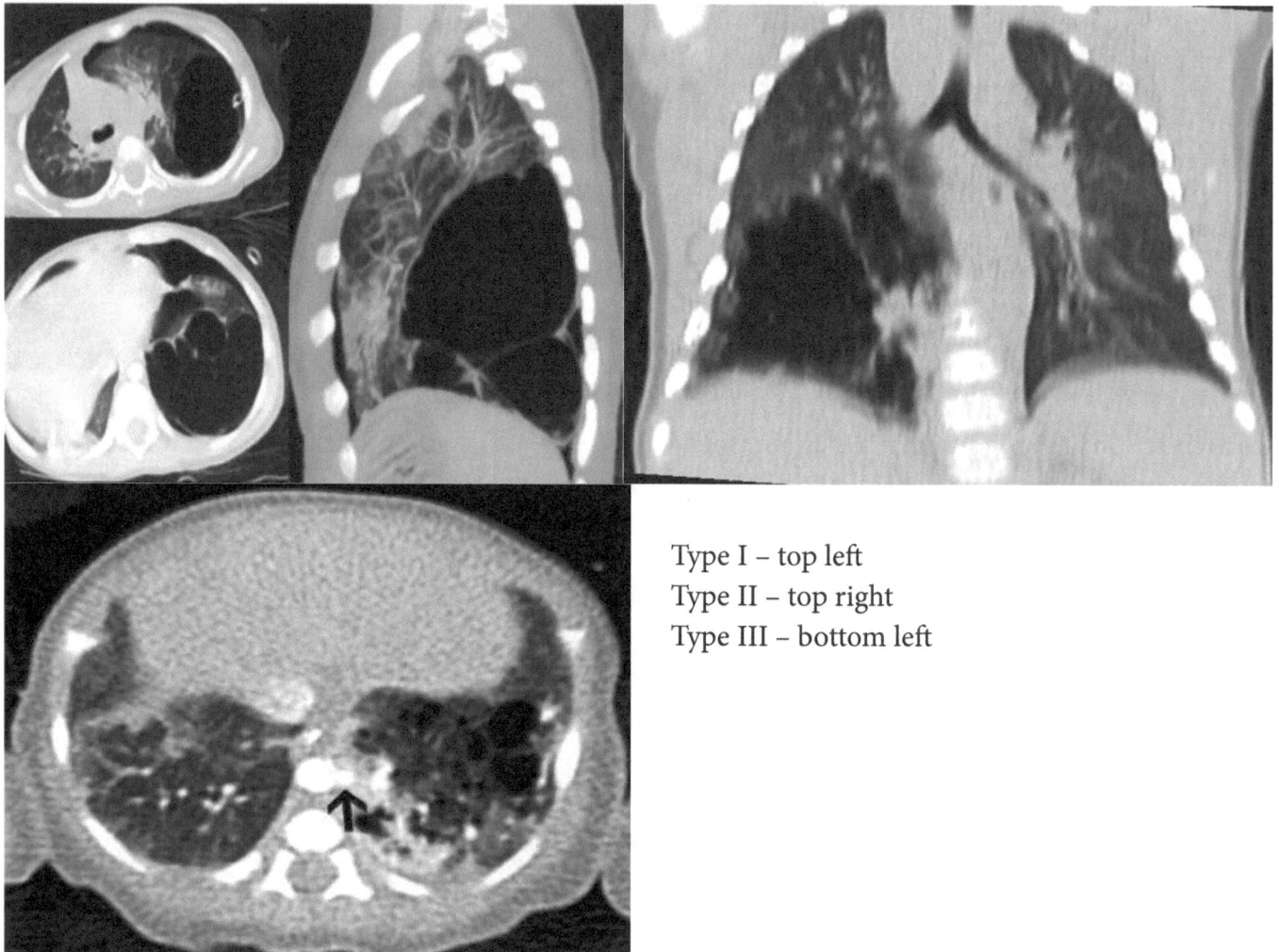

Type I – top left
Type II – top right
Type III – bottom left

Heterotaxy Syndromes: these are a disturbance in the usual left and right distribution of thoracic and abdominal organs. Use the bronchial anatomy to help guide you to the right diagnosis.

Hyparterial bronchi – below the pulmonary artery and supply the bi–lobed left lung Eparterial bronchi – above the artery and supply the tri–lobed right lung

Left sided isomerism:

- two hyparterial bronchi with two left lungs
- short, horizontal bronchi with widened carina
- two left atria
- midline liver
- **polysplenia**
- interrupted IVC with azygous continuation

Right sided isomerism:

- two eparterial bronchi with two right lungs
- long vertical bronchi with narrow carina
- two right atria
- **no spleen**

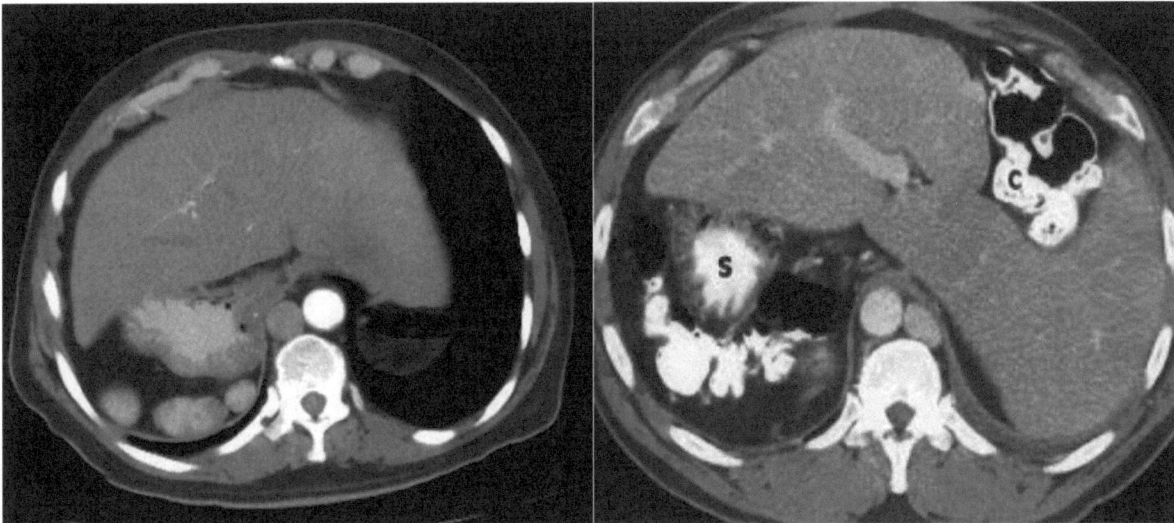

Left Isomerism   Right Isomerism

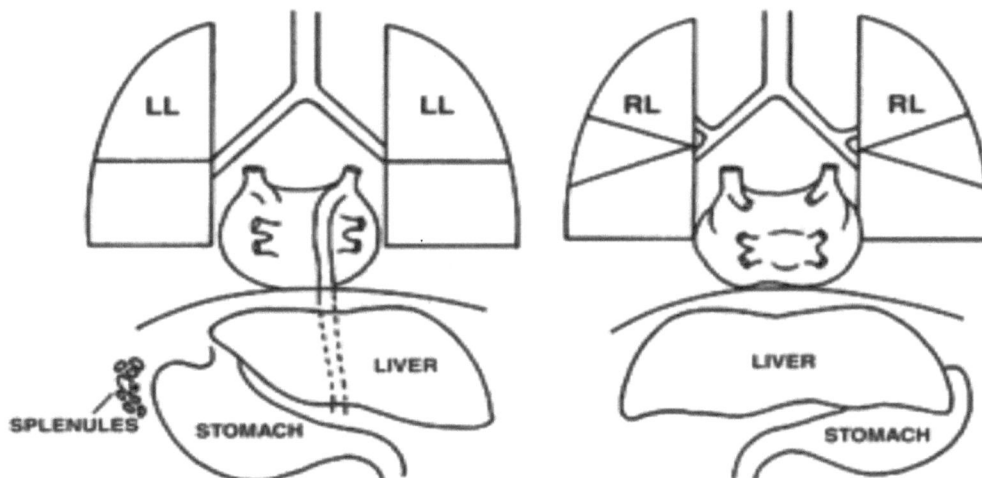

CONGENITAL HEART DISEASE: this stuff is tough yo, but the most basic approach consists of three things:

1. Cyanotic vs. acyanotic
2. Increased or decreased pulmonary vascularity
3. Big or normal sized heart

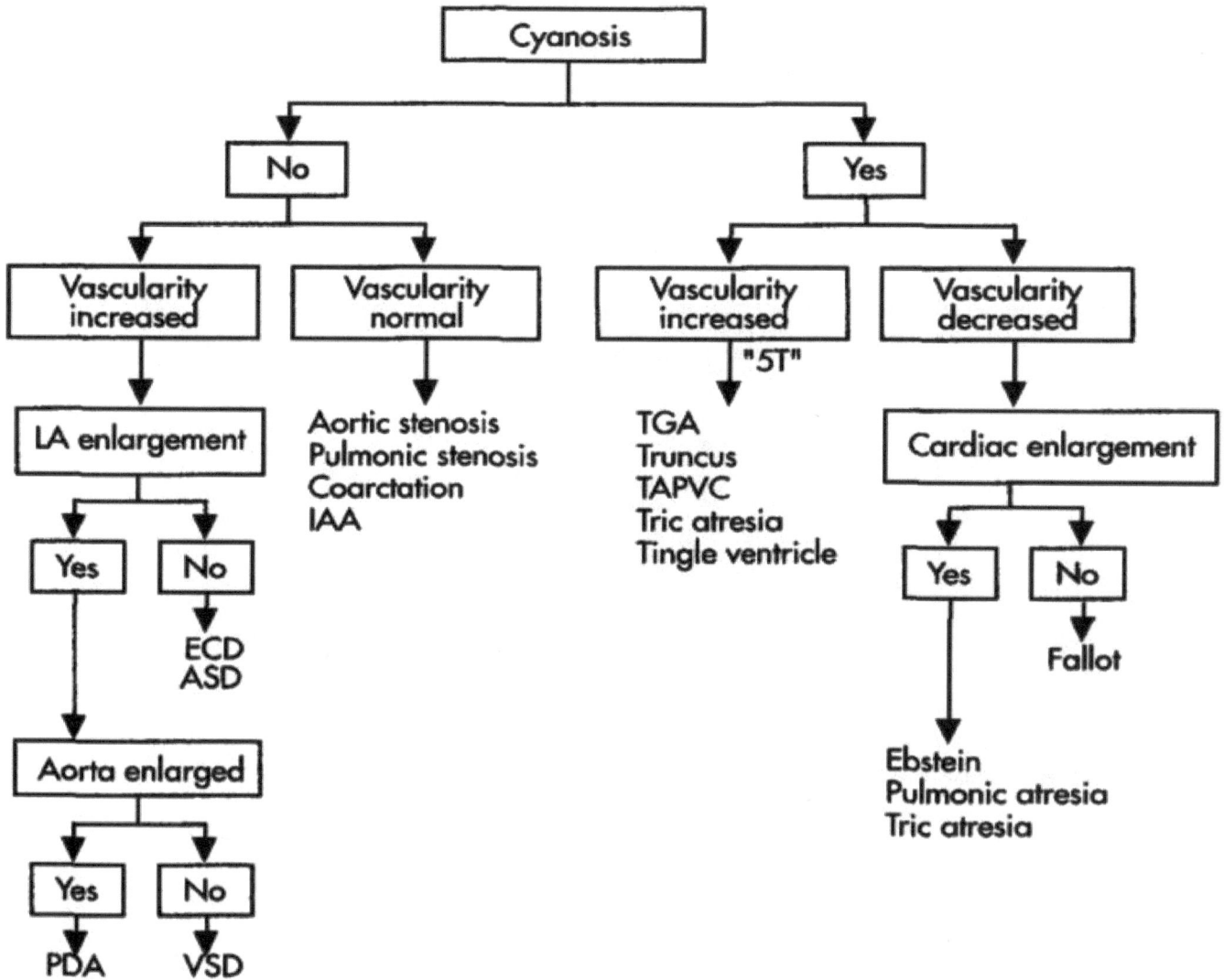

1. The most common set of defects involves an acyanotic patient with increased blood flow (L →→ R shunt). At this point there are two things to address, is the LA enlarged and is the aorta enlarged. Differential of L →→ R shunts is: ASD, VSD, PDA, ECD. Of these, the VSD is the most common. ASD is most likely to be discovered incidentally in a middle aged-female.

ASD: the ostium secundum is most common type (located most inferior) and remains asymptomatic until adulthood because of the low-pressure system. A sinus venosus defect is at the entrance of the SVC and always associated with a PAPVR (right upper lobe pulmonary vein).

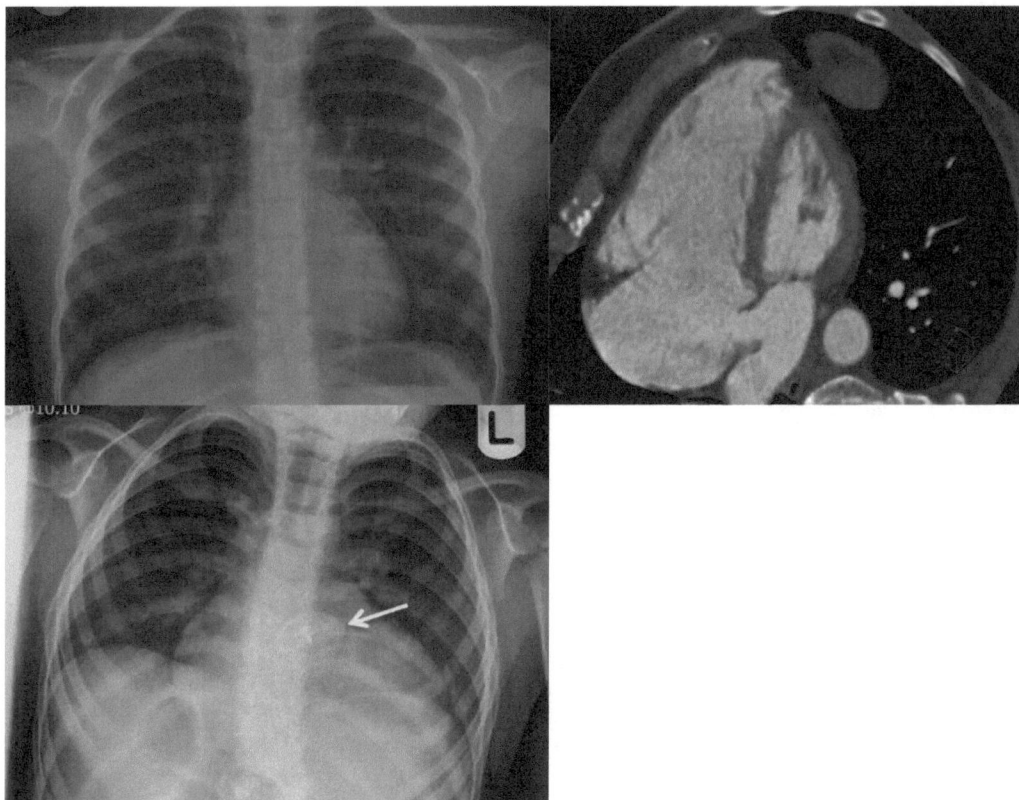

X-Rays show increased vascularity with normal sized heart. CT shows an ostium secundum defect. Bottom x-ray shows closure device (arrow).

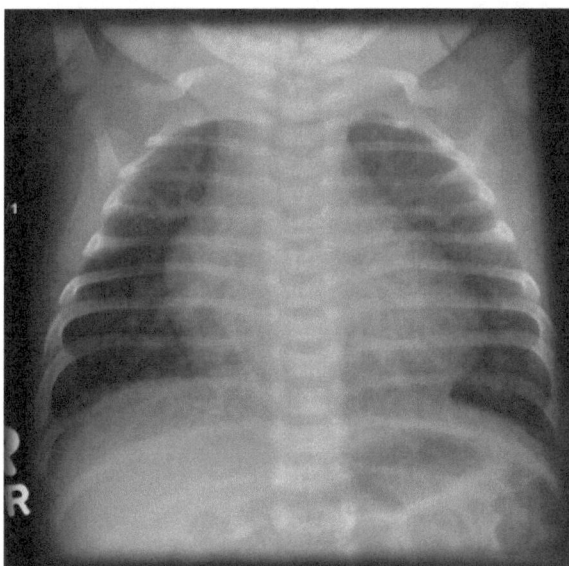

VSD: the most common congenital defect and is often associated with other findings. Membranous defect is the most common. Other associations: TOF, Truncus, tricuspid atresia, etc. Larger defects cause cardiac enlargement and increased pulmonary vascularity.

PDA: persistent patency of the ductus arteriosus which allows left-sided aortic blood to flow into the pulmonary artery. Prostaglandin E1 keeps the ductus open and indomethacin is used to close it. Duct can be ligated surgically or can be treated endovascularly with a closure device.

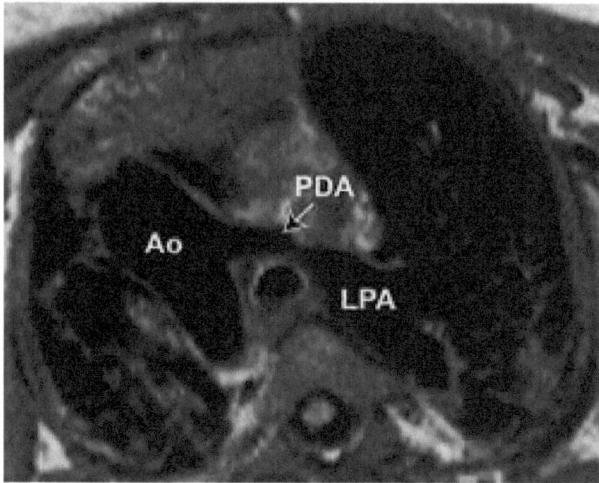

ECD: comprise a relatively wide range of defects involving the atrial septum, ventricular septum and one or both tricuspid and mitral valves. Associated with Down's syndrome.

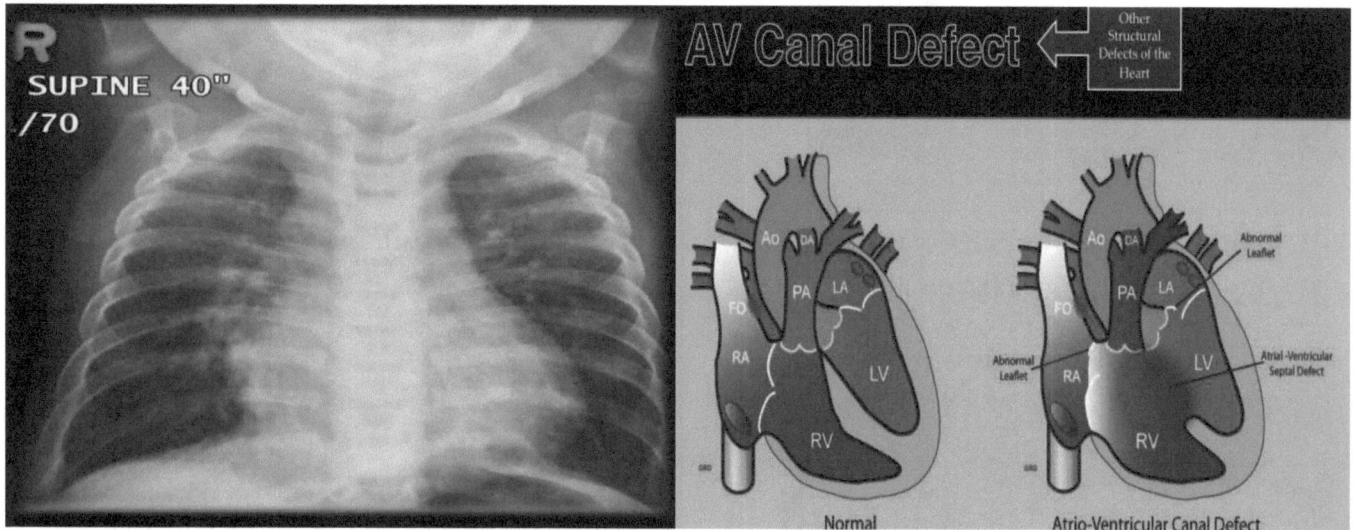

1. The next set of defects involves a cyanotic patient with normal to decreased pulmonary blood flow and a normal heart size.

TOF: the most common disease in this category. It consists of:

–

–

–

VSD

Aorta that overrides the VSD

RV Hypetrophy

- Pulmonic stenosis (the severity of the disease is based on the degree of stenosis) – most often **infundibular stenosis**
- R-aortic arch in 25% of patients

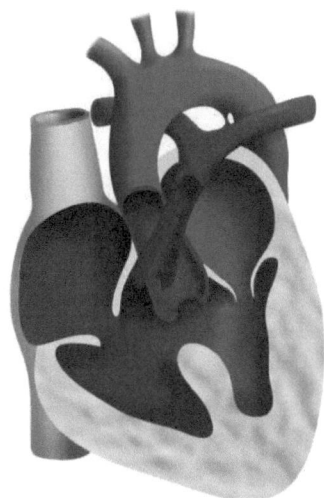

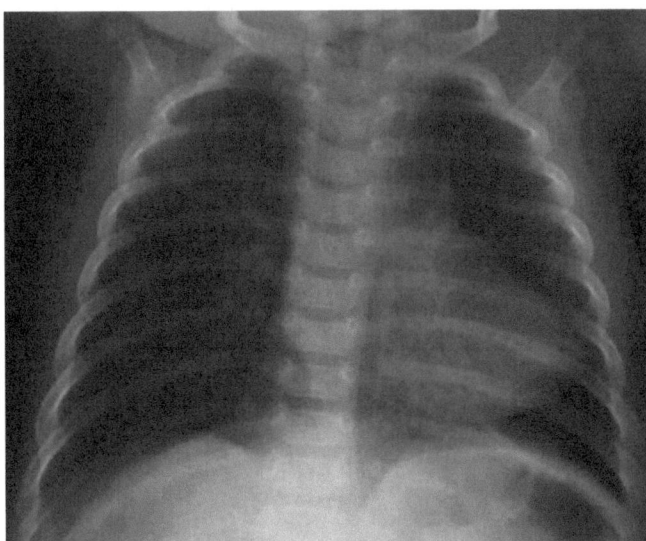

1. This group of diseases covers the cyanotic patients with big hearts and normal to decreased flow (think heart outflow problems).

Ebstein's Anomaly: The main abnormality is an abnormal anterior tricuspid leaflet displaced down into the right ventricle ("atrialization of the ventricle"). Can be associated with tricuspid regurgitation (black streaks in RA on MRI below).

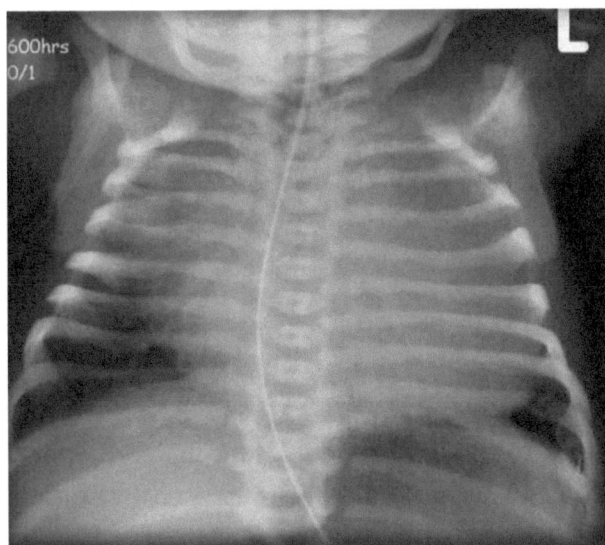

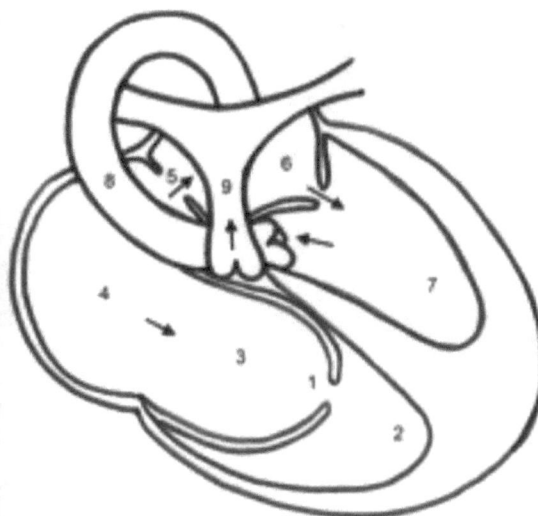

Drawing shows the pattern of blood flow (arrows) caused by downward displacement of the tricuspid valve *(1)*, with resultant formation of a common chamber *(3)* consisting of the right ventricle *(2)* and the dilated right atrium *(4)*, and by the right-to-left shunt of blood through a defect at the atrial level *(5)*. 6 = left atrium, 7 = left ventricle, 8 = aorta, 9 = pulmonary artery.

IV. Cyanotic diseases with increased pulmonary blood flow. This is because of mixing of oxygenated and de-oxygenated blood flow. T-Lesions: TGA, TAPVR, Tricuspid atresia, Tingles (HLH and HRH). When differentiating these, look at the superior mediastinum to see if it is enlarged or small.

1. Normal superior mediastinum with enlarged heart – TGA
2. Widened superior mediastinum with enlarged heart – TAPVR

TGA: is one of the commonest congenital lesions. L-type (live) is a congenitally corrected TGA. D-type (die) is transposition of the arteries – this is incompatible with life unless there is a left →→ right shunt. Treatment is via an arterial switch procedure.

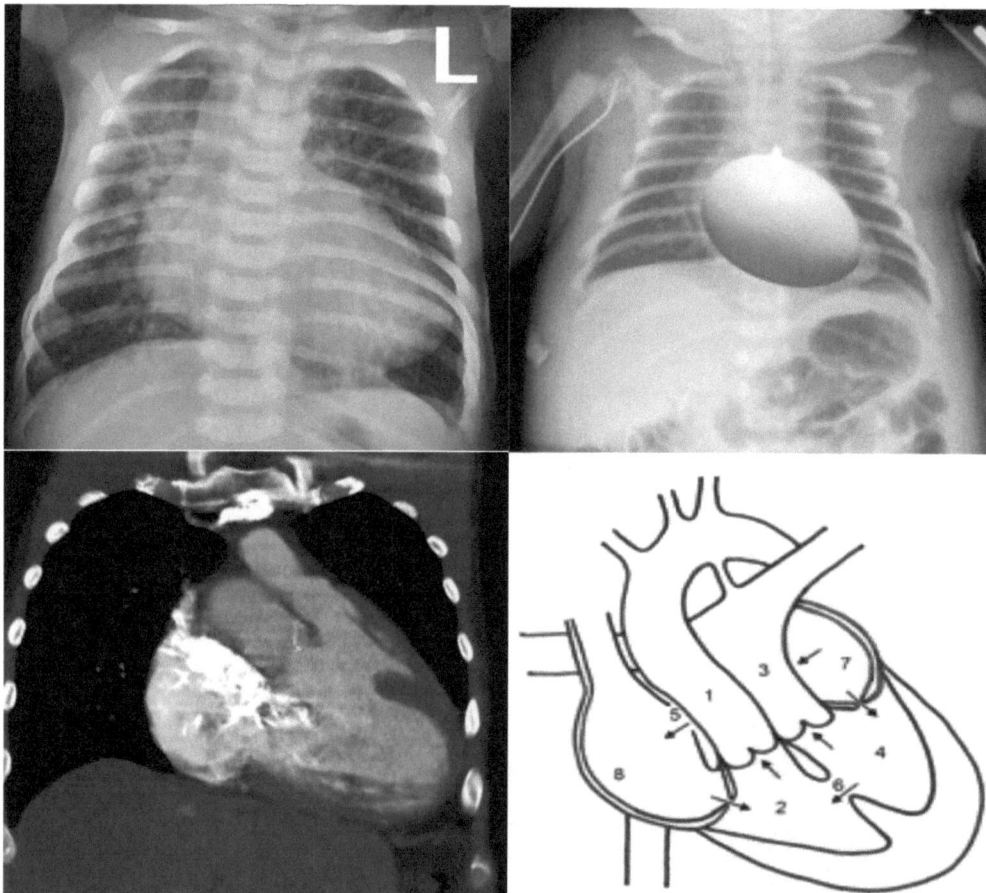

Drawing shows the pattern of blood flow (arrows) through the heart with transposition of the great arteries. The aorta *(1)* arises from the right ventricle *(2)*, and the pulmonary artery *(3)* arises from the left ventricle *(4)*. Communication between the systemic and the pulmonary circulation—an interatrial septal defect *(5)*, an interventricular septal defect *(6)*, or both—sustains life by allowing oxygenated blood from the left atrium *(7)* to mix with deoxygenated blood from the right atrium *(8)* before it flows via the right ventricle to the aorta and via the left ventricle to the pulmonary artery.

TAPVR: all the systemic and pulmonary blood flow enters the RA and nothing drains into the left atrium (mixing of oxy and de-oxy blood). A R →→ L shunt is needed to survive and occurs via a patent foramen ovale. Infants have cyanosis and CHF early on.

Type I – supracardiac (commonest) with anomalous veins returning into the left vertical vein which goes into SVC or azygous. This is shows in the images below.

Type II – cardiac (2nd commonest) with venous connection at the cardiac level and blood draining into the coronary sinus and then RA.

Type III – infracardiac with blood returning below the level of the heart. Usually the vein passes through the esophageal hiatus (obstructive) and joins the portal system or IVC.

Scimitar syndrome: hypoplastic right lung with infracardiac **partial** anomalous return via a large curved draining vein. Also small RPA and has a RLL systemic arterial supply.

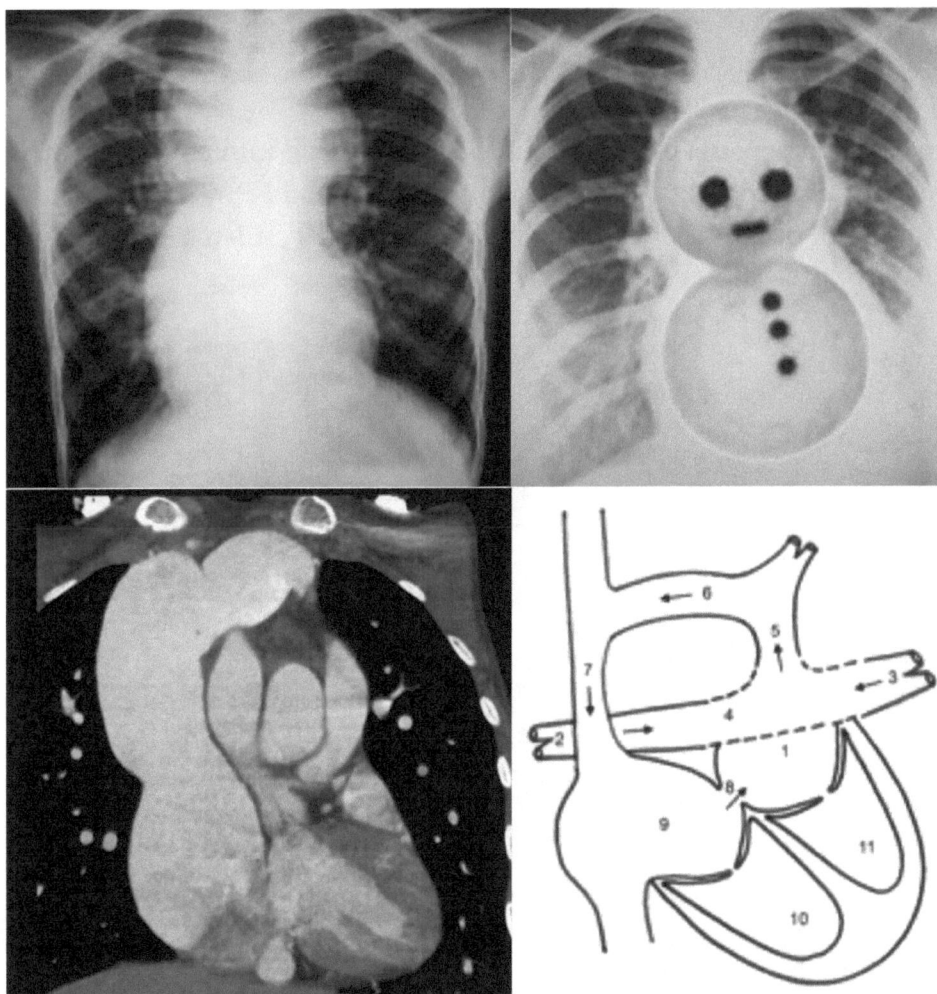

Drawing shows the return of venous blood (arrows). Instead of draining into the LA (1), the pulmonary veins (2,3) converge behind the heart to form a common vein (4) that drains into the left vertical vein (5) which then drains into the innominate vein (6). The left innominate drains into the SVC (7). A R →→ L shunt (8) has to be presents since all blood drains into the right side.

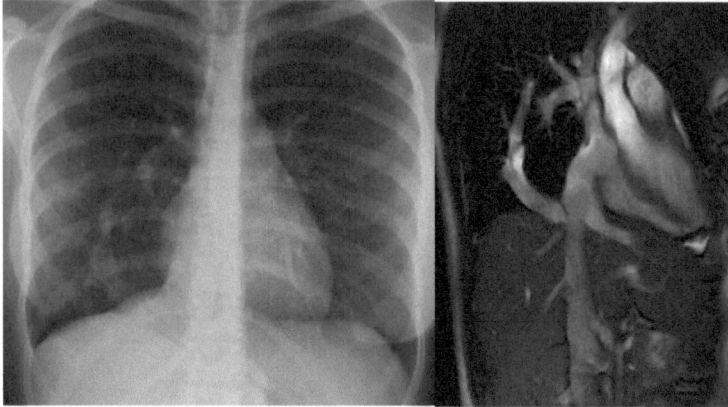

Scimitar syndrome

1. Cyanotic heart diseases with pulmonary edema (indistinct vessels) and signs of heart strain. Think of infracardiac TAPVR, HLH, and sever aortic coarctation. More commonly it's because of severe anemia and asphyxia.

Hypoplastic Left Heart: characterized by hypoplasia or absence of the left ventricle with an atretic aortic and mitral valve. The valve atresias require large inter-atrial left to right shunt and PDA (right to left) to sustain life. Radiographically there will be cardiac enlargement with pulmonary edema. The RV and pulmonary artery will be enlarged.

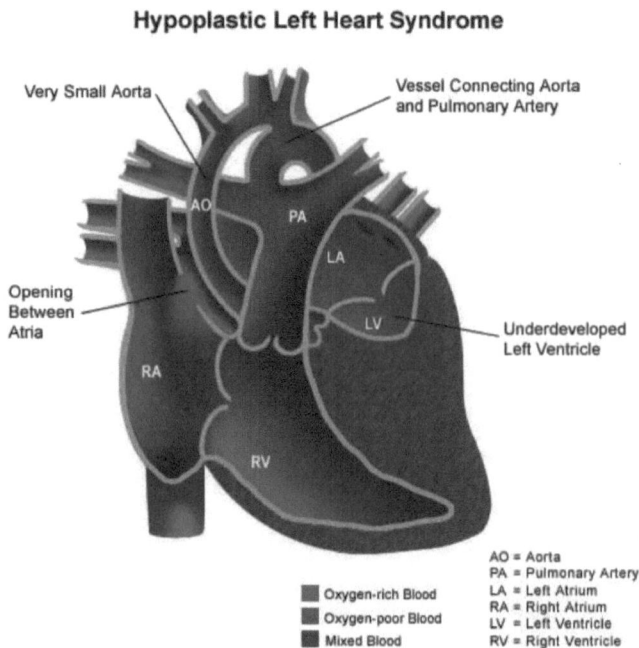

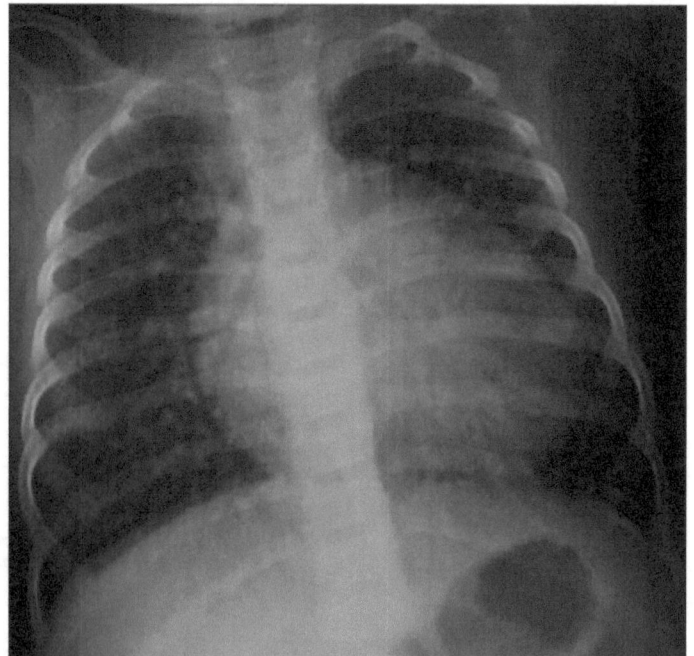

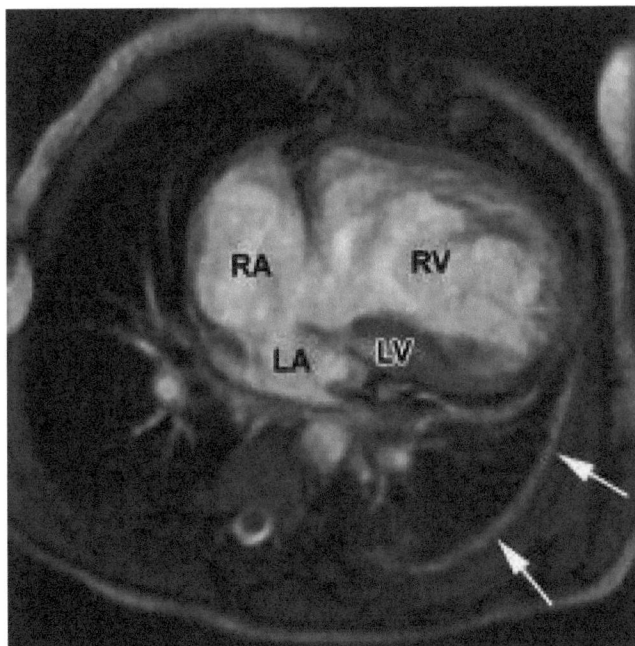

FUN FACTS:

1. Most common cause of papillary muscle rupture is ischemia or infarction.
2. PV pressure > 18 – Kerley B lines, PV pressure > 25 – batwing appearance
3. Most common intracardiac mass overall is a thrombus and it usually forms in LA appendage in patients with A-fib.
4. Pressure gradient across a valve = $4v^2$
5. Most common site of true LV aneurysm is antero-apical, false is infero-posterior
6. Pericardium calcifications are due to chronic pericarditis or more commonly TB. Pericardial thickening and septal bounce = constrictive pericarditis
7. The most common primary malignant cardiac tumor is angiosarcoma.
8. The most common benign cardiac tumor is myxoma.
9. The most common tumor of papillary muscle is a myxopapillary fibroma.
10. In congenital pulmonic stenosis the main and LPA are dilated, but the RPA is normal.
11. Persistent LSVC results when the left anterior cardinal vein persists
12. Most common PAPVR is RUL pulmonary vein to the SVC (can be seen with a sinus venosus defect)
13. Cardiac lipoma most often occurs in the right atrium
14. Interposition of lung between the aorta and the pulmonary artery is partial absence of pericardium – dangerous because heart can herniate through and torse
15. An enlarged calcified LA is indicative of mitral stenosis
16. After a lobectomy, if the pleural space isn't completely filled with fluid, or if air starts to show up on a later date, think broncho-pleural fistula (bad)
17. Empyema necessitates – empyema that invades through the chest wall. Often due to osteomyelitis of an adjacent rib.

GASTROINTESTINAL

Esophageal Atresia: an absence in the continuity of the esophagus due to inappropriate foregut division. This is the most common congenital anomaly of the esophagus. Several findings are clinically suspicious: the inability to swallow or pass an NGT are two of the most common. Frequently associated with a trachea–esophageal fistula. Pure atresia will show a paucity of bowel air but fistula will allow air into bowels. Fetal US has polyhydramnios. Associated with VACTERL.

The most common TE fistula is **proximal atresia with distal fistula**

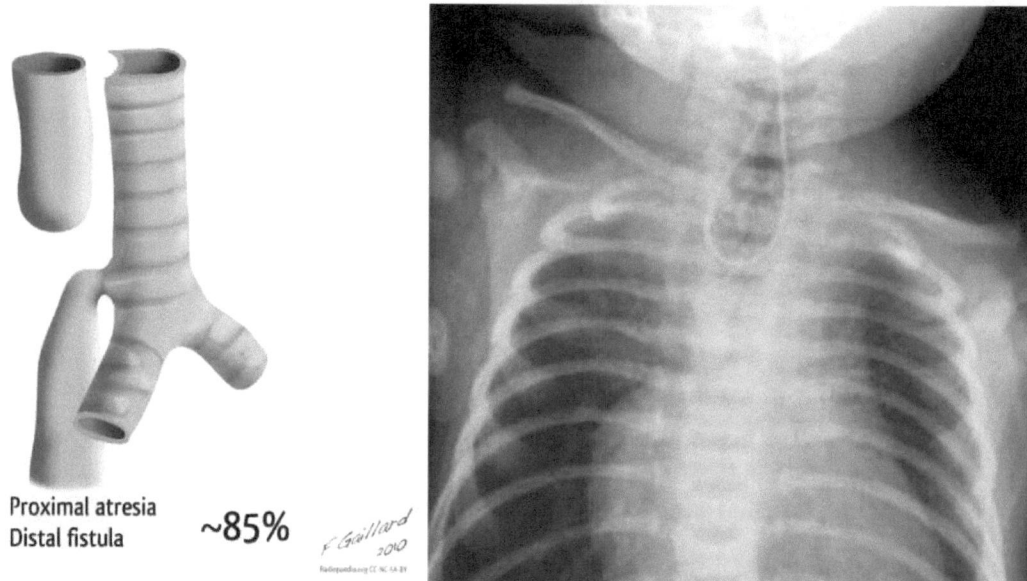

Proximal atresia
Distal fistula   ~85%

4% of the time there is no atresia, just an H–type fistula distally running in an oblique upwards course.

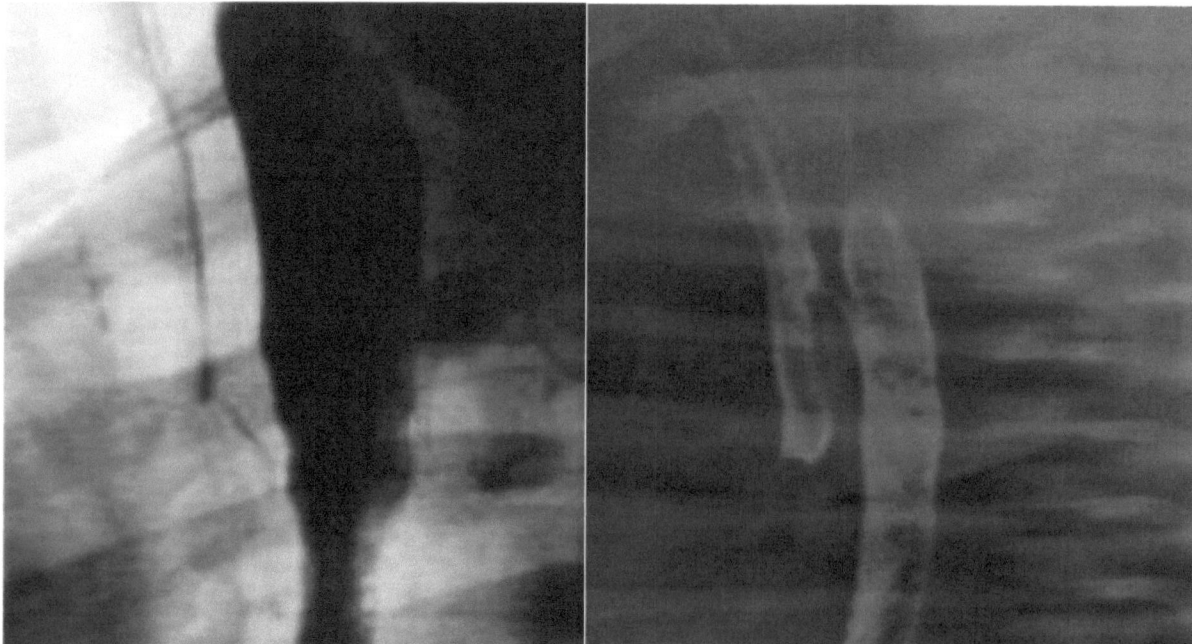

Gastric Atresia/Antral Web: atresia will present early in life, the web will present with non–bilious vomiting.

Hypertrophic Pyloric Stenosis: presents with non–bilious vomiting in the 2nd – 6th weeks of life, has a male predominance, and is caused by hypertrophy of the circular muscle fibers of the pylorus. Ultrasound is the initial test of choice. A thickness of > 3 mm from the echogenic mucosa to the serosa and a pyloric channel length of > 16 mm are diagnostic. If the US is negative, get an UGI.

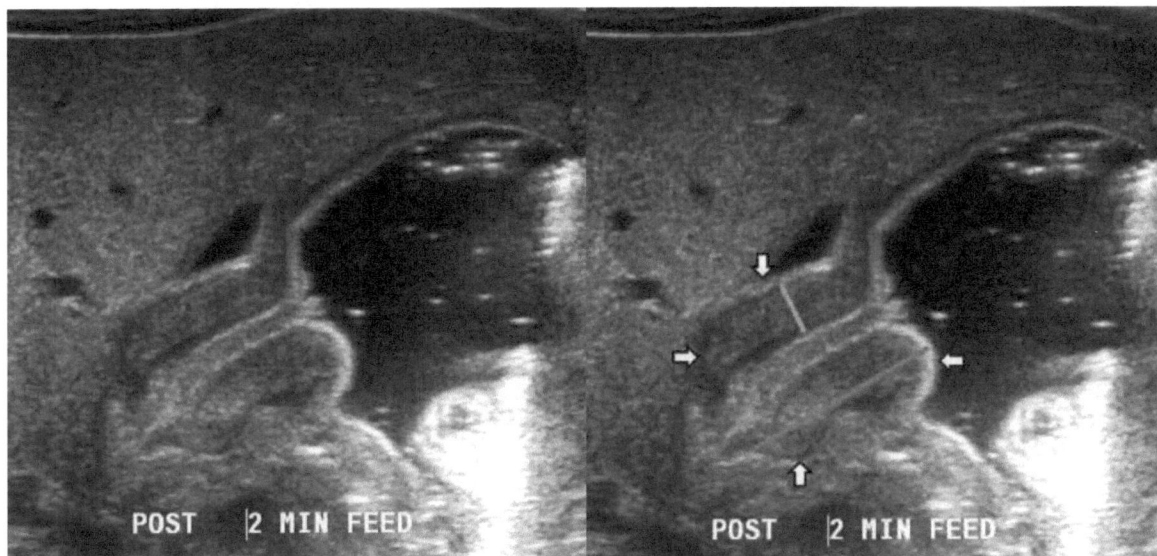

Duodenal Atresia: congenital malformation of the duodenum and is one of the commonest forms of neonatal bowel obstruction. Associated with Down's Syndrome and VACTERL. Patients present early in life with abdominal distention and absent bowel movements and bilious vomiting. Often time it is diagnosed in utero on US with the classic double bubble sign.

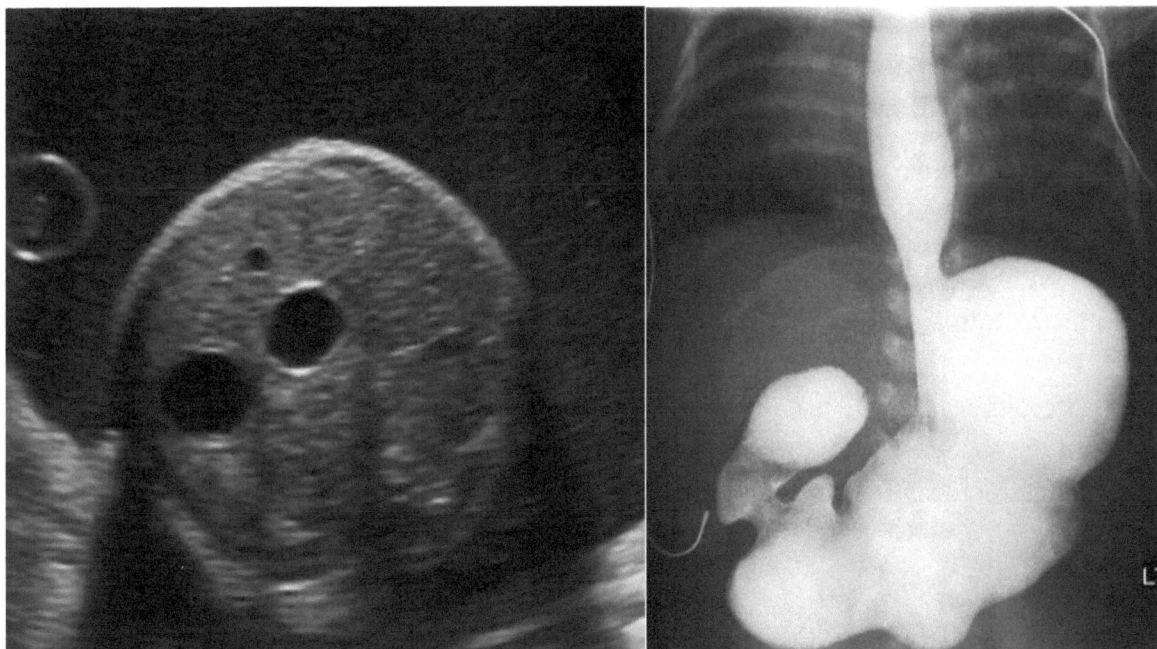

With double bubble also think of annular pancreas and duodenal web (intermittent symptoms).

Jejunal Atresia: thought to be related to an ischemic injury in utero. Radiographs show distended loops of small bowel with paucity of air in the colon.

Ileal Atresia: congenital abnormality with stenosis or complete absence of a portion of the ileum – due to vascular insult. Can be discovered prenatally, like any of the above atresias, these kids have polyhydramnios and upstream fluid filled lumens.

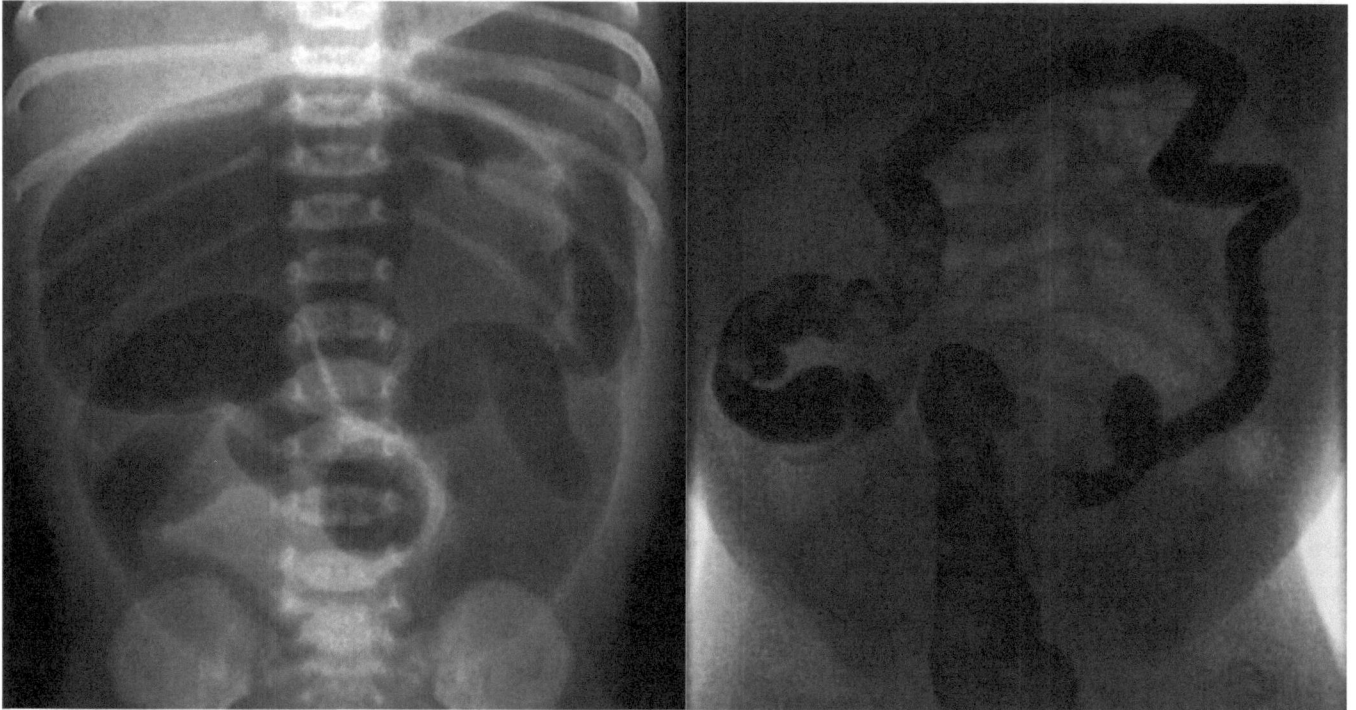

Plain film shows numerous dilated bowel loops. The barium enema shows a normal rectum with an unused appearing colon with multiple filling defects. Contrast refluxed into a normal appearing terminal ileum but would go no further indicating atresia.

Hirschsprung Disease: most common cause of neonatal colonic obstruction. Typical presentation is the failure to pass meconium in the first 1–2 days after birth. This is characterized by aganglionic segment of bowel most often in the rectum and sigmoid. Total colonic is uncommon.

On fluoroscopy the affected segment is usually small with proximal dilation. Look at the rectosigmoid ratio – the diameter of the rectum divided by the diameter of the sigmoid colon during contrast enema filling. Normal kids have rectums that are larger than the sigmoid (>1), while in HIrschsprung's the ratio is < 1.

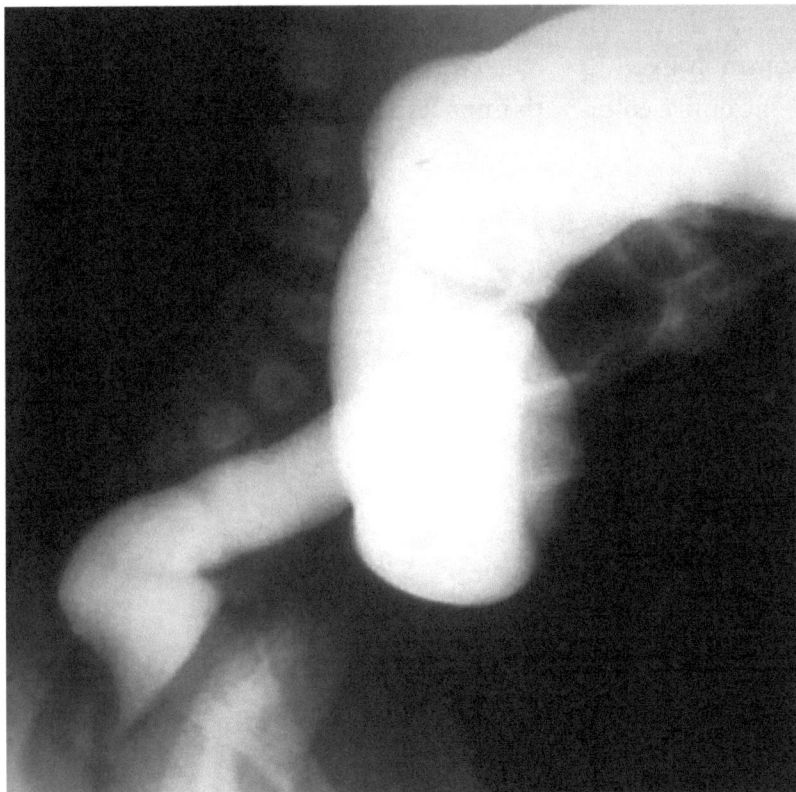

Functional Immaturity of the Colon: seen in children of mothers on MgSO4 and diabetics. The appearance is of a narrow descending colon starting abruptly at the splenic flexure with upstream dilation.

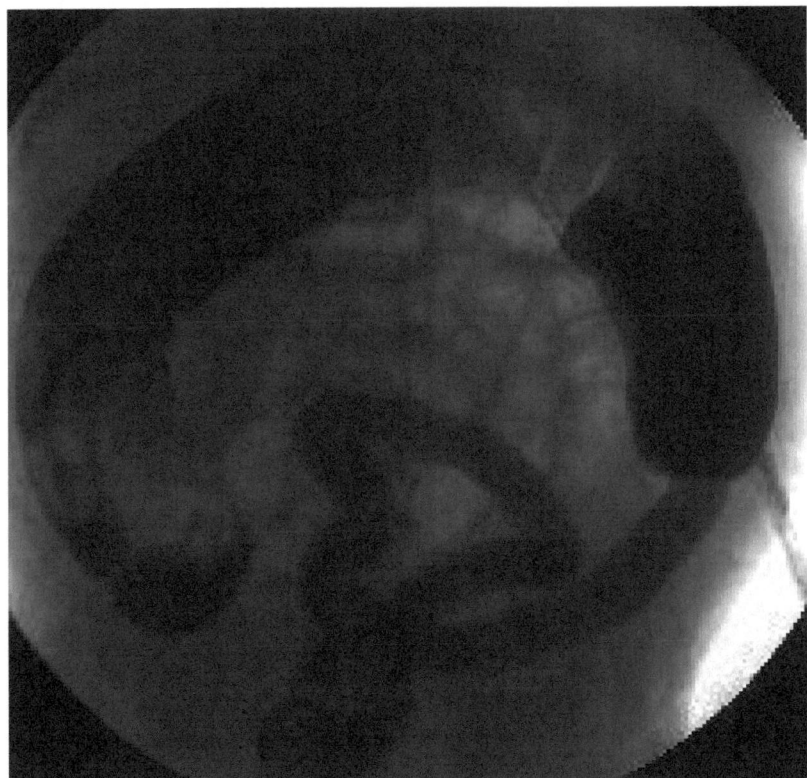

Meconium Ileus: bowel obstruction of the distal ileum due to thick impacted meconium. This is often a manifestation of CF and as such is more common in whites. Dilated loops of small bowel are noted on x– ray. Enema shows a microcolon involving the entire colon with impacted meconium pellets in the right colon or distal ileum.

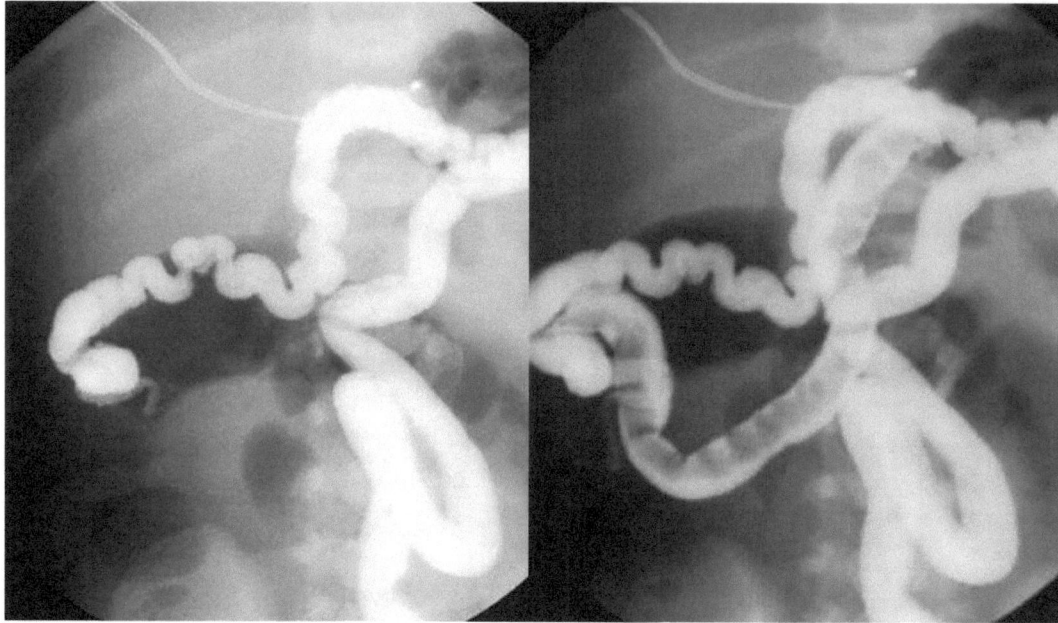

Meconium Peritonitis: sterile chemical perotinitis due to intra–uterine bowel perforation and spill of meconium into the peritoneal cavity. Commonly a cause of peritoneal calcifications. The bowel perforates as a result of obstruction (atresia or meconium ileus).

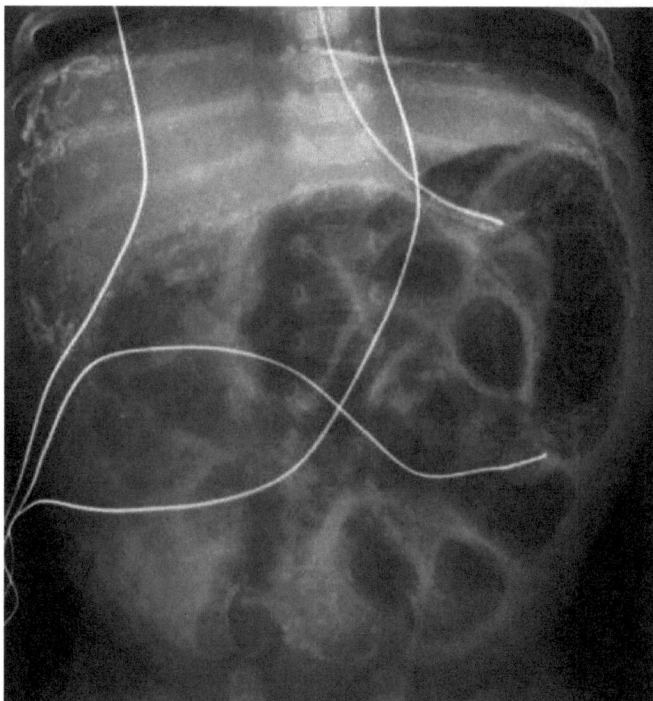

Complications include: ascites, bowel obstruction, meconium pseudocyst formation.

Meconium Plug Syndrome: is a functional colonic obstruction in a newborn due to an obstructing meconium **plug in the left colon.** The bowel distal to the plug is small (microcolon). Higher prevalence in children of diabetic mothers. X–ray will show non–specific dilated loops of bowel. On fluoro look for filling defects in the left colon with distal small colon.

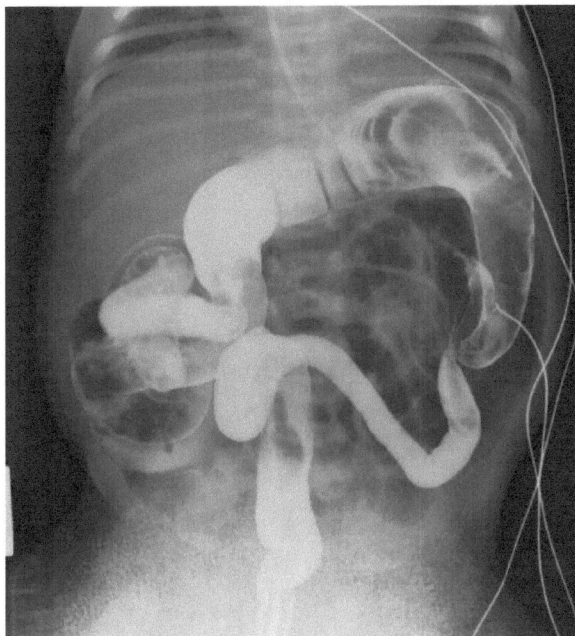

Midgut Volvulus: is a malrotated small bowel around the mesenteric axis and is a surgical emergency. The neonate is typically asymptomatic initially, and then develops bilious vomiting. If there isn't spontaneous resolution, the venous obstruction created by the SMV being wrapped around the SMA causes ischemia and necrosis. This is an easy diagnosis on the UGI – corkscrew appearance of duodenum with dilated stomach.

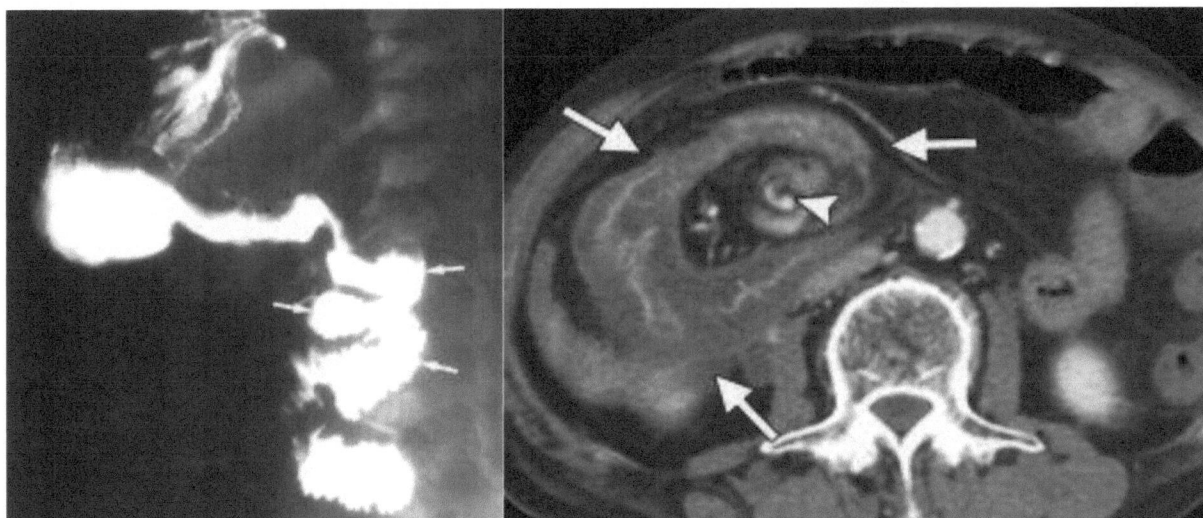

Intussusception: occurs when one segment of bowel telescopes into another causing obstruction. This is an emergency as well. 90% of the time, no lead point mass is seen in kids, in 90% of adults a lead point is noted. There is a predilection for the ileocecal region.

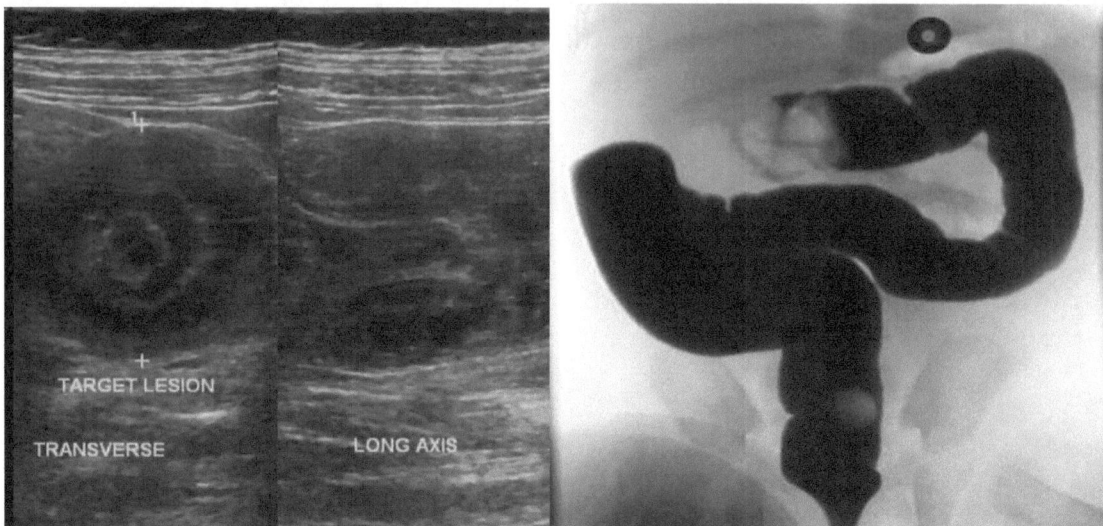

The US shows a classic target pattern of one bowel + mesentery inside another bowel. This has been described as the "pseudokidney" appearance as well. The fluoroscopy image shows retrograde contrast filling of colon coming to a halt at the mid transverse colon due to a filling defect from a loop of bowel.

Necrotizing Enterocolitis: seen in premature babies as bowel ischemia related to hypoxic event. Bacteria invade the wall of the bowel and cause pneumatosis. Earliest sign is abnormal bowel dilation – long tubular loops. Bloody stools are common. Affects the RLQ most often.

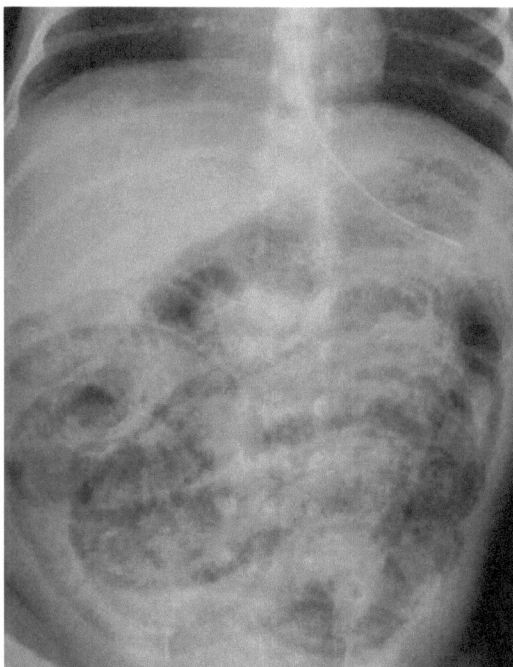

Neonatal Hepatitis: between weeks 1–4 of age. The patient will have jaundice and a coarsened liver echogenicity. The liver does not take up mebrofenin well so the blood pool is delayed, but there will be excretion after 24 hours.

Biliary Atresia: is a congenital disorder characterized by jaundice and increased bilirubin. An early diagnosis is key so that a Kasai procedure can be performed. The intra or extrahepatic ducts can be obstructed and this leads to fibrosis. Transplant is the cure. Diagnosed on cholescintigraphy. Prior to exam give baby 5mg/kg phenobarbital for 5 days. Look for persistent activity in the liver after 24–hours.

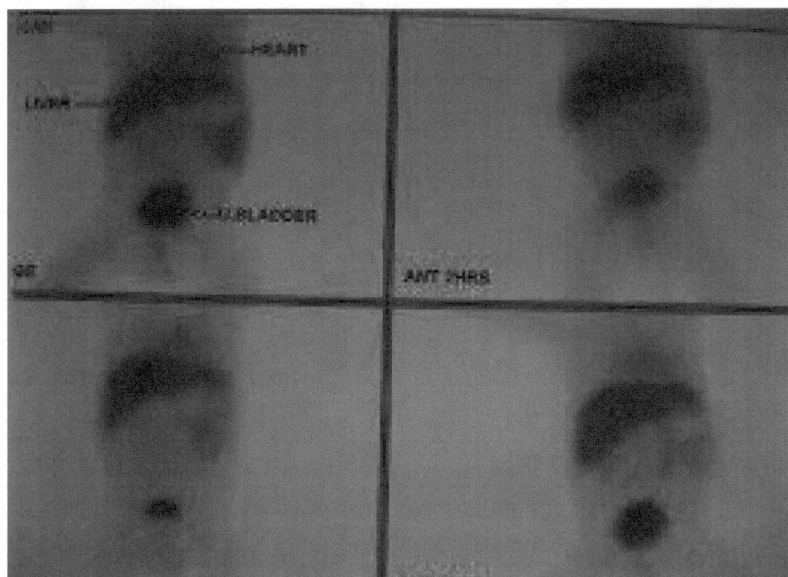

Hepatoblastoma: is **the number one liver tumor of childhood**. It presents as a large, solid, solitary right hepatic lobe mass. Kids will have abdominal pain, vomiting, and a palpable mass.

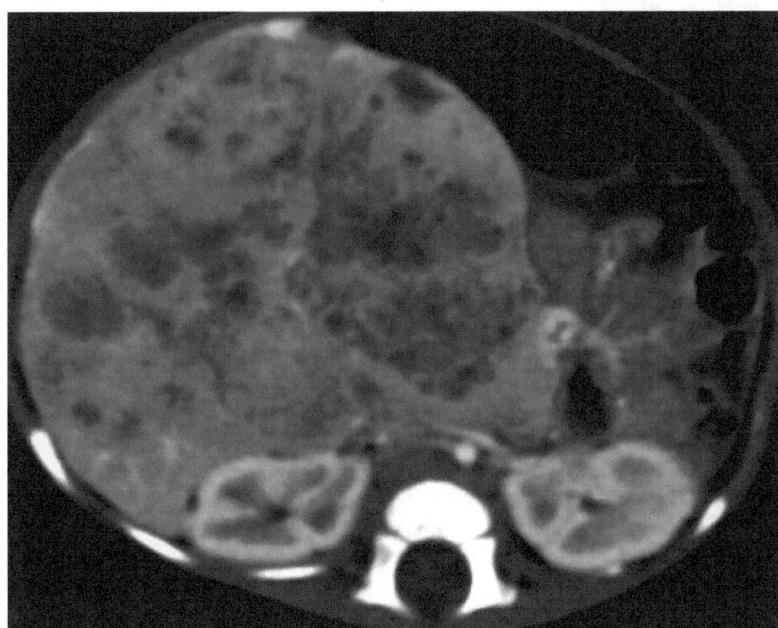

Mesenchymal Hamartoma: multilocular cystic hepatic mass most often seen in kids younger than 2 years of age. In utero this can cause fetal hydrops and respiratory distress from mass effect.

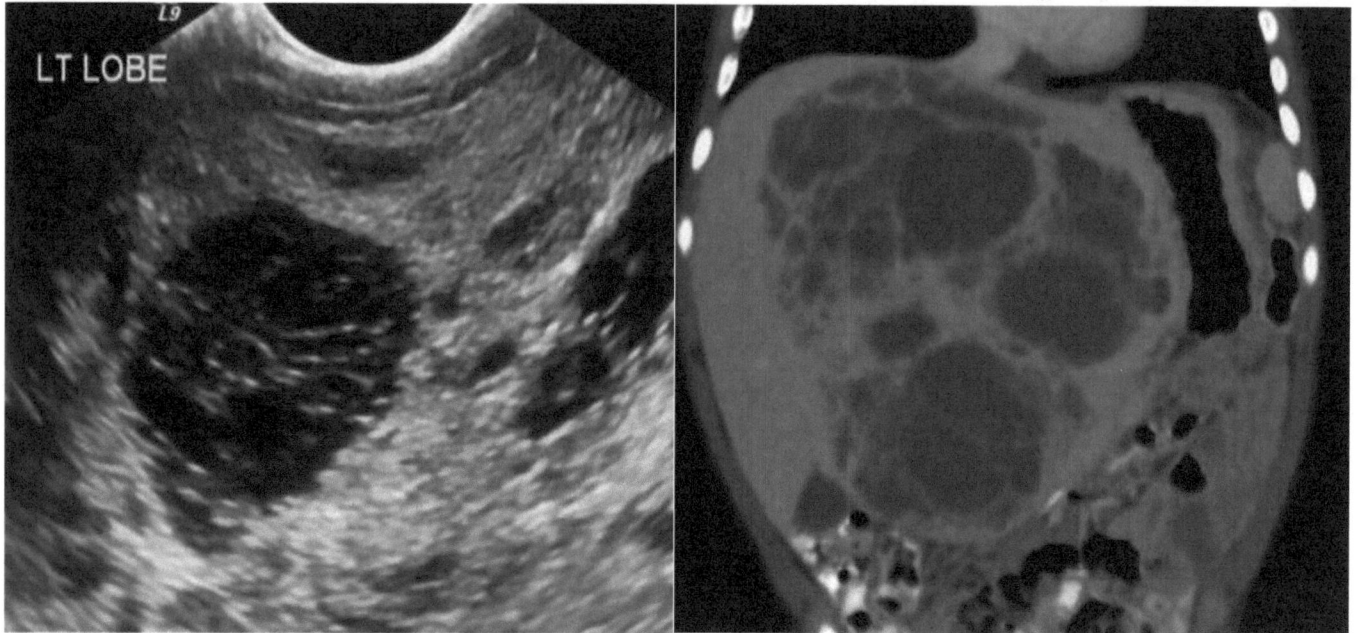

Hemangioendothelioma: a liver lesion composed of large endothelial–lined vascular channels seen in fetuses and neonates. It has substantial AV shunting and may lead to fetal cardiac compromise and hydrops. This like a giant hemangioma can sequester platelets leading to Kasabach–Merritt Syndrome – thrombocytopenia. Its natural course is to rapidly enlarge in the first six months of life and then regression and involution.

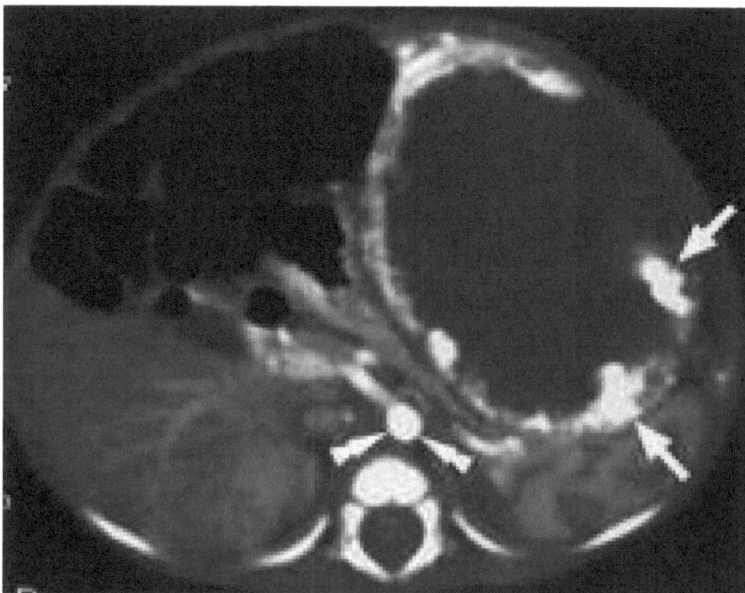

This is a hypodense mass typically seen with calcifications, eccentric enhancement and cystic components.

GENITOURINARY

Vesicoureteral Reflux: causes scarring of the kidneys due to repeated infections and abscesses. Primary is caused by a short submucoasl intravesicle distal ureter and secondary is because of bladder outlet obstruction.

I – ureter only
II. – into the calyces without blunting
III – blunted calyces
IV – dilated tortuous ureter V – loss of papilla

Use DMSA scans to look for pyelonephritis and scarring – areas of photopenia

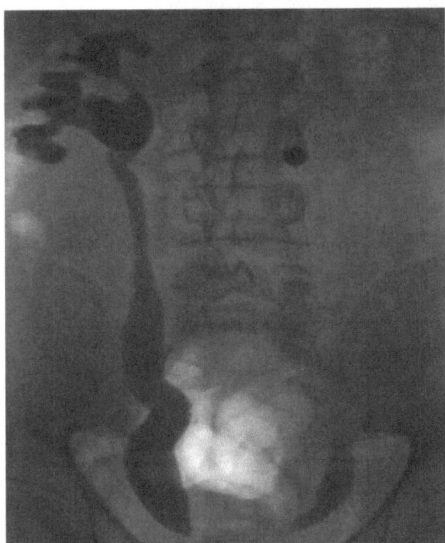

Grade IV right and Grade I left

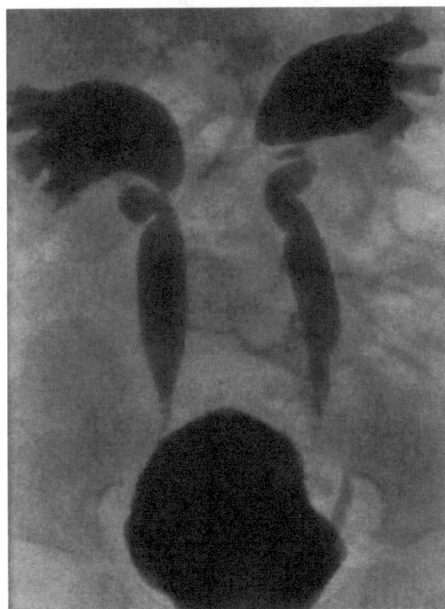

Bilateral Grade IV–V

Posterior Urethral Valves: this is the number one cause of bladder outlet obstruction in male infants, look for **abrupt narrowing of the bulbous urethra**. Often discovered in utero in babies with oligohydramnios.

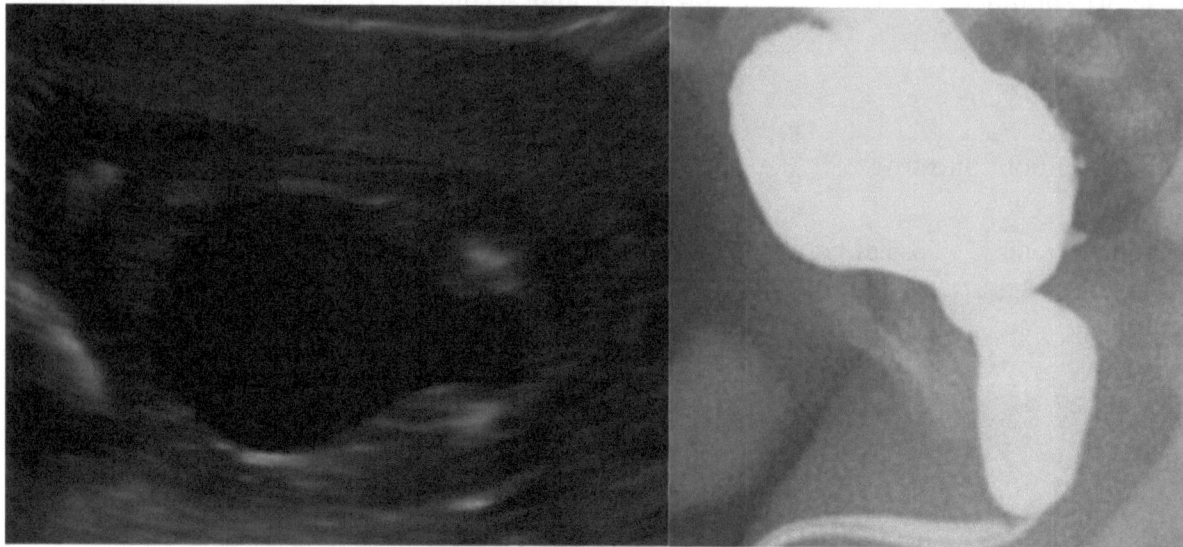

US shows a keyhole sign with a dilated bladder and dilated posterior urethra. Similar findings seen on fluoroscopy.

Duplicated Collecting System: 50% of the time this is bilateral. Upper pole obstructs because of ureterocele and the lower pole refluxes. Follows Weigert–Meyer rule – upper pole ureter inserts inferior and medial to the normally inserting ureter. The duplication doesn't have to be complete; the two ureters can fuse before inserting into the bladder.

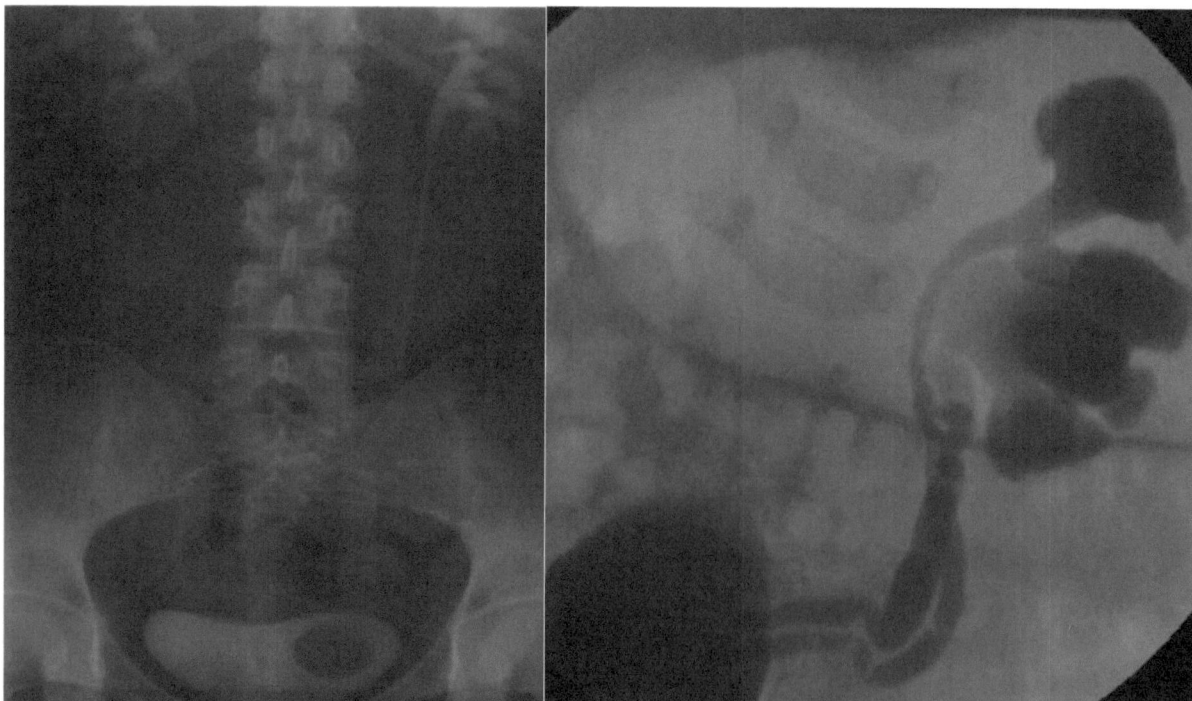

Image on the left shows filling defect from an ureterocele and right image shows duplicated system with contrast filling of both ureters.

Fun Fact: Ureteroceles are best seen on early filling phase of the VCUG

Fun Fact: In men the ectopic ureter typically inserts above the external sphincter, in women it inserts below the sphincter leading to incontinence

UPJ Obstruction: is the most common cause of obstructive uropathy and can be congenital or acquired. Often unilateral, but if present, the contralateral kidney has reflux or UVJ obstruction. It can be caused by a variant crossing renal artery or by fibrosis.

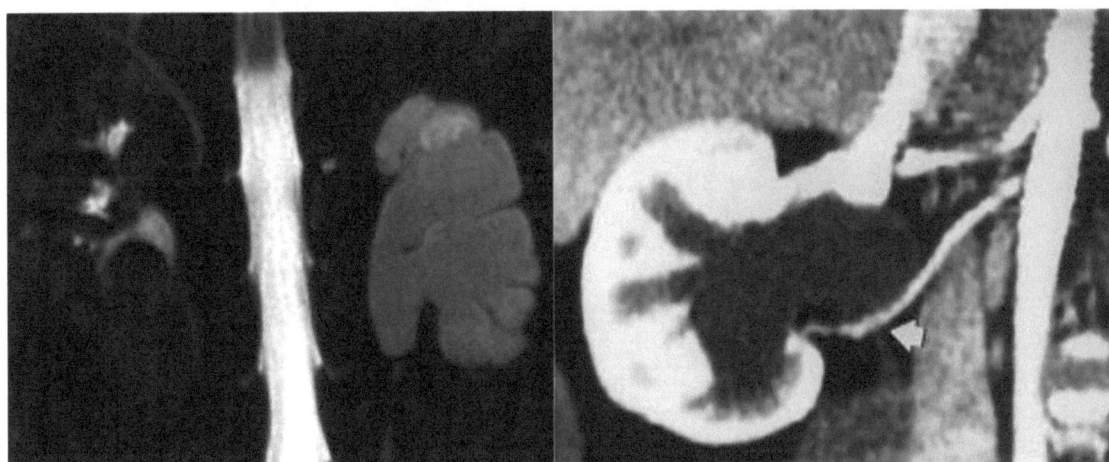

Urachal Remnant: refers to a series of potential anomalies that can occur in association with the urachus. The urachus connects the dome of the bladder to the umbilicus duct during fetal life and is located behind the abdominal wall and anterior to the peritoneum in the space of Retzius.

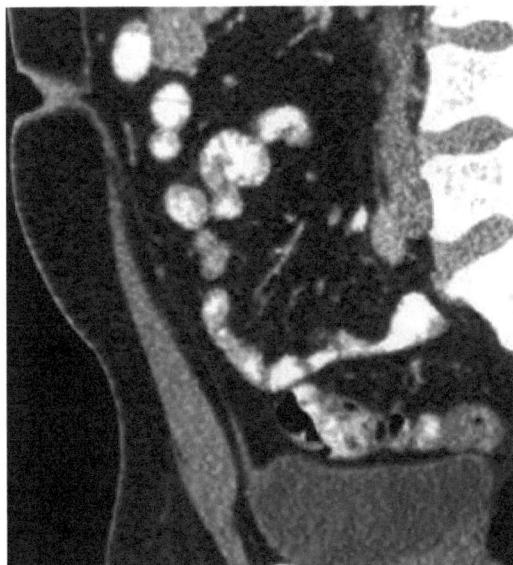

Patent urachus – most common (50%) seen in the image on the left Urachal cyst – 30% Urachal–umbilical sinus – 15% Vesicourachal diverticulum – 5%

Urachal remnants are associated with a higher rate of malignancy – Adenocarcinoma

Fun Fact: Hydronephrosis is the number one cause of a neonatal abdominal mass

Prune Belly Syndrome: rare anomaly comprising of three major findings 1) gross bladder and ureteric dilation 2) anterior abdominal wall underdevelopment 3) bilateral undescended testicles. Death usually occurs in the 1st year of life.

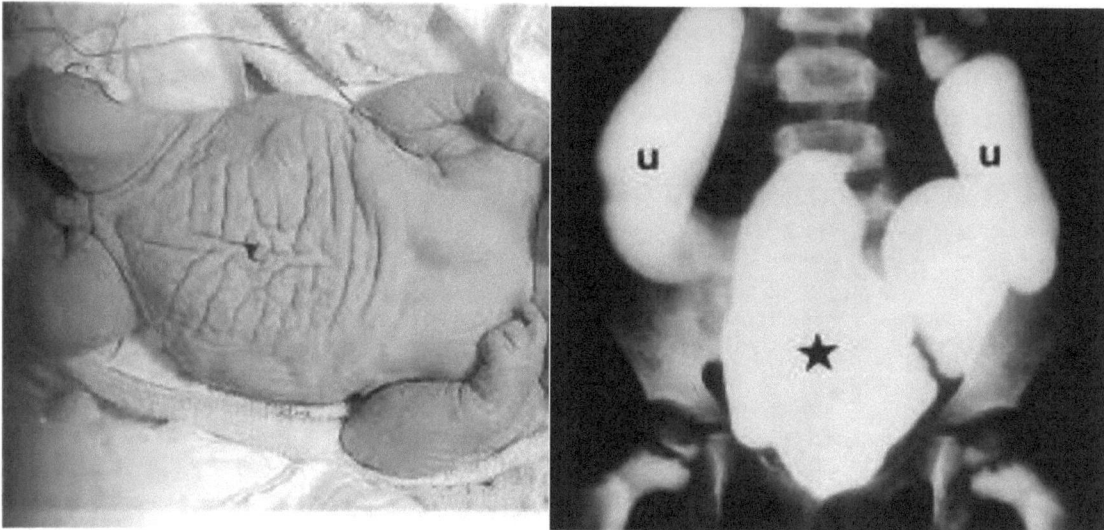

MCDK: most common cystic renal disease in children and number one cause of a renal mass in the 1st week of life. Multiple different sized cysts with no working renal parenchyma. Shrinks down over time.

Most common contralateral abnormality is VUR and next most common is UPJ obstruction.

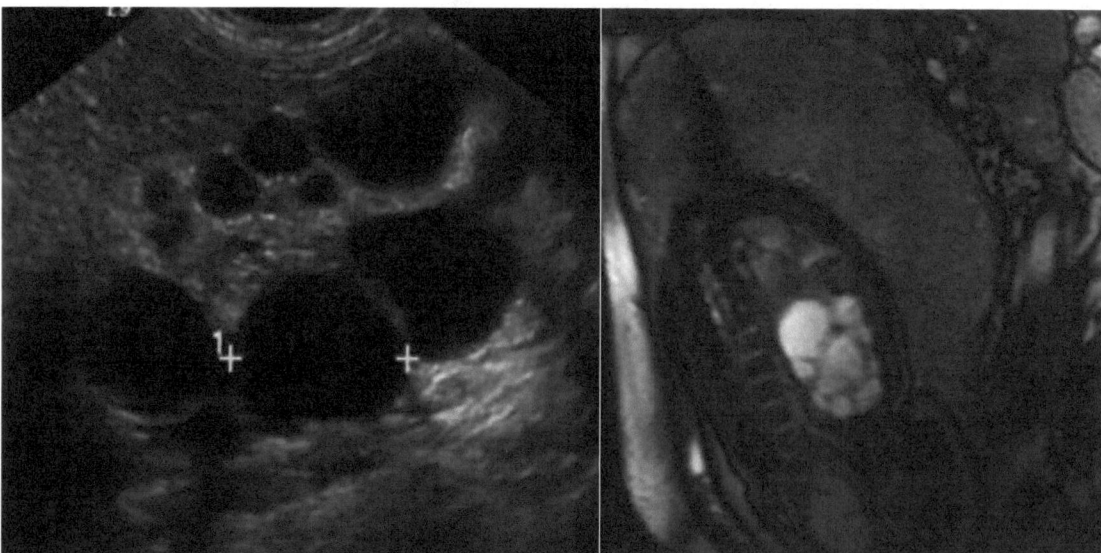

US and fetal MRI show varying sized cysts.

ARPCKD: this is a cystic disease of the kidney; the severity is inversely related to the amount of involved hepatic fibrosis. Kids who present early have more renal disease and kids who present at an older age have more hepatic fibrosis. Associated with oligohydramnios because the baby can't pee. The oligohydramnios can cause pulmonary hypoplasia.

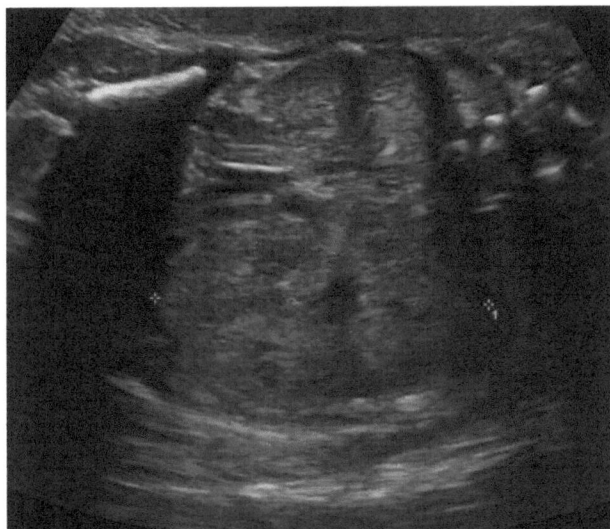

US showing bilateral enlarged **echogenic** kidneys

Hemorrhagic Cystitis: early chemotherapy (cyclophosphamide) can cause desquamation of the bladder mucosa and lead to hemorrhagic cystitis. Imaging shows abnormal bladder wall with irregular thickening and spasticity. Chronic phase shows a small fibrosed bladder with wall calcifications.

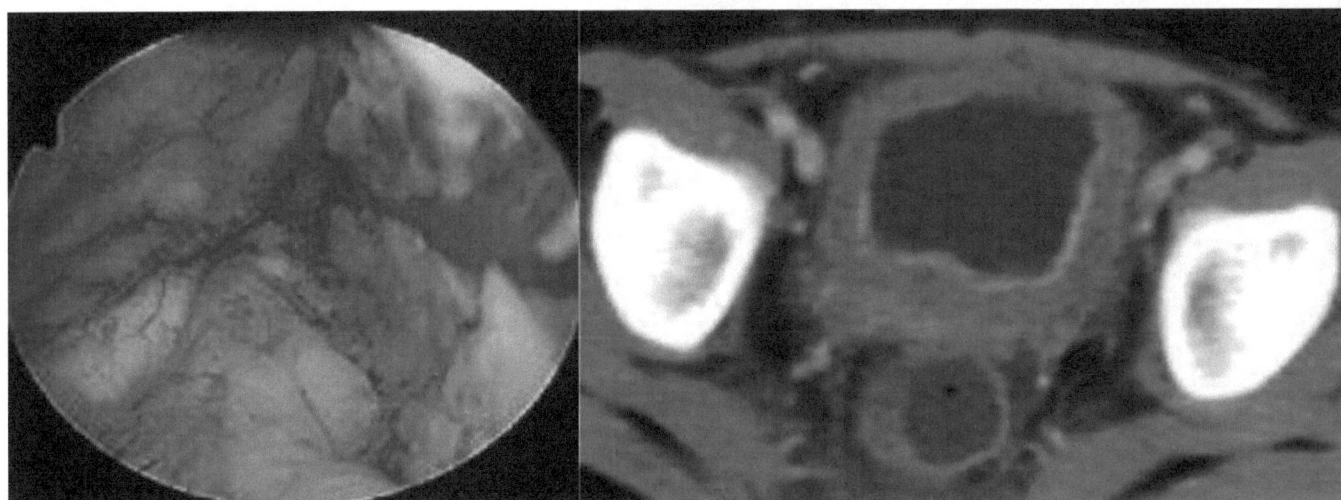

Treatment is with copious bladder irrigation, drainage, and discontinuing the offending agent.

Bladder Exstophy: refers to a herniation of the urinary bladder through an anterior abdominal wall defect with variable severity. Caused by a developmental defect of the cloacal membrane.

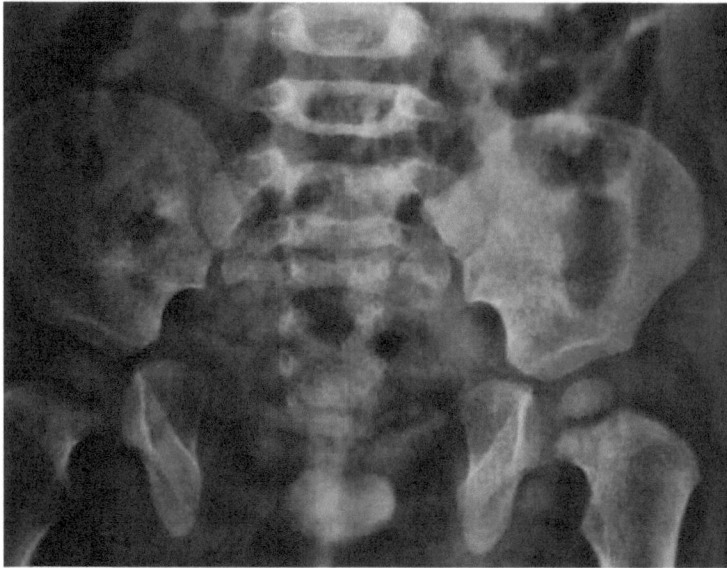

NEOPLASMS:

Wilm's Tumor: the most common pediatric abdominal mass. Associated with aniridia, genital abnormalities, and mental retardation (WAGR). Other associations are Beckwidth–Weidemann Syndrome (hemihypertrophy). Peak incidence is 3–4 years of age. Likes to invade the renal veins and IVC, make sure to look for the "claw" of renal tissue around the mass.

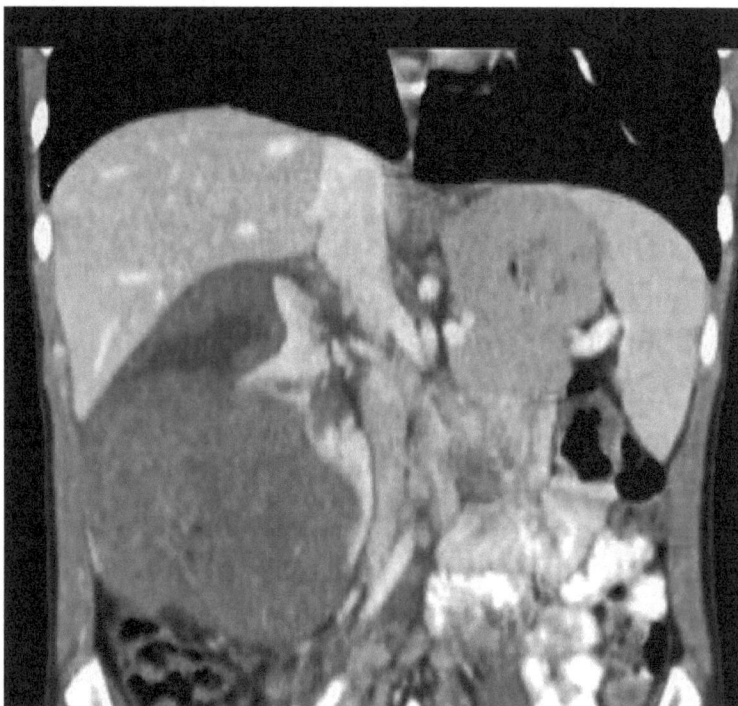

Neuroblastoma: this is the 2nd most common abdominal mass after Wilm's tumor. It presents as a large, palpable RP mass arising from the adrenal gland. Metastases are to the liver, lungs, and bones are common. Tumor can occur anywhere along the sympathetic chain.

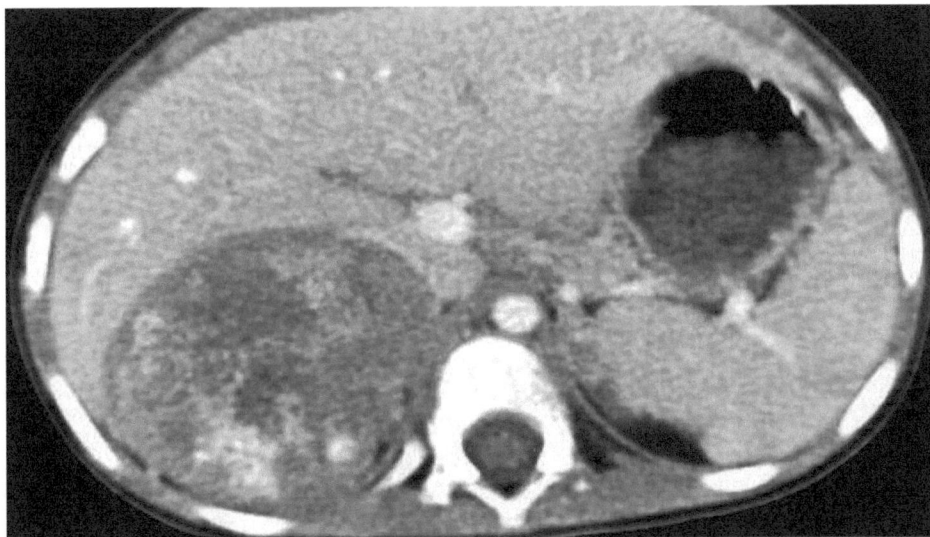

Nephroblastomatosis: persistent metanephric blastema which can be bilateral. Precursor to Wilm's tumor, suspicious if changing appearance. Look for large hypodense confluent masses making the kidneys look huge.

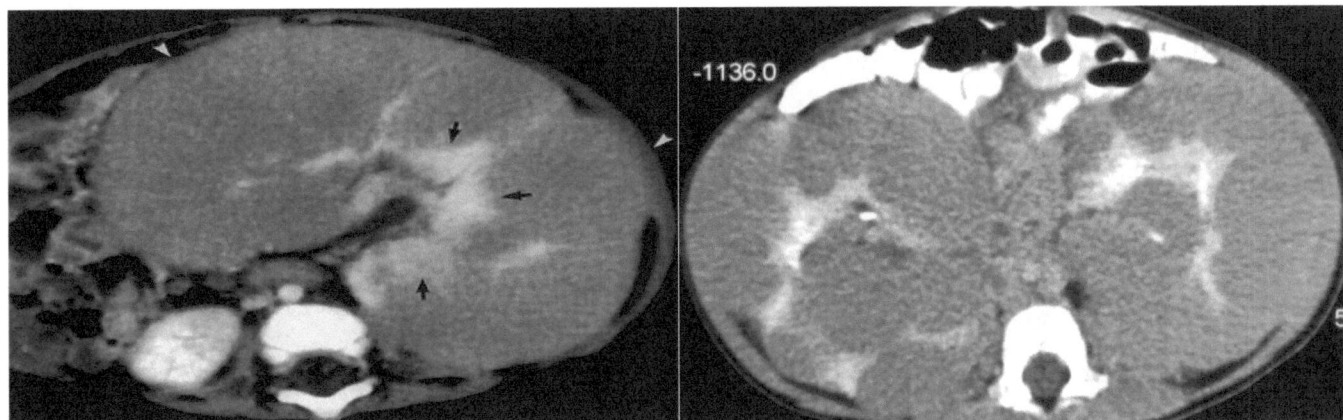

Multilocular Cystic Nephroma: common tumor in young boys and older women. Characteristic finding is a tumor that herniates into the renal sinus. Causes pain and hematuria. It has to be removed to exclude cystic renal cell cancer.

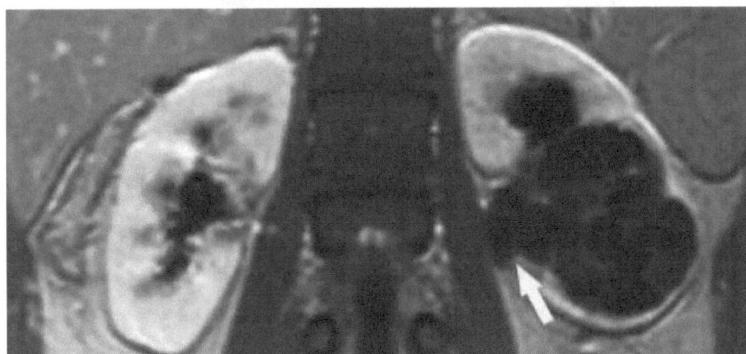

Mesoblastic Nephroma: this is the number on tumor in **children younger than 3 months** of age. Heterogeneous appearing solid mass on US and MRI, tends to be large and deforms the kidney. This tumor is associated with polyhydramnios.

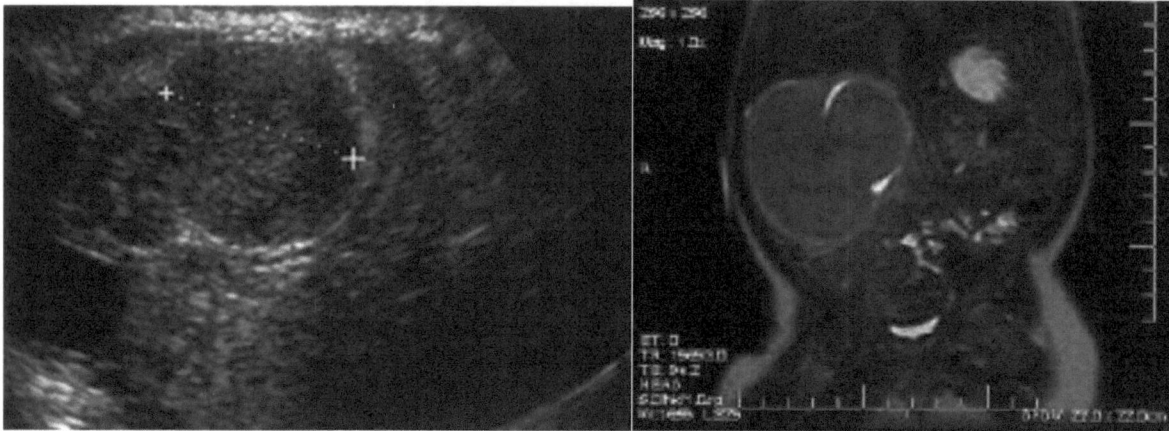

Fun Fact: Renal cell carcinoma is rare in pediatrics, so if it is there think about VHL and look at the other kidney.

Fun Fact: Rhabdoid tumors are rare aggressive tumors that arise from the renal medulla.

MSK
Salter–Harris Classification:

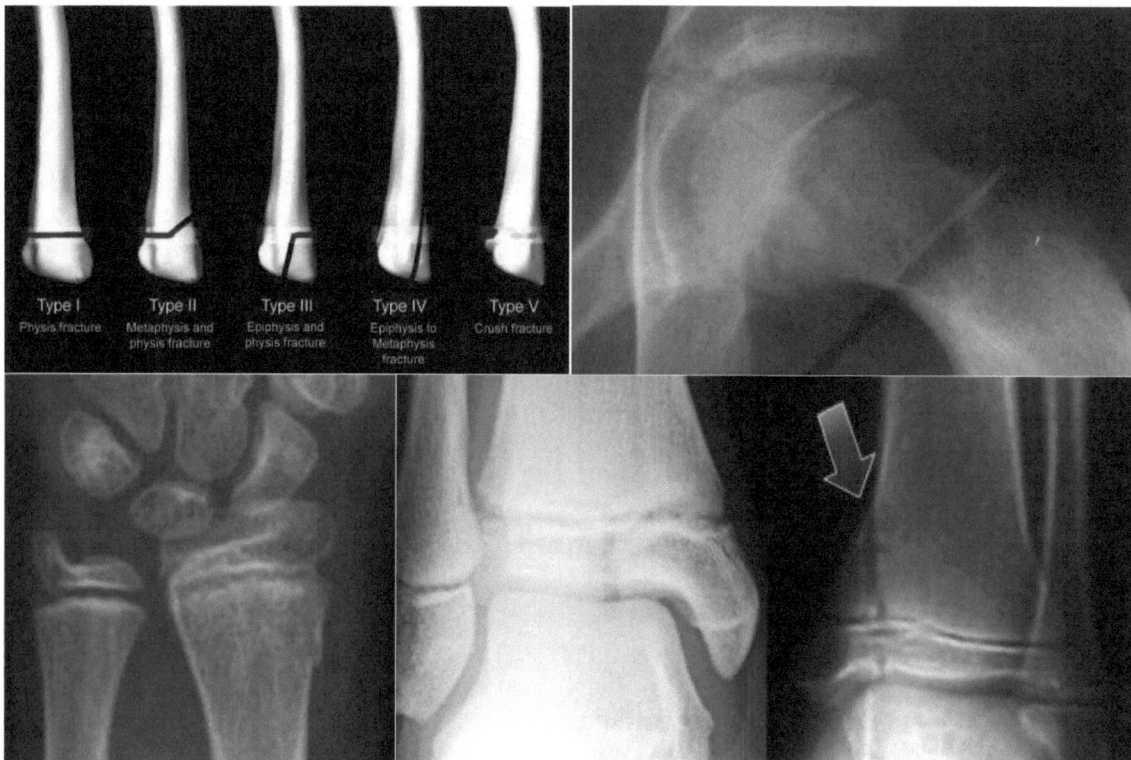

Eponym	SH Class
SCFE	I
Juvenile Tillaux	III
Triplane	Type IV

SCFE: this is a type I SH injury and presents with knee and thigh pain. Kids tend to be black, fat, and male. Earliest sign is a lucent wide physis. Weight bearing has to be stopped immediately and orthopod needs to be consulted. The goal is to catch it early, fix it and keep it from slipping further.

Image is above – top right

LCP Disease: idiopathic AVN of a growing femoral epiphysis in kids typically seen between ages 4–8. Earliest signs are asymmetrical femoral epiphyseal size and increased density of the affected femoral head. The physis collapses and the goal is to treat early and avoid severe degenerative changes.

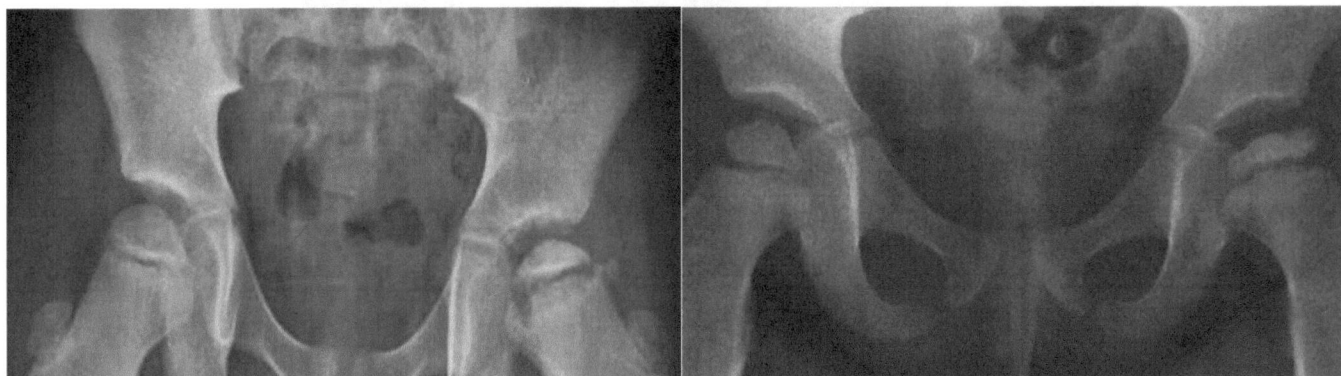

Juvenile–Tillaux: is a fracture through the lateral aspect of the distal tibial epiphysis with variable amounts of displacement. This occurs laterally because the physis fuses medial to lateral. This is a SH type 3 injury. Surgeons will try to do a closed reduction but no displacement is accepted – otherwise go on to surgery.

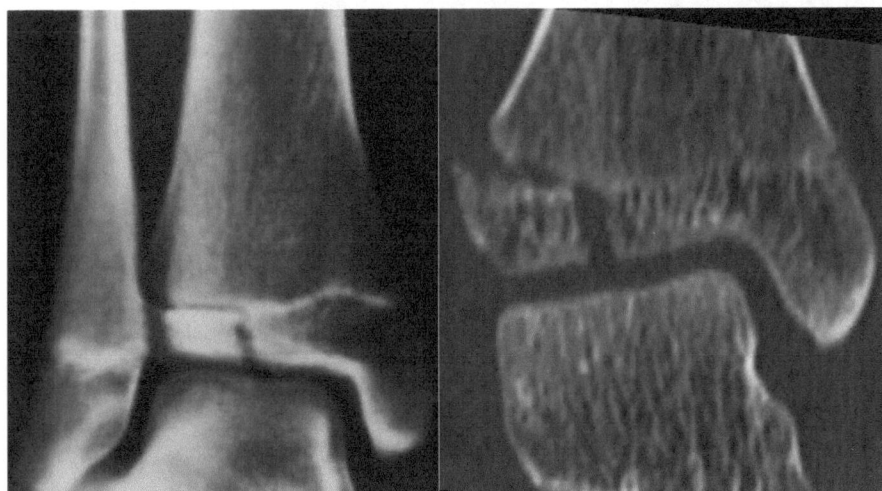

Triplane Fracture: is a fracture of the distal tibia in skeletally immature patients. The lateral half of the distal tibia epiphysis and physeal plate and the posterior tibial metaphysis are involved. "Triplane" means the fracture happens in all three geometric planes. A fracture that causes more than 2–mm of articular incongruity requires reduction.

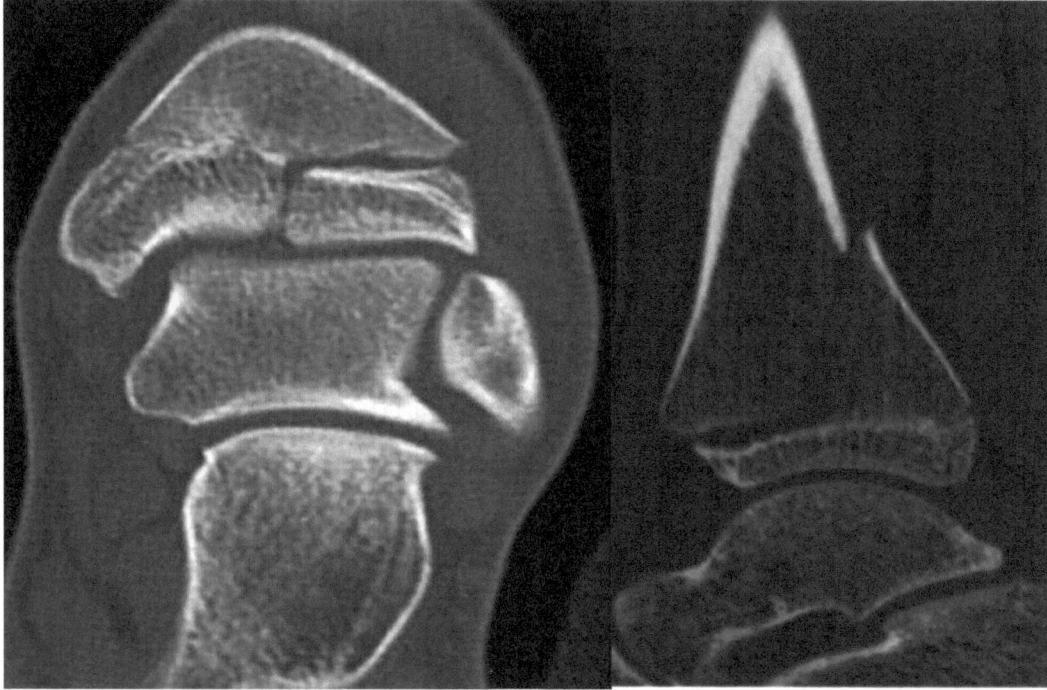

Little Leaguer's Elbow: is a medial epicondyle avulsion due to acute valgus stress.

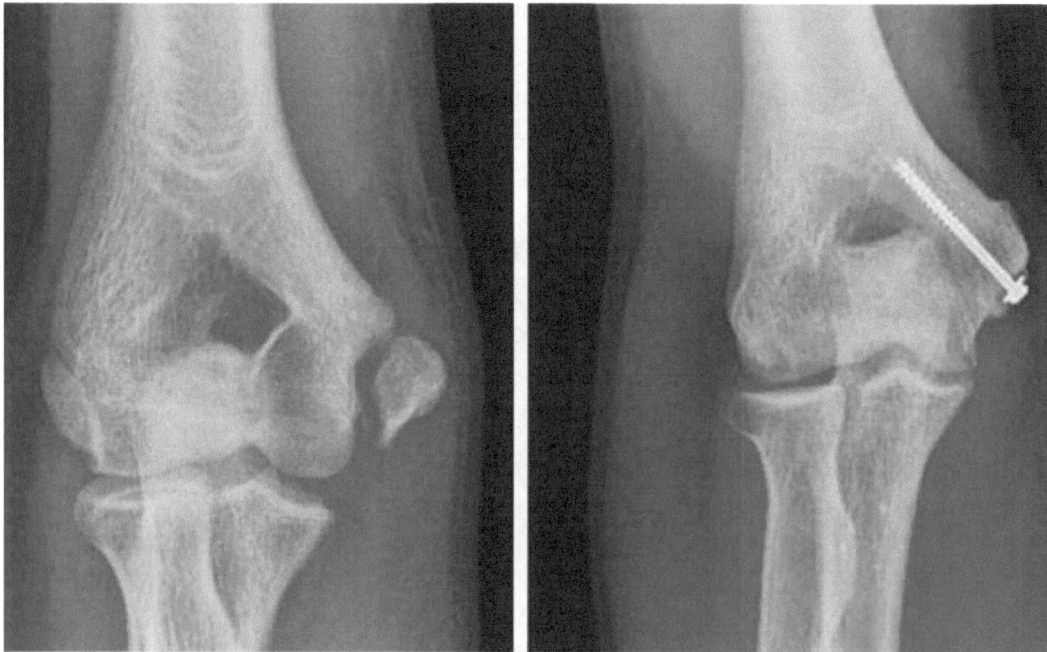

Panner Lesion: osteochondrosis of the capitellum which is typically seen in children 5–10 years of age. It is seen in throwers due to repeated trauma but should be distinguished from osteochondritis dissecans which also affects the capitellum. The key differentiator is the age, Panner (5–10) involves the entire capitellum while osteochondritis (12–16) involves part of or the whole bone.

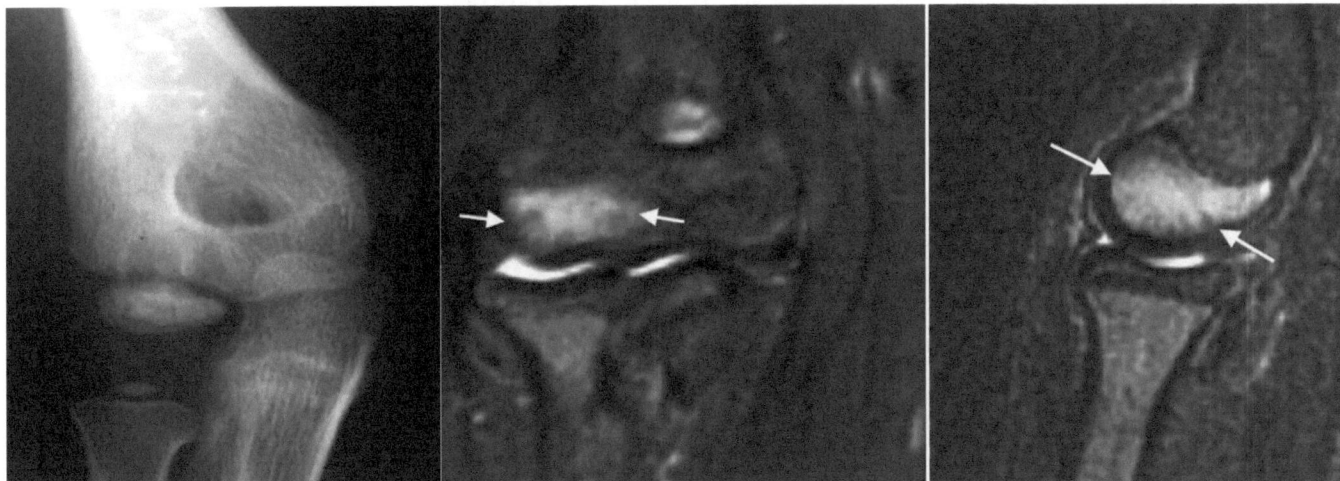

The other important thing to remember is that Panner has no intra–articular loose bodies but osteochondritis dessicans can. Also, osteochondritis dessicans can happen elsewhere – knee and patella.

Osteochondritis is unstable when joint fluid tracks under the cartilage fragment – this is a surgical lesion. Stable lesions can be watched.

Chondrodysplasia Punctata: this is an Aunt Minnie, look for calcifications around the hips in the tri–radiate cartilage in a baby. Also in other areas of fibrocartilage (TFC).

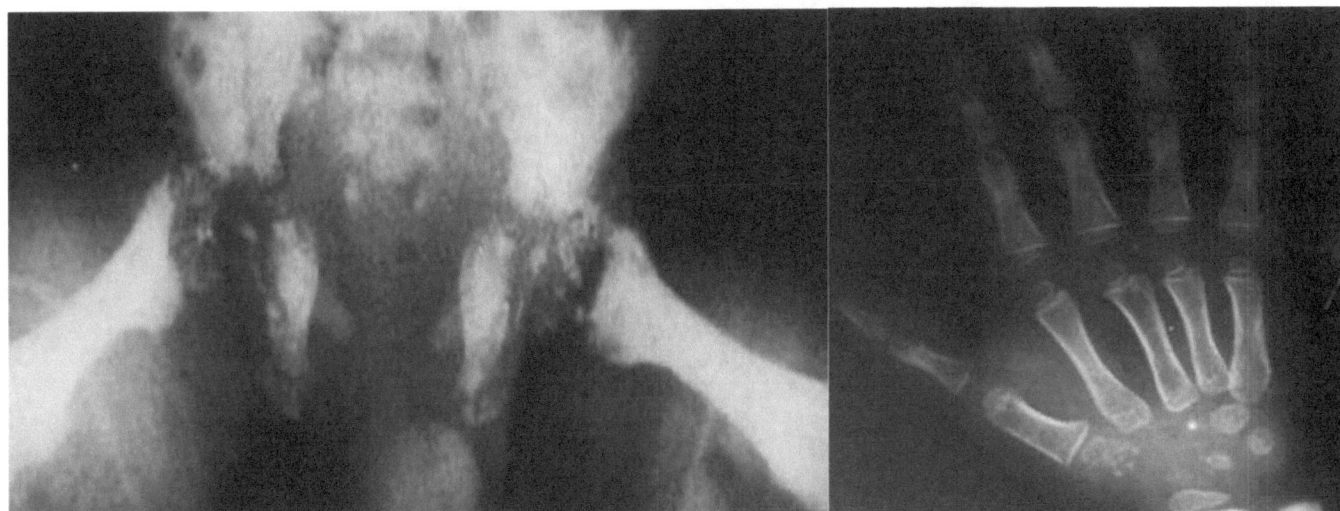

Madelung Deformity: epiphyseal growth plate arrest that occurs after a distal radius injury with a v–shaped carpus and volar tilt of the articular surface. It is also seen with Turner syndrome.

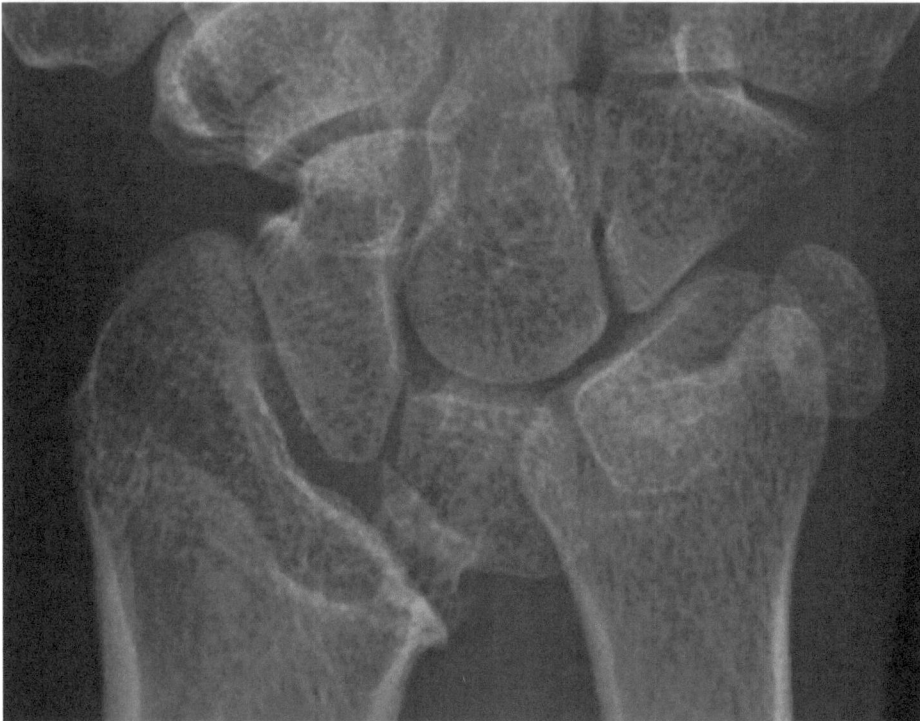

Lucent Metaphyseal Bands: are seen often in NICU babies, Rickets, infection, and leukemia.

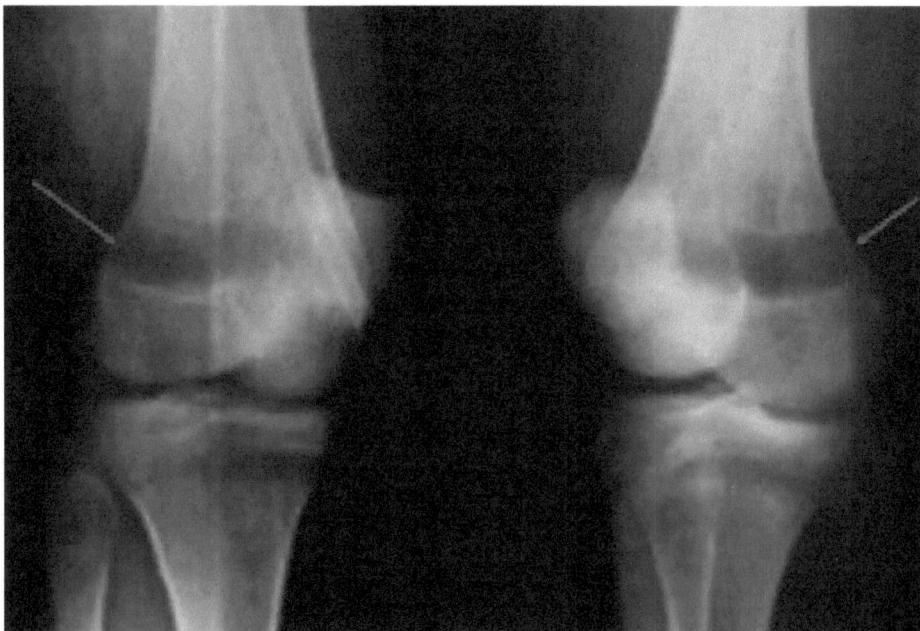

Dense Metaphyseal Bands: these are growth recovery lines, healing SH 1 fracture, lead poisoning, and scurvy. Lead poisoning is visible as dense bands when the lead levels are > 70 micrograms/deciliter. Lead inhibits osteoclast activity leading to uninhibited osteoblast activity. The dense line is the Wimberger sign. Lead causes axonal degeneration in the spinal cord and replaces Ca2+ in areas of rapid bone growth... I remember eating paint chips when I was little.

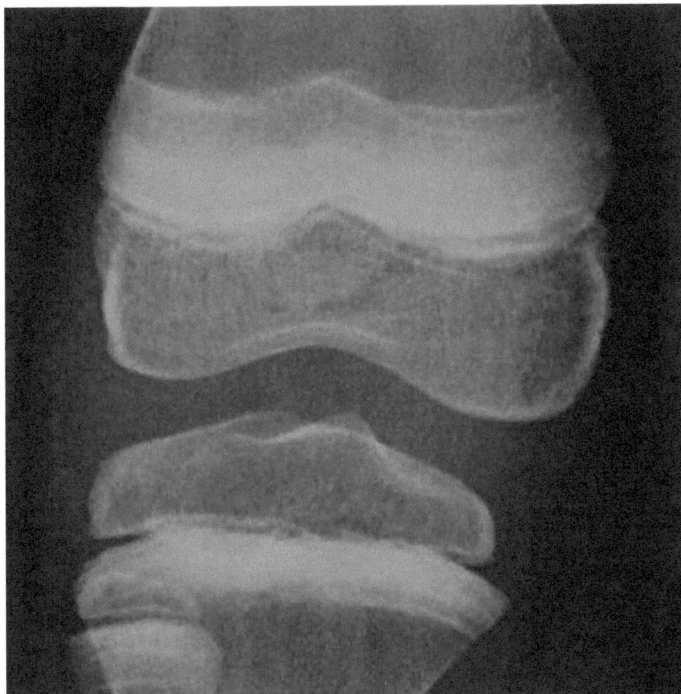

Tibial Bowing	
Anterolateral	NF, pseudoarthrosis
Anteromedial	Fibular hemimelia
Posteromedial	Congenital

Plastic Fracture: almost exclusively seen in kids 2–5 years of age. Produced by microfractures on the concave surface of bones with intact cortex on the convex side. Most common in the forearm.

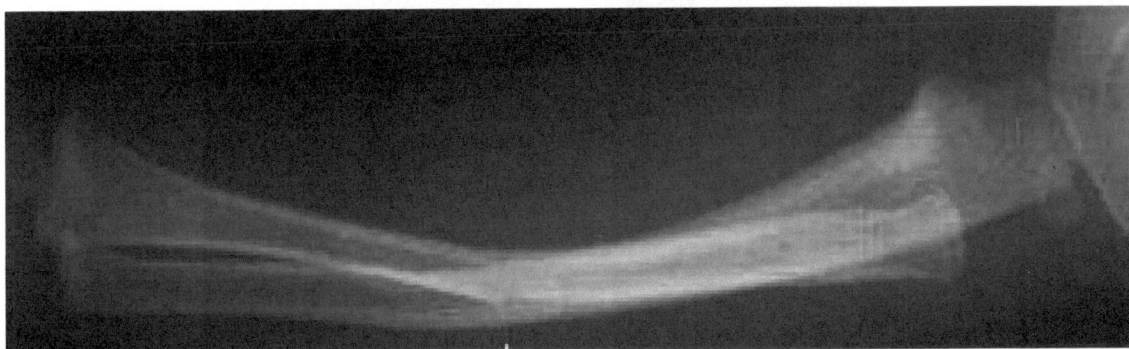

Toddler's Fracture: is a spiral fracture of the tibia in a walking child, if the kid is not ambulating, then it is child abuse.

Non–Accidental Trauma: classic signs of child abuse include: metaphyseal corner fractures, bilateral subdurals, posterior rib fractures, fractures in different staged of healing, get skeletal survey.

Hip Dysplasia: abnormal relationship of the femoral head ossification center with the acetabulum. The femoral head ossification center should fall in the inferior–medial quadrant of the Hilgenreiner's and Perkin's line intersection.

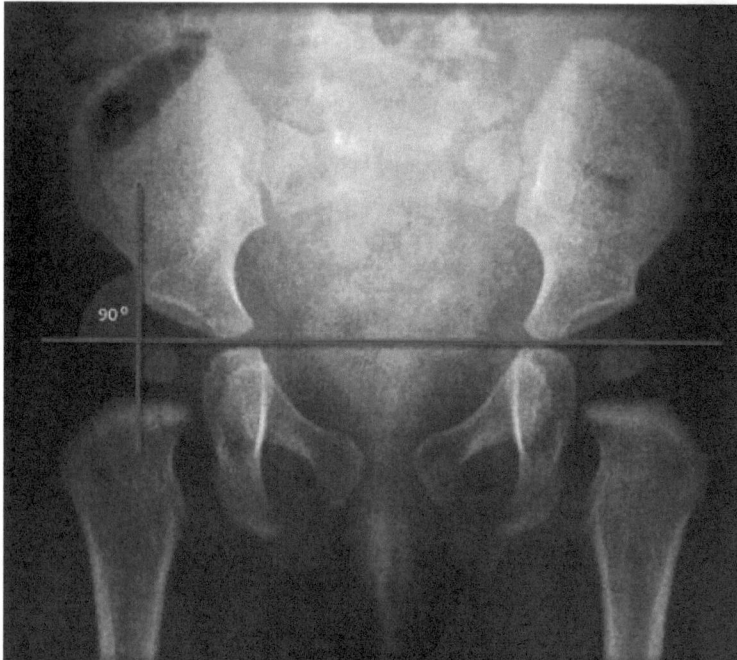

Hilgenreiner's line (horizontal) drawn through the triradiate cartilage and Perkin's line (vertical) drawn 90–deg to Hilgenreiner's line.

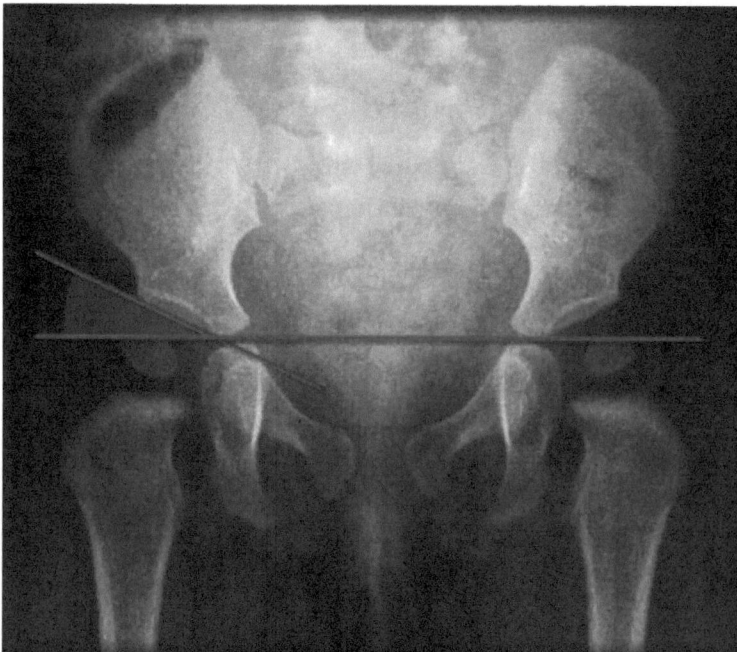

Acetabular angle is formed by the intersection of a line tangential to the acetabular roof and Hilgenreiner's line, should be 30–degrees at birth and regress as patient ages.

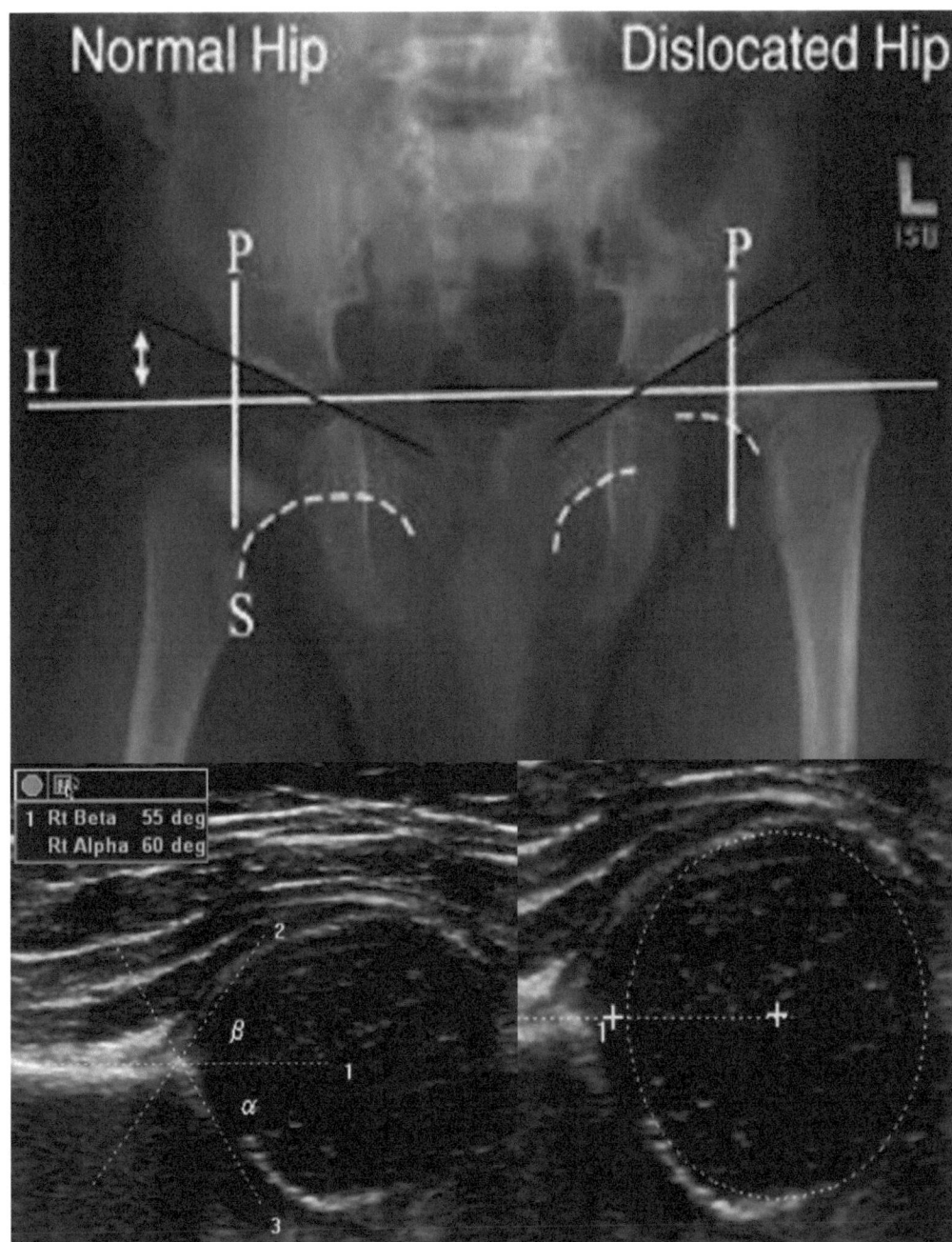

The left hip is dislocated as seen by a femoral head ossification center in the upper–outer quadrant and elevated femoral metadiaphysis. The US shows normal appearing hips. The alpha–angle should be greater than or equal to 60–degrees (bottom left) and the bony coverage by the acetabulum should be 50% of the femoral head (bottom right). For children with hip dysplasia the Pavlik harness is used first in kids < 6 months of age and closed or open reduction is used in older kids.

Septic Arthritis: is due to hematogeneous spread of infection and can present as knee pain. Patient will refuse to bear weight, have a SED rate > 40, WBC > 12,000, and fever. Surgical drainage and antibiotics are needed.

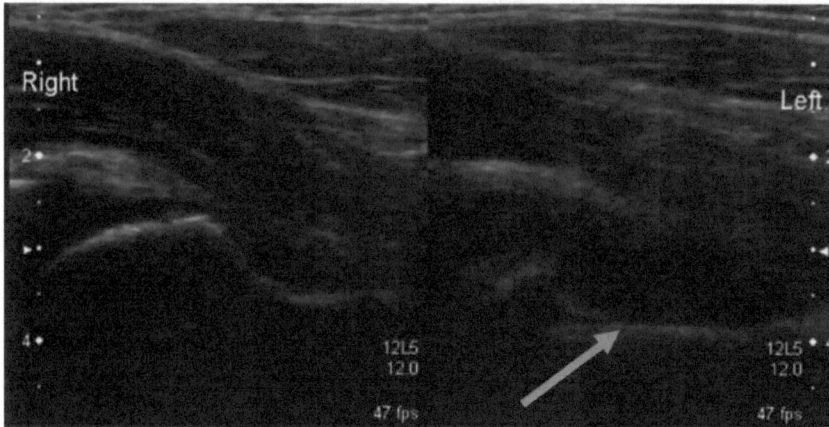

Arrow points to a joint effusion on the left, note lack of fluid on the right.

Toxic Synovitis: short lived acute inflammatory process in children, usually seen in boys ages 2–10. This is the most common cause of painful hip in the pediatric population. This is a diagnosis of exclusion; you have to rule out septic hip first. Same presenting symptoms as septic hip, aspirate fluid to rule out infection.

Proximal Focal Femoral Deficiency: congenital absence of the femoral head and may also involve parts of the proximal femur, patella, and ACL. Whole limb is shortened.

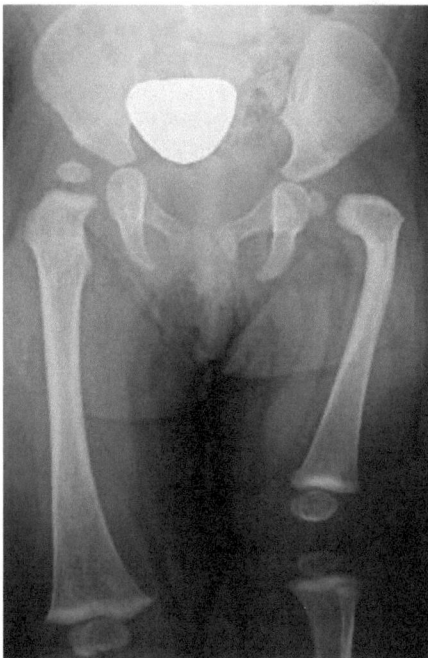

Trevor Disease: occurrence of intra–articular osteochondroma–like lesions from the epiphysis. Usually unilateral and more common in the lower extremity – ankle is the most common site; in the femur it arises more often from the medial condyle.

Rhizomelic Dwarfism: the dominant feature is proximal limb shortening
Mesomelic Dwarfism: shortening of the middle portion of a limb

Ewing's Sarcoma: the second most common childhood bone tumor after osteosarcoma. Typically in children between 10–20 years of age with a slight male predominance. It is a small round blue cell tumor and most commonly located in the lower limbs (femur). Look for a permeative lesion in the diaphysis or metadiaphysis of a long bone with periosteal reaction, codmans triangle, and with a large **soft tissue component**.

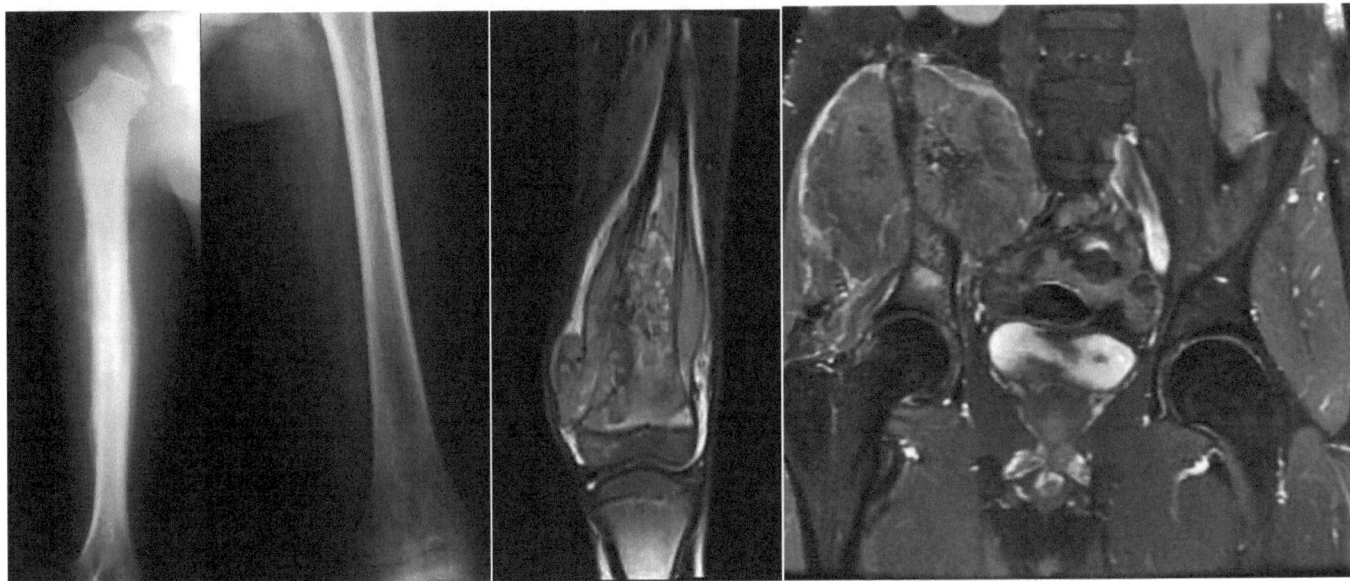

Osteosarcoma: the commonest primary bone tumor of childhood. Typically occurs in the metaphysis of long bones with exuberant periosteal reaction in a sunburst pattern. This is a permeative lesion with tumor matrix and ossification prone to pathologic fracture.

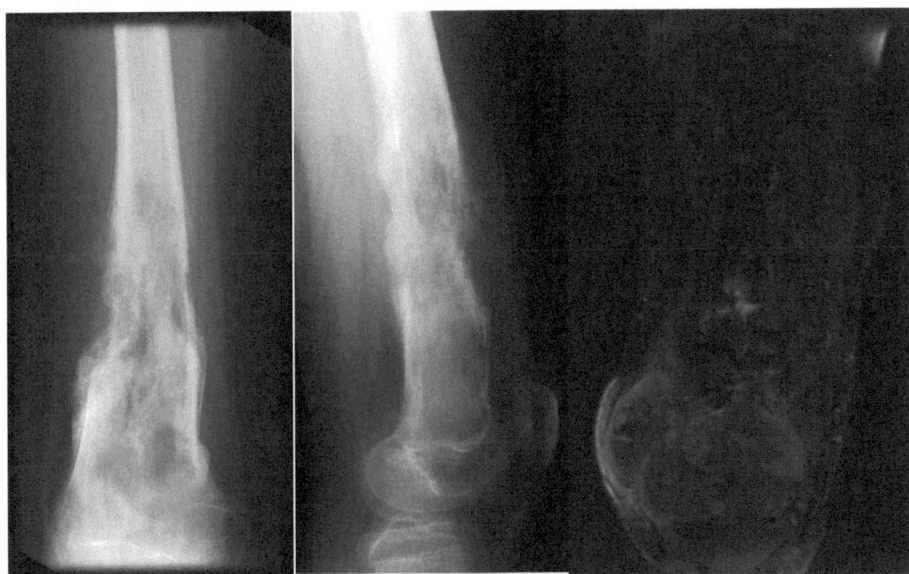

DEMOlish: **D**iaphysis **E**wing's and **M**etaphysis **O**steosarcoma – both demolish bone

Ultrasound

SCROTAL US: The key with scrotal masses is to decide if they are intra–testicular (malignant) or extra– testicular (benign). Of the intra–testicular lesions there are three broad categories:

Solid	Cystic	Ca2+
Neoplasm	Cystic Teratoma	Burned out GCT
Adrenal Rest	Cyst	Microliths
Sarcoid	Epidermoid	Granuloma
Lymphoma	Tubular ectasia of Rete Testis	

Neoplasms: seen in younger males and have a variable prognosis. The majority (90%) are germ cell tumors (GCT) and of those 50% are Seminomas (phew).

Seminoma: is a well–defined hypoechoic intra–testicular mass with homogeneous texture and a good prognosis. 70% present as stage 1 disease and it is very radiation sensitive. It should demonstrate Doppler flow. Below is a small seminoma, they can be big and replace a lot of the testicle. Bigger lesions can have heterogeneity.

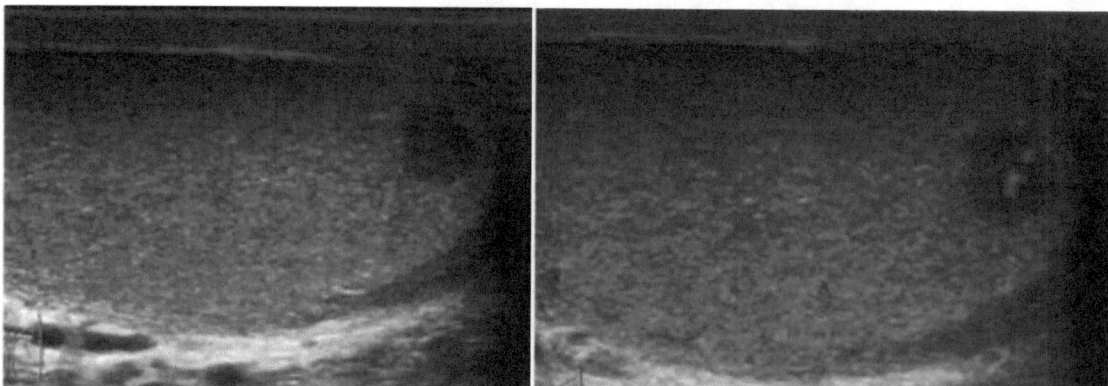

Non–Seminomatous GCT: mixed cell types ranging from teratoma → → choriocarcinoma. 60% are stage 2–3 at diagnosis. These are heterogeneous, contain Ca2+, cystic spaces from necrosis and have blood flow. They look ugly compared to the seminoma.

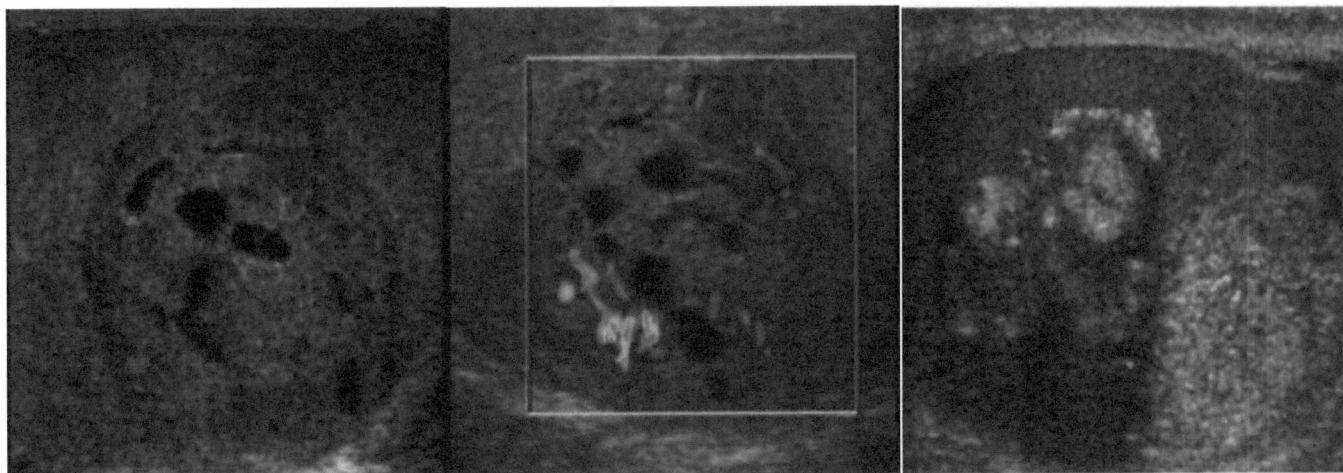

When you see dystrophic calcifications in a testis with a heterogeneous parenchyma think of burned out GCT – this is bad, it's widely metastasized at this point. Look for RP LAD.

Stromal Tumors (Sertoli and Leydig): the presence of these tumors cannot be suggested by imaging alone, they look like a bad malignancy, but 40% are hormonally active, so if given that history we can suggest these. 90–95% are benign but cannot tell from imaging so they have to come out.

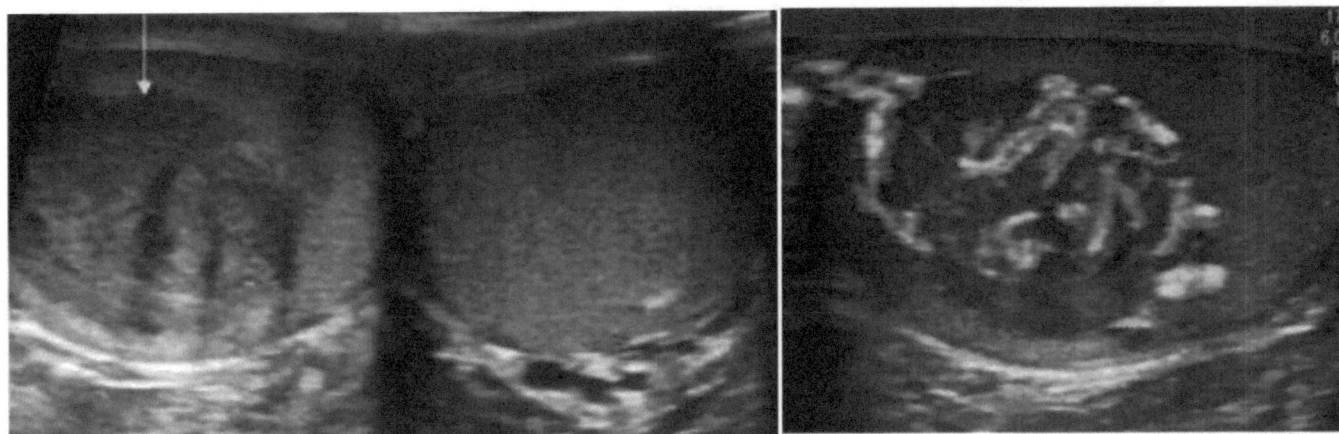

Lymphoma: this is the number one testicular tumor in men over the age of 60 and it is the number one bilateral tumor as well. Patient usually has a prior history of lymphoma and the tumor hides there, the patient gets chemo, then the drugs stop and tumor comes back. Testicular lymphoma is common in the HIV population. Imaging shows bilateral, large, very vascular testes.

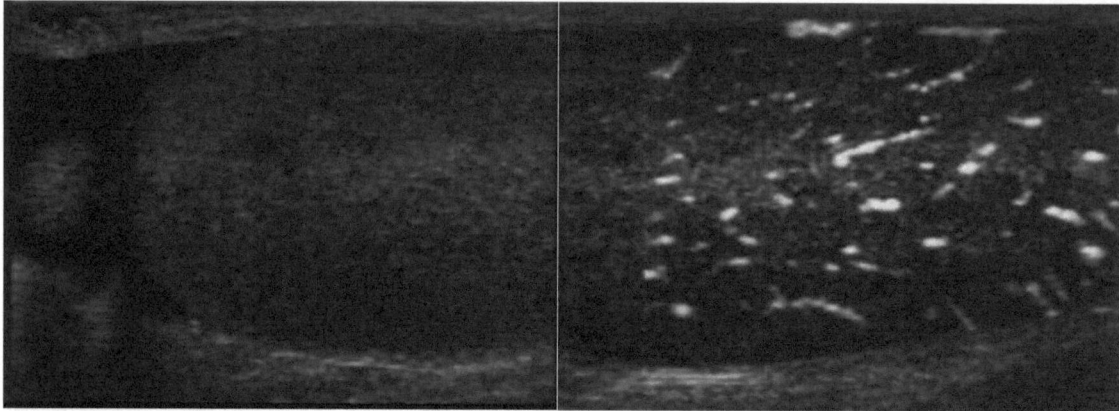

Adrenal Rests: are usually asymptomatic but when exposed to increased levels of ACTH they can enlarge to form a mass. These are often identified in patients with adrenal hyperplasia and Cushing's syndrome. Sonographic appearance is variable, but lesions are typically bilateral, multiple and eccentrically located.

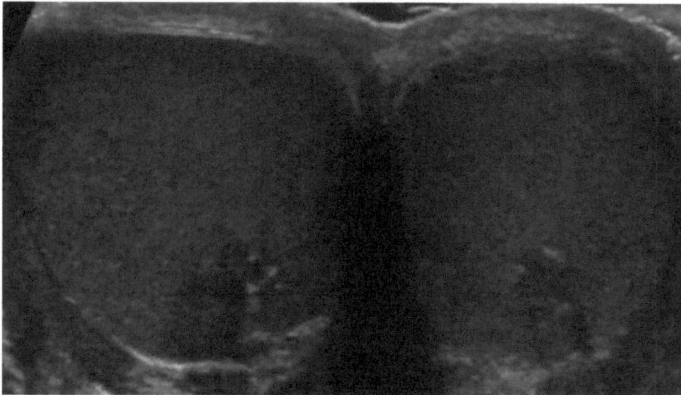

Cystic Teratoma: this accounts for 50% of childhood testicular cancer and when seen in kids it is a benign finding, however, in adults it is malignant. This is a cystic mass with Ca2+, thick septa and complexity.

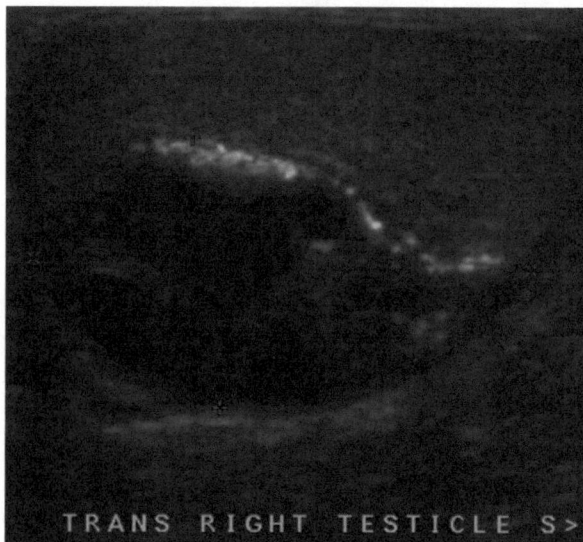

Testicular Cyst: benign anechoic, avascular lesion.

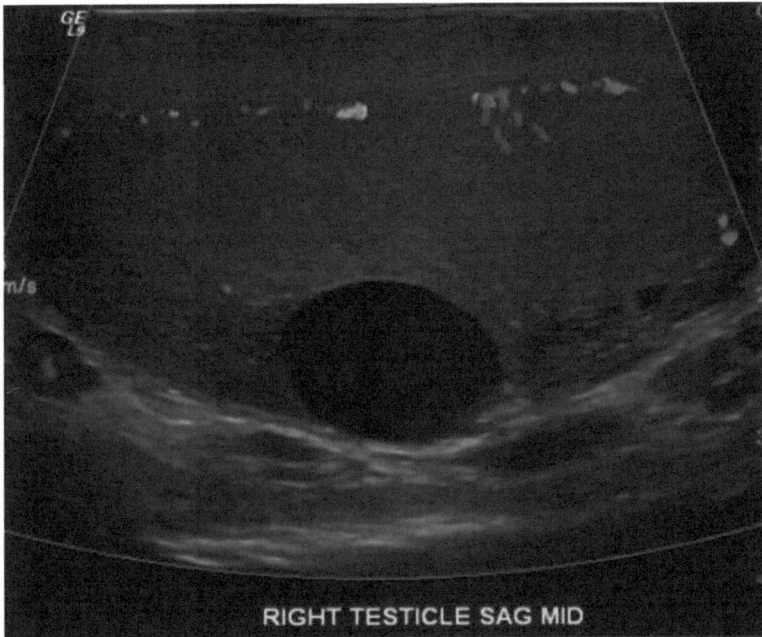

RIGHT TESTICLE SAG MID

Epidermoid: rare benign tumors filled with keratin. They have an echogenic rim and a classic "onion skin" appearance (arrow).

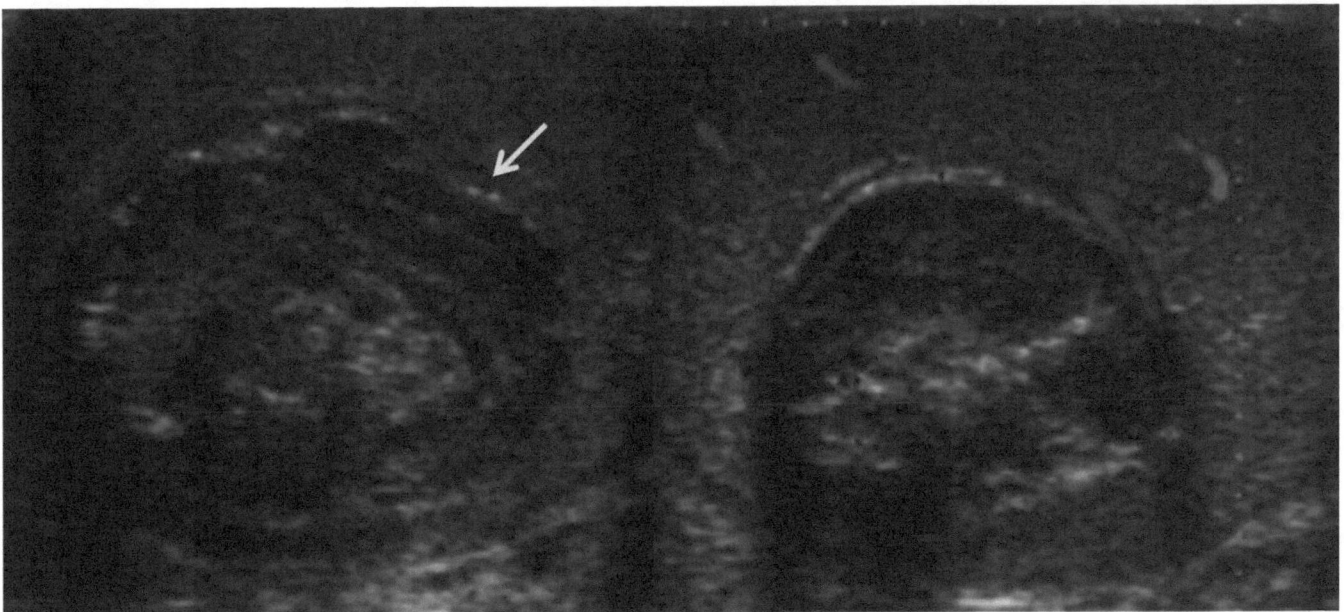

Tubular Ectasia of the Rete Testes: this is due to obstruction of the outflow of sperm (obliterated efferent duct) and dilation of the mediastinal tubules. Look for multiple small cystic spaces in the testicular mediastinum.

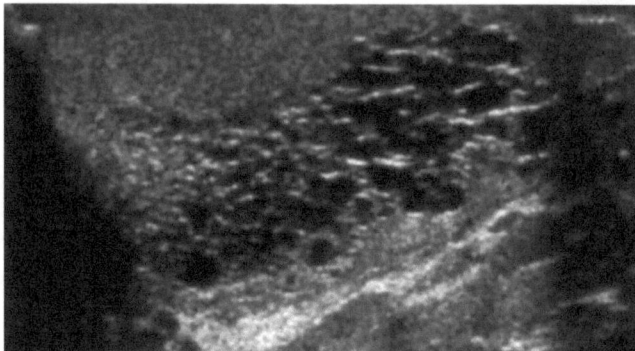

Microlithiasis: this is defined as > 5 punctate calcifications on a single image without shadowing. This has an association with cryptorchidism and neoplasm. Microlithiasis tends to be diffuse and bilateral.

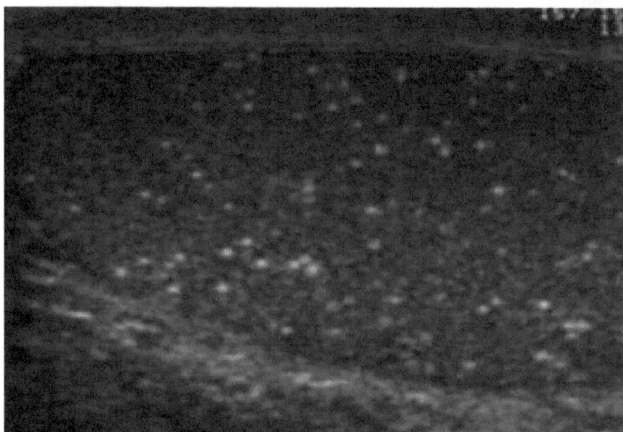

EXTRA–TESTICULAR (SOLID):

Adenomatoid Tumor: is the most common epididymal tumor and is a benign finding. It is a round, homogeneous, isoechoic mass with blood flow. More often these are seen in the lower pole.

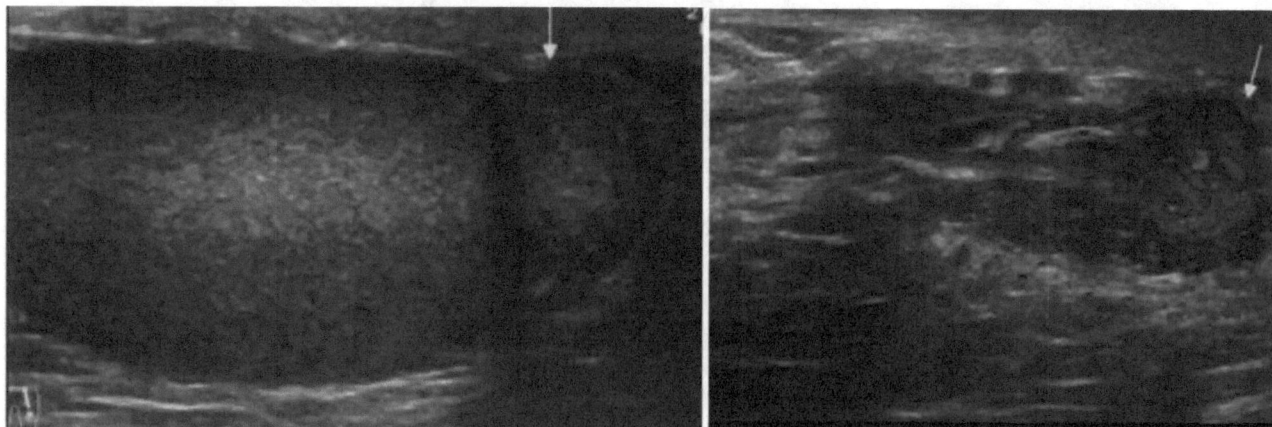

EXTRA–TESTICULAR (CYSTIC):

Spermatocele: this is associated with tubular ectasia of the rete testis. It is a large fluid filled dilation of the efferent tubules in the head of the epididymis. These can be very large but will not surround the testicle like a hydrocele will, in fact, if you see the largest hydrocele you've ever seen, it's probably a spermatocele (UCSF). The internal echoes are debris and spermatozoa. Small spermatoceles cannot be distinguished from epididymal head cysts.

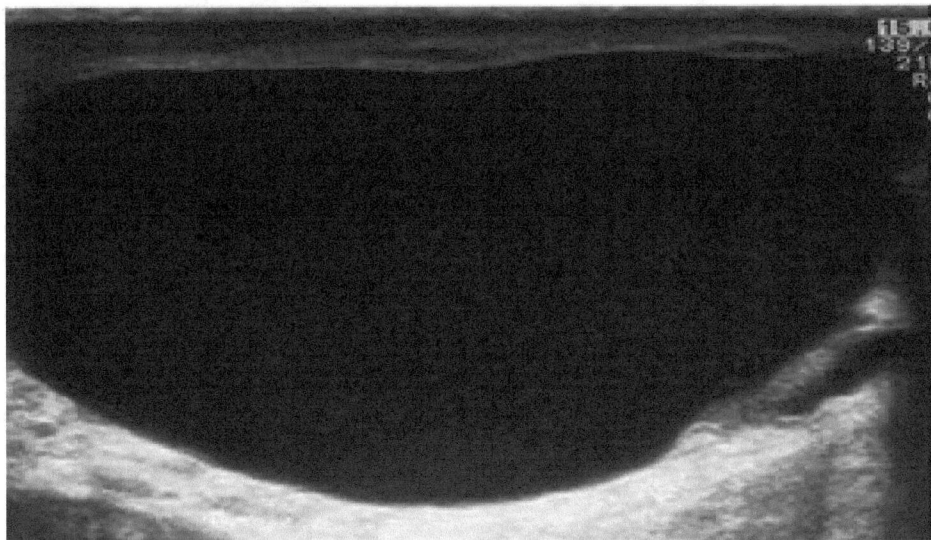

Hydrocele: acquired congenital fluid collection within the layers of the tunica vaginalis. These present as enlarging painless scrotal masses. They surround the testis. Can become infected, but more often than not, it is a simple collection. Note the acute angles between the fluid and the inferior margin of the testis.

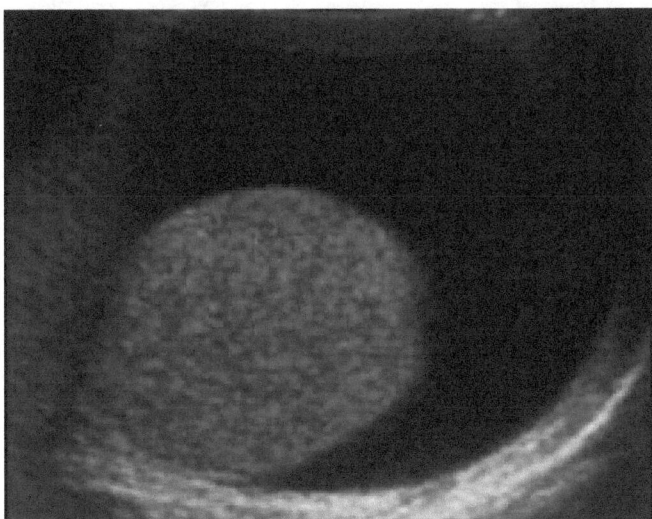

Varicocele: is a dilation of the pampiniform plexus and is associated with infertility. On US, veins > 3-mm that enlarge with valsalva is the diagnostic finding. This is far more common on the left than on the right. Actually, if you see a right sided varicocele, or the development of a new varicocele, look up in the RP for a tumor!

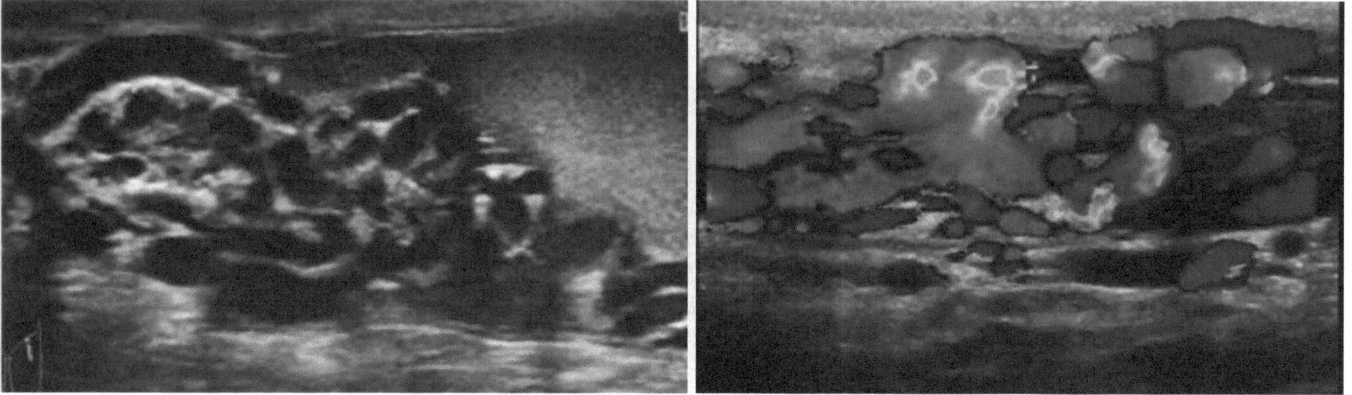

SCROTUM:

Inguinal Hernia: solid mass with dirty shadowing that demonstrates peristalsis. If there is no peristalsis, then it's probably a spermatic cord tumor and you should get an MRI.

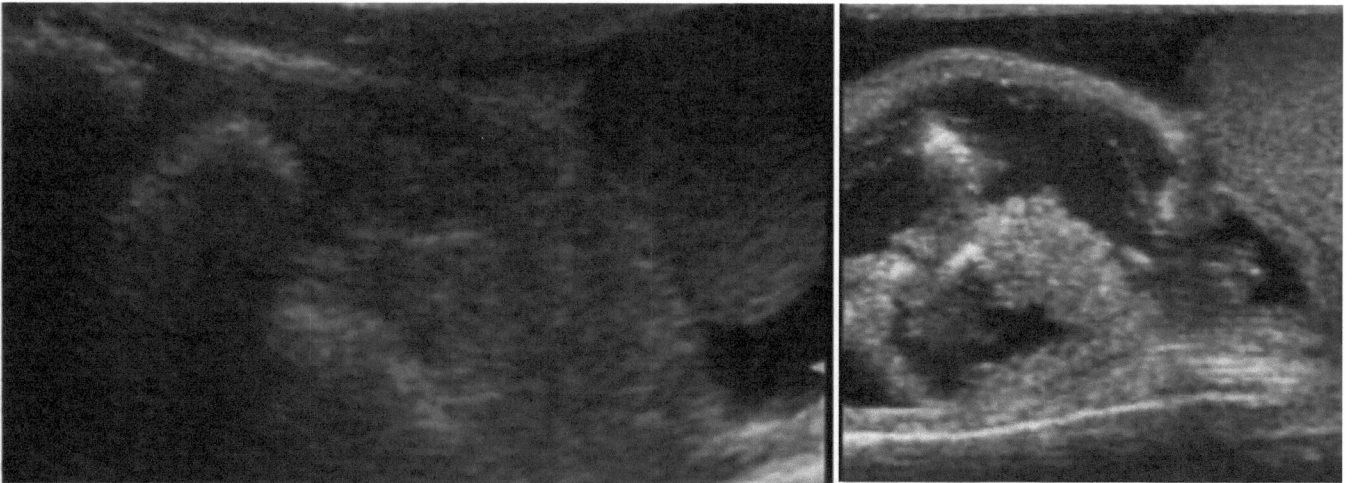

Indirect – more common than direct and is more common in males. This enters the inguinal canal at the deep ring **lateral to the inferior epigastric vessels**.

Direct – arises due to a weakness in the posterior wall of the inguinal canal **medial to the inferior epigastric vessels** (Hasselbach's triangle). It is called direct because the sac directly protrudes through the inguinal canal wall. These are less susceptible to strangulation than indirect hernias and less likely to go into the scrotum.

Scrotal Pearl: floating calcification due to prior torsion of the testicular appendix. In kids it can be a calcification due to meconium peritonitis.

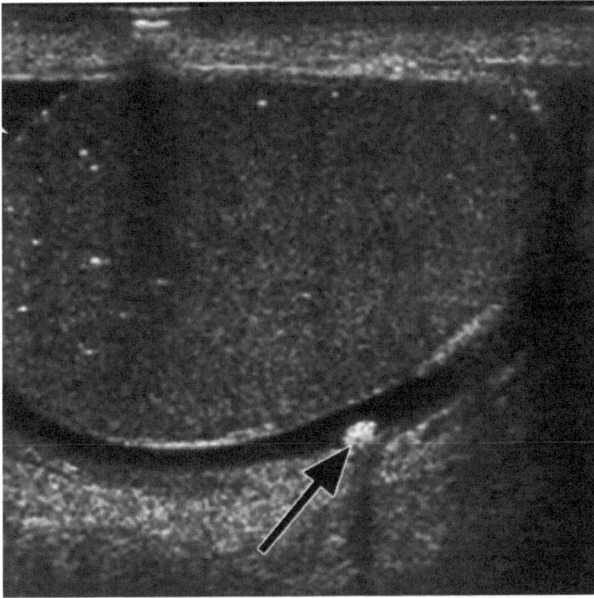

Epididymo–Orchitis: is due to a retrograde infection. Hyperemia is the earliest sign. Can be associated with pyocele and if you see scrotal wall thickening and air in the subcutaneous tissues and in the scrotum (yellow arrow), start to worry about gas gangrene (Fornier's) – more common in diabetics.

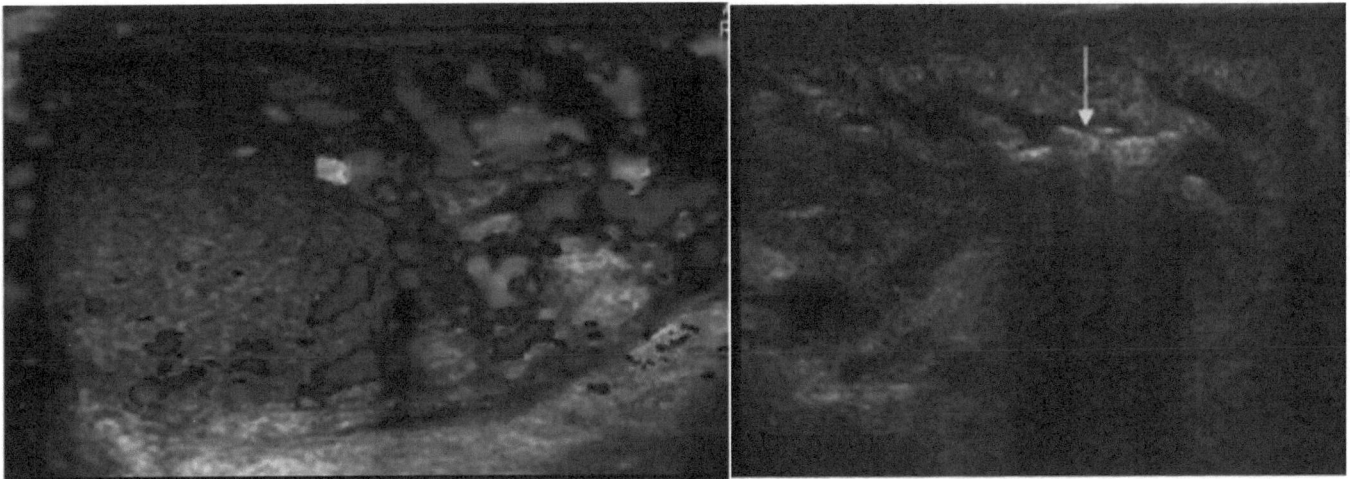

Torsion: surgical emergency, viable testicle if ischemic for less than 4 hour and infarcted after 10 hours. Initially there is venous compromise so the testicle swells and becomes hypoechoic. Then we lose arterial flow. Patients will have horrible pain, but this can be relapsing and remitting – intermittent torsion.

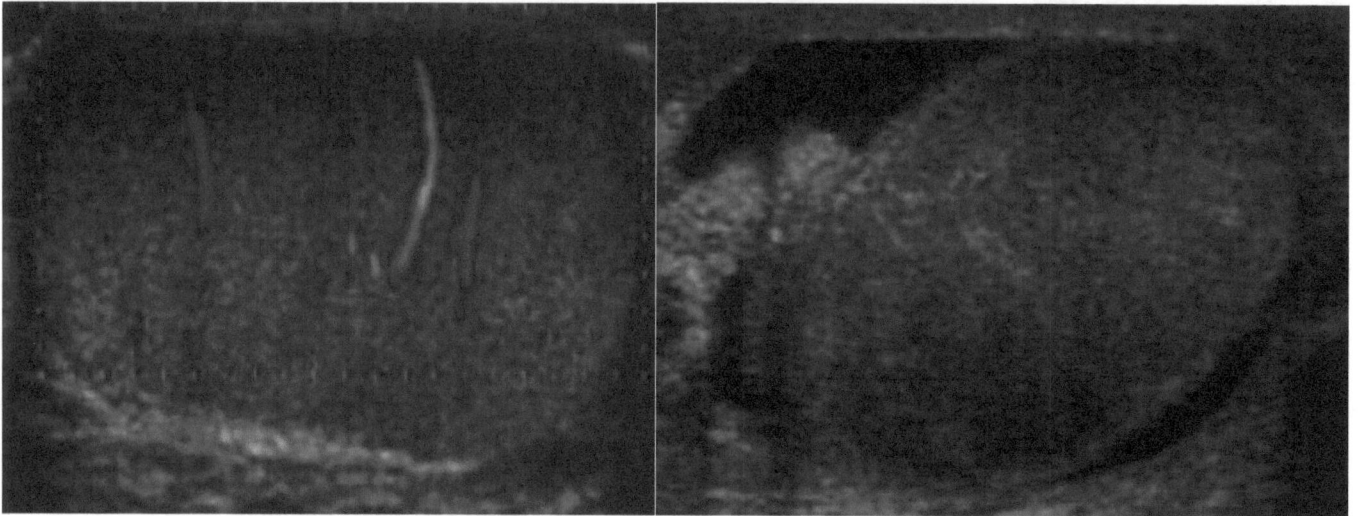

Normal flow is seen in the right testis. The left testis looks edematous, has no flow, and there is a hydrocele.

Vascular and IR

ngiography is essentially "lumenography" giving us excellent information about the lumen of the vessel but not much else. Other findings can be inferred from the luminal appearance. So try and think about it like this:

Pathology	Angiogram
Wall thickening/compression	Stenosis
Wall weakened	Aneurysm/dissection
Wall rupture	Extravasation/pseudoaneurysm/AVF
Occlusion	Stasis

The **size of vessel** involved as well as regional location can help guide your differential. Some conditions just affect certain areas:

2. Thoracic aorta and great vessels – Giant Cell arteritis (women > 50) and Takayasu's (women < 50)
3. Abdominal aorta – AAA
4. Visceral vessels – Polyarteritis nodosa, FMD
5. Lower extremity – atherosclerosis, Buerger's disease

Atherosclerosis: causes thickening and loss of vessel elasticity. Related to smoking, DM, poor diet, genetics, etc. The plaques enlarge over time causing stenosis, ulcerations, and rupture from aneurysm formation.

Embolic Disease: causes sudden onset ischemic symptoms in distal structures, always go looking for a proximal source. Atheroemboli do not respond to tPA, the treatment of choice is heparin.

FMD: this is a non-inflammatory, non-atherosclerotic disease of medium sized vessels. Most often seen in women between the ages of 30-50. If symptomatic, the patients will have HTN from RAS or ischemia from narrowing of other vessels i.e. CVA from ICA disease. Most common location in descending order: renal arteries > extracranial ICA > vertebral arteries > iliac arteries. Can have spontaneous dissection, embolism, and aneurysm rupture.

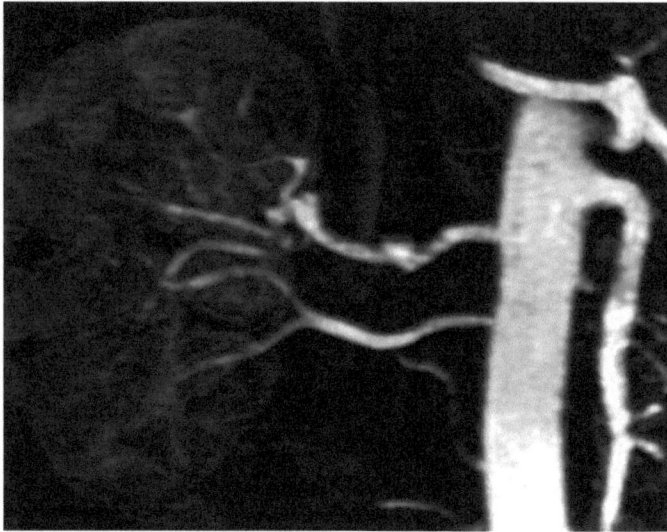

Remember that in the renal arteries, this will be at the midportion not at the ostium (atherosclerosis). This responds to balloon angioplasty, stent not needed.

Dissection: linear filling defects caused by blood entering the media through a tear in the intima. Forms a second blood–filled channel (false lumen) and can occlude blood flow to organs. Associated with HTN, Marfan's, atherosclerosis, and iatrogenic causes.

Fun Fact: if iatrogenic and if in the lower extremity (iliac) and it happens against the flow of blood, it'll fix itself because the blood will flow over it pressing the flap against the wall.

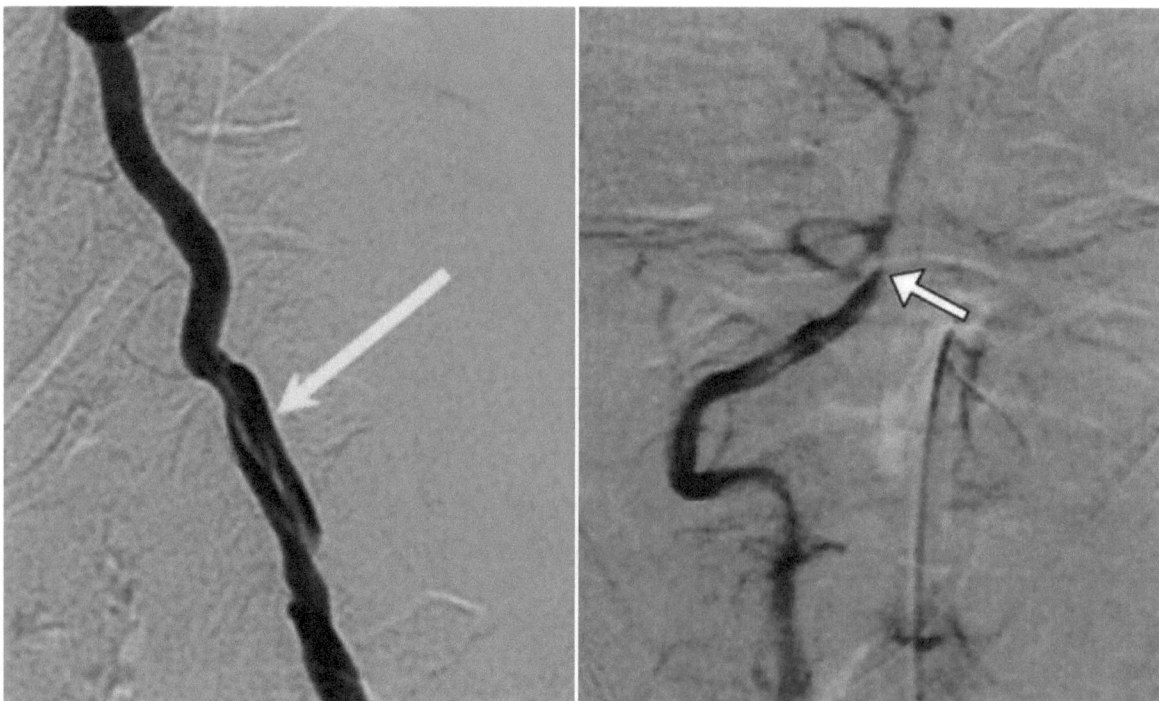

Pseudoaneurysm: is a weakness in the wall not containing all three layers "false aneurysm". Often caused by trauma, iatrogenic, repeated inflammation of vessel (pancreatitis), etc. Look for a narrow neck and big vascular sac rather than fusiform dilation.

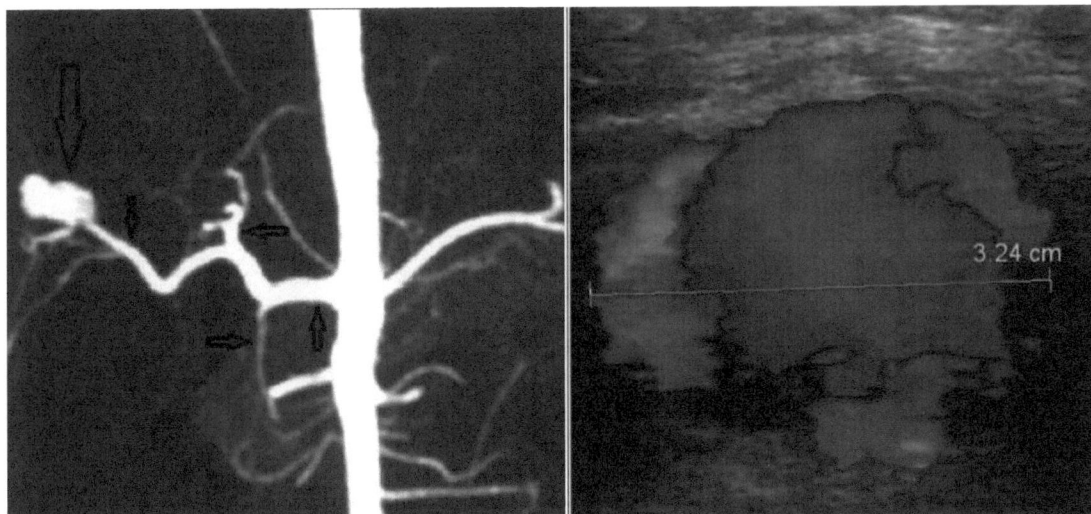

These are inherently weak structures and can bleed (leak slowly or fast hemorrhage). They can have thrombus. When it occurs in a femoral artery after groin puncture – most will thrombose on their own, if it starts to get bigger or doesn't go away, we can do US guided thrombin injection or compression. Look for the classic "yin–yang" sign (right).

AVF: is an abnormal connection between the arterial and venous system bypassing the capillary beds. They tend to be asymptomatic, but they can be large and cause arterial steal or high–output cardiac failure. They are usually iatrogenic or post–traumatic. Look for venous filling during arterial phase of contrast injection.

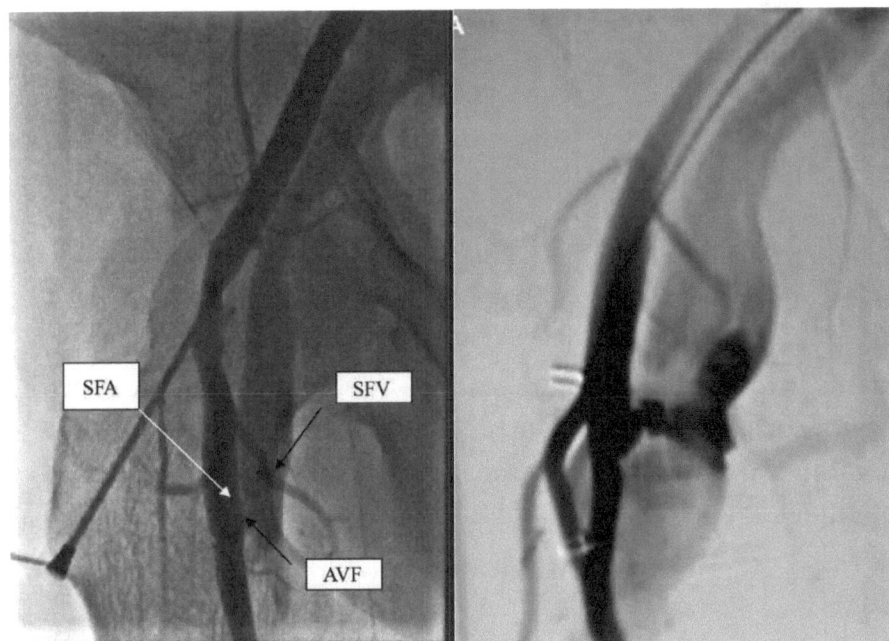

Vasculitis: infiltration of the media by histiocytes causing stenosis, thrombus, aneurysm, pseudoaneurysm, and extravasations. Can affect almost any organ system but let's split them up by vessel size involved and explore a few common ones.

Large Vessel	Takayasu, Giant Cell
Medium Vessel	Polyarteritis nodosa, Wegner's, Churg–Strauss
Small Vessel	Henoch–Schonlein Purpura
Random Conditions	Buerger's Disease, Kawasaki, Bechet
Secondary	Infection related, connective tissue disease (SLE, RA)

Takayasu – large vessel disease primarily affecting the aorta and the great vessels and major aortic branches with increased prevalence in young Asian women. Clinical symptoms are due to stenosis of vessels.

Giant Cell – the most common systemic vasculitis, tends to affect older women (> 50). Like Takayasu, it likes the aorta and major branches (particularly the extracranial branches of the carotid artery). Diagnosis is with a temporal artery biopsy. Treat with steroids.

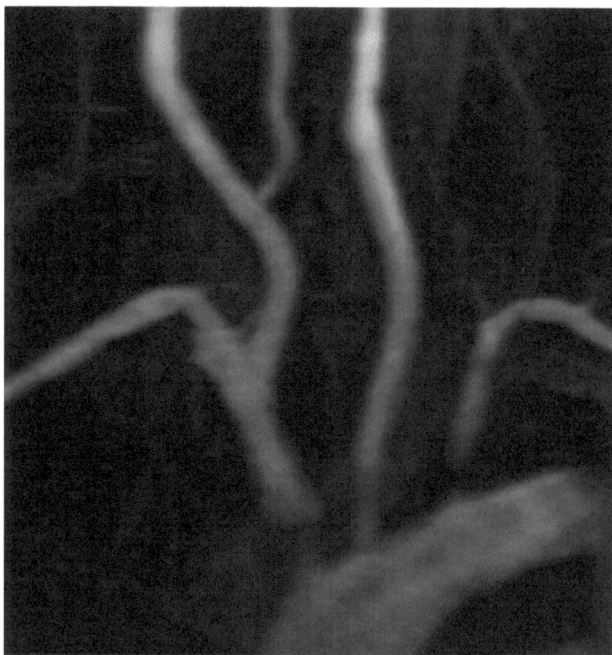

Note the areas of stenosis involving the origins of the great vessels.

Polyarteritis Nodosa – systemic vasculitis involving the medium sized vessels, more common in males and seen in the 5th–7th decades. Strong association with Hepatitis B antigen positivity, pANCA levels correlate with disease activity. Look for it in the renal arteries, coronaries, GI tract, hepatic arteries most often. Also causes, intracranial complications 20–40% of the time. Fatal unless treated with steroids and cyclophosphamide.

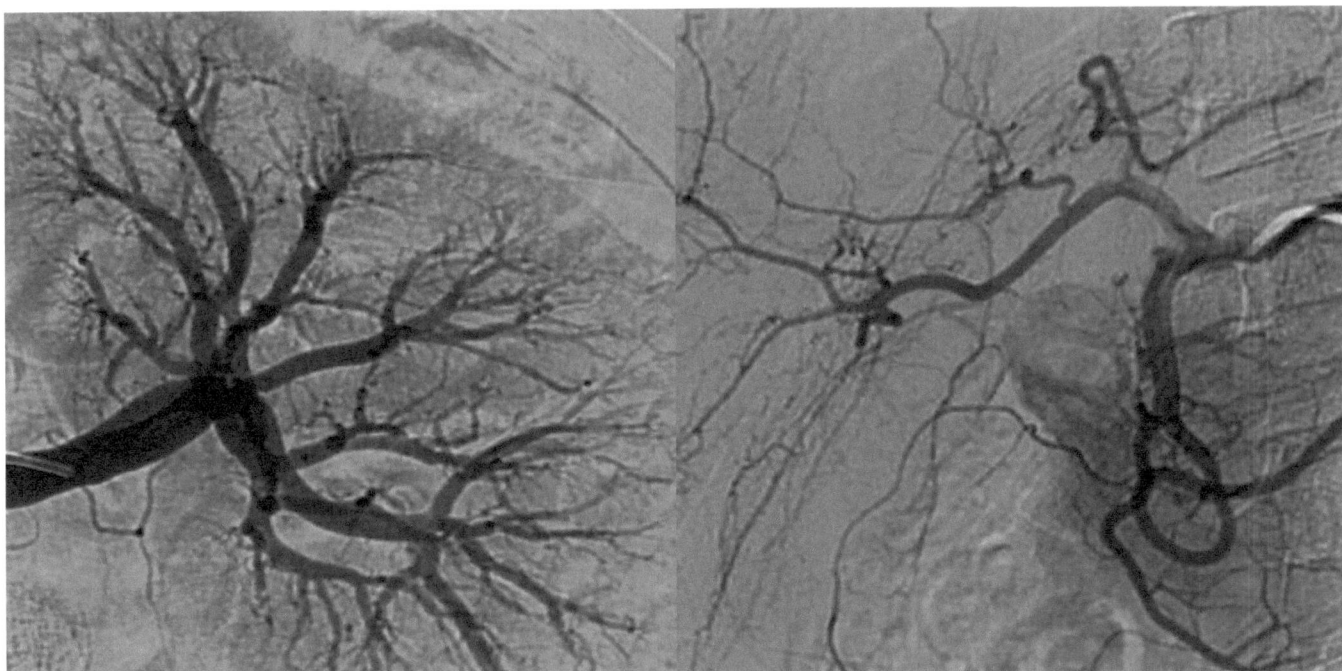

Look for multiple microaneurysms in the interlobar and arcuate arteries of the kidney, can hemorrhage

Buerger Disease (thromboangitis obliterans): is an obliterative process seen in heavy smokers affecting medium and small vessels of the lower extremities. Patients present with hand and foot claudication progressing to ischemia and necrosis. Tips of fingers and toes can just fall off (according to Goljan from med school pathology review lectures). Angiography shows extensive arterial **occlusion** and **corkscrew** collaterals.

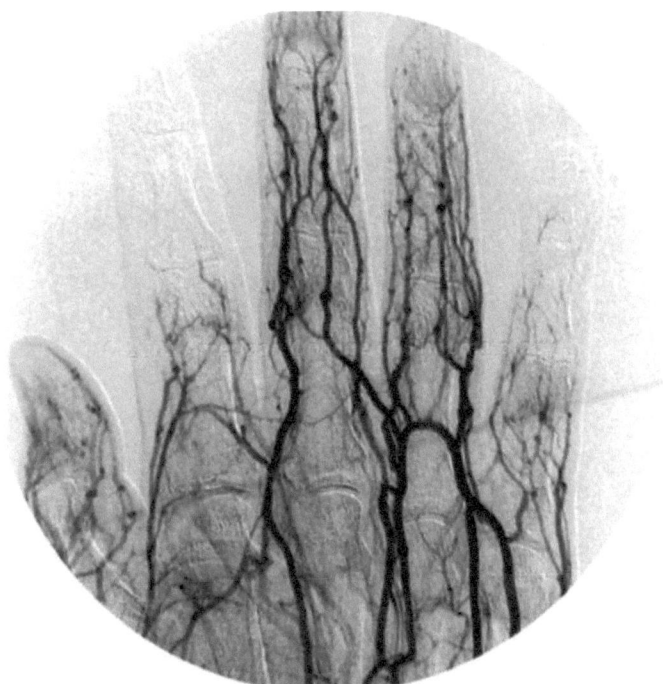

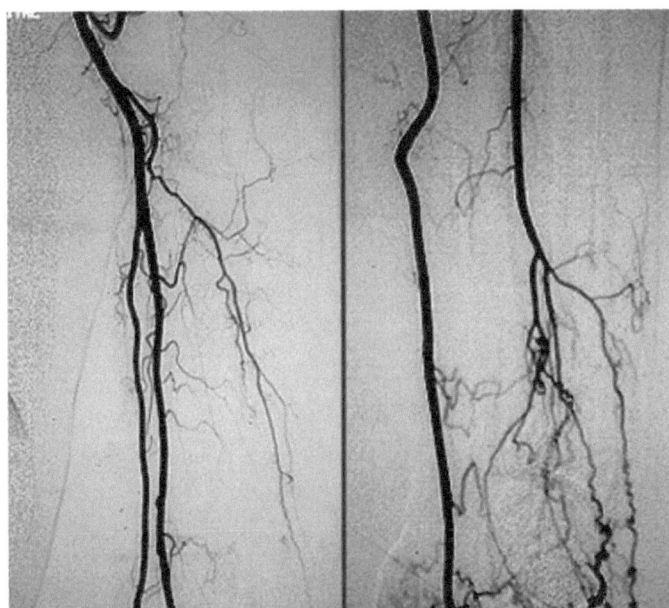

▲ normal angiogram   ▲ abnormal angiogram

Midaortic Syndrome: uncommon entity affecting children and young adults characterized by narrowing of the abdominal aorta and its major branches. Symptoms begin in early adulthood – hypertension, claudication, and renal failure. Look for enlarged collateral branches: IMA, arc of Riolan, marginal artery of Drummond.

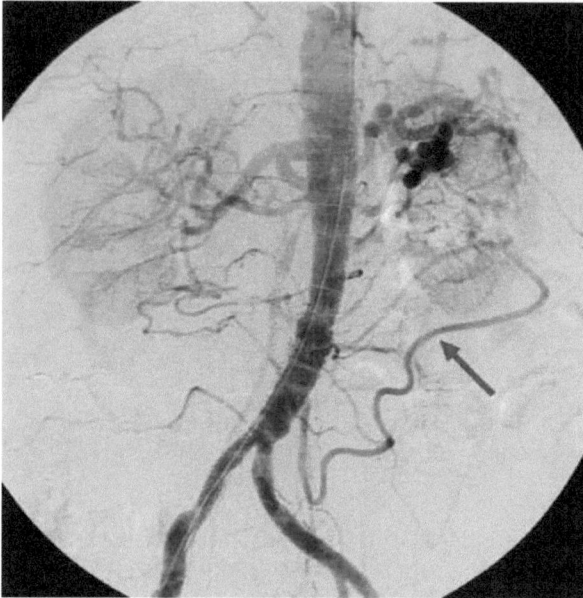

Arc of Riolan – connects the IMA to the SMA or a branch of the SMA. In proximal SMA occlusion it provides collateral from IMA to SMA and in IMA occlusion it provides collaterals from SMA t o IMA.

Marginal artery of Drummond – is a continuous circle formed by the anastomoses of the ileocolic, right colic, middle colic, left colic, and sigmoid branches of the IMA. This arc passes the vasa recta to the colon. Weak point is at the splenic flexure.

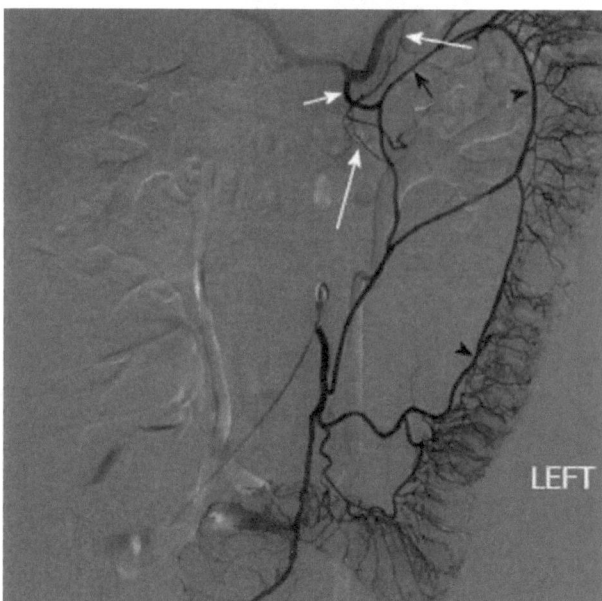

Leriche Syndrome: complete occlusion of the aorta distal to the renal arteries with classic findings of: buttock claudication, impotence, and absent femoral pulses. A large network of collaterals forms to bypass the occlusion and the most common pathway is: SMA →→ IMA →→ hemorrhoidal arteries →→ external iliac arteries. Treat with aorto–biiliac bypass or kissing balloon stents.

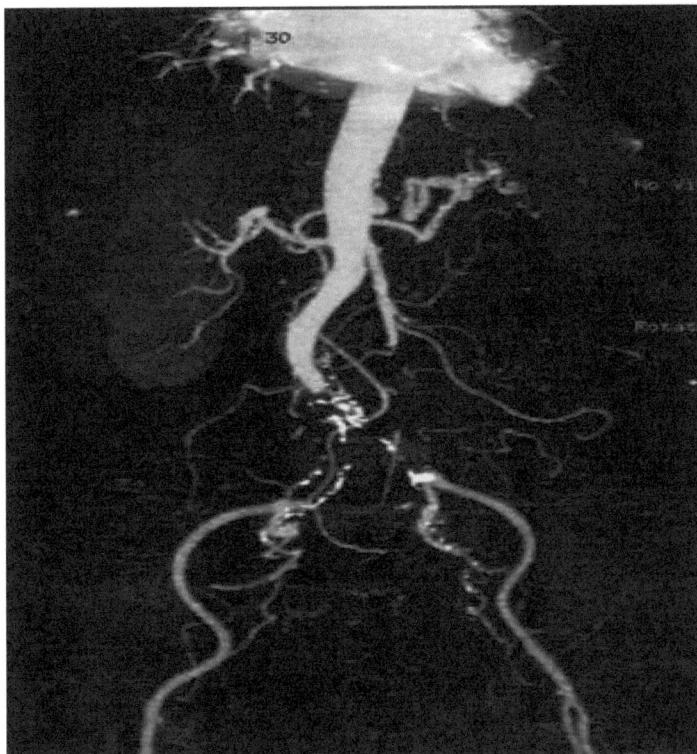

Arcuate Ligament Syndrome: caused by impression upon the celiac axis by the median arcuate ligament inserting in an abnormally low position. Radiographic appearance **gets worse on expiration.** Look for a focal stenosis at the celiac origin with upward hooking of the post–stenotic dilated portion. Treated surgically by decompressing the ligament.

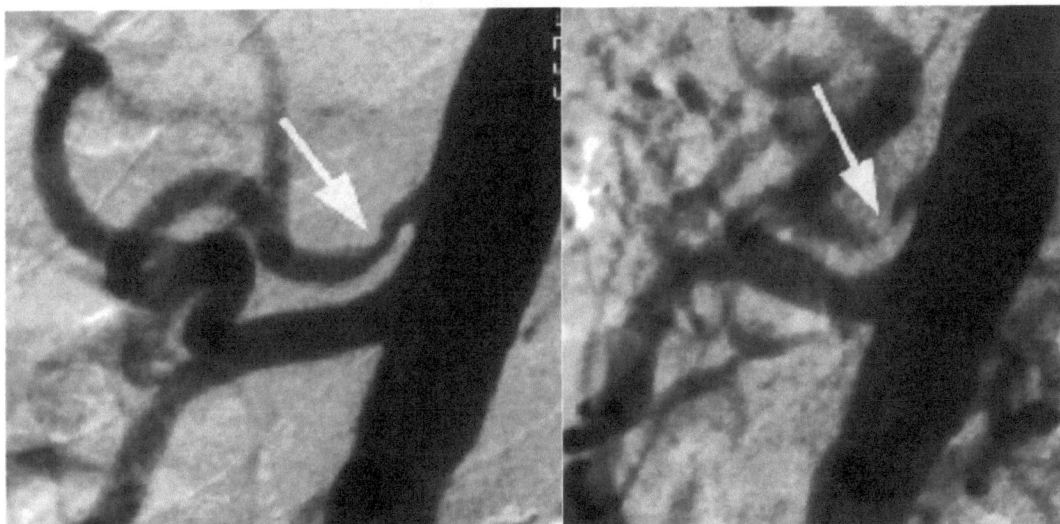

Inspiration – Left
Expiration – Right

Popliteal Entrapment: refers to compression of the popliteal artery due to an abnormal relationship with the **medial head of the gastrocnemius**. The compression can lead to chronic microvascular trauma and thrombus formation and ischemia. Stenosis and turbulent flow lead to ectasia and aneurysm formation. Limb threatening thrombosis will require bypass surgery, intermittent occlusion can be treated by release of the artery or saphenous vein bypass.

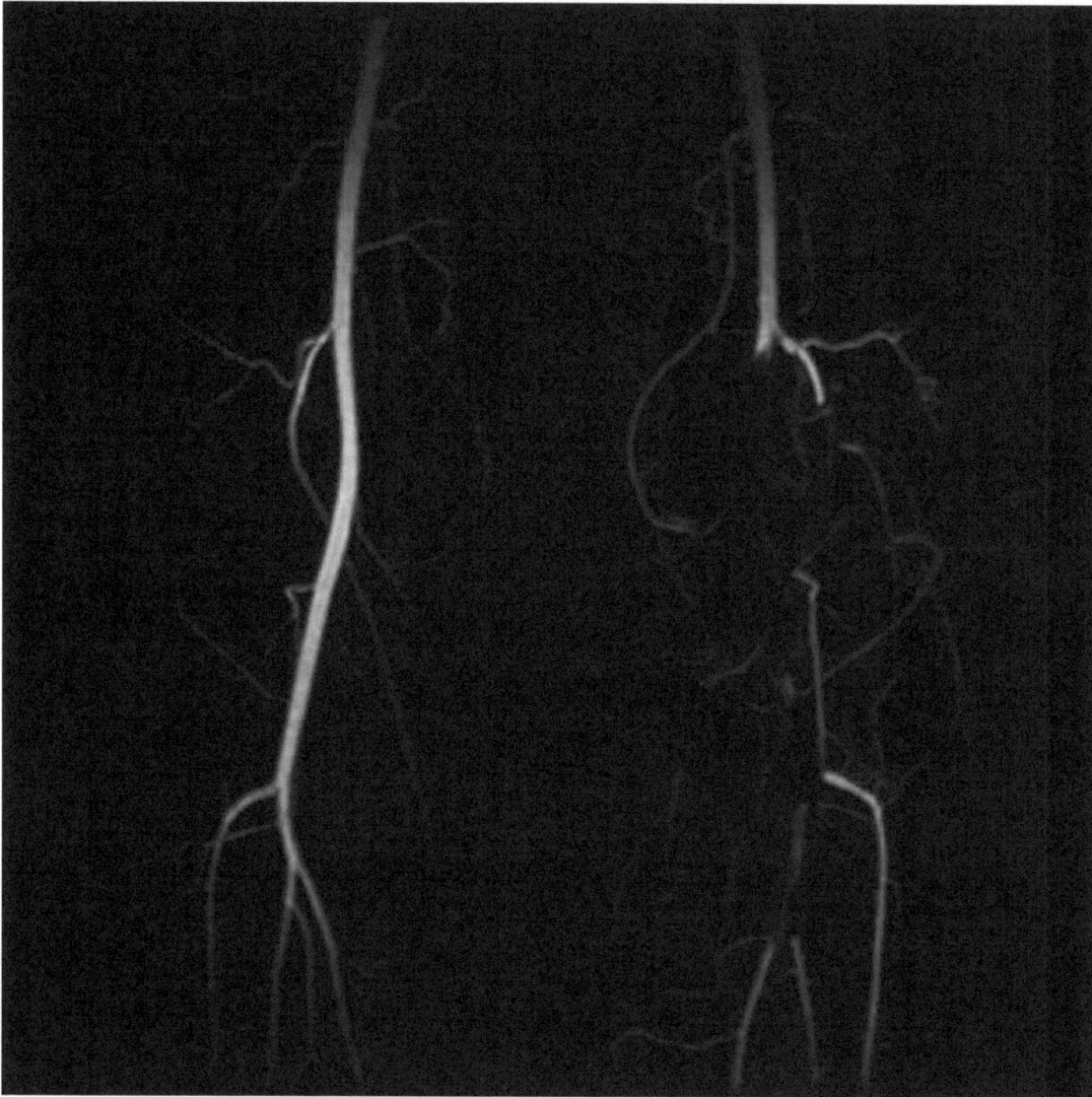

The patient has a normal right popliteal artery, but the left artery demonstrates signs of wall irregularity and cut off.

Hypothenar Hammer Syndrome: occurs from trauma to the distal ulna artery or proximal portion of the superior palmar arch as a result of repeat blows to the hypothenar eminence. Patients have a cold sensation in the palm of the hand and 4th and 5th digit ischemia. Look for a beaded appearane of the distal ulnar artery +/− aneurysm formation and occlusion.

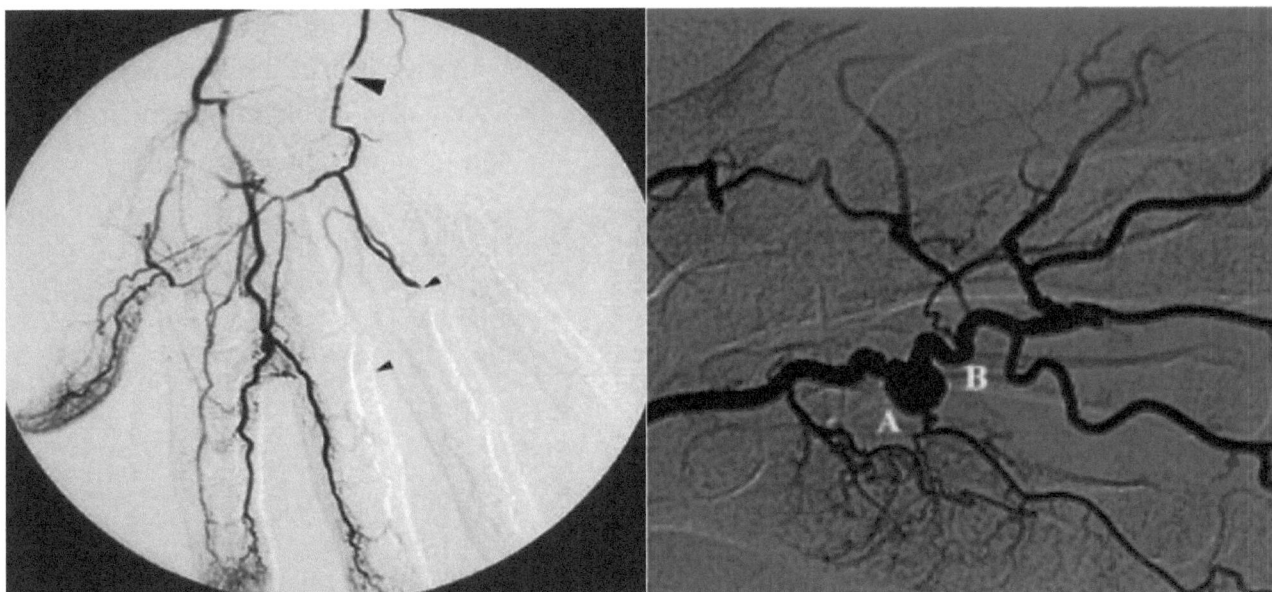

May–Thurner Syndrome: deep venous thrombosis resulting from chronic compression of the left common iliac vein by the right common iliac artery. First line treatment is with thrombolysis and stenting.

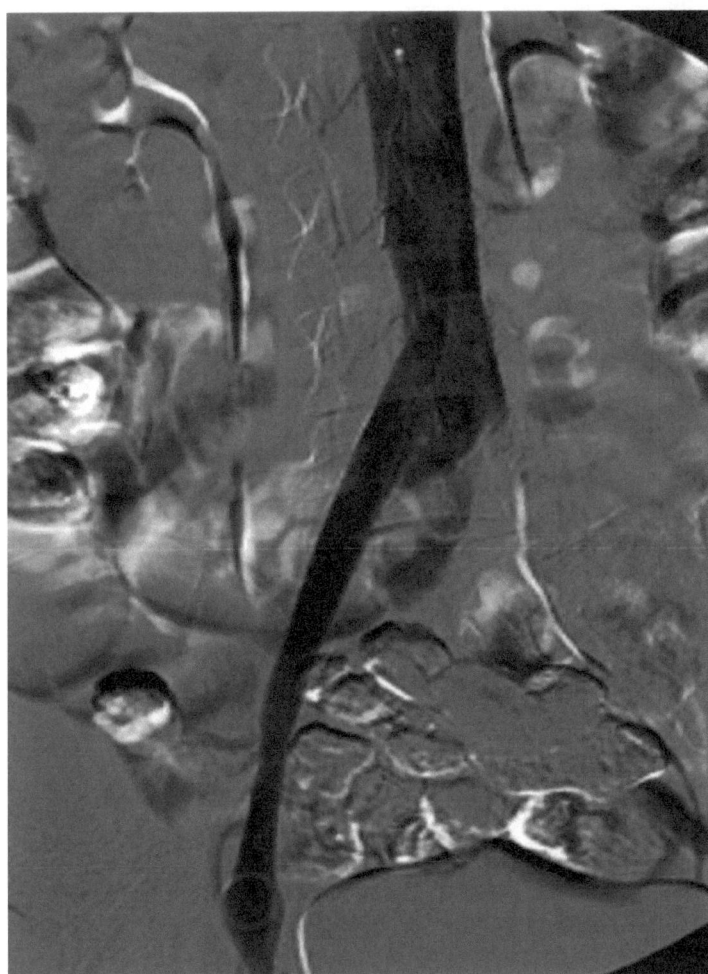

Nutcracker Syndrome: compression of the left renal vein between the SMA and aorta leading to renal venous hypertension causing hematuria. Can also occur in people with a retroaortic or circumaortic renal vein. This causes intermittent gross hematuria and flank pain. The hematuria should only come from the left ureter orifice when seen on cystoscopy.

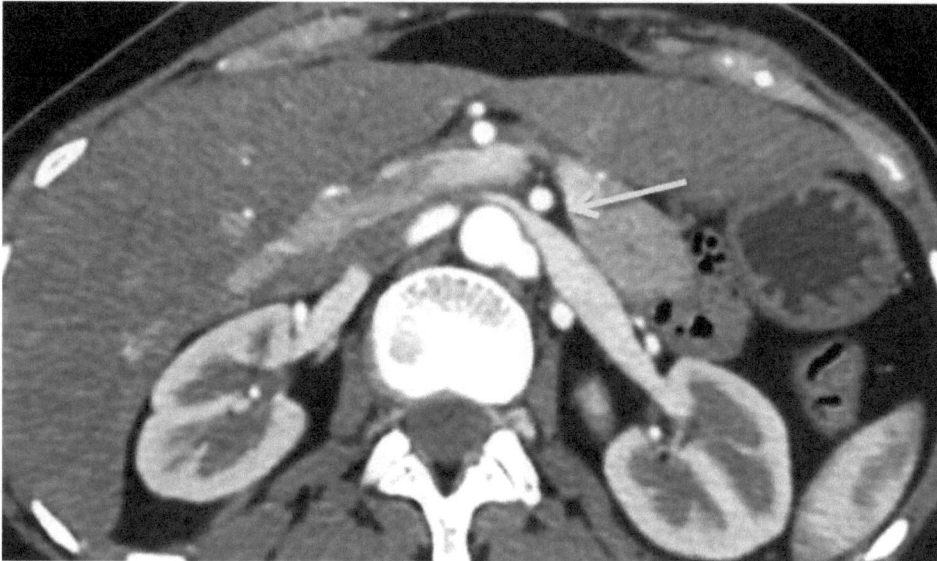

Paget–Schroetter Syndrome: subclavian vein thrombosis due to mechanical compression in the costoclavicular space. This is also known as effort thrombosis and is associaed with forced abduction of the upper arm seen in young athletes. Signs and symptoms of upper limb DVT (arm pain and swelling). Thrombus is treated with anticoagulation and catheter–directed thrombolysis after which surgical decomression is performed. Look for multiple collaterals.

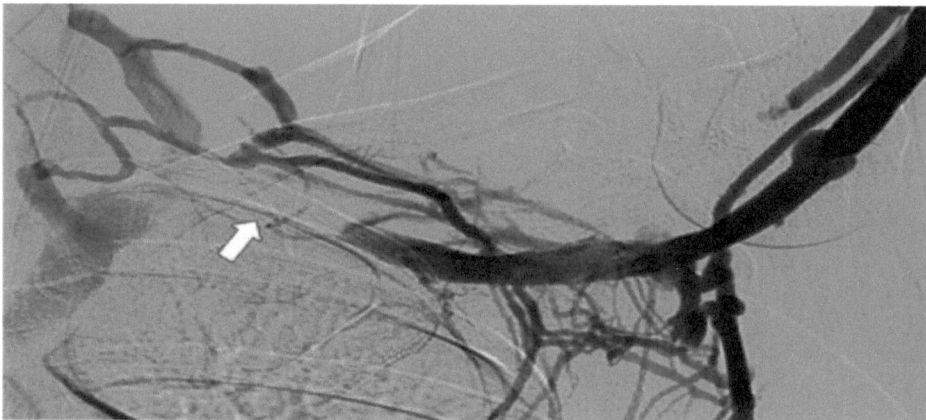

Subclavian Steal Syndrome: results from the occlusion or severe stenosis of the left subclavian artery origin causing retrograde flow of blood down the left vertebral artery into the left arm. This causes syncope, vertigo, etc. Most often caused by atherosclerosis or a vasculitis. On US look for a **biphasic left vertebral artery pulse**. Treated with endovascular angioplasty and stenting or it can be treated with a carotid subclavian bypass.

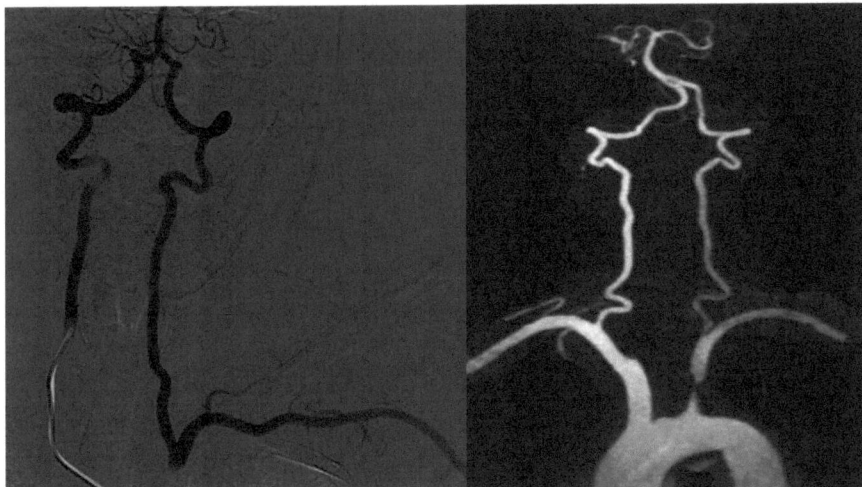

Thoracic Outlet Syndrome: compression of the brachial plexus (majority of cases) and/or subclavian vessels seen most commonly at the scalene triangle. The usual cause is an abnormally inserting anterior scalene muscle onto the 1st rib. Other causes include: cervical ribs, muscle hypertrophy, and fibrous bands. Patients present with pain, parasthesias, ischemia of the upper limb. Angio diagnosis is made with the Adson's maneuver – patient arm abducted and head turned to other side. Treatment is directed at the underlying cause with surgical decompression and angioplasty. Try not to place a stent.

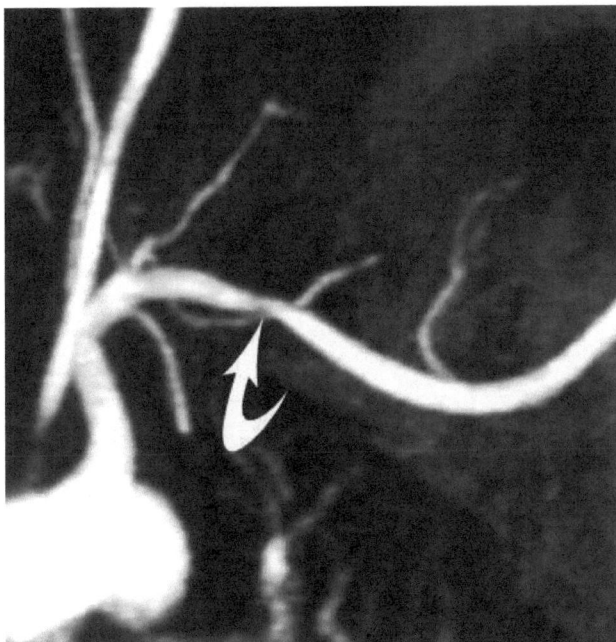

Abdominal Aortic Aneurysm: this is a dilation of the aorta that is 50% greater than the normal segment or > 3cm in diameter. Can cause abdominal pain and present as a pulsatile mass. More seriously, they can rupture and patient presents with severe back pain and hypotension. The nautral history is that of slow progression in size with a marked increase in probability of rupture when the aneurysm is > 5 cm in women and 6 cm in men. An aneurysm **expanding at more than 10 mm** per year needs to be treated.

BC often extends into the ilaic arteries and most patients with iliac aneurysms have AAA. Another common association is that 10% of patients with AAA have popliteal artery aneurysms, and 50% of patients with popliteal artery aneurysms have an AAA. 50–70% of popliteal aneurysms are bilateral. Treatment of AAA is with endovascular repair or open surgical repair. Iliac arteries are treated with kissing stents. Popliteal aneurysms are treated if asymptomatic and greater than 2–cm or if symptomatic. Stenting is difficult because of movement at the knee, surgical repair is the preferred choice with vein graft.

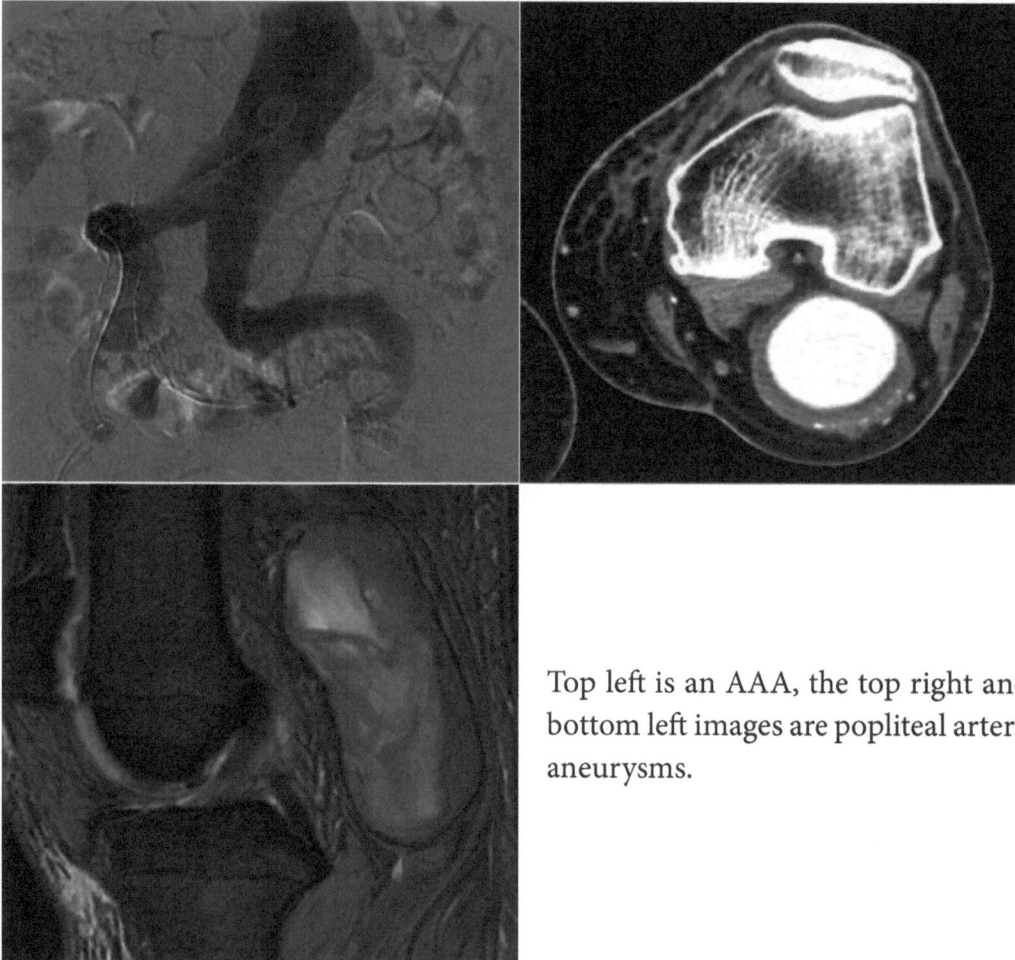

Top left is an AAA, the top right and bottom left images are popliteal artery aneurysms.

Endoleaks: occur after treatment of an aneurysm with an endoluminal stent. Image below is an example of an endoleak.

Type 1	A. proximal B. distal
Type 2	Sac continues to fill by a collateral – lumbar or IMA
Type 3	Graft defect
Type 4	Porous graft
Type 5	Endotension – sequential studies show increase in size of lumen without signs of extravasation

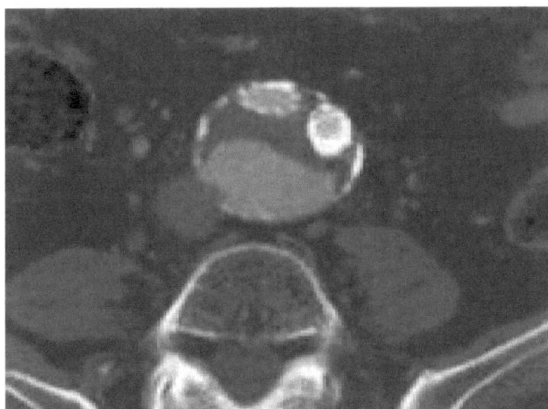

Hemobilia: follwing PTC or PBD 2–10% of patients can develop hemobilia which can be life–threatening. Patients should be instructed to contact the Radiologist if they notice bloody output from the drain or around the skin site. Most bleeding is transient and resolves, catheter repositioning or upsizing might be needed. Severe hemobilai is the result of a bile duct communicating with the hepatic artery branch or major venous branch. If an arterial bleed is suspected, emergent angiography is needed and once localized coiling should be done.

Fun Fact: Rest pain occurs with ABI < 0.4
Fun Fact: Effort claudication occurs with ABI 0.5–0.9

Penetrating Aortic Ulcer: as discussed in the Chest section, this is on a spectrum of diseases from hematoma to dissection. It presents with pain and acute aortic syndrome. It is seen as a focal outpouching of contrast into the thickened aortic wall with signs of atherosclerosis. Treatment can be surgical or endovascular.

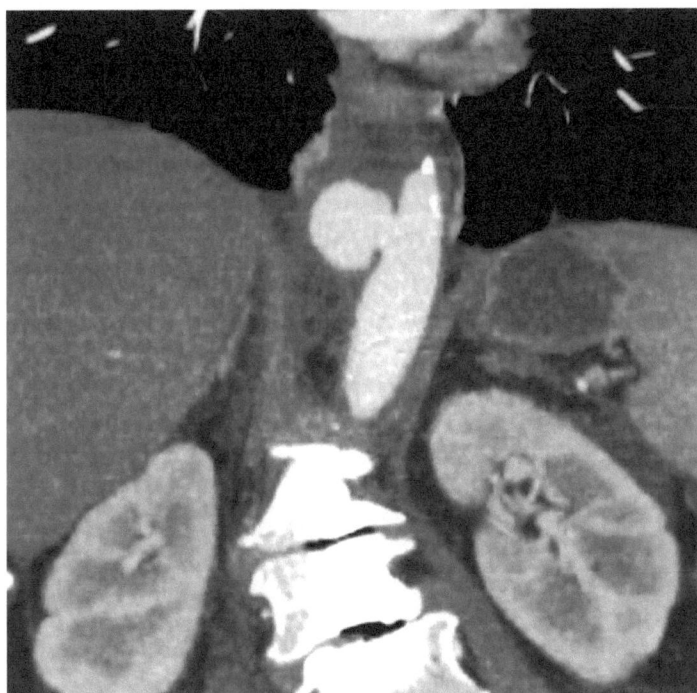

INTERVENTIONS: below is some information regarding types of interventions – high yield

Endovascular treatment is better for **shorter, unilateral lesions,** and in patients too sick for surgery
Surgical therapy is better for **larger, multiple lesions**

When placing a stent across a joint use a Nitinol stent – self expanding

If post balloon angioplasty there is failure to reduce the stenosis to less than 30% of original, a persistent pressure gradient > 10–mmHg across the lesion, or if it recurs, place a stent.

Fibrinolysis: done for acute or subacute thrombosis in native vessels or grafts < 2 weeks old. This is not to be done in patients with a threatened limb, those patients need surgical embolectomy. Fibrinolysis cannot be done in patients with recent GI bleed, intracranial bleed, stroke, recent surgery. The dose is 1 mg per hour; have to look for a source.

Embolization: is used to control active bleeding from trauma or used prior to surgery. Common agents are: coils, gelfoam, spheres, PVA, glue, and EtOH.
–
–
–

UAE is done with 300–500 micron particles
Lower GI bleed should be treated with superselctive coil embolization, if not possible, use vasopressin – don't use vasopressin on UGI bleeds
Simple AVM can be treated with coil embolization of feeding artery only

Indications for Thrombolysis:

4. Young patient with LEDVT
5. Phlegmasia cerulia dolens – venous obstrution impairs arterial inflow
6. Severe pain or morbidity from DVT
7. To maintain access i.e. dialysis access
8. Prevent post–thrombotic syndrome

IVC Filter Indications:

2. Patient with DVT with contraindication to anticoagulation
3. Patient with DVT and complication with anticoagulation
4. Patient with DVT who fails anticoagulation
5. Free floating thrombus in the IVC
6. DVT in setting of severe cardiopulmonary disease
7. Poor compliance with anticoagulation regimen

Prior to placement do an IVC-gram to look for: renal vein anatomy, duplication of IVC, size of IVC (to look for megacava > 28mm).

Stainless steel filters need 3–6 months before MRI can be performed, Nitinol filters are MRI safe.

Indications for Suprarenal Vein Placement:

2. Renal vein thrombus
3. IVC thrombus above renal veins
4. Thrombus above previously placed filter
5. Placement in pregnancy

Abscess Drains: have replaced surgical debridement and placing a drain can cause bacteremia so the patient should have antibiotics on board prior to the procedure. Can traverse liver and stomach as well as use a transvaginal or transrectal approach, but never through bowel. Use the shortest possible route.

Contraindications are: coagulopathy and lack of a safe path between skin and abscess
Safest transgluteal approach is as low as possible and as close to the sacrum to avoid the sciatic nerve.

Percutaneous Transhepatic Biliary Drain:

2. Relief of malignant obstruction
3. Biliary stricture or leak
4. Access for stone retrieval

Contraindications: ascites, colon in the way, liver cysts and coagulopathy

Two types of drains: metal stents are only for terminal patients with < 6 months to live, benign diseases get plastic stent by ERCP or internal–external drains.

3. External – anywhere in the biliary tract
4. Internal–external – from biliary tree into the bowel

Cholecystostomy Tube: done in very sick patients with acalculous cholecystitis. Can remove the tube after 6 weeks because a tract has to form to avoid bile peritonitis. Also there should be no stones and cystic duct has to be patent.

Nephrostomy Tubes: done for obstruction or leaks, done emergently in patients with obstruction and sepsis. Puncture the subcostal tip of the 12th posterior rib and place into the lower pole calyx, 8–10 Fr tube is used. Contraindications are: renals cysts, bowel in the way, and coagulopathy.

Ureteral Stents: are usually to relieve obstruction or to cross a leak.

Key Points:

2. Splenic abscesses are risky to drain because the spleen bleeds a lot, usually treat with antibiotics alone.
3. Do not drain pancreatic pseudocysts as a first line option, they should be emptied into the stomach by GI.
4. Never place a drain into a necrotic neoplasm, these people will get drains for life.
5. Tubo–ovarian abscess is not treated with a drain 1st, they are treated with antibiotics first.

Indication for TIPS:

18. Refractory ascites
19. Bleeding varices with failed endoscopic therapy
20. Hydrothorax

Contraindications to TIPS:

2. Heart failure or cardiac valvular insufficiency
3. Rapidly progressive liver failure and clinically significant encephalopathy (worsens with TIPS)
4. Systemic infection or sepsis
5. Liver malignancy
6. Coagulopathy

For the patients with malignant ascites or ascites caused by heart failure, place a tunneled peritoneal catheter instead.

TIPS is placed to decrease portal venous pressure by creating a conduit for blood to bypass the hepatic parenchyma and into the systemic circulation. A long curved needle is passed through the hepatic parenchyma from the right hepatic vein into the right portal vein. The hepatic tract is dilated and a stent graft is inserted. Post–TIPS portal vein and right atrial pressures are then acquired. The goal is to reduce the portosystemic gradient to less than 12–mm Hg to decrease the risk of variceal bleeding. The pressure needs to drop between 6–8–mm Hg to treat intractable ascites. TIPS stenosis happens at the hepatic venous end.

Catheters: we can place an entire gamut of central catheters

1. PICC – small caliber catheters that are used for short–term (2–6 weeks) of venous access
2. Nontunneled or tunneled – long–term access for giving blood transfusions, antibiotics, and parenteral medications
3. Nontunneled or tunneled pheresis catheters
4. Nontunneled or tunneled hemodialysis catheters
5. Implantable ports for intermittent access

The internal jugular vein is the preferred access site for long–term access. IJ spares the subclavian veins which may be important in patients with ESRD who will need dialysis. For nontunneled catheters the subclavian vein is preferred because the chest wall exit sites are associated with less infection than neck or groin. Tip of the catheter should be in the distal SVC.

A common problem with catheters is the formation of a **fibrin sheath**. This leads to **the inability to aspirate**, but preservation of the ability to inject.

Uterine Artery Embolization:

1. To control postpartum bleeding refractory to medical management
2. To control postoperative bleeding after cesarean section
3. To treat trauma–related pelvic hemorrhage
4. To improve symptoms in women with uterine fibroids
5. To palliate bleeding pelvic malignancies

Prior to the procedure there should be a thorough evaluation of the patient by a gynecologist, pelvic US MRI, and pregnancy test. Uterine artery arises from the anterior division of the internal iliac artery. The artery is embolized with PVA (300–500 microns) or embospheres. After procedure give IVF and pain control and anti–pyretics. Patients can get *post-embolization syndrome* – fever, nausea, pain within the first 72 hours. It is not a sign of infection, it is common and resolves in 72 hours. Pre and post embolization images are below.

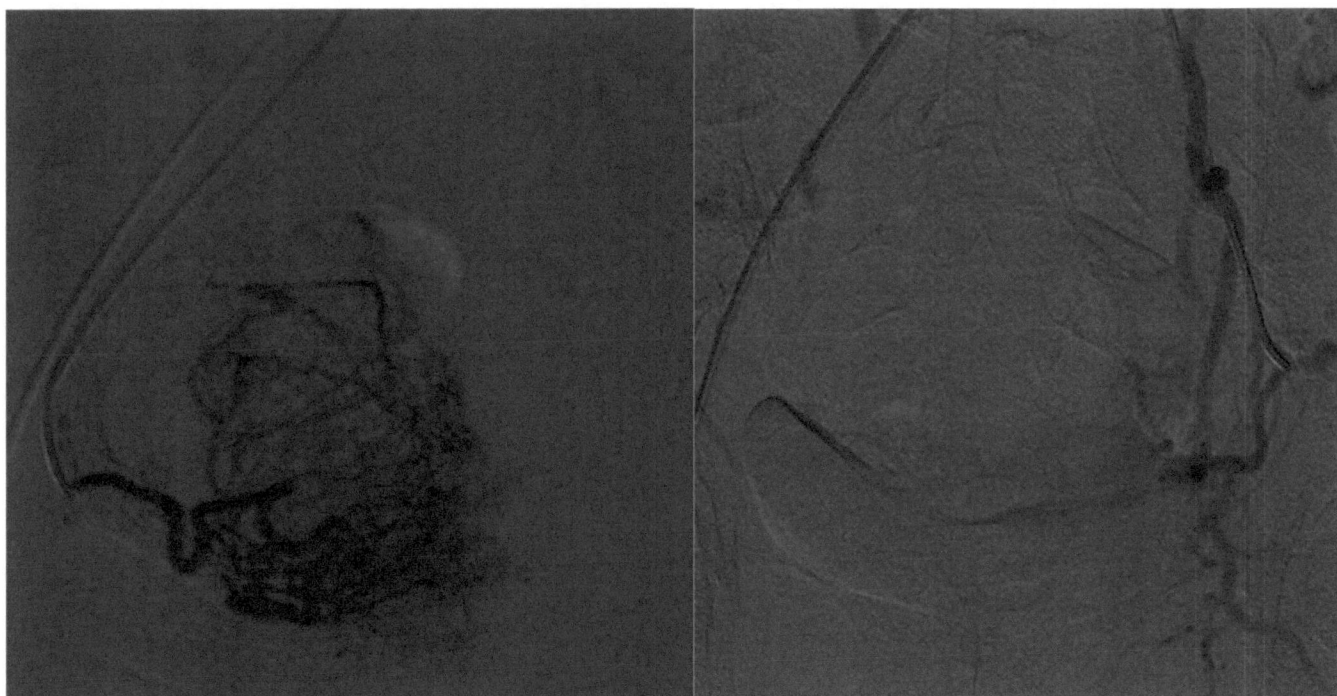

Y–90 Chemoembolization: is an FDA approved therapy for treating unresectable hepatocellular carcinoma and metastatic colorectal cancer. The microspheres are delivered to the tumor through the hepatic artery. Prior to the procedure, the patient undergoes a Tc–99 MAA study to check for any abnormal shunting, especially to look for a right to left shunt. After optimizing arterial anatomy (embolizing the GDA to prevent duodenal reflux of spheres – catastrophic) the microcatheter tip is placed in the planned position for delivery. Dose delivery is monitored carefully, delivery is stopped when flow slows down, do not let it reach stasis.

Important Anatomy: know the branches of the celiac axis

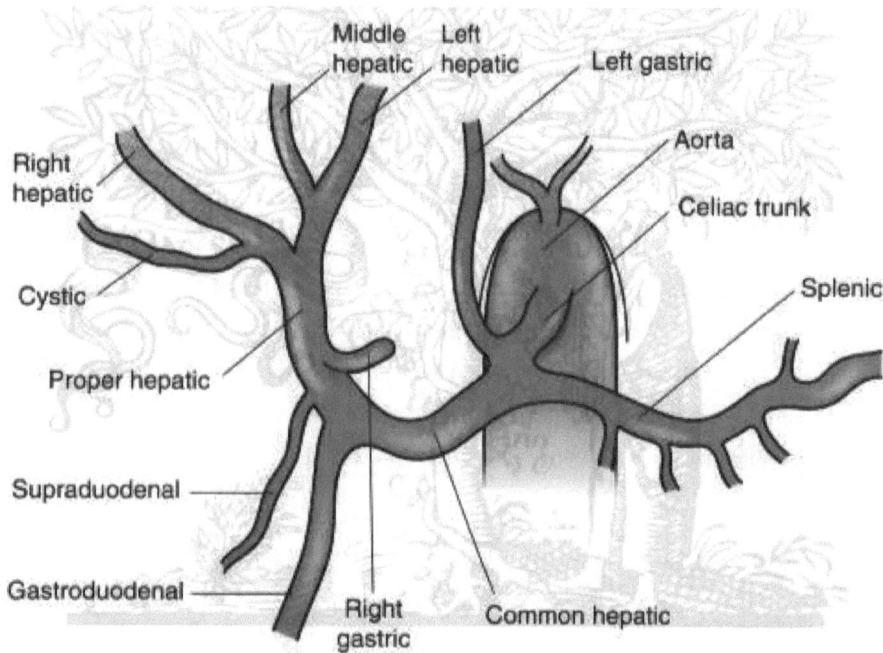

VASCULAR ULTRASOUND:
Common Carotid Arteries – sharp upstroke with a normal PSV < 125 cm/sec

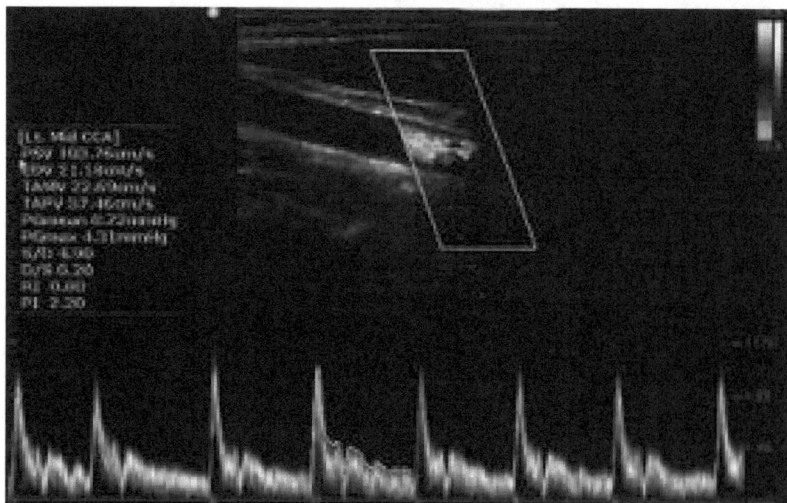

Carotid stenosis:

6.50% stenosis: PSV < 125 cm/sec with visible sonographic plaque 50–69% stenosis: PSV between 15–230 cm/sec with visible plaque 70% stenosis: PSV > 230 cm/sec with plaque and luminal narrowing Near Occlusion: velocities may not apply because they can be high or low

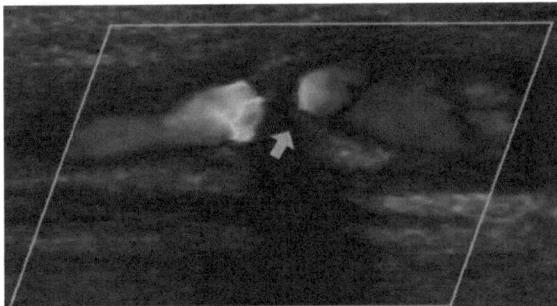

Vertebral Arteries and Subclavian Steal: normal vertebral artery waveform should be a brisk upstroke during systole with broad diastolic component (image 1). With subclavian steal the flow reverses direction and is below the baseline (image 2). This is more common on the left than on the right.

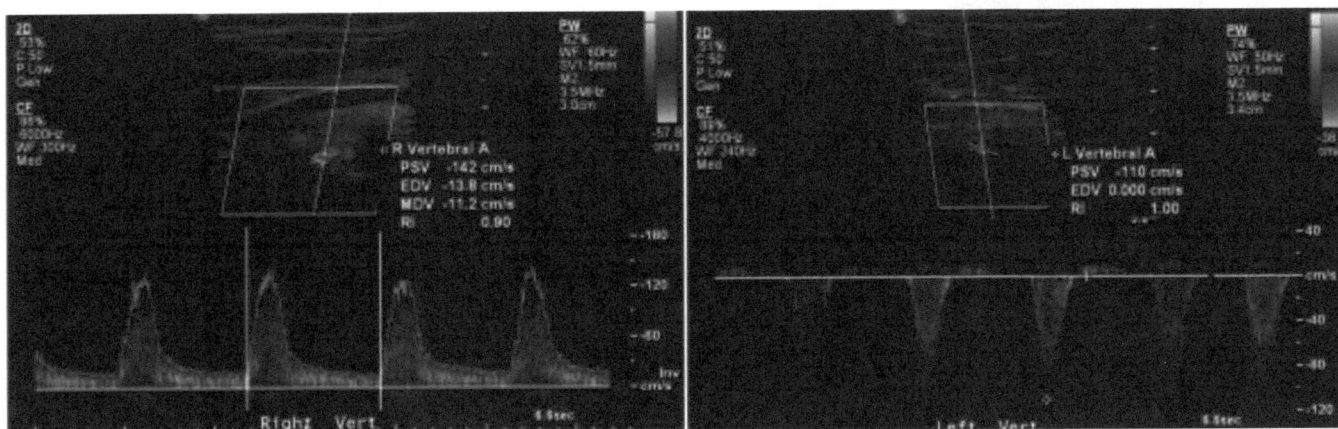

BD 95% below the renal arteries, strong association with smoking, atherosclerosis, and HTN. Any dilation > 3–cm is an aneurysm.

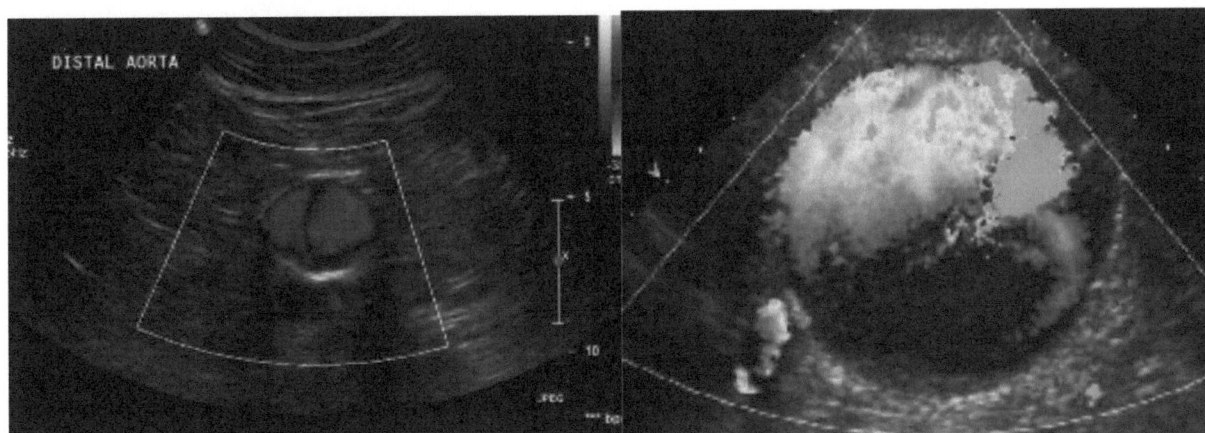

The area of no color flow on the right is thrombus within the aneurysm.

PV – flow should be red signifying towards the transducer – smooth waveform
HV – flow should be blue, away from the transducer – triphasic waveform like the IVC

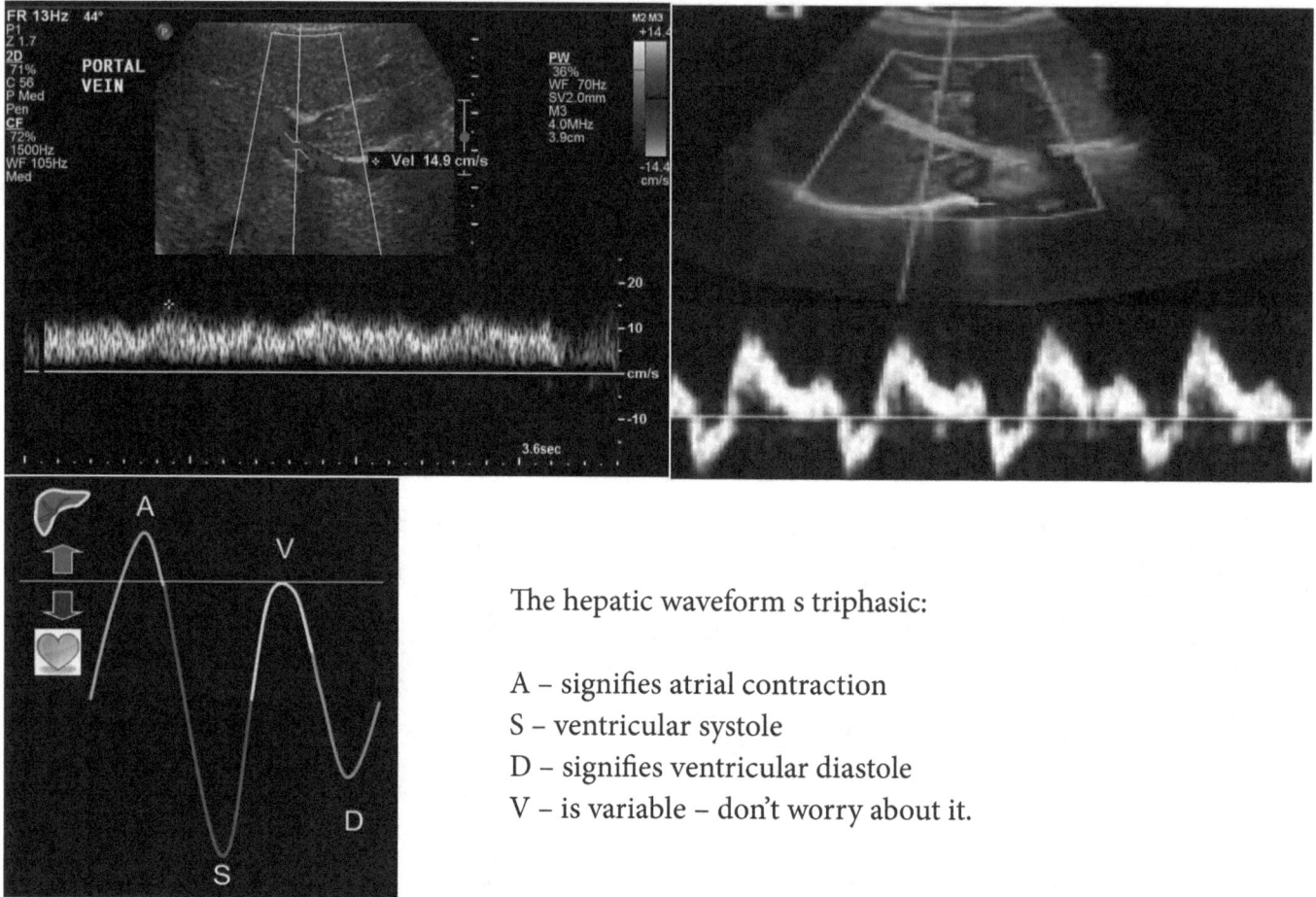

The hepatic waveform s triphasic:

A – signifies atrial contraction
S – ventricular systole
D – signifies ventricular diastole
V – is variable – don't worry about it.

Portal Hypertension: cirrhotic patients, look for reversal of flow as a late sig of portal HTN. Often these patients will have a rencalized umbilical vein (seen in the ligamentum teres) as a collateral. Flow reversal is more common in the right portal vein. Remember this will also cause flow reversal in the splenic vein. Normal PV velocity is 15–30 cm/sec.

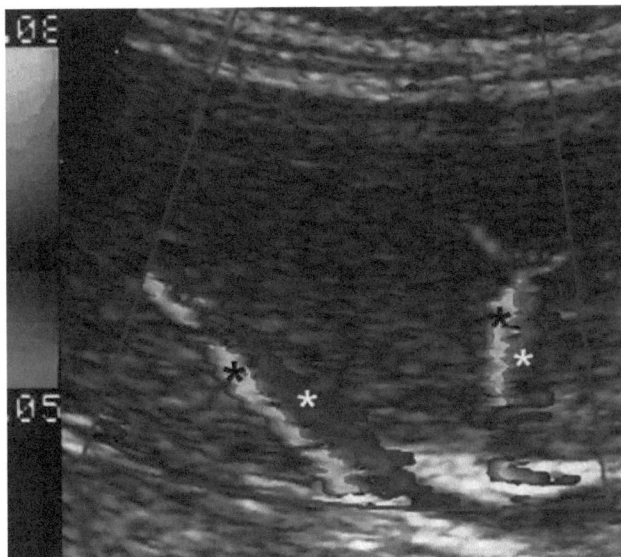

This image shows a portal vein (blue) and hepatic artery (red) side by side. Normally both of these vessels should have hepatopetal (flow towards transducer/into liver), but in this case the portal vein has reversed flow.

Portal Vein Thrombus: can be bland thrombus or tumor thrombus (look for vein expansion and vascularity of thrombus). There will be no flow in the portal vein. Caused by hypercoagulable states, mets, trauma, pregnancy, and infections.

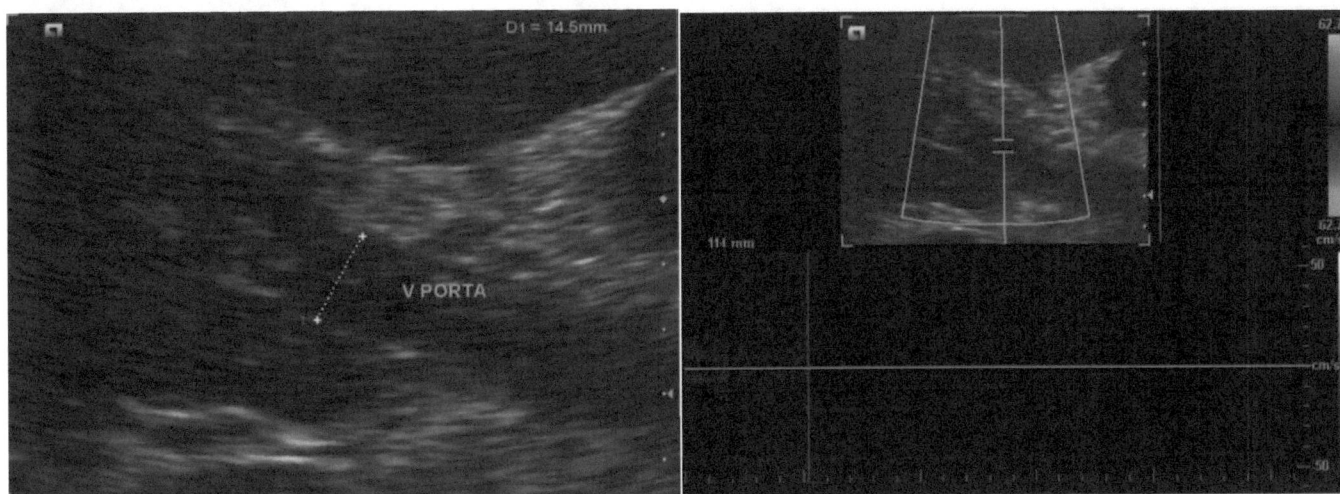

Renal Artery Stenosis: There are two ways to evaluate the renal arteries 1) just like the carotids – try to find the artery and get peak systolic velocities or 2) look at the waveforms of the distal vessels to see what they are doing. The upper limit of normal for **renal arteries is 180–200 cm/sec**. A resistive index 9.0.7 is considered bad. The distal arteries should should a tardus waveform – slow upstroke, broadened or rounded systolic peak.

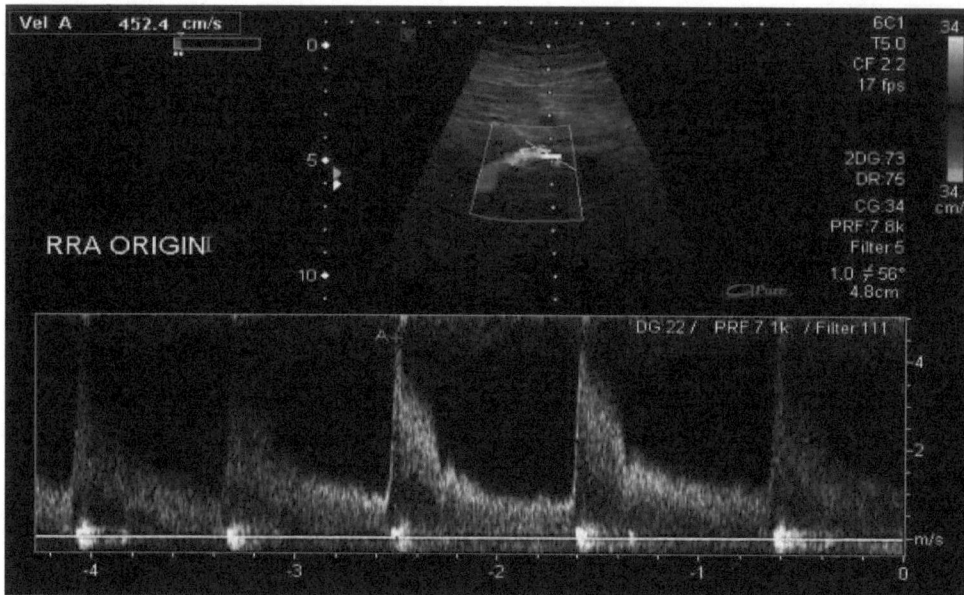

Abnormal elevated velocity > 400 cm/sec consistent with stenosis

Parvus Tardus: means that there is upstream stenosis

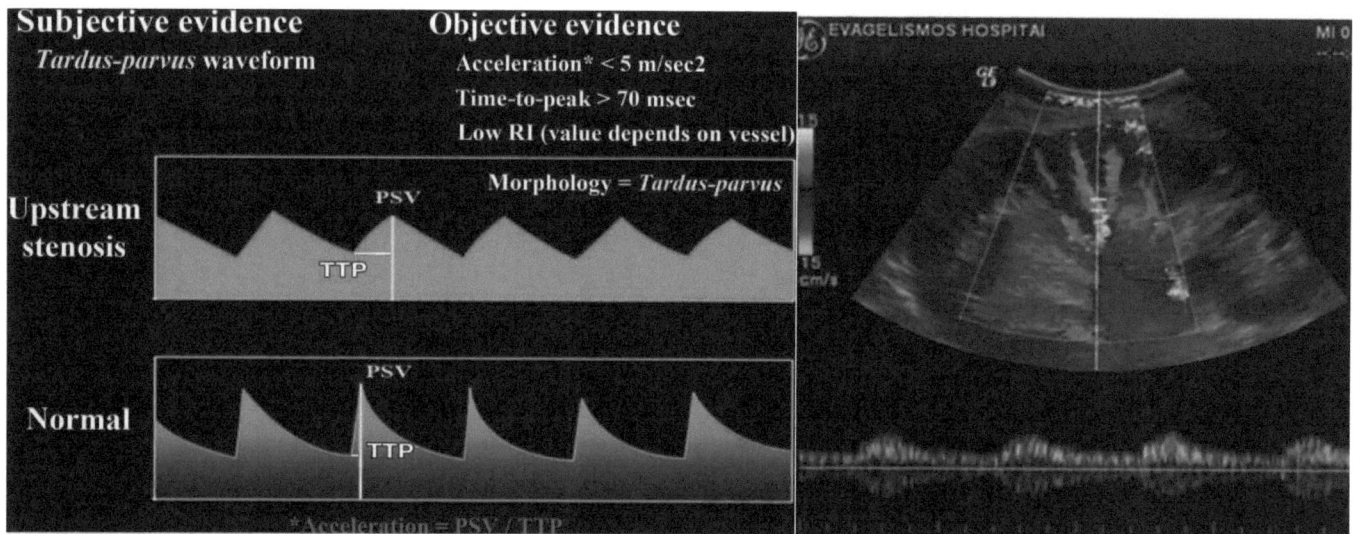

Deep Vein Thrombosis: US is the procedure of choice to diagnose this, normally the deep veins should be completely compressible with the transducer, DVT is when the vein fails to compress fully. Low–level echoes are commonly seen in veins – this is probably artifact. A clot can also be hypoechois, so we cannot use echogenicity to predict the presence of a thrombus.

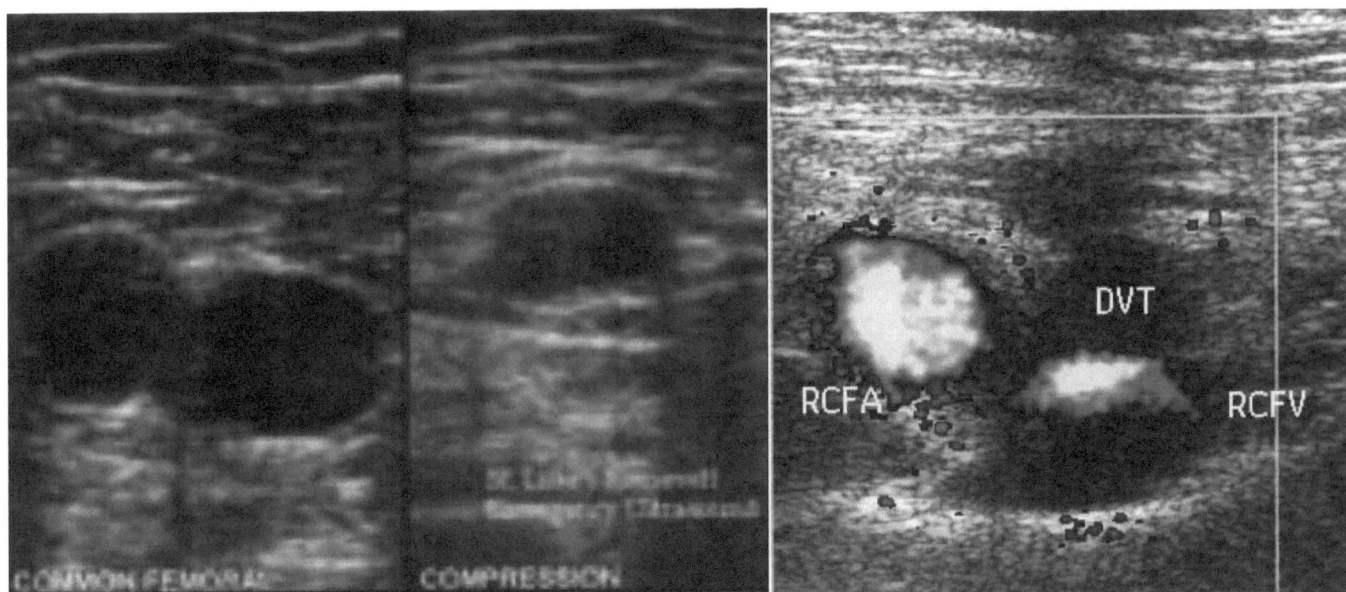

Image on left shows normal compressibility of a vein while the image on the right shows a low level clot with some flow an lack of full compressibility consistent with a DVT.

Replaced Right Hepatic Artery: arises from the superior mesenteric artery and travels behind the MPV ascending into the liver in the hepatoduodenal ligament.

Replaced Left Hepatic Artery: arises from the left gastric artery and enters the liver through a fissure for the ligamentum venosum.

Liver Transplant: Ultrasound is used to assess for complications of liver transplant. For example, these patients do not have a GB, so any fluid in the GB fossa is abnormal and represents some sort of pathology.
-
-
-
-

Hematoma, seroma, biloma, abscess
HA stenosis or aneurysm
IVC/PV stenosis or thrombosis
Neoplasm

Hepatic artery thrombosis is the most common vascular complication following liver transplantation (10% of cases). Look for blunting (tardus) waveforms and low RI < 0.4, however, if the RI is > 0.5 thrombosis is unlikely. Hepatic artery thrombosis can lead to bile duct ischemia, so a cholangiogram would show strictures.

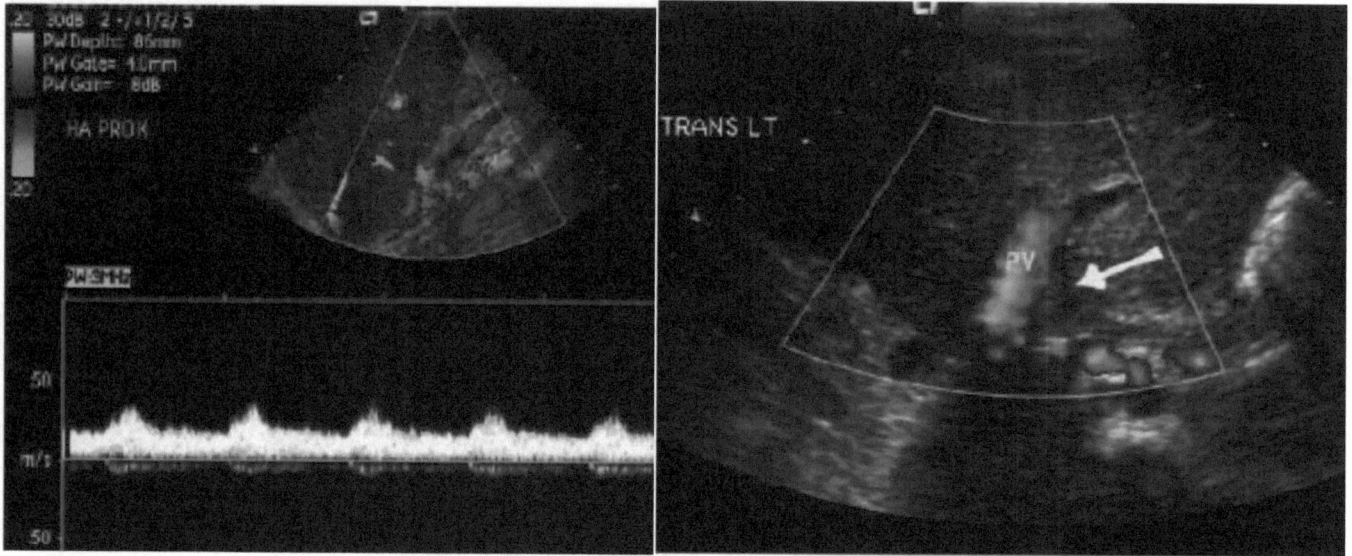

Image on the left shows a tardus parvus waveform in the hepatic artery with dampened flow. The image on the left shows absent flow in a thrombosed hepatic artery right next to the portal vein.

Renal Transplant: this is a pretty important topic since US is really the only tool we have to fully evaluate a transplanted kidney. A renal transplant is going to be much easier to image because it is in the RLQ of the abdomen and fairly superficial. There are two types of anastomoses:

-

-

End–to–side arterial anastomosis with the common iliac artery End–to–end arterial anastomosis with the external iliac artery

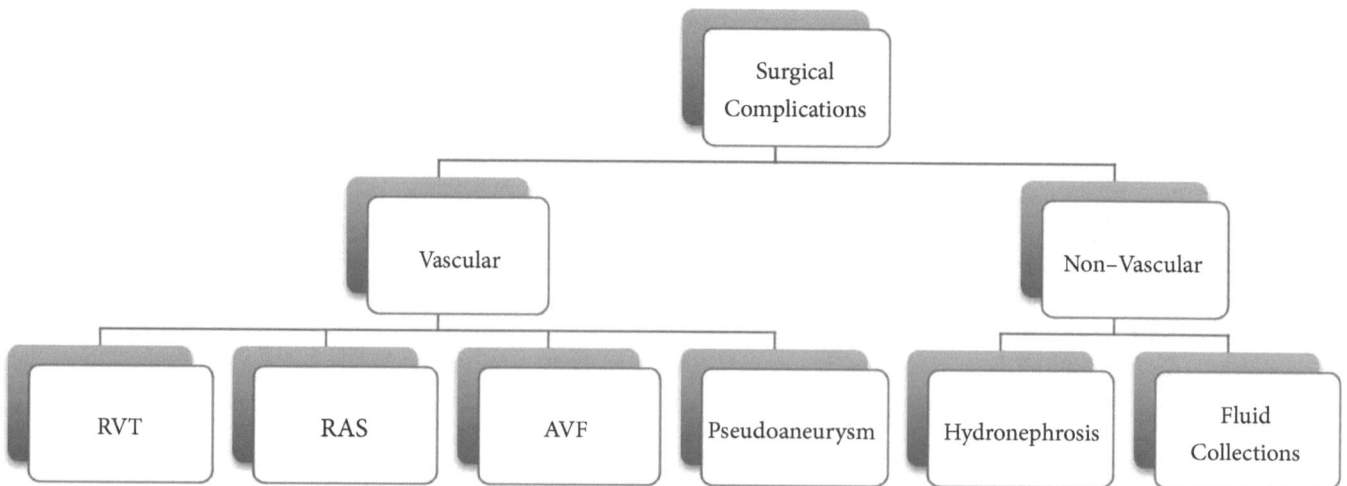

Fluid Collections occur in 50% of transplants and the timing of the fluid collection is key:

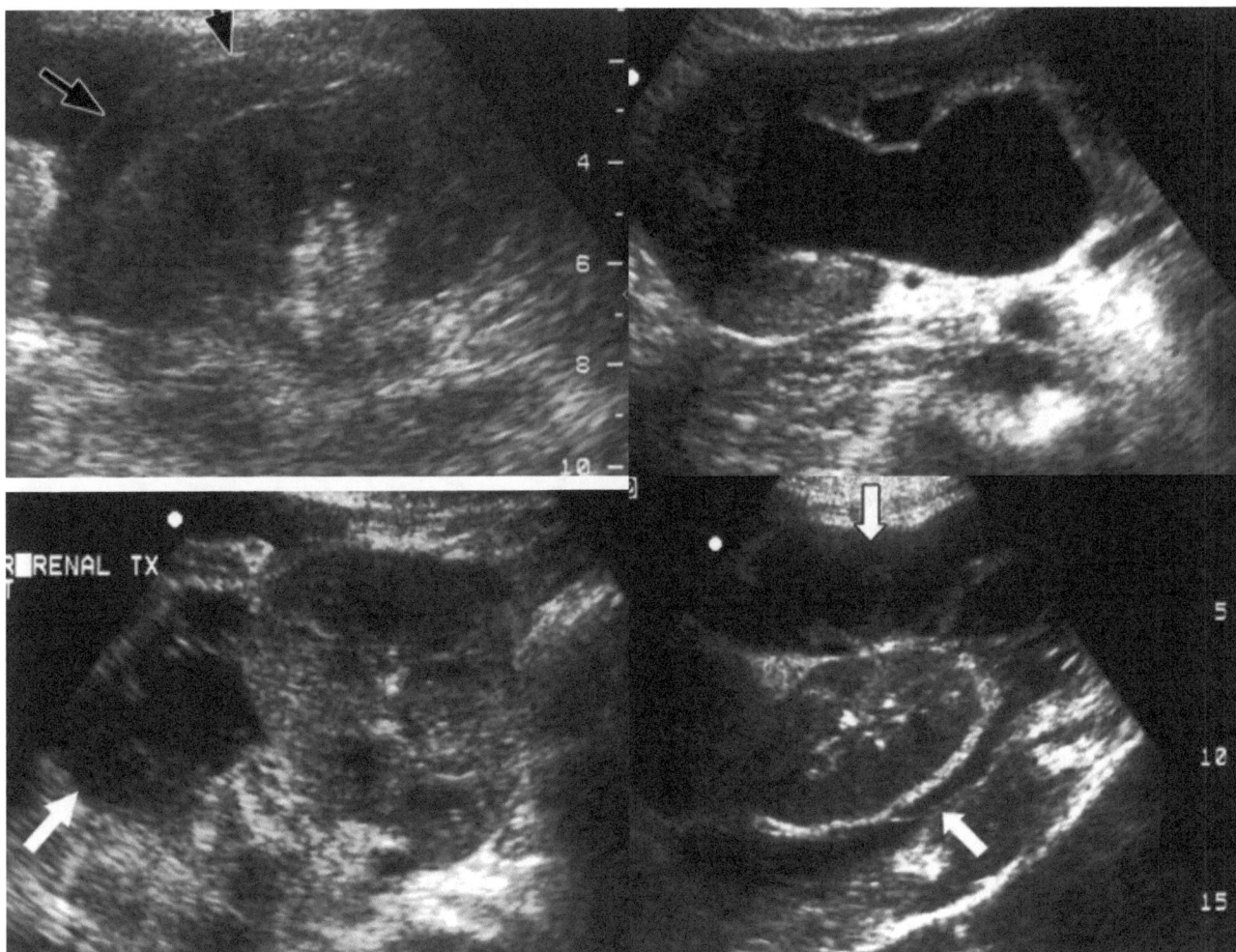

8. Immediate post–op – Hematoma
9. 1–2 weeks – Urinoma
10. 3–5 weeks – Abscess

Hydronephrosis is usually a functional issue in renal transplants due to edema at the anastomosis, kink in the ureter, or can be obstructive due to clots, fungus balls (remember these people are on immunosuppresants), and stones.

Renal Vein Thrombus: this can occur due to technical problems but is more likely due to compression or kinking related to a long vein or graft mobility. It typically occurs in the first few days following graft placement and the patient will demonstrate decreased or absent urine output, elevated creatinine, hematuria, and pain. Since the transplant hasn't had time to develop collaterals, it is more likely to infarct and this is a surgical emergency.

Doppler features are pandiastolic flow reversal and lack of detectable venous flow in the parenchyma and hilum. Notice below how all of the diastolic flow is below the line!

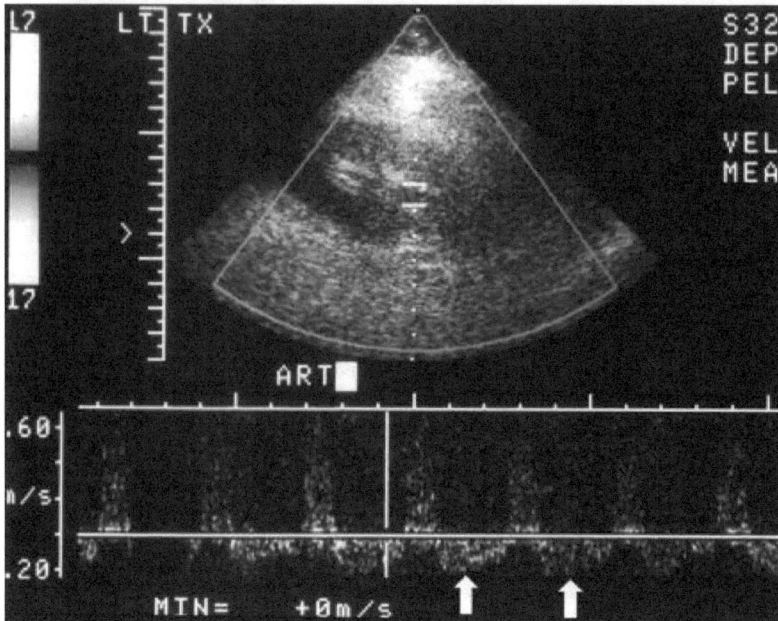

Renal Artery Stenosis: was discussed above. Just know that in the setting of a transplant it is a late complication and the stenosis occurs at the anastomosis with the main RA PSV > 200 cm/sec. As seen above, look for main RA turbulence and distal tardus parvus.

Pseudoaneuysm: a renal transplant should NOT have any cysts – these are essentially perfect kidneys when transplanted, the appearance of a cyst is a bad sign, have to worry about pseudoaneurysm, especially if there was a biopsy. Look for the classic yin–yang appearance which signifies blood swirling inside the aneurysm sac.

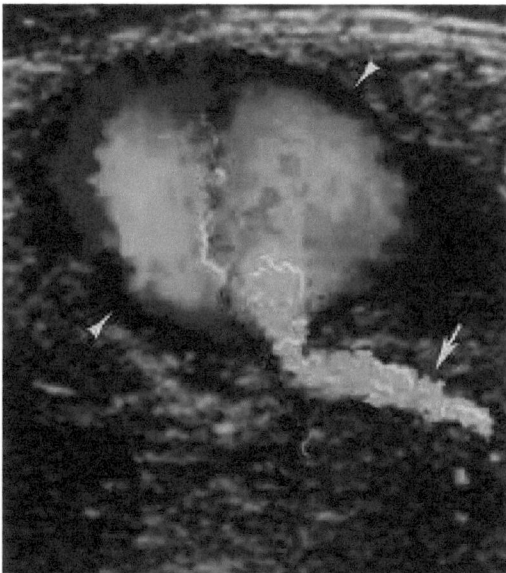

A few words about post–catheterization pseudoaneurysms: these are seen in the groin as a hypoechoic pulsatile mass. The Doppler waveform will lose the normal triphasic characteristics and have diastolic reversal. These can be watched and most will spontaneously resolve. However, if they become symptomatic or enlarge, then we can do US–guided thrombin injection.

AVF: high velocity lesion where the artery feeds the vein. Look for a pulsatile venous wave form and aliasing on Doppler. The color images look smudgy with blue and red just mixing all over the place.

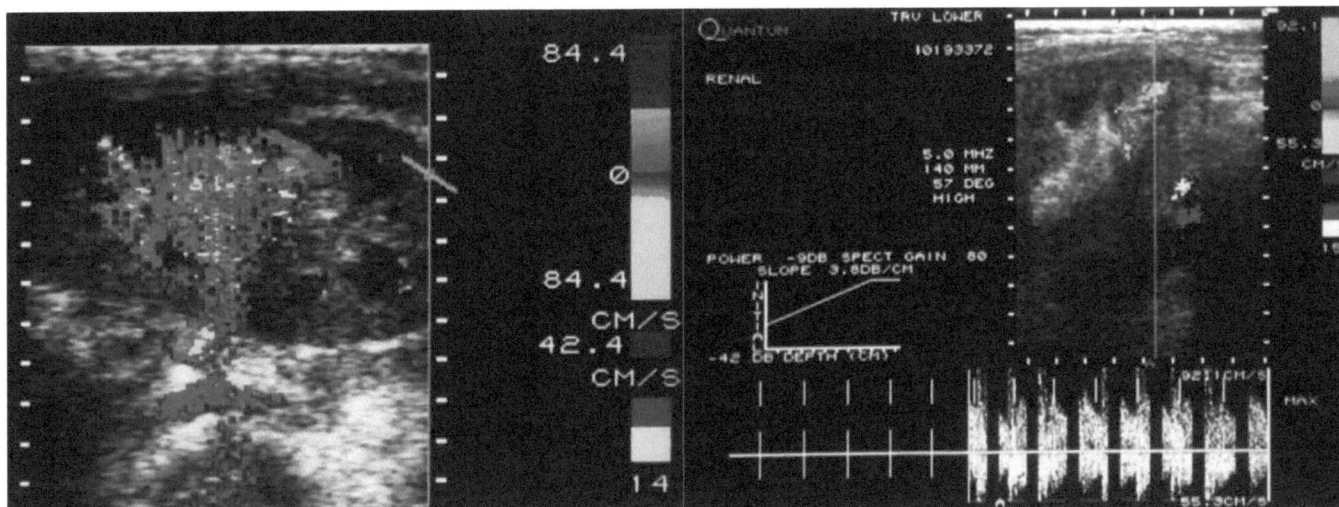

Medical Complications:

6. Acute Tubular Necrosis – happens between days 1–3; the kidney maintains perfusion, but function drops
7. Rejection
    - Hyperacute – occurs in less than 24 hours, sometimes the surgeons can see it happening in the OR
    - Acute – 1 week to 3 months
    - Chronic – after 1 year; no recovering from this

US will show a swollen kidney with prominent pyramids and a high RI (> 0.7).

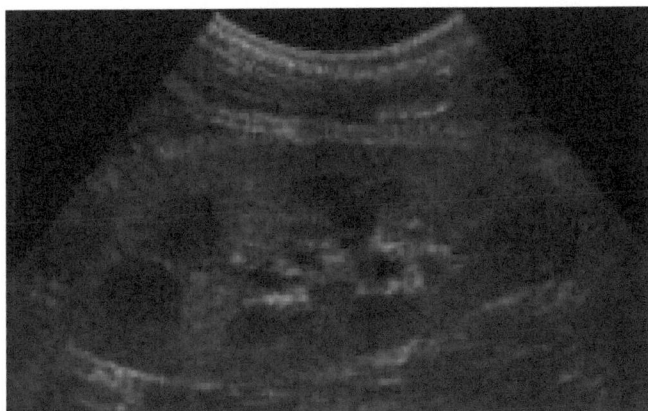

Post Transplant Lymphoproliferative Disorder: is an intra– or extra–renal solid mass often situated near the hilum caused by EBV infection in the setting of T–Cell suppression. Looks like a peri–transplant fluid collection with internal vascularity.

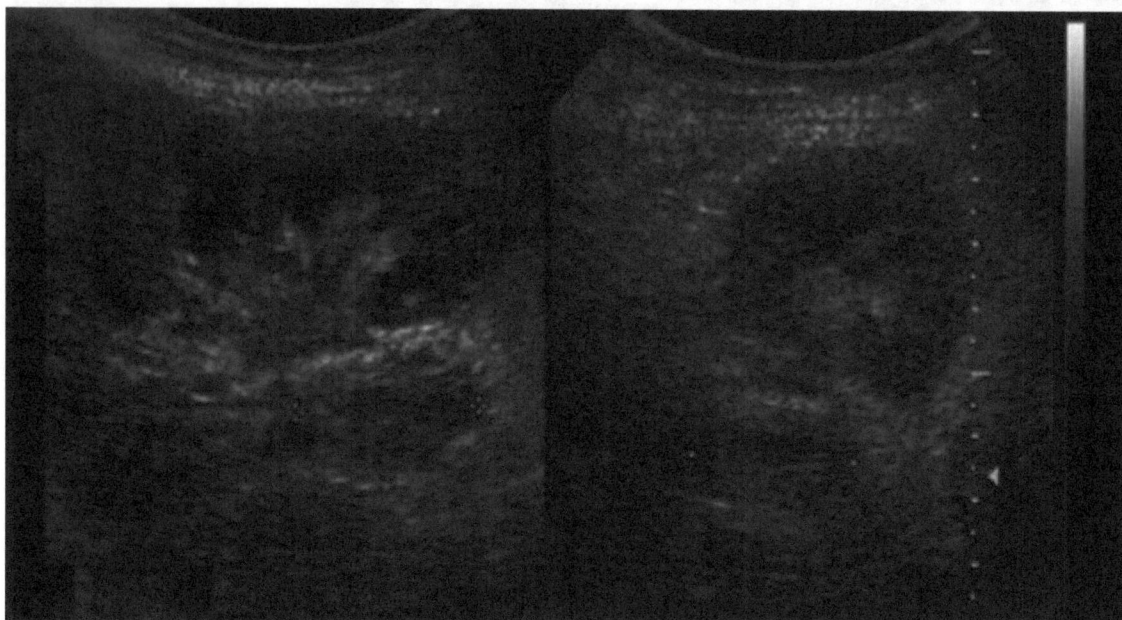

Obstetrics

FETAL ULTRASOUND: the easiest way to approach this is to break the topic down by trimester and then think about what you're looking for in the normal baby, how to measure it, and then what pathology can happen

1st Trimester: this is the first 13 weeks of pregnancy following the last menstrual period. US during this phase is concerned with *dating the pregnancy, signs of early pregnancy failure,* and *confirming intra- or extra-uterine pregnancy.*

A yolk sac should be seen with a gestational sac measuring 8-mm and a fetal pole should be visible when the sac is 12-mm.

Dates: the most accurate measurement of gestational age in the 1st trimester, especially after 6 weeks is the crown rump length (CRL). The normal CRL is measured from the top of the head to the bottom of the buttocks.

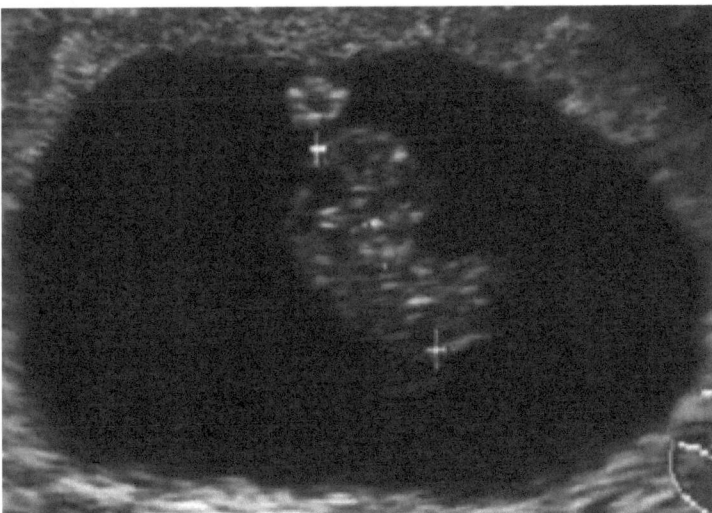

Assessment of fetal cardiac activity is important, not only to confirm a viable baby, but also an abnormal heart rate can be a sign of impending failure. Normal 1st trimester **heart rate is > 120 to < 160 bpm**.

Cardiac activity should be visible at 6 weeks gestation or with a fetal pole of 5–mm, if not seen here, reimage in one week and follow with b–HCG.

Nuchal lucency (1st trimester) is not to be confused with nuchal thickness (2nd trimester). This is performed between 11–13 weeks and if increased is considered to be due to dilated lymphatic channels – badness. It can be associated with aneuploidy (trisomies and Turners). It is measured on a sagittal view, and **the normal thickness is 2.5–3.0 mm**; if abnormal, correlate with AFP, amniocentesis, or CVS. It can regress over time or evolve into a cystic hygroma.

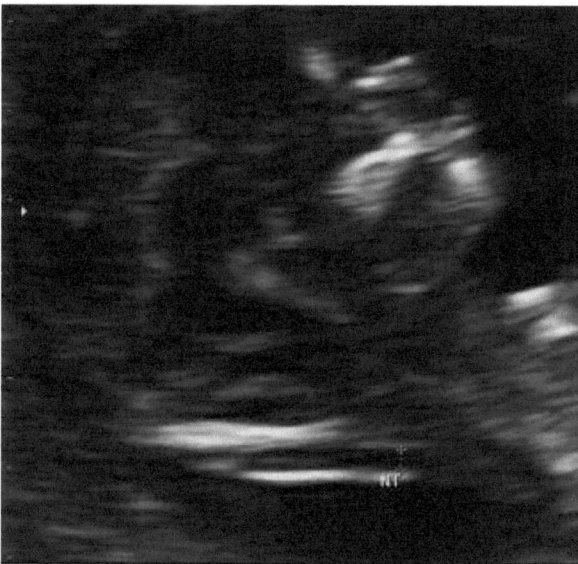

An IUP should be confirmed on US, if one is not seen then the patient should have serial b–HCG and repeat US done until an IUP is established, an ectopic is visualized, or the the b–HCG starts to trend down suggesting miscarriage.

Definitions:

1. Threatened abortion – refers to pain, bleeding or contractions during the 1st twenty weeks of gestation with a **closed cervical os.**
2. Inevitable abortion – open cervix in the presence of bleeding during the 1st trimester.
3. Missed abortion – non–viable fetus without expulsion of contents from womb (CRL > 7–mm without a heart beat – ACOG)
4. Complete abortion – all products of conception have been passed from the uterus

RPOC: following a spontaneous abortion or after a D&C and endometrial stripe < 5–mm is a good predictor of complete evacuation. Any collection > 5–mm or thickening of the endometrium suggests RPOC. A hyperechoic mass > 15–mm is the best predictor. The differential includes molar pregnancy and endometritis (look for air and patient with fever). The b–HCG should fall with RPOC but will increase with molar pregnancy. This tissue should have vascularity and a waveform that would be absent in decidua or hemorrhage. However, absence of a vascular endometrial mass doesn't exclude RPOC.

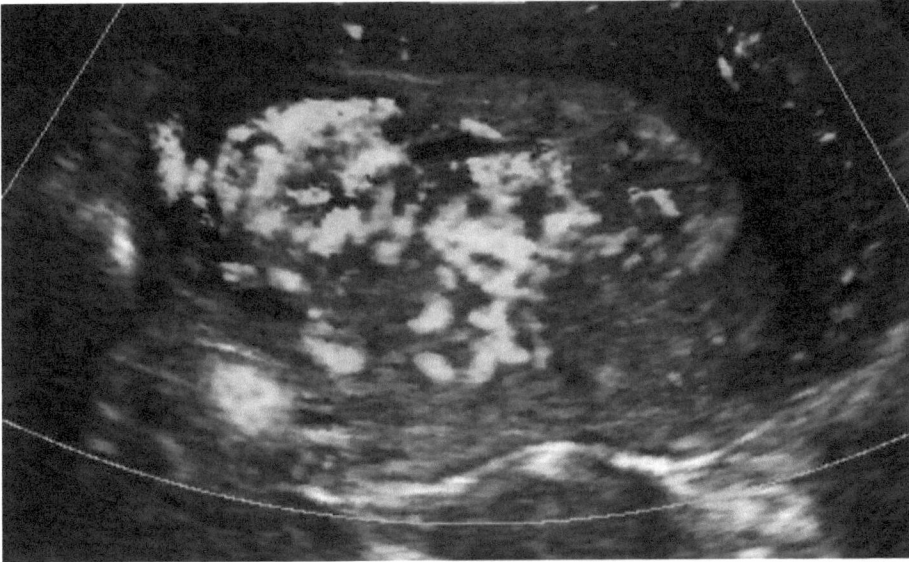

Ectopic Pregnancy: is the presence of an embryo outside of the uterus and is an emergency. The classic presentation is acute abdominal pain and bleeding in a young female (although the ER's criteria is just a young female). For US, a serum b–HCG should be over 1000, but we do see these at lower levels. Most common location for an ectopic is in the fallopian tube, specifically at the ampulla. They can occur almost anywhere though, cesarean section scars, ovary, cervix, and abdominal cavity. There is an increased incidence in women undergoing IVF, IUD in place, those with prior ectopics and PID. It is important to be able to differentiate these from the corpus luteum cyst. Look for an echogenic mass adjacent to the ovary with a ring of fire blood supply, whereas a CL cyst will be an intra–ovarian mass with ring of fire.

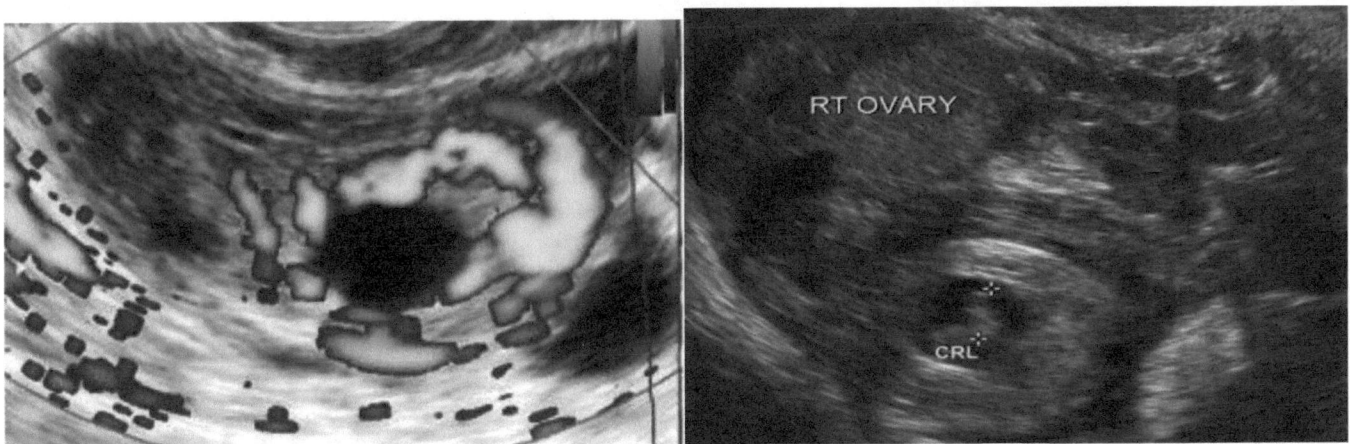

Cervical Ectopic: implantation of the ovum in the cervix rather than the uterus, look for a fetal heart rate to distinguish from abortion in progress. Do not do D&C because that will result in life–threatening hemorrhage, instead MTX, uterine artery ligation, and then D&C. This is overall rare, but increasing in incidence because of IVF.

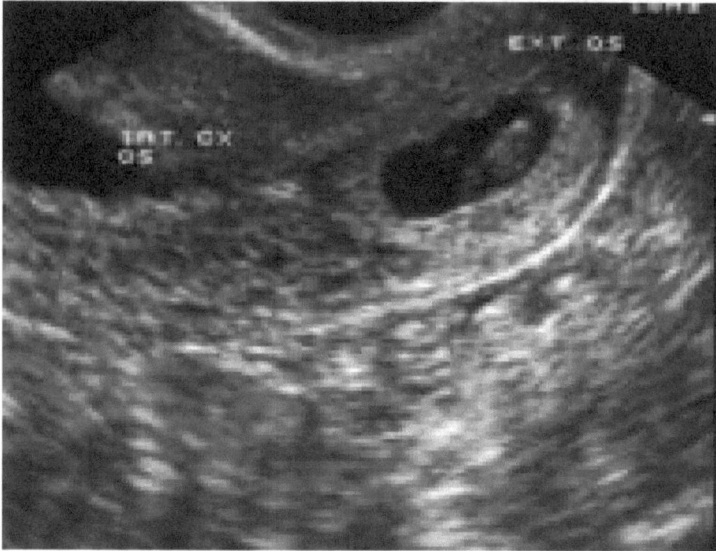

2nd Trimester: falls between 13 weeks and 27 weeks of gestation. US in this phase is mostly concerned with *fetal anatomy*. Basic things to look for are: number of fetuses and their position, fetal heart rate, location of placenta, AFI and an anatomic survey. The anatomy should include: cerebral ventricles and posterior fossa, 4–chamber heart view (with the cardiac axis at 45–degrees to the left), fetal spine, stomach, kidneys, urinary bladder, umbilical artery, and extremities.

Biparietal Diameter: is one of the most accurate 2nd trimester measurements of gestational age and is measured from the outer cortex of the closest parietal bone to the inner cortex of the other parietal bone at the level of the cavum septum pellucidum.

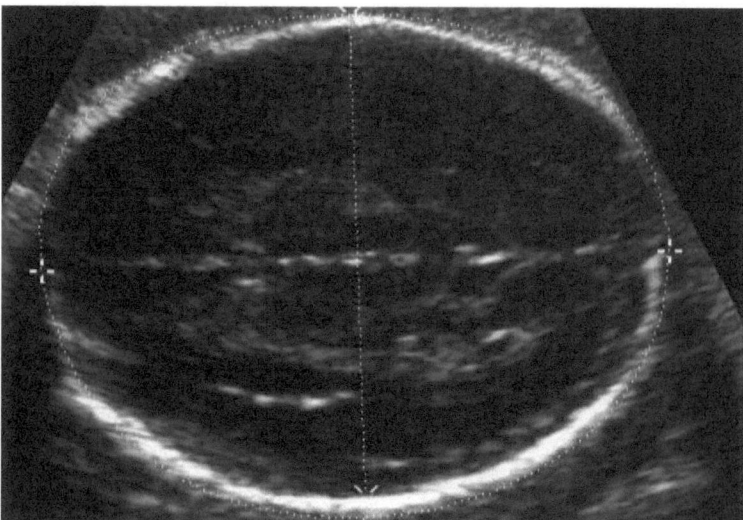

AFI < 8 cm implies oligohydramnios and > 20 implies polyhydramnios.

Nuchal Thickness is measured between 18–22 weeks of gestation. Increased thickness implies cardiac defects or lymphatic malformations both of which are associated with aneuploidy. Unlike the translucency (measured in sagittal plane), this is measured in the axial plane from the surface of the skin to the outer cortex of the occipital bone and is **abnormal if > 6-mm** in thickness – associated with

Down's, also look for intracardiac echogenic focus (papillary muscle calcification – most common in LV) and an absent nasal bone.

Cervical Incompetence: refers to a painless spontaneous dilation of the cervix and is a common cause of pregnancy failure in the 2nd trimester. A normal cervical length is > 3 cm and < 2 cm is abnormal. Patients at risk include those with DES exposure, uterine anomalies, prior abortions, and multifetal pregnancies. The cervix begins to funnel as it opens and the shape of the funnel holds prognostic value. As the internal os dilates > 6 mm the cervix will look like a T, Y, V, or U. V–shaped cervix has the worst prognosis.

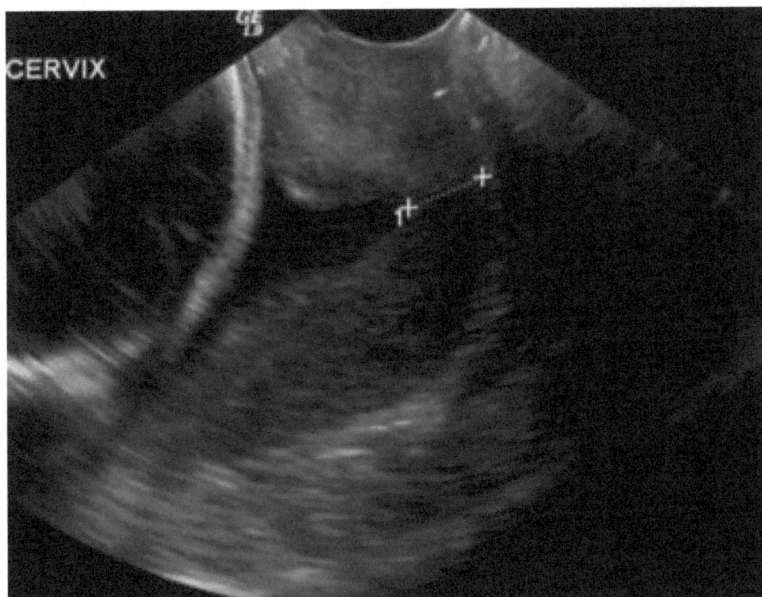

3rd Trimester: looking for fetal position, placenta, and growth.

Umbilical Artery Doppler: this study is indicated if we see oligohydramnios and IUGR. A waveform should be obtained at the fetal end, mid artery, and placental end and the S:D ratio is obtained at each point. **With increasing gestational age, the S:D should decrease.** Absence or reversal of diastolic flow has been associated with intrauterine growth restriction, fetal asphyxia, perinatal mortality, and long- term neurological issues.

When fetal hypoxia occurs due to decreased diastolic flow, the fetal circulation responds by performing a brain–sparing maneuver and redistributes blood to the brain. We can look for this by performing an MCA

Doppler and if the MCA pulse index is normal, then there has been redistribution of flow. If this pulse index decreases, the baby is decompensating. **MCA peak systolic velocity increases in anemia.**

Placental Abruption: a retroplacental hemorrhage that separates the placenta from the uterine wall, it can be partial or complete. Risk factors include maternal HTN, cocaine, smoking, and trauma. Patient presents with pain and bleeding. The fetal prognosis depends on the amount of hemorrhage and placental separation.

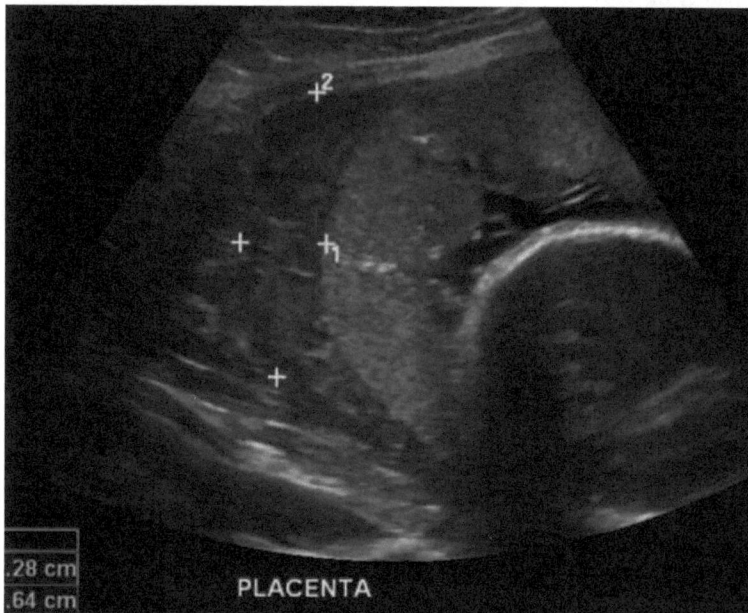

Fetal Neuro: evaluation of the fetal nervous system should include BPD, HC, entire spine, septum pellucidum, falx, upper lip, ventricles, and posterior fossa: cerebellum, cisterna magna. A lot of the neuro pathology is covered in the peds neuro section of this study guide, so I didn't delve too deep into it.

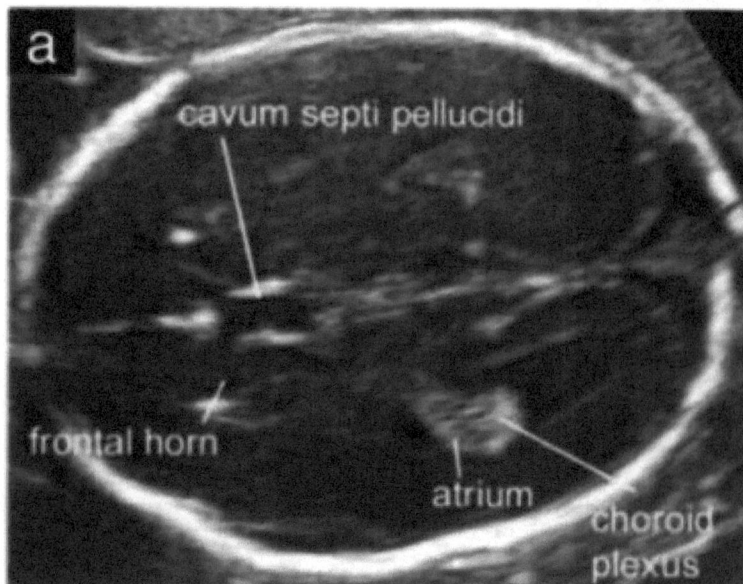

Ventriculomegaly is a guarded prognosis and when we see it, we have to look for a cause. It's easy to identify as the normal ventricle should measure < 1 cm throughout gestation, also subjectively, look for the "dangling choroid". It is associated with neural tube defects, **aqueductal stenosis** (20% of in utero hydro), infection, and hemorrhage. When mild (10–15–mm) it can be an isolated finding and baby can be screened further with MRI to make sure nothing is wrong. When > 15–mm we start to worry about some of the stuff mentioned above.

Anencephaly: this is the most common neural tube defect and is lethal as there is absence of brain tissue above the orbits. There is an elevated AFP and this has a female predominance. Do not be confused by angiomatous stroma.

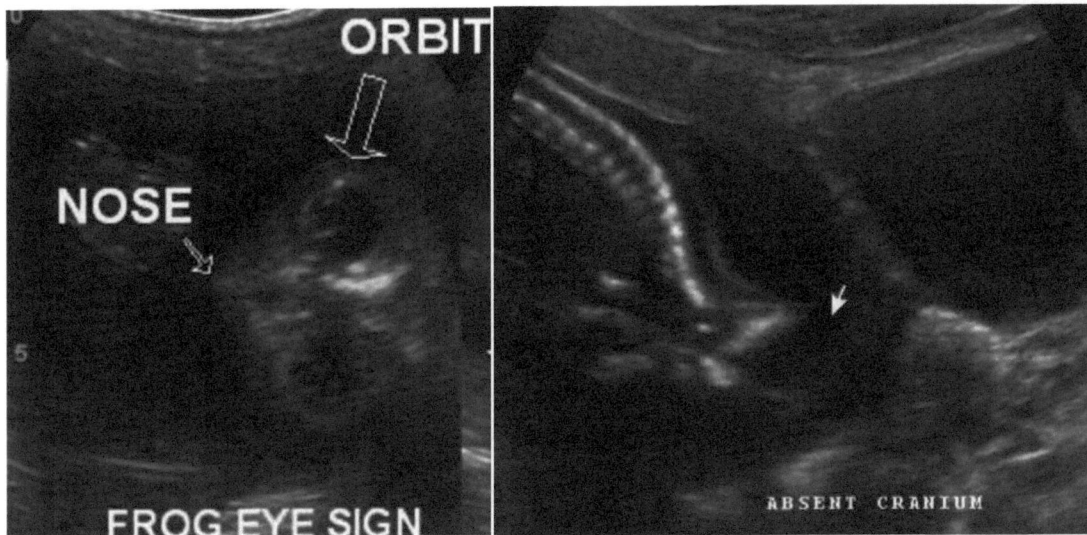

Cephalocele	Cystic Hygroma
Acute angles with scalp	Obtuse angles with scalp
Skull defect	Nuchal ligament thickened
Abnormal brain	Normal brain

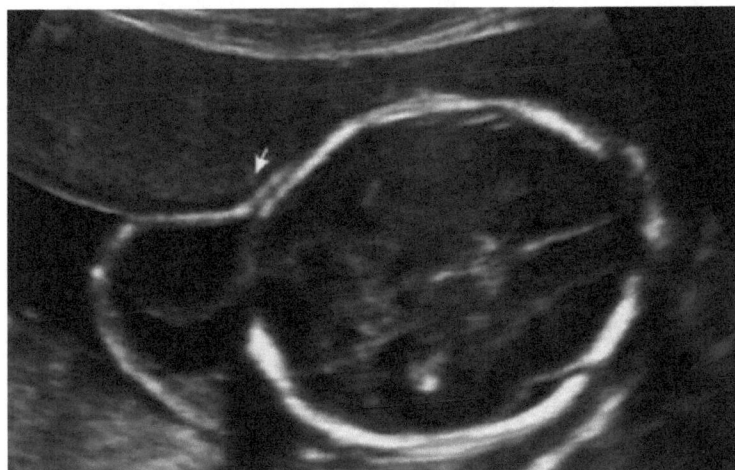

This is a classic example of a cystic hygroma, it has all of the features above and you can see the thick band of tissue down the midline, which is the nuchal ligament.

Cephalocele is associated with Chiari III and there is an image of it in the pediatric neuro study guide.

Dandy–Walker Malformation: look for an absent vermis with a dilated cisterna magna that communicates with the fourth ventricle.

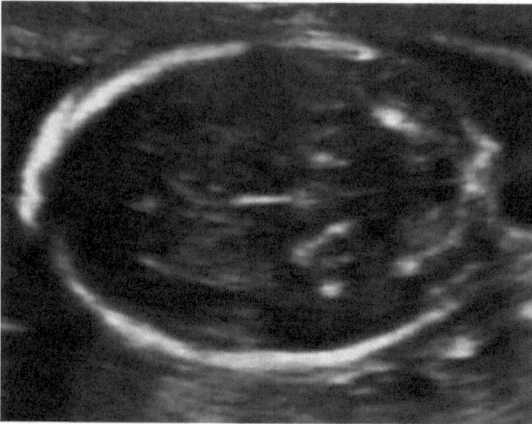

Agenesis of the CC: this is associated with tons of other stuff, look for high riding 3rd ventricle, parallel configuration of ventricles, and a tear drop atrium (shown below).

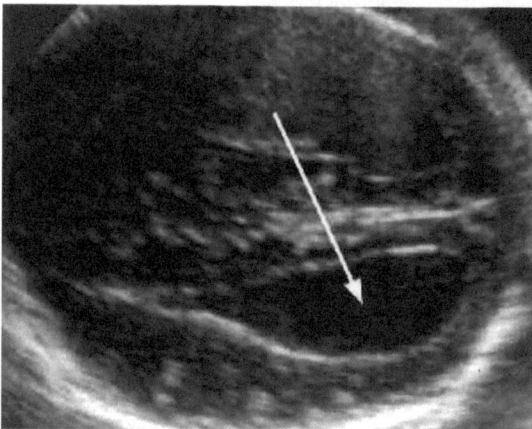

Choroid Plexus Cyst: are often benign and transient, especially when solitary. They are present in almost 1% of fetuses and are just spaces in the choroid plexus filled with CSF as they have no epithelial lining. There is a soft association with Trisomy 18 – look for overlapping digits, CHD, rocker bottom feet. If no other abnormalities noted, and the cyst is solitary, no follow up needed.

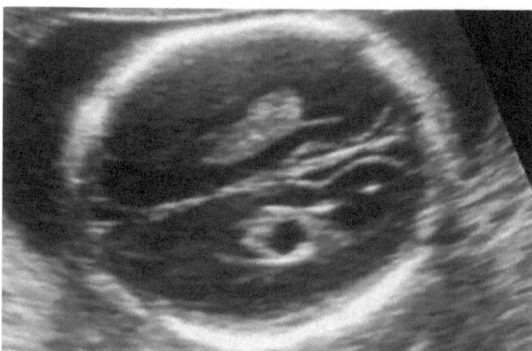

Vein of Galen Malformation: an abnormal connection between the deep choroidal arteries and median prosencephalic vein (precursor to VoG). The MPV fails to regress and drains into the straight sinus or a persistent falcine sinus. Discovered early in life as it can cause high output cardiac failure.

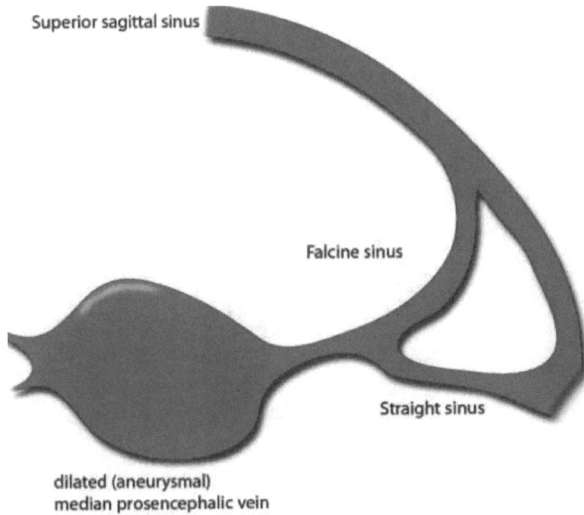

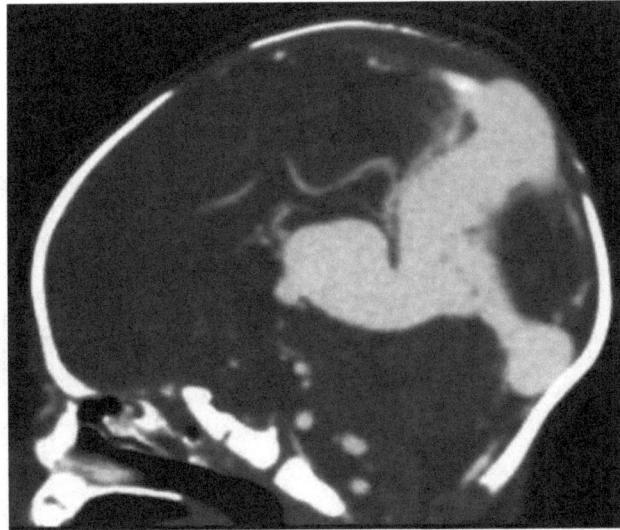

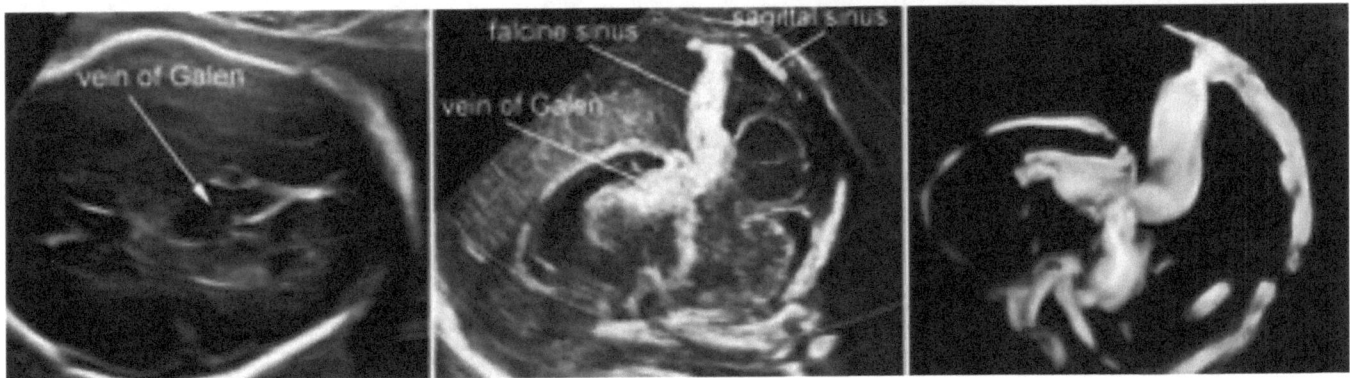

Spalding Sign: describes overlapping skull bones on a fetal ultrasound, which correlates with fetal demise. The overlapping bones are due to autolysis.

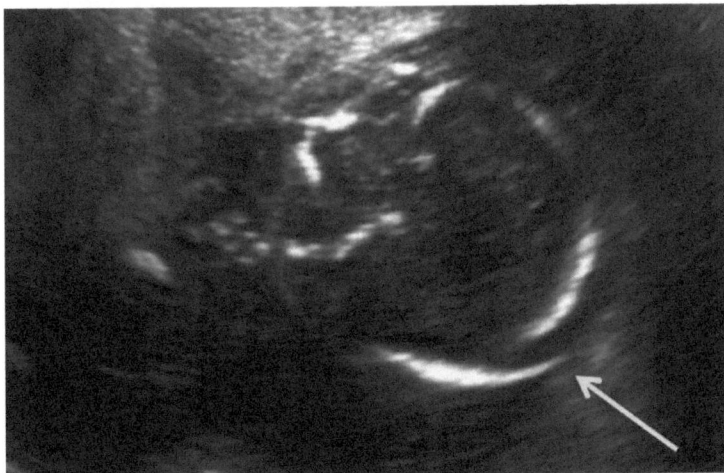

Cleft Lip: is the most common facial anomaly and is associated with cleft palate in 80% of cases. Isolated cleft lip has a better prognosis and when isolated it is usually on the left.

Type 1 – cleft lip only
Type 2 – **unilateral cleft lip and palate** – most common finding Type 3 – bilateral cleft lip and palate
Type 4 – midline cleft lip and palate – poorer prognosis because associated with Trisomy 13 Type 5 – facial defects associated with amniotic bands or a limb–body–wall complex

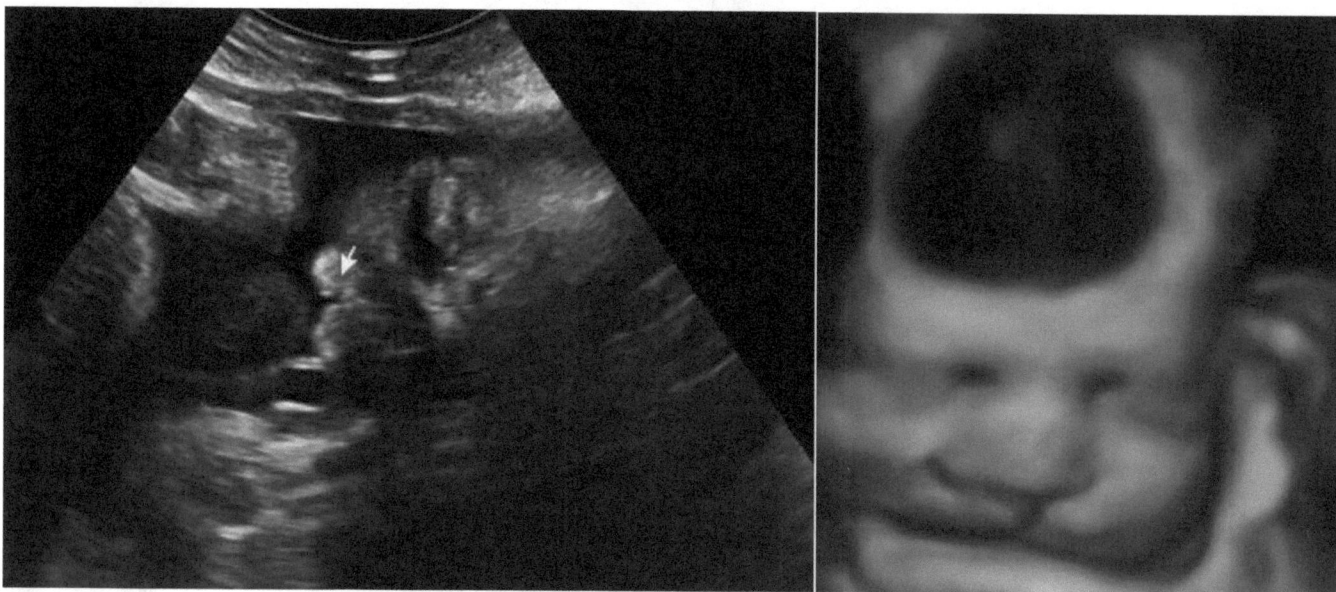

Chest:

Chest Mass	
CPAM	Solid echogenic mass on US with prognosis dependent on degree of mass effect on fetal lung
CDH	Usually left–sided, echogenic intrathoracic mass on US, poor prognosis if liver is herniated
Sequestration	LLL with separate parietal pleura and arterial supply, can be fluid–filled or echogenic
Tracheal Agenesis	Bilateral enlarged echogenic lungs with fluid–filled bronchi

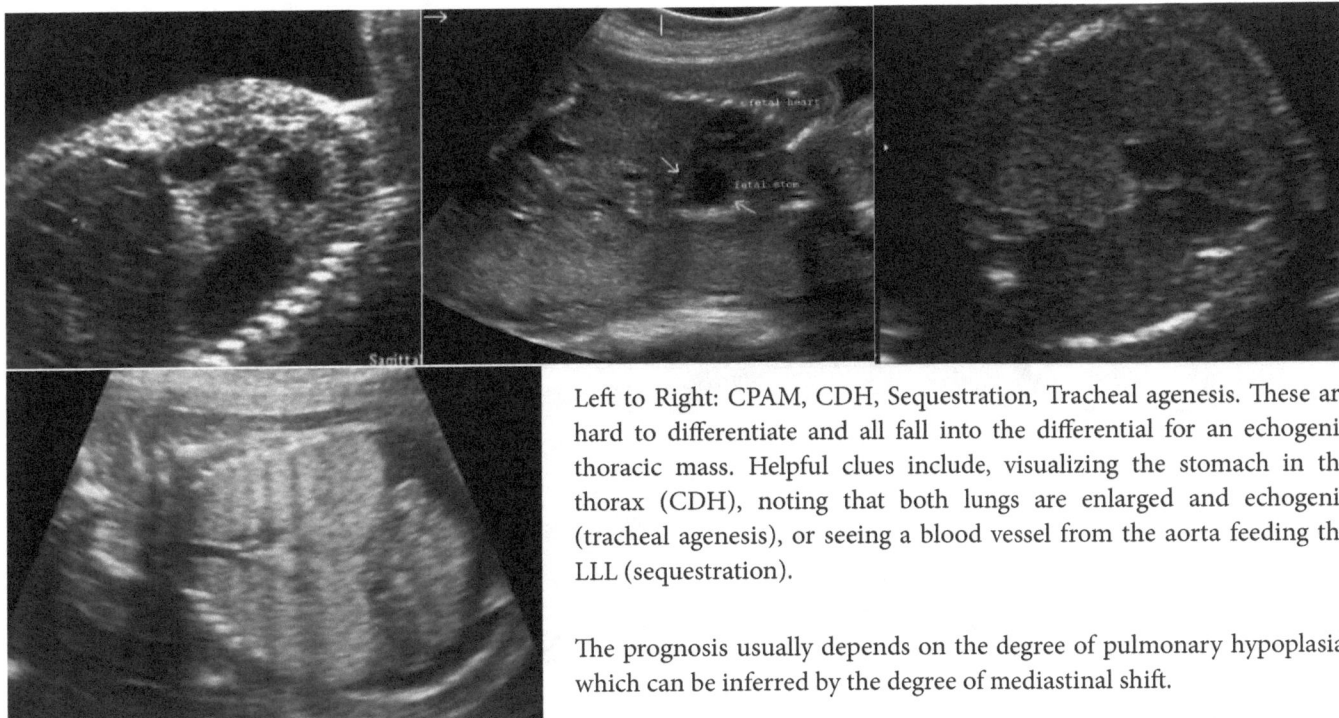

Left to Right: CPAM, CDH, Sequestration, Tracheal agenesis. These are hard to differentiate and all fall into the differential for an echogenic thoracic mass. Helpful clues include, visualizing the stomach in the thorax (CDH), noting that both lungs are enlarged and echogenic (tracheal agenesis), or seeing a blood vessel from the aorta feeding the LLL (sequestration).

The prognosis usually depends on the degree of pulmonary hypoplasia, which can be inferred by the degree of mediastinal shift.

Fun Fact: Isolated pleural effusions in the womb are associated with Trisomy 21 and Turner's. Isolated ascites with no other abnormality is seen with CMV infection.

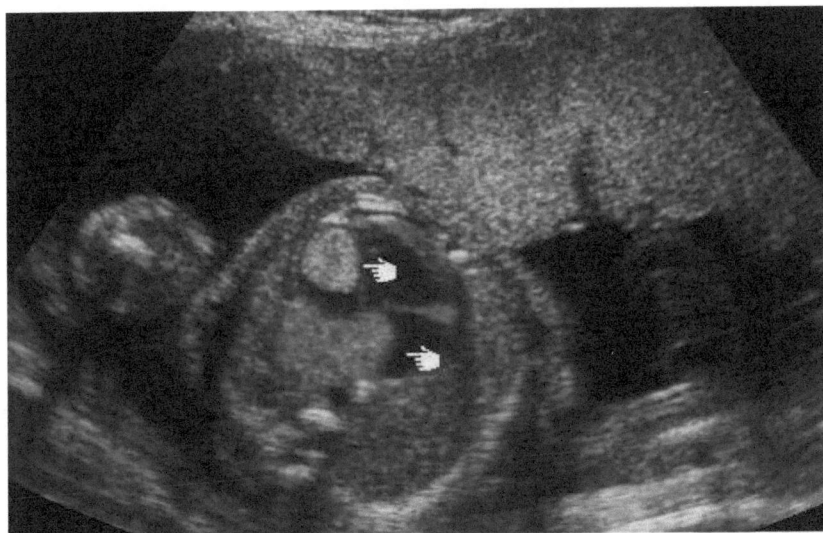

Cardiac Rhabdomyoma: is the most common cardiac mass in the fetus, infant, and in childhood. Ninety percent are multiple and of those diagnosed with rhabdomyoma, ¾ have tuberous sclerosis. They appear as hyperechoic masses in the right or left ventricles. They are histologically benign and if small cause no obstruction. Most will regress by 4 years of age.

Gastrointestinal: a lot of the very common pathology here was discussed in the pediatric GI section (esophageal atresia, GI atresias, meconium syndromes, etc.)

Gastroschisis: is the extra-abdominal herniation of fetal bowel loops without an overlying membrane through a para-umbilical wall defect (usually right-side). The small intestine always herniates, with variable herniation of colon, stomach, and liver. Most cases are sporadic and there is less of an association with other abnormalities in this condition than there is in omphalocele. Maternal serum AFP may be elevated. The condition of the bowel at birth is the single most important predictor of prognosis.

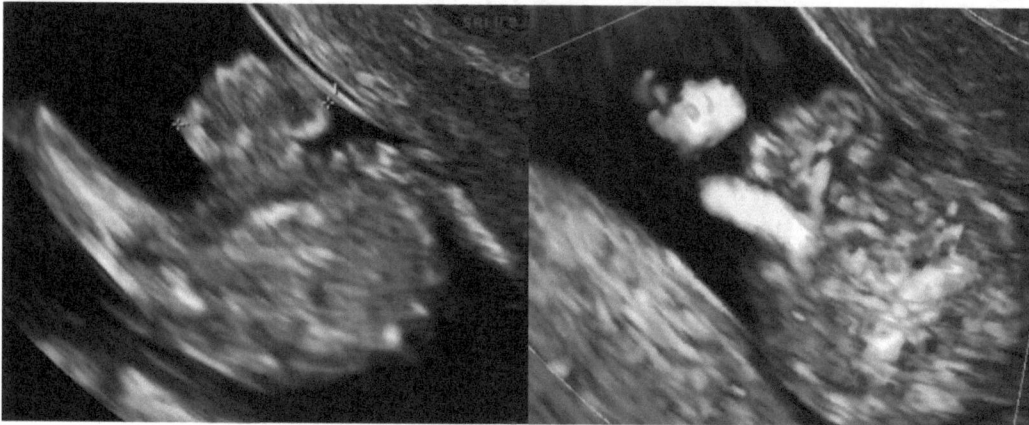

Umbilical cord to the left of the defect

Omphalocele: is a congenital midline abdominal wall defect at the base of the umbilical cord with herniation of the gut into a membrane covered sac. Bowel loops and liver herniate most often. There is a high incidence of associated anomalies: trisomies, Turner, congenital heart defect, etc. Higher overall morbidity and morality than gastroschisis primarily due to the association with other abnormalities. Don't forget that because of normal midgut herniation, this diagnosis has to wait until after 12 weeks (the bowel can be out, the liver cannot!).

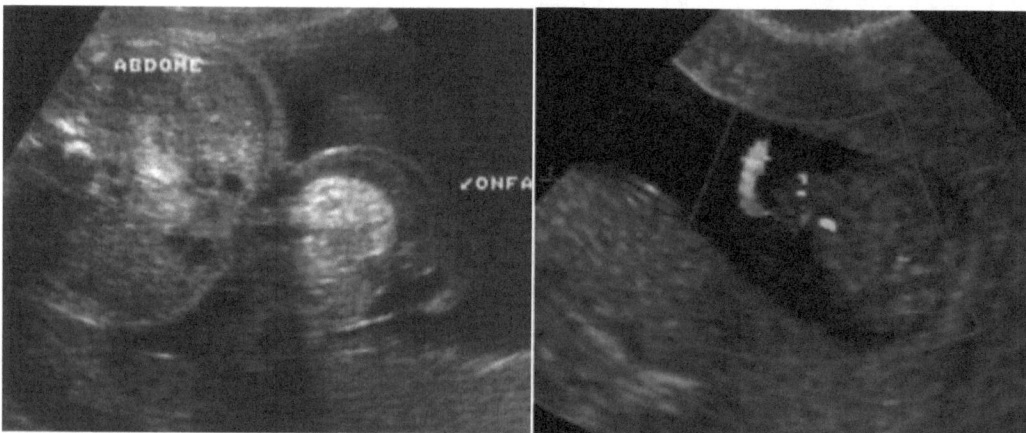

Umbilical cord on the defect

Genitourinary: suspect a GU abnormality in patients with oligohydramnios if there isn't PROM. Biggest things to think about are causes for bladder outlet obstruction (males with PUV), MCDK, renal agenesis, or ARPCKD. All of these are discussed in detail in the pediatric GU section.

Remember that it is never normal to see cysts in a fetal kidney; this is a sign of damage. The most common cause of hydronephrosis is UPJ obstruction.

Oligohydramnios (AFI < 8–cm)	Polyhydramnios (AFI > 20–cm)
PROM	CNS anomalies – impaired swallowing mechanism
IUGR	High GI obstruction
GU Anomaly	Twin Syndromes – TTT, TRAP
Low GI obstruction	

MSK:

Clubfoot: common congenital anomaly that can be bilateral and be associated with trisomies 13 and 18. However, the most common cause is idiopathic. Extrinsic causes like olighydramnios and amniotic band syndrome can lead to clubfoot. This is also called talipes equinovarus.

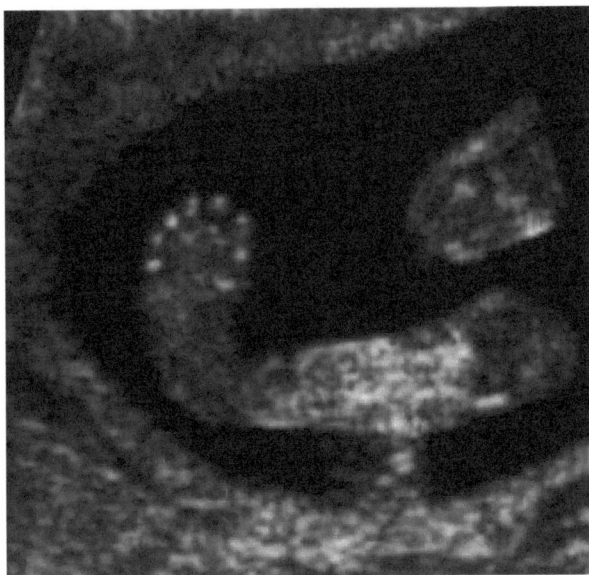

Osteogenesis Imperfecta: is a connective tissue disorder attributed to a type 1 collagen defect. The ultrasound diagnosis relies on the detection of in utero fractures, bowing of the long bones, and decreased bone brightness.

Type 1 – Autosomal dominant, non–lethal, mild fragility without significant deformity Type 2 – Autosomal dominant –lethal, demineralization and fractures

Type 3 – Autosomal recessive – non–lethal, presents with fractures of bone and spine Type 4 – Autosomal dominant – mild severity

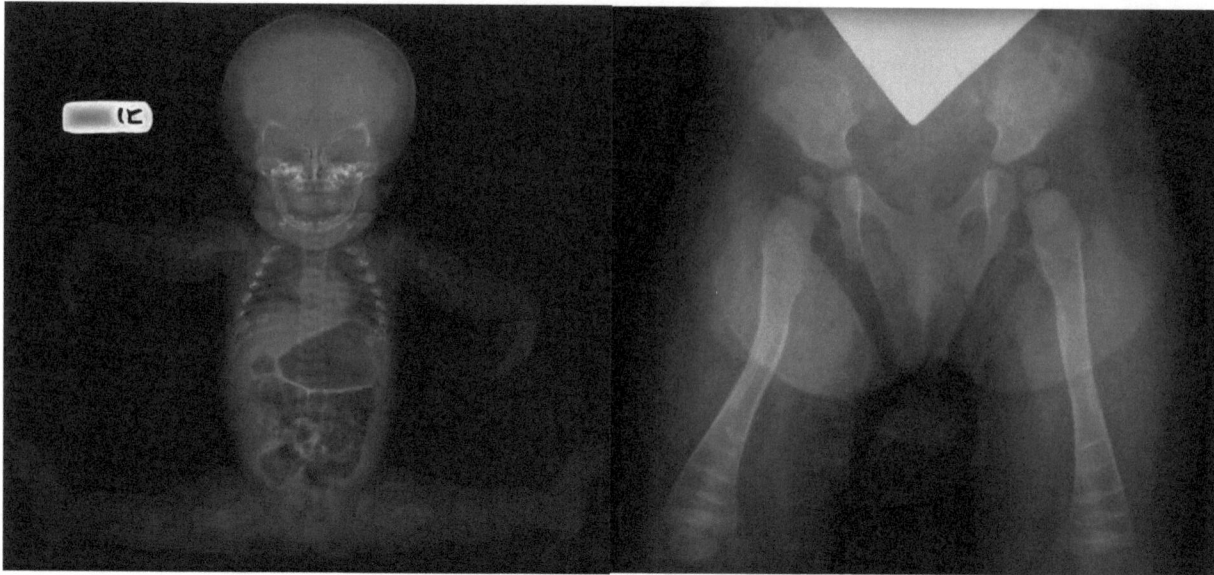

Twin Pregnancies: are more prone to suffer complications. The type of twin pregnancy depends on the type of fertilization that took place and the day on which the egg splits after fertilization.

Dizygotic – two sperm fertilizing two eggs – all dizygotic twins have two placentas (dichorionic)
Monozygotic – two sperm fertilizing one egg

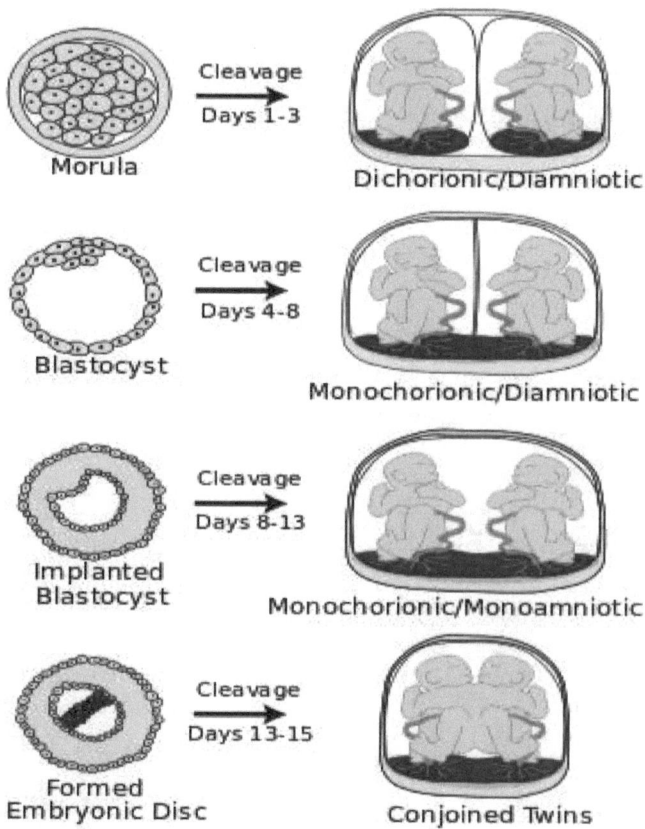

Of the monochorionic twins, the most common is the monochorionic/diamniotic

Dizygotic twins have a characteristic "twin peak" sign and all dizygotic twins are diamnionic

Twin–Twin Transfusion Syndrome (TTTS): most common complication of monochorionic twinning due to an abnormal AV connection in the placenta with the smaller twin pumping blood into the recipient twin. Both the donor and recipient twin have a poor prognosis. Always have to give the % growth discordance.

Donor	Recipient
Oligohydramnios	Polyhydramnios
Stuck and often in a non–dependent position	Floating in a sea of fluid
Smaller	Bigger
	Can have hydrops

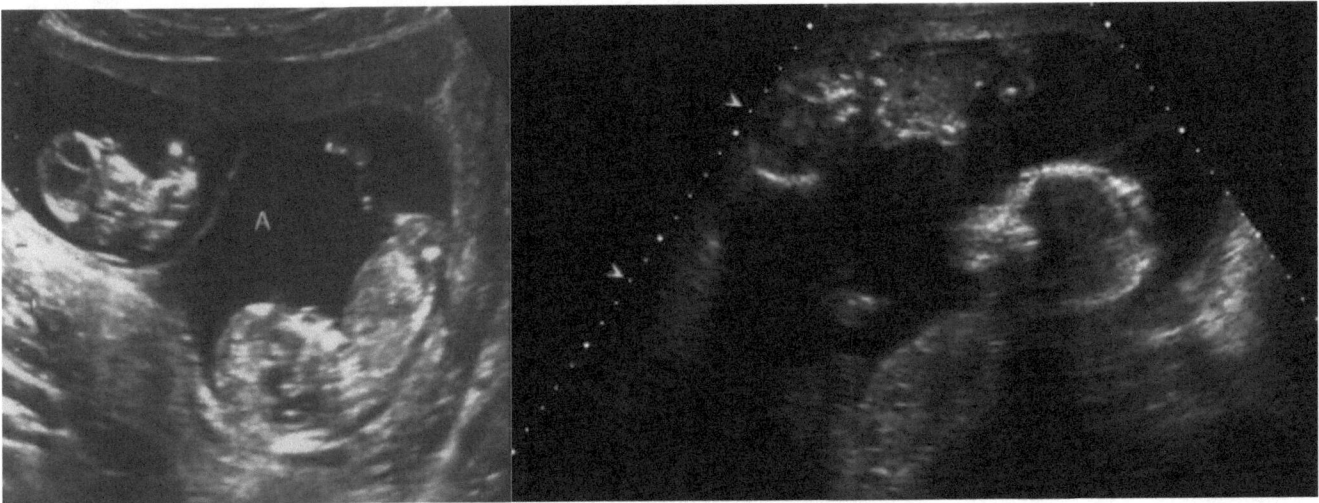

Twin Embolization Syndrome: rare complication of a monozygotic twin pregnancy following in utero demise of the co–twin. The surviving twin bleeds into the placental territory of the dead twin and this leads to ischemia.

Acardiac Twin (TRAP): consists of a viable and non–viable twin. The non–viable twin is anencephalic with a cystic hygroma, no upper extremities, normal lower extremities, and lacks a heart (perfused by other twin). The normal twin experiences high output cardiac failure. The normal twin is also at risk for early delivery and hydrops. Treatment is by RFA of the abnormal vascular connection.

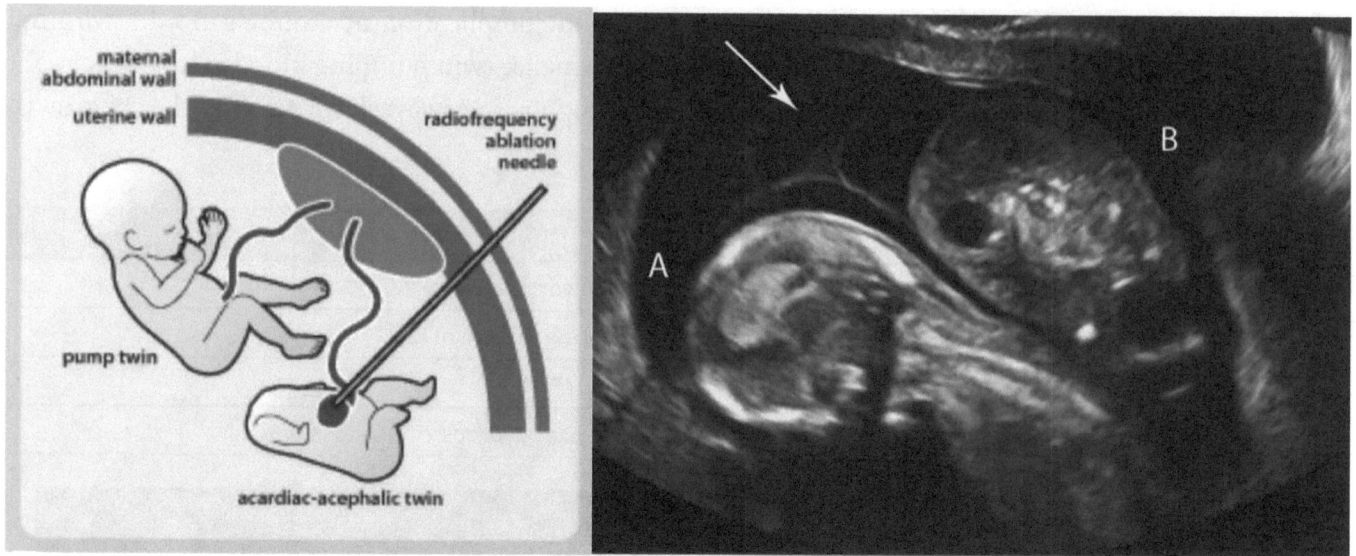

Conjoined Twins: result from a failure of the zygote to split by 13 weeks. Conjoined twins are monochorionic, monoamniotic, and monozygotic. Conjoined twins are classified based on the most prominent site of connection with thoracopagus (thorax) being the commonest. Higher incidence of congenital malformations.

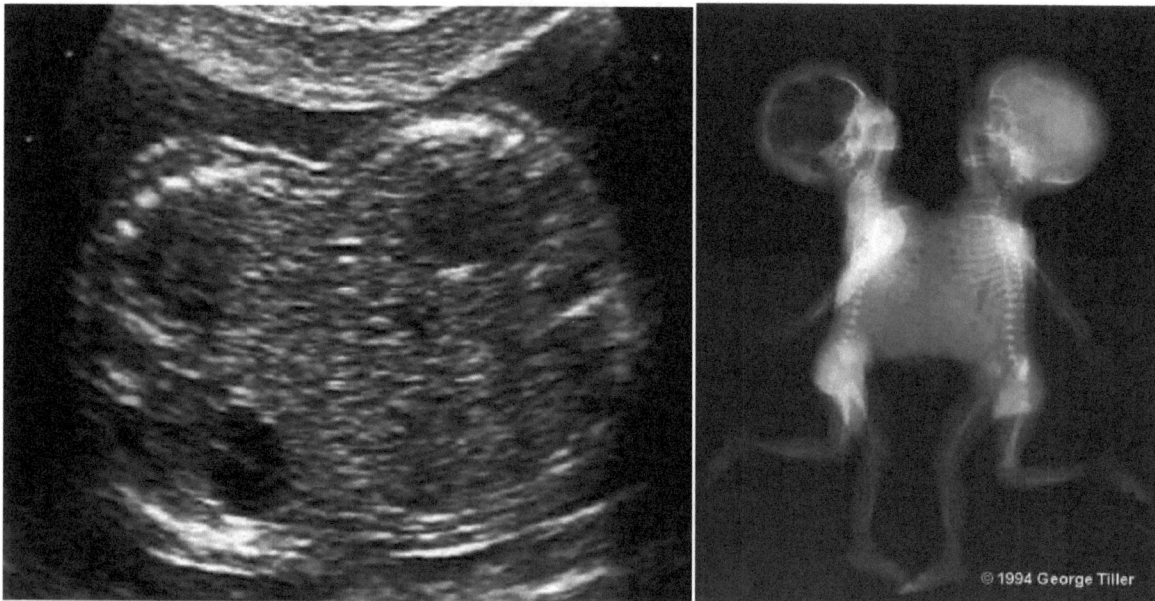

US shows two abdominal cavities with two stomachs in these thoracopagus twins

Trisomy 21	AV canal defects, echogenic focus in the ventricle, short humerus and femur, widening of the iliac angle with pelvic flaring
Trisomy 18	Choroid plexus cysts, omphaloceles, **clenched fists, rocker bottom feet**, CHD, radial ray abnml
Trisomy 13	Holoprosencephaly, cleft lip/palate, **polydactyly, clubfoot**

Gestational Trophoblastic Disease: several pathologies comprise the spectrum that is gestational trophoblastic disease. The most common is hydatidiform mole followed by invasive mole, and choriocarcinoma. On ultrasound this is going to appear as an enlarged uterus with an irregular shape. The endometrium is expanded with a snowstorm appearance that is caused by tiny vesicles that have increased through transmission. US documentation of myometrial penetration is key – look for myometrial nodules. "Bunch of grapes".

Complete mole usually confined to endometrium
Invasive mole goes into myometrium
Look for bilateral theca lutein cysts as a result of hyperstimulation from increased b–HCG

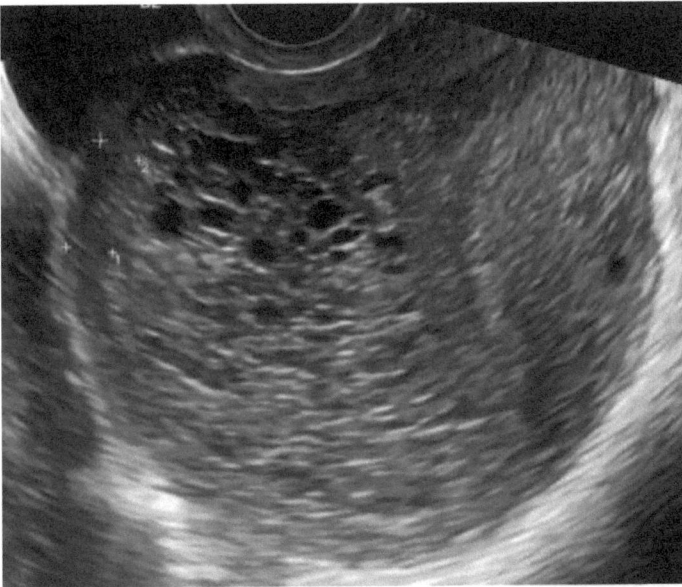

Hydrops: the abnormal collection of fluid involving at least two fetal compartments. This may manifest as: pleural effusions, pericardial effusion, anasarca, or ascites.

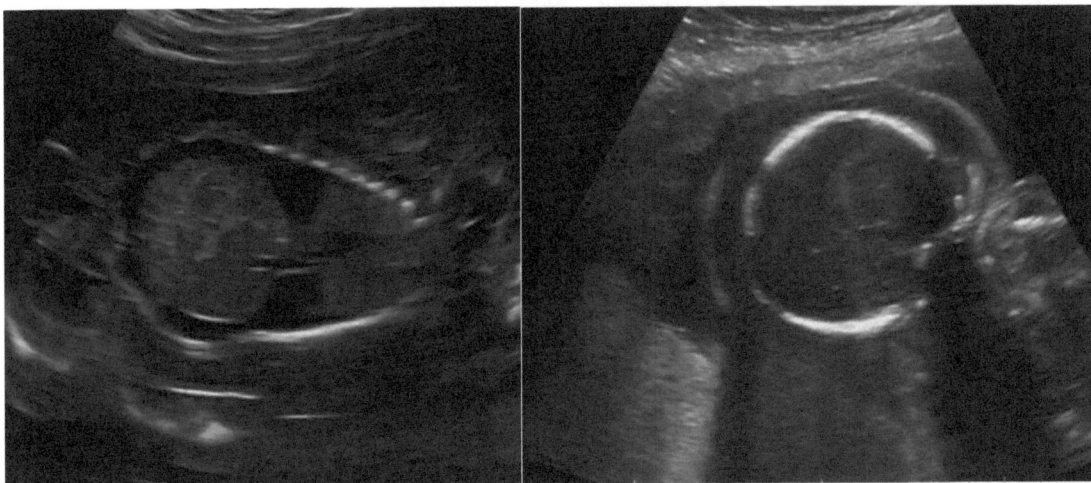

Left – pleural effusions and ascites

Right – scalp edema

Hydrops can be caused by a variety of factors (80 to be exact). The most common is non–immune hydrops:

Chromosomal abnormalities (1st trimester due to lymphatic obstruction – earliest sign increased nuchal lucency > 3–mm)
Cardiac defects
Twin pregnancy complications
TORCH infections
Tumors (sacrococcygeal teratomas, hemangioendotheliomas)
Metabolic disease (Gaucher)
High output (Vein of Galen)

Placenta Previa: is the implantation of the placenta over the cervix and can be marginal (placenta tip at the edge near the os), partial (placenta partially covers the os), and complete (placenta totally covers the os). Low–lying placenta is < 2–cm from the os. This can be problematic during delivery because it can lead to significant hemorrhage. Fetuses are at risk for IUGR and cerebral palsy. Most cases, resolve as the placenta remodels throughout pregnancy. Imaging at 30 weeks is necessary to assess and if persistent, planned c–section is done.

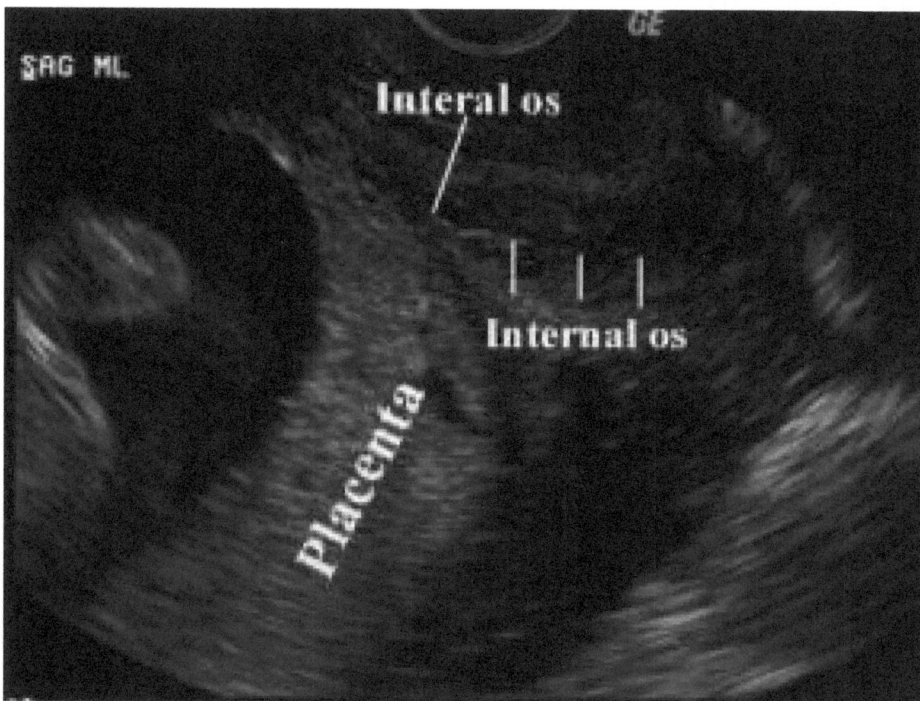

Complete Previa

Subchorionic Hemorrhage: think of this in a pregnant patient who present with vaginal bleeding and pain. On US a 1st trimester hemorrhage appears as a crescent or oval fluid collection adjacent to the gestation sac in the endometrial canal. In the 2nd and 3rd trimesters the hemorrhage appears as a crescent or ovoid mass projecting into the amniotic space. Early 1st trimester hemorrhages have worse prognosis and so do large bleeds.

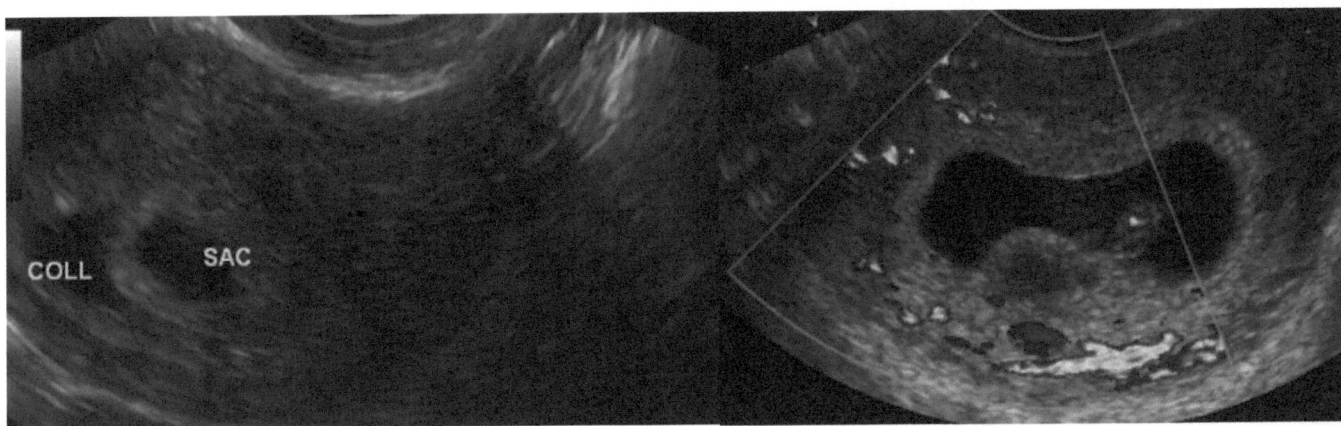

2-Vessel Cord: results when there is a congenital absence of one umbilical artery (usually the left). Most of the time this is an isolated finding but the US should be used to exclude any other anomalies: marginal and vilamentous cord insertions have been associated. Anomalies including holoprosencephaly and hydrocephalus have been seen and Trisomy 18 is the most common chromosomal abnormality. IUGR is common.

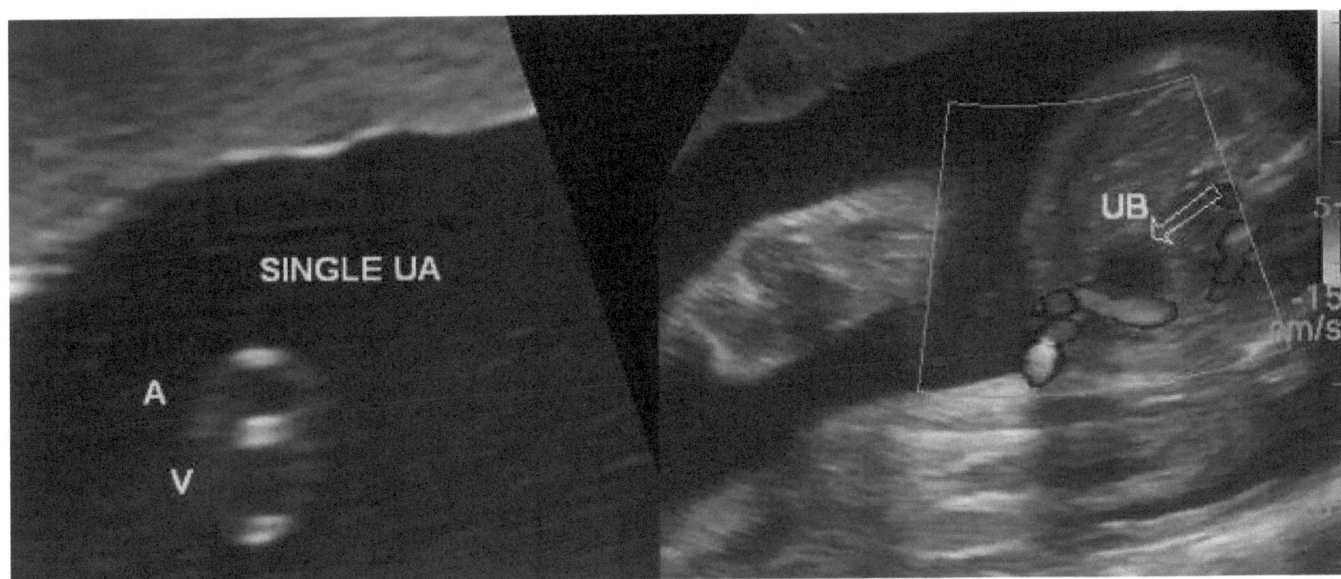

Placenta Accreta: the placental villi extend beyond the confines of the endometrium and implant into the myometrium without deep invasion. Risk factors include: placenta previa, advanced maternal age, prior c-section.

Placenta Increta: invasion into the myometrium without serosal contact.

Placenta Percreta: invasion through the myometrium with serosal contact.

Look for an anterior, low–lying placenta near the lower uterine segment. The invasion can go into the bladder with subsequent bladder rupture.

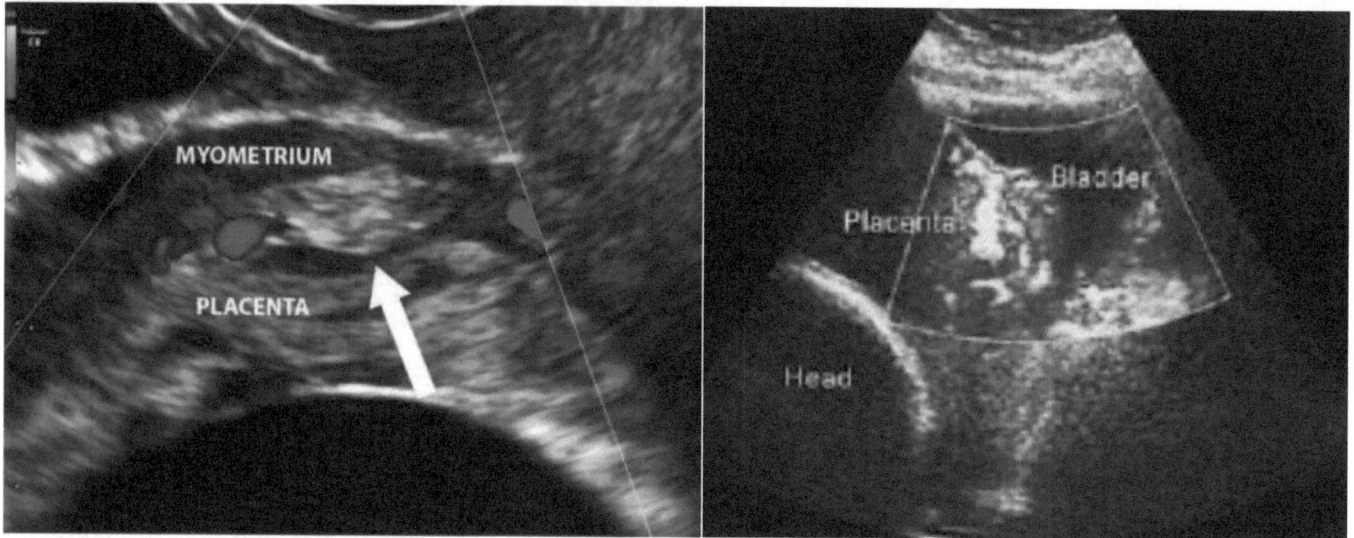

The placental tissue is seen extending into the myometrium (left) and the increased vascularity carried by the placenta is seen abutting the bladder (right) consistent with myometrial invasion.

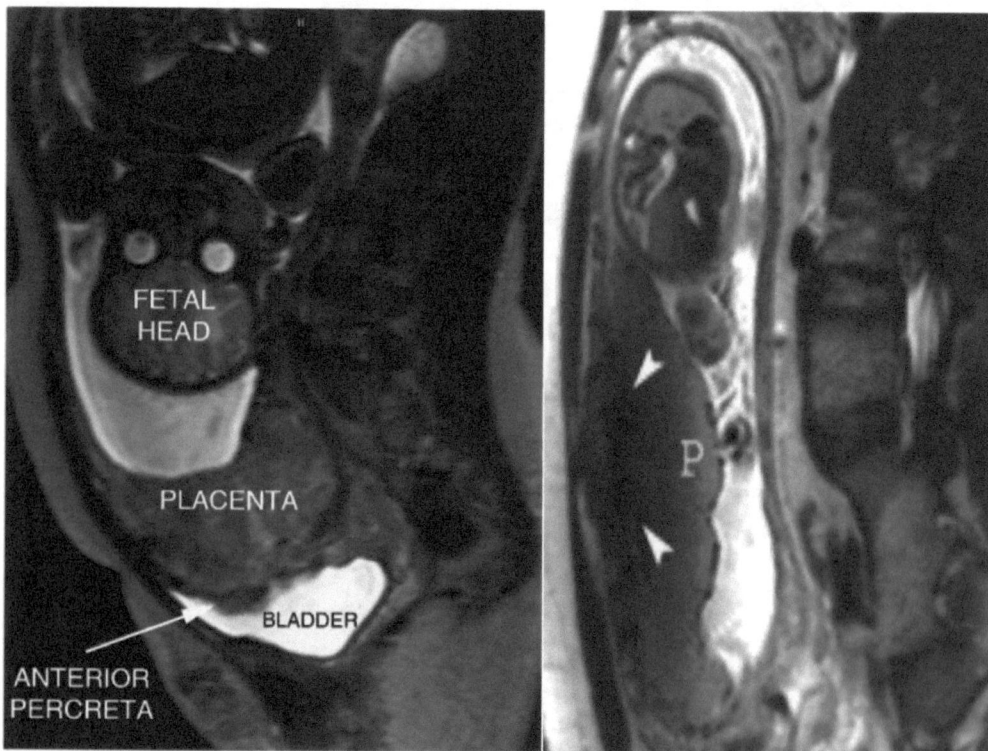

Sagittal MRI images demonstrate a placenta previa (left) with percreta – tissue extending into the bladder wall. On the right, there is an anterior placenta with myometrial invasion.

Always remember to look for Vasa Previa, which is the abnormal course of fetal vessels within the amniotic membranes crossing the internal os. Can lead to catastrophic hemorrhage either spontaneous or during vaginal delivery.

Succenturiate Lobe: is a small accessory lobe of the placenta that retains vascularity and results from failure of villous atrophy. It can lead to hemorrhage either prior to term or during delivery. If not delivered, it can lead to post-partum hemorrhage or infection.

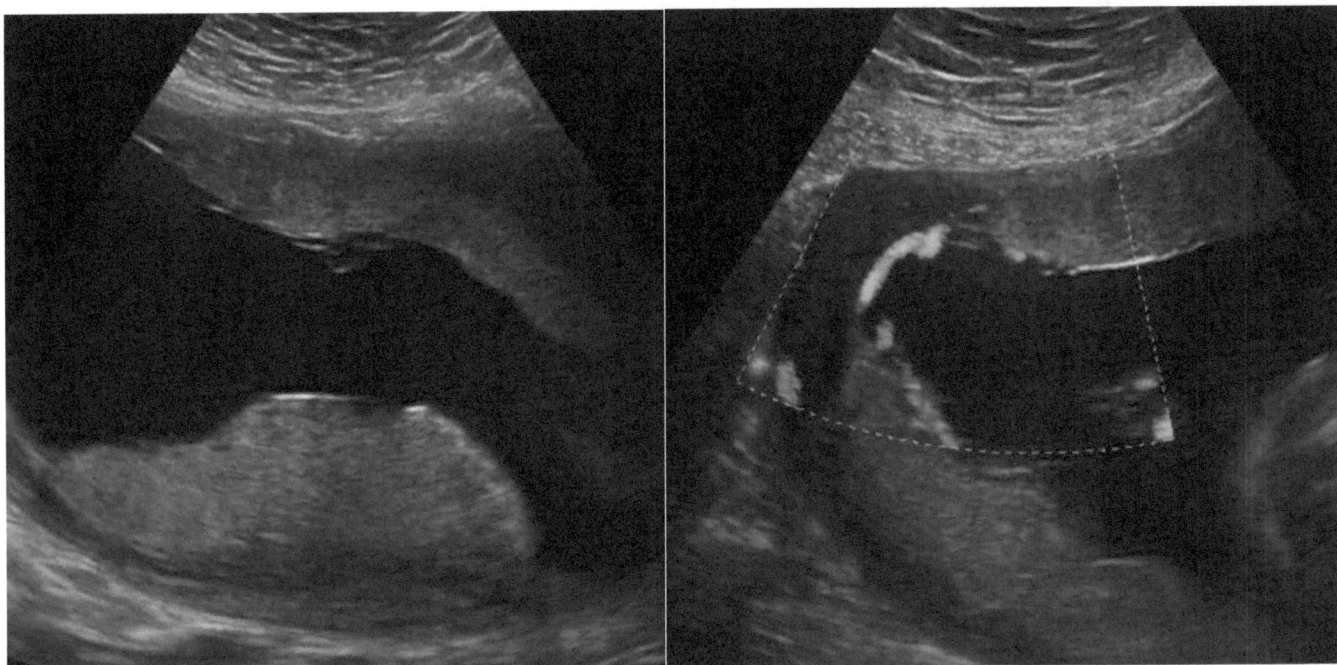

PCOS: is a clinical syndrome consisting of hirsutism, infertility, and oligomenorrhea in an obese female. The imaging findings are bilateral enlarged ovaries with peripherally distributed follicles. Also called Stein-Leventhal Syndrome. Lab analysis will show elevated LH:FSH ratio. The therapy is clomiphene citrate.

Endometrium: measured from the echogenic line to the echogenic line at the thickest point.

Menstrual 1–4 mm (thin)
Proliferative 4–8 mm (trilaminal)
Secretory 8–16 mm (bulbous)
Post-menopausal, if bleeding, > 5 mm is abnormal
If < 5 mm it is atrophic
Post-menopausal fluid in the endometrial cavity is never normal, usually because of cervical stenosis or obstructing cancer

Tamoxifen: causes hyperplasia, cystic changes, and **polyps** – we cannot differentiate between hyperplasia and cancer on imaging alone, need history and biopsy.

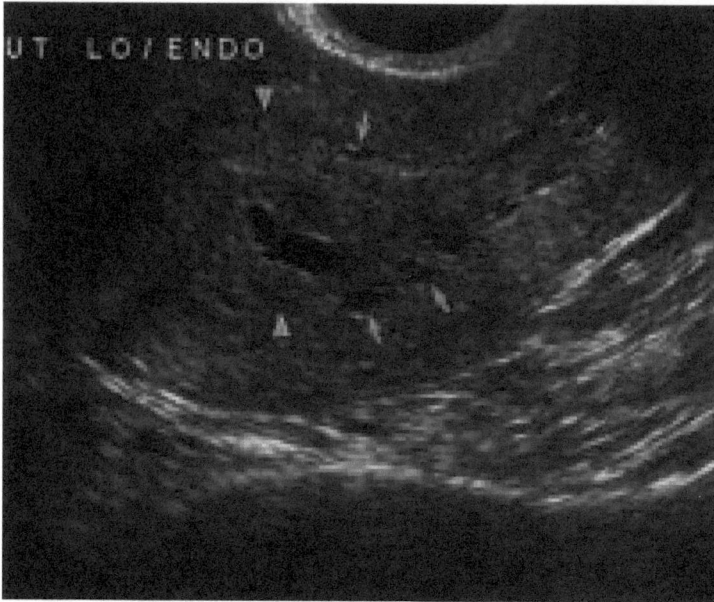

Dermoid: the most common ovarian neoplasm composed of mature elements (teratoma). Identified in younger women around the age of 30, usually asymptomatic but it can predispose the ovary to torsion. Look for the classic Rokitansky nodule (dermoid plug). Can contain ectopic thyroid tissue – struma ovarii tumor – patient presents with thyrotoxicosis.

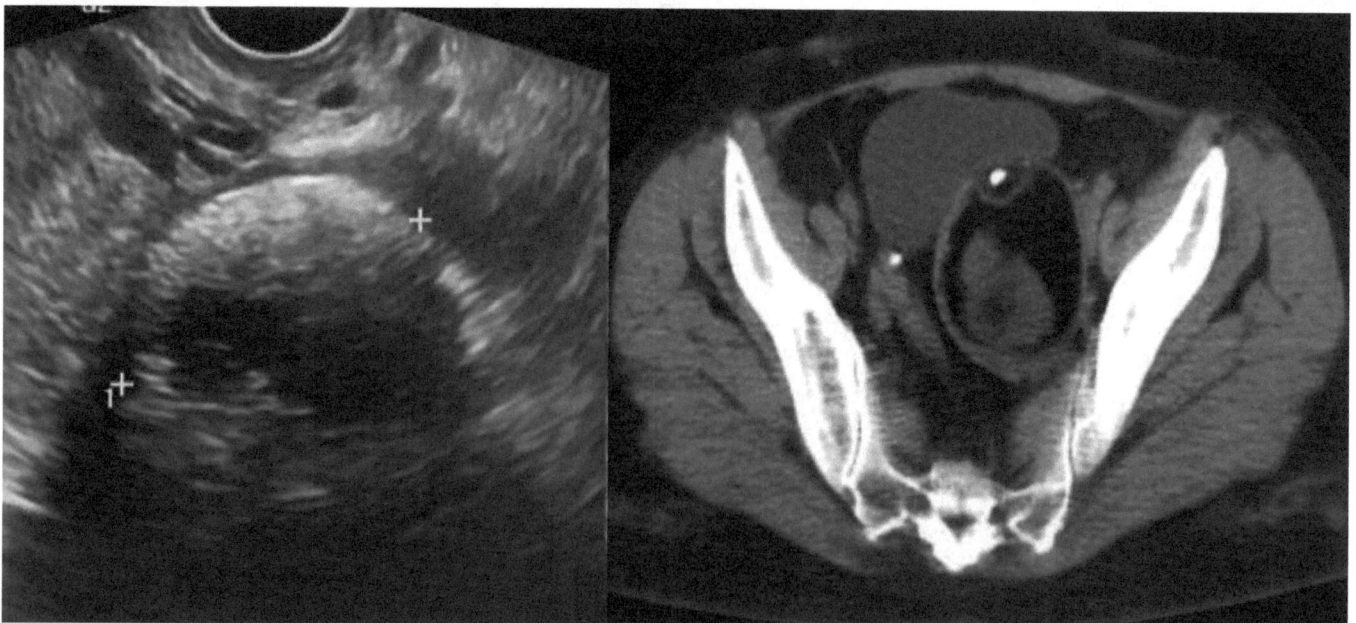

Made in United States
Troutdale, OR
04/23/2024